Eleventh Edition

LAST'S ANATOMY
Regional and Applied

CHUMMY S. SINNATAMBY FRCS

Surgical Anatomy Tutor, Royal College of Surgeons of England
Director of Studies in Anatomy, St Catharine's College and Hughes Hall, Cambridge

Formerly:
Head of Anatomy, Royal College of Surgeons of England
Member of Court of Examiners, Royal College of Surgeons of England
Examiner in Anatomy, Royal College of Surgeons in Ireland
External Examiner in Anatomy, University of Cambridge
External Examiner in Anatomy, Trinity College, University of Dublin

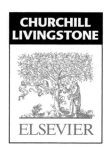

CHURCHILL LIVINGSTONE

ELSEVIER

EDINBURGH LONDON NEW YORK OXFORD PHILADELPHIA ST LOUIS SYDNEY TORONTO 2006

CHURCHILL
LIVINGSTONE

First edition 1954
Second edition 1959
Third edition 1963
Fourth edition 1966
Fifth edition 1972
Sixth edition 1978
Seventh edition 1984
Eighth edition 1990
Ninth edition 1994
Tenth edition 1999
Eleventh edition 2006

Standard Edition ISBN 10: 0 443 10033 0   ISBN 13: 978-0-443-10033-8
International Student Edition ISBN 10: 0 443 10032 2   ISBN 13: 978-0-443-10032-1

British Library Cataloguing in Publication Data
A catalogue record for this book is available from the British Library

Library of Congress Cataloging in Publication Data
A catalog record for this book is available from the Library of Congress

Note

Medical knowledge is constantly changing. Standard safety precautions must be followed, but as new research and clinical experience broaden our knowledge, changes in treatment and drug therapy may become necessary or appropriate. Readers are advised to check the most current product information provided by the manufacturer of each drug to be administered to verify the recommended dose, the method and duration of administration, and contraindications. It is the responsibility of the practitioner, relying on experience and knowledge of the patient, to determine dosages and the best treatment for each individual patient. Neither the Publisher nor the author assume any liability for any injury and/or damage to persons or property arising from this publication.

The Publisher

ELSEVIER   your source for books,
journals and multimedia
in the health sciences
www.elsevierhealth.com

Working together to grow
libraries in developing countries
www.elsevier.com | www.bookaid.org | www.sabre.org

ELSEVIER   BOOK AID International   Sabre Foundation

The
publisher's
policy is to use
**paper manufactured
from sustainable forests**

Printed in China

Preface to the eleventh edition

In response to innumerable requests, all the illustrations in the eleventh edition appear in full colour. Care has been taken in the choice of and consistency in use of colours for similar structures to facilitate ease of recognition and enhance the reader's appreciation of the illustrations as a meaningful adjunct to the text. Some of the illustrations in the first edition of R. J. Last's *Anatomy, Regional and Applied* were partly coloured as they appeared in relation to the text. In the seventh edition several partly coloured illustrations were collectively positioned as plates at the front of the book, but these were then omitted from subsequent editions. It has been gratifying to be able to restore colour to *Last's Anatomy* and extend its application to full colour for all the illustrations as they remain integrated with the text.

Several new illustrations, including clinical photographs, radiographs and magnetic resonance images, have been added, depicting normal anatomy and lesions that have an anatomical basis.

The text has been extensively revised with several additions to the clinical and applied aspects of anatomy and textual changes in the interests of clarity and accuracy.

I am grateful to the many readers, postgraduate and undergraduate, in the UK and abroad, who have communicated their appreciation of and comments on the tenth edition. Their input has encouraged and aided the preparation of the eleventh edition.

Chummy S. Sinnatamby
2005

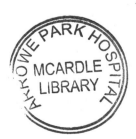

Preface to the tenth edition

In 1954, after seven years of association with postgraduate students of anatomy at the Royal College of Surgeons of England, R. J. Last published the first edition of *Anatomy, Regional and Applied*. Forty-five years later Last's 'approach to the study of anatomy' is still of value to undergraduate and postgraduate students of anatomy. The chief assets of *Last's Anatomy* were epitomised in its title. In the assessment and treatment of patients' lesions, clinicians encounter the anatomy of the human body on a regional basis, and the book presented applied anatomy data regionally arranged. When R. M. H. McMinn took over the editorship in 1990 he retained 'the flavour of earlier versions' and added to the applied aspects of the subject.

In preparing the tenth edition of *Last's Anatomy*, I have maintained the overall structure and arrangement of the book. The entire text, however, has undergone comprehensive revision directed towards a reduction of its volume and greater clarity. Anatomical detail of no clinical relevance, phylogenetic discussion and comparative anatomy analogies have been omitted. Within the constraints of conciseness, clinically correlated topographical anatomy relevant to the expanding frontiers of diagnostic and surgical procedures has been included. Surface anatomy pertaining to physical examination is presented. Histological features and developmental aspects have been mentioned only where they aid the appreciation of the gross form or function of organs and the appearance of the commoner congenital anomalies.

In keeping with the extensive textual changes in this edition, the illustrations have also undergone major revision. While several figures which appeared in previous editions but did not significantly contribute to or enhance the text, have been removed, 97 new illustrations have been added. The latter include original artwork specially commissioned for this edition, figures reproduced from *Gray's Anatomy* (with the kind permission of the publishers) on account of their anatomical accuracy and clarity, and examples of current diagnostic imaging techniques.

Throughout the preparation of this edition the curricular reforms of undergraduate education and the restructuring of surgical training have been borne in mind. Time constraints and the interdisciplinary integration pertaining to both have restricted the study of anatomy. Nevertheless, anatomical knowledge is required for performing physical examination and diagnostic tests, interpreting their results and instituting treatment, particularly surgical procedures. In his preface to the second edition Last stated that: 'While the text was written chiefly to help students who are revising their anatomy for an examination, it is particularly gratifying to find that so many clinicians and surgeons have found the book of value in their practice.' It is hoped that the clinically relevant anatomical information presented in the tenth edition, in as concise a form as its content concedes, will be of use to students preparing for examinations, participants in basic and higher surgical training programmes, and practising surgeons.

Thirty-seven years ago I purchased a copy of the second edition of *Last's Anatomy* while preparing for the primary fellowship examination, in the oral section of which I was examined by Professor Last himself. Little did I imagine then that it would one day be my privilege to prepare the tenth edition of *Last's Anatomy*, thereby maintaining the linkage between the editorship of this publication and the headship of anatomy at the Royal College of Surgeons of England.

Chummy S. Sinnatamby
1998

Acknowledgements

I thank Timothy Horne of Churchill Livingstone, an imprint of Elsevier Limited, for inviting me to prepare another edition of Last's Anatomy and I acknowledge the assistance given to me for this task by Hannah Kenner and Frances Affleck. My grateful appreciation is extended to Bruce Hogarth and his team of illustrators for the diligence and skill with which they have coloured the illustrations in the eleventh edition.

I am indebted to Dr Gina Brown of the Royal Marsden Hospital, Sutton, and Drs Richard Coulden and Ruchi Sinnatamby of the Cambridge University Hospital for the new radiographs and magnetic resonance images included in this edition.

I am grateful to my wife, Selvi, for her unconditional support throughout the period of my editorial involvement with Last's Anatomy.

Contents

CHAPTER 4

Thorax

CHAPTER 5

Abdomen

CHAPTER 6
Head and neck and spine

CHAPTER 7

Central nervous system

CHAPTER 8

Osteology of the skull and hyoid bone

Introduction to regional anatomy

PART ONE

Tissues and structures

The body is composed of four basic tissues—epithelium, connective tissue, muscle and nerve—and every part of the body can only be made up of one or more of these four elements.

Skin

Skin consists of two components: epidermis and dermis (Fig. 1.1). The surface epithelium of the skin is the **epidermis** and is of the keratinized stratified squamous variety. The various skin appendages—sweat glands, sebaceous glands, hair and nails—are specialized derivatives of this epidermis, which is ectodermal in origin. The deeper **dermis** is mesodermal in origin and consists

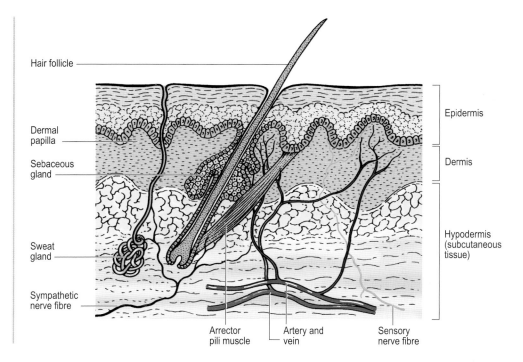

Fig. 1.1 Structure of the skin and subcutaneous tissue.

Hair follicle

Dermal papilla

Sebaceous gland

Sweat gland

Sympathetic nerve fibre

Arrector pili muscle

Artery and vein

Sensory nerve fibre

Epidermis

Dermis

Hypodermis (subcutaneous tissue)

mainly of bundles of collagen fibres together with some elastic tissue, blood vessels, lymphatics and nerve fibres.

While partly due to its thickness and blood flow, the main factor determining the colour of skin is the degree of pigmentation produced by melanocytes, which are mainly found in the basal layer of the epidermis. Melanocyte numbers are similar in all races. In darker skins the melanocytes are more active and produce more pigment. There are also racial differences between melanins which can vary in colour from yellows to browns and blacks.

Sweat glands are distributed all over the skin except on the tympanic membranes, lip margins, nipples, inner surface of prepuce, glans penis and labia minora. The greatest concentration is in the thick skin of the palms and soles, and on the face. Sweat glands are coiled tubular structures that extend into the dermis and subcutaneous tissue. They are supplied by cholinergic fibres in sympathetic nerves. **Apocrine glands** are large, modified sweat glands confined to the axillae, areolae, periumbilical, genital and perianal regions; their ducts open into hair follicles or directly on to the skin surface. Their odourless secretion acquires a smell through bacterial action. They enlarge at puberty and undergo cyclic changes in relation to the menstrual cycle in females. They are supplied by adrenergic fibres in sympathetic nerves.

Sebaceous glands are small saccular structures in the dermis, where they open into the side of hair follicles. They also open directly on to the surface of the hairless skin of the lips, nipples, areolae, inner surface of prepuce, glans penis and labia minora. There are none on the palms or soles. They are particularly large on the face. Androgens act locally on these glands which have no motor innervation.

Hair and nails are a hard type of keratin; the keratin of the skin surface is soft keratin. There is no new development of hair follicles after birth. Each hair is formed from the hair matrix, a region of epidermal cells at the base of the hair follicle, which extends deeply into the dermis and subcutaneous tissue. As the cells move up inside the tubular epidermal sheath of the follicle they lose their nuclei and become converted into the hard keratin hair shaft. Melanocytes in the hair matrix impart pigment to the hair cells. The change with age is due to decreasing melanocyte activity. Most follicles have an arrector pili muscle attached to the connective tissue of the base of the follicle and passing obliquely to the upper part of the dermis. When this smooth muscle, with a sympathetic innervation, contracts to make the hair 'stand on end', it may also squeeze the sebaceous gland that lies between the muscle and the hair follicle. Hair follicles are richly supplied by sensory nerves.

Nails consist of nail plates lying on nail beds on the dorsum of the terminal segment of fingers and toes. Compacted keratin-filled squames form the nail plate, which develops from the epidermal cells of the nail matrix deep to its proximal part. Here the nail plate is overlapped by the skin of the proximal nail fold. Blood vessels and sensory nerve endings are plentiful in the nail bed.

The **arteries** of the skin are derived from a tangential plexus at the boundary between the dermis and the subcutaneous connective tissue. Branches from this plexus form a subpapillary network in the dermis (Fig. 1.1). Arteriovenous anastomoses are abundant in the skin. The **veins** have a similar arrangement to the arteries. From a meshwork of lymphatic capillaries in the papillary layer of the dermis, **lymphatics** pass to a network between the dermis and hypodermis and thence run centrally with the blood vessels. Cutaneous **nerves** carry afferent somatic fibres, mediating general sensation, and efferent autonomic (sympathetic) fibres, supplying smooth muscle of blood vessels, arrector pili muscles and sweat glands. Both free sensory nerve endings and several types of sensory receptors are present in the skin.

The proportionate **surface area** of the skin over different regions of the body can be estimated by the 'rule of nines' and this is useful in assessing the need for fluid replacement after burns. This rule is a guide to the size of body parts in relation to the whole: head 9%; upper limb 9%; lower limb 18%; front of thorax and abdomen 18%; back of thorax and abdomen 18%.

Tension lines of the skin, due to the patterns of arrangement of collagen fibres in the dermis, run as shown in Figure 1.2. Skin tension is also dependent on the protrusion of underlying bones and cartilage, the contraction of muscles and joint movements. Wrinkle lines are caused by the contraction of underlying muscles; they do not always correspond to tension lines. Flexure lines over joints run parallel to tension lines. The cleavage lines originally described by Langer in 1861 on cadavers do not entirely coincide with the lines of greatest tension in the living. Incisions made along skin tension lines heal with a minimum of scarring (Fig. 1.3).

Superficial fascia

The skin is connected to the underlying bones or deep fascia by a layer of loose areolar connective tissue. This layer, usually referred to as superficial fascia, is of variable thickness and fat content. Flat sheets of muscles are also present in some regions. These include both skeletal muscles (platysma, palmaris brevis) and smooth muscles (subareolar muscle of the nipple, dartos,

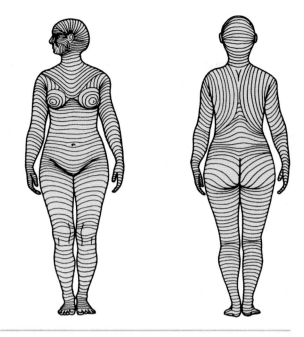

Fig. 1.2 Tension lines of the skin, front and back.

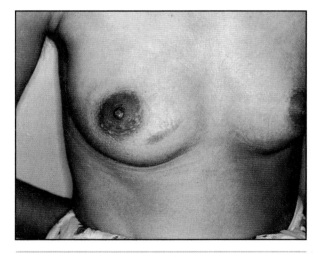

Fig. 1.3 An incision over the medial part of the right breast has crossed tension lines and resulted in excess scar formation. An incision at the lower margin of the areola along a tension line has healed with minimal scarring.

corrugator cutis ani). The superficial fascia is most distinct on the lower abdominal wall where it differentiates into two layers. Strong connective tissue bands traverse the superficial fasica binding the skin to the underlying aponeurosis of the scalp, palm and sole.

Deep fascia

The limbs and body wall are wrapped in a membrane of fibrous tissue, the deep fascia. It varies widely in thickness. In the iliotibial tract of the fascia lata, for example, it is very well developed, while over the rectus sheath and external oblique aponeurosis of the abdominal wall it is so thin as to be scarcely demonstrable and is usually considered to be absent. In other parts, such as the face and the ischioanal fossa, it is entirely absent. Where deep fascia passes directly over bone it is always anchored firmly to the periosteum. In the neck, as well as the investing layer of deep fascia, there are other deeper fascial layers enclosing neurovascular structures, glands and muscles. Intermuscular septa are laminae of deep fascia which extend between muscle groups and frequently become continuous with the periosteum of bones. Transverse thickenings of deep fascia over tendons, attached at their margins to bones, form retinaculae at the wrists and ankles and fibrous sheaths on the fingers and toes.

Deep fascia is very sensitive. Its nerve supply, and that of subcutaneous periosteum, is that of the overlying skin. The nerves to muscles supply the intermuscular septa and deep periosteum.

Ligaments

Ligaments are composed of dense connective tissue, mainly collagen fibres, the direction of the fibres being related to the stresses which they undergo. In general ligaments are unstretchable, unless subjected to prolonged strain. A few ligaments, such as the ligamenta flava between vertebral laminae and the ligamentum nuchae at the back of the neck, are made of elastic fibres, which enables them to stretch and regain their original length thereafter. Ligaments are usually attached to bone at their two ends.

Tendons

Tendons have a similar structure to collagenous ligaments, and attach muscle to bone. They may be cylindrical or flattened into sheet-like **aponeuroses**. Tendons have a blood supply from vessels which descend from the muscle belly and anastomose with periosteal vessels at the bony attachment.

Synovial sheaths

Where tendons bear heavily on adjacent structures, and especially where they pass around loops or pulleys of fibrous tissue or bone and change the direction of their pull, they are lubricated by being provided with a synovial sheath. The parietal layer of the sheath is firmly attached to the surrounding structures, the visceral layer is firmly fixed to the tendon, and the two layers glide on each other, lubricated by a thin film of synovial fluid secreted by the lining cells of the sheath. The visceral and parietal layers join each other at the ends of their extent. Usually they do not enclose the tendon cylindrically; it is as though the tendon was pushed into the double layers of the closed sheath from one side. In this way blood vessels can enter the tendon to reinforce the longitudinal anastomosis. In other cases blood vessels perforate the sheath and raise up a synovial fold like a little mesentery—a mesotendon or vinculum—as in the flexor tendons of the digits (see Fig. 2.44C, p. 94).

Cartilage

Cartilage is a type of dense connective tissue in which cells are embedded in a firm matrix, containing fibres and ground substance composed of proteoglycan molecules, water and dissolved salts. There are three types of cartilage. The most common is **hyaline cartilage** which has a blue-white translucent appearance. Costal, nasal, most laryngeal, tracheobronchial, articular cartilage of typical synovial joints and epiphyseal growth plates of bones are hyaline cartilage.

Fibrocartilage is like white fibrous tissue but contains small islands of cartilage cells and ground substance between collagen bundles. It is found in intervertebral discs, the labrum of the shoulder and hip joints, the menisci of the knee joints and at the articular surface of bones which ossify in membrane (squamous temporal, mandible and clavicle). Both hyaline cartilage and fibrocartilage tend to calcify and they may even ossify in old age.

Elastic cartilage has a matrix that contains a large number of yellow elastic fibres. It occurs in the external ear, auditory (Eustachian) tube and epiglottis. Elastic cartilage never calcifies.

Fibrocartilage has a sparse blood supply, but hyaline and elastic cartilage have no capillaries, their cells being nourished by diffusion through the ground substance.

Muscle

There are three kinds of muscle—skeletal, cardiac and smooth—although the basic histological classification is into two types: *striated* and *non-striated*. This is because both skeletal and cardiac muscle are striated, a structural characteristic due to the way the filaments of actin and myosin are arranged. The term striated muscle, however, is usually taken to mean skeletal muscle. Smooth muscle, also known as visceral muscle, is non-striated. Smooth muscle also contains filaments of actin and myosin, but they are arranged differently. The terms 'muscle cell' and 'muscle fibre' are synonymous. Smooth and cardiac muscle fibres, like most cells, usually have a single nucleus, but skeletal muscle fibres are multinucleated cells.

Smooth muscle consists of narrow spindle-shaped cells, usually lying parallel. They are capable of slow but sustained contraction. In tubes that undergo peristalsis they are arranged in longitudinal and circular fashion (as in the alimentary canal and ureter). In viscera that undergo a mass contraction without peristalsis (such as urinary bladder and uterus) the fibres are arranged in whorls and spirals rather than demonstrable layers. Contractile impulses are transmitted from one cell to another at sites called *nexuses* or *gap junctions*, where adjacent cell membranes lie unusually close together. Innervation is by autonomic nerves, and because of the gap junctions many muscle fibres do not receive nerve fibres.

Cardiac muscle consists of much broader, shorter cells that branch. Cardiac muscle is less powerful than skeletal muscle, but is more resistant to fatigue. Part of the boundary membranes of adjacent cells make very elaborate interdigitations with one another (at the 'intercalated discs' of light microscopy) to increase the surface area for impulse conduction. The cells are arranged in whorls and spirals; each chamber of the heart empties by mass contraction. Innervation, like that of visceral muscle, is by autonomic nerves.

Skeletal muscle consists of long, cylindrical non-branching fibres. Individual fibres are surrounded by a fine network of connective tissue, the endomysium. Parallel groups of fibres are surrounded by less delicate connective tissue, the perimysium, to form muscle bundles or fasciculi. Thicker connective tissue, the epimysium, envelops the whole muscle. The collagen fibres of these connective tissue sheaths fuse with those of attached tendons and aponeuroses. Neurovascular structures pass along the sheaths.

The orientation of individual skeletal muscle fibres is either parallel or oblique to the line of pull of the whole muscle. The range of contraction is long with the former arrangement, while the latter provides increased force of contraction. Sartorius is an example of a muscle with parallel fibres.

Muscles with an oblique disposition of fibres fall into several patterns:

- **Unipennate muscles**, where all the fibres slope into one side of the tendon, giving a pattern like a feather split longitudinally (e.g. flexor pollicis longus).
- **Bipennate muscles**, where muscle fibres slope into the two sides of a central tendon, like an intact feather (e.g. rectus femoris).

- **Multipennate muscles**, which take the form of a series of bipennate masses lying side by side (e.g. subscapularis), or of a cylindrical muscle within which a central tendon forms. Into the central tendon the sloping fibres of the muscle converge from all sides (e.g. tibialis anterior).

The attachment of a muscle, where there is less movement, is generally referred to as its origin, and the attachment, where there is greater movement, as its insertion. These terms are relative; which end of the muscle remains immobile and which end moves depends on circumstances and varies with most muscles. Simple usage of 'attachment' for both sites of fixation of a muscle avoids confusion and inaccuracy.

Movements are the result of the coordinated activity of many muscles, usually assisted or otherwise by gravity. Bringing the attachments of a muscle (origin and insertion) closer together is what is conventionally described as the 'action' of a muscle (isotonic contraction, shortening it). If this is the desired movement the muscle is said to be acting as a *prime mover*, as when biceps is required to flex the elbow. A muscle producing the opposite of the desired movement—triceps in this example—is acting as an *antagonist*; it is relaxing but in a suitably controlled manner to assist the prime mover. Two other classes of action are described: fixators and synergists. *Fixators* stabilize one attachment of a muscle so that the other end may move, e.g. muscles holding the scapula steady are acting as fixators when deltoid moves the humerus. *Synergists* prevent unwanted movement; the long flexors of the fingers pass across the wrist joint before reaching the fingers, and if finger flexion is the required movement, muscles that extend the wrist act as synergists to stabilize the wrist so that the finger flexors can act on the fingers. A muscle that acts as a prime mover for one activity can of course act as an antagonist, fixator or synergist at other times. Muscles can also contract isometrically, with increase of tension but the length remaining the same, as when the rectus abdominis contracts prior to an anticipated blow on the abdomen. Many muscles can be seen and felt during contraction, and this is the usual way of assessing their activity, but sometimes more specialized tests such as electrical stimulation and electromyography may be required.

Muscles have a rich blood supply. Arteries and veins usually pierce the surface in company with the motor nerves. From the muscle belly vessels pass on to supply the adjoining tendon. Lymphatics run back with the arteries to regional lymph nodes.

Embedded among the ordinary skeletal muscle cells are groups of up to about 10 small specialized muscle fibres that constitute the *muscle spindles*. The spindle fibres are held together as a group by a connective tissue capsule and are called intrafusal fibres (lying within a fusiform capsule), in contrast to ordinary skeletal muscle fibres which are extrafusal. Spindles act as a type of sensory receptor, transmitting to the central nervous system information on the state of contraction of the muscles in which they lie.

Skeletal muscle is supplied by somatic nerves through one or more motor branches which also contain afferent and autonomic fibres. The efferent fibres in spinal nerves are the axons of the large α anterior horn cells of the spinal cord which pass to extrafusal fibres, and of the small γ cells which supply the spindle (intrafusal) fibres. The motor nuclei of cranial nerves provide the axons for those skeletal muscles supplied by cranial nerves.

The nerves supplying the ocular and facial muscles (third, fourth, sixth and seventh cranial nerves) contain no sensory fibres. Proprioceptive impulses are conveyed from the muscles by local branches of the trigeminal nerve. The spinal part of the accessory nerve and the hypoglossal nerve likewise contains no sensory fibres. Proprioceptive impulses are conveyed from sternocleidomastoid and trapezius by branches of the cervical plexus, and from the tongue muscles probably by the lingual nerve (trigeminal).

Bone

Bone is a type of vascularized dense connective tissue with cells embedded in a matrix composed of organic materials, mainly collagen fibres, and inorganic salts rich in calcium and phosphate.

Macroscopically, bone exists in two forms: compact and cancellous. **Compact bone** is hard and dense, and resembles ivory. It occurs on the surface cortex of bones, being thicker in the shafts of long bones, and in the surface plates of flat bones. The collagen fibres in the mineralized matrix are arranged in layers, embedded in which are osteocytes. Most of these lamellae are arranged in concentric cylinders around vascular channels (Haversian canals), forming Haversian systems or osteons, which usually lie parallel to each other and to the long axis of the bone. Haversian canals communicate with the medullary cavity and each other by transversely running Volkmann's canals containing anastomosing vessels. **Cancellous bone** consists of a spongework of trabeculae, arranged not haphazardly but in a very real pattern best adapted to resist the local strains and stresses. If for any reason there is an alteration in the strain to which cancellous bone is subjected there is a rearrangement of the trabeculae. The moulding of bone results from the resorption of existing bone by phagocytic osteoclasts and the deposition of new bone by osteoblasts. Cancellous bone is found in the interior of bones and at the articular ends of long bones. The organization of cancellous or trabecular bone is also basically lamellar but in the form of branching and anastomosing curved plates. Blood vessels do not usually lie within this bony tissue and osteocytes depend on diffusion from adjacent medullary vessels.

The medullary cavity in long bones and the interstices of cancellous bone are filled with red or yellow marrow. At birth all the marrow of all the bones is red, active haemopoiesis going on everywhere. As age advances the red marrow atrophies and is replaced by yellow, fatty marrow, with no power of haemopoiesis. This change begins in the distal parts of the limbs and gradually progresses proximally. By young adult life there is little red marrow remaining in the limb bones, and that only in their cancellous ends; ribs, sternum, vertebrae and skull bones contain red marrow throughout life.

The outer surfaces of bones are covered with a thick layer of vascular fibrous tissue. This layer is the **periosteum** and the nutrition of the underlying bone substance depends on the integrity of its blood vessels. The periosteum is osteogenic, its deeper cells differentiating into osteoblasts when required. In the growing individual new bone is laid down under the periosteum, and even after growth has ceased the periosteum retains the power to produce new bone when it is needed, e.g. in the repair of fractures. The periosteum is united to the underlying bone by collagen (Sharpey's) fibres, particularly strongly over the attachments of tendons and ligaments. Periosteum does not, of course, cover the articulating surfaces of the bones in synovial joints; it is reflected from the articular margins to join the capsule of the joint.

The single-layered **endosteum** that lines inner bone surfaces (marrow cavity and vascular canals) is also osteogenic and contributes to new bone formation.

One or two nutrient arteries enter the shaft of a long bone obliquely and are usually directed away from the growing end. Within the medullary cavity they divide into ascending and descending branches. Near the ends of bone they are joined by branches from neighbouring vessels and from periarticular arterial anastomoses. Cortical bone receives blood supply from the periosteum and from muscular vessels at their attachments. Veins are numerous and large in the cancellous red marrow bones (e.g. the basivertebral veins). Lymphatics are present, but scanty; they drain to the regional lymph nodes of the part.

Subcutaneous periosteum is supplied by the nerves of the overlying skin. In deeper parts the local nerves, usually the branches to nearby muscles, provide the supply. Periosteum in all parts of the body is very sensitive. Other nerves, probably vasomotor in function, accompany nutrient vessels into bone.

Bone develops by two main processes, intramembranous and endochondral ossification (ossification in membrane and cartilage). In general the bones of the vault of the skull, the face and the clavicle ossify in membrane, while the long bones of the skeleton ossify in cartilage.

In **intramembranous ossification**, osteoblasts simply lay down bone in fibrous tissue; there is no cartilage precursor. As well as the bones of the skull vault, face and the clavicle, it should be noted that growth in the thickness of other bones (subperiosteal ossification) is also by intramembranous ossification.

In **endochondral ossification** a pre-existing hyaline cartilage model of the bone is gradually destroyed and replaced by bone (Fig. 1.4). Most bones are formed in this way. It is essential to appreciate that the cartilage is not converted into bone; it is destroyed and then replaced by bone. During all the years of growth there is constant remodelling with destruction (by osteoclasts) and replacement (by osteoblasts), whether the original development was intramembranous or endochondral. Similarly endochondral ossification, subperiosteal ossification and remodelling occurs in the callus of fracture sites.

The site where bone first forms is the primary centre of ossification, and in long bones is in the middle of the shaft (*diaphysis*), the centre first appearing about the eighth week of intrauterine life. The ends of the bone (*epiphyses*) remain cartilaginous and only acquire secondary ossification centres much later, usually after birth. The growing end of the diaphysis is the *metaphysis*, and the adjacent epiphyseal cartilage is the *epiphyseal plate*. When ossification occurs across the epiphyseal plate, the diaphysis and epiphysis fuse and bone growth

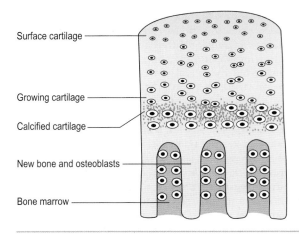

Surface cartilage

Growing cartilage

Calcified cartilage

New bone and osteoblasts

Bone marrow

Fig. 1.4 Endochondral ossification in the epiphysis at the end of a long bone.

ceases. The more actively growing end of a bone starts to ossify earlier and is the last to fuse with the diaphysis.

In the metaphysis the terminal branches of the nutrient artery of the shaft are end arteries, subject to the pathological phenomenon of embolism and infarction; hence osteomyelitis in the child most commonly involves the metaphysis. The cartilaginous epiphysis has, like all hyaline cartilage, no blood supply. As ossification of the cartilaginous epiphysis begins, branches from the periarticular vascular plexus penetrate to the ossification centre. They have no communication across the epiphyseal plate with the vessels of the shaft. Not until the epiphyseal plate ossifies, at cessation of growth, are vascular communications established. Now the metaphysis contains no end arteries and is not subject to infarction from embolism; therefore osteomyelitis no longer has any particular site of election in the bone.

Sesamoid bones

Sesame seed-like sesamoid bones are usually associated with certain tendons where they glide over an adjacent bone. They may be fibrous, cartilaginous or bony nodules, or a mixture of all three, and their presence is variable. The only constant examples are the patella, which is by far the largest, and the ones in the tendons of adductor pollicis, flexor pollicis brevis and flexor hallucis brevis. In the foot they can also occur in the peroneus longus tendon over the cuboid, the tibialis anterior tendon against the medial cuneiform and the tibialis posterior tendon opposite the head of the talus. A sesamoid bone in the lateral head of gastrocnemius (the fabella) is not associated with a tendon. The reasons for the presence of sesamoids are uncertain. Sometimes they appear to be concerned in altering the line of pull of a tendon (patella in the quadriceps tendon) or with helping to prevent friction (as in the peroneus longus tendon moving against the cuboid bone).

Joints

Union between bones can be in one of three ways: by fibrous tissue; by cartilage; or by synovial joints.

Fibrous joints occur where bones are separated only by connective tissue (Fig. 1.5A) and movement between them is negligible. Examples of fibrous joints are the sutures that unite the bones of the vault of the skull and the syndesmosis between the lower ends of the tibia and fibula.

Cartilaginous joints are of two varieties, primary and secondary. A **primary cartilaginous joint (synchondrosis)** is one where bone and hyaline cartilage meet (Fig. 1.5B). The junction of bone and cartilage in ossifying hyaline

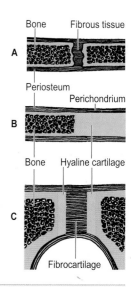

Fig. 1.5 Fibrous and cartilaginous joints in section: **A** fibrous joint; **B** primary cartilaginous joint; **C** secondary cartilaginous joint.

cartilage provides an example. Thus all epiphyses are primary cartilaginous joints, as are the junctions of ribs with their own costal cartilages. All primary cartilaginous joints are quite immobile and are very strong. The adjacent bone may fracture, but the bone–cartilage interface will not separate.

A **secondary cartilaginous joint (symphysis)** is a union between bones whose articular surfaces are covered with a thin lamina of hyaline cartilage (Fig. 1.5C). The hyaline laminae are united by fibrocartilage. There is frequently a cavity in the fibrocartilage, but it is never lined with synovial membrane and it contains only tissue fluid. Examples are the pubic symphysis and the joint of the sternal angle (between the manubrium and the body of the sternum). An intervertebral disc is part of a secondary cartilaginous joint, but here the cavity in the fibrocartilage contains a gel (p. 440).

A limited amount of movement is possible in secondary cartilaginous joints, depending on the amount of fibrous tissue within them. All symphyses occur in the midline of the body.

Typical **synovial joints**, which include all limb joints, are characterized by six features: the bone ends taking part are covered by *hyaline cartilage* and surrounded by a *capsule* enclosing a joint *cavity*, the capsule is reinforced externally or internally or both by *ligaments*, and lined internally by *synovial membrane*, and the joint is capable of varying degrees of *movement*. In atypical synovial joints the articular surfaces of bone are covered by *fibrocartilage*.

The synovial membrane lines the capsule and invests all non-articulating surfaces within the joint; it is attached round the articular margin of each bone. Cells of the membrane secrete a hyaluronic acid derivative which is responsible for the viscosity of synovial fluid, whose main function is lubrication. The viscosity varies, becoming thinner with rapid movement and thicker with slow. In normal joints the fluid is a mere film. The largest joint of all, the knee, only contains about 0.5 mL.

The extent to which the cartilage-covered bone-ends make contact with one another varies with different positions of the joint. When the surfaces make the maximum possible amount of contact, the fully congruent joint is said to be *close-packed* (as in the knee joint in full extension). In this position the capsule and its reinforcing ligaments are at their tightest. When the surfaces are less congruent (as in the partly flexed knee), the joint is *loose-packed* and the capsule looser, at least in part.

Intra-articular fibrocartilages, discs or menisci, in which the fibrous element is predominant, are found in certain joints. They may be complete, dividing the joint cavity into two, or incomplete. They occur characteristically in joints in which the congruity between articular surfaces is low, e.g. the temporomandibular, sternoclavicular and knee joints.

Fatty pads are found in some synovial joints, occupying spaces where bony surfaces are incongruous. Covered in synovial membrane, they probably promote distribution of synovial fluid. The Haversian fat pad of the hip joint and the infrapatellar fold and alar folds of the knee joint are examples.

Mucous membranes

A mucous membrane is the lining of an internal body surface that communicates with the exterior directly or indirectly. This definition must not be taken to imply that all mucous membranes secrete mucus; many parts of the alimentary and respiratory tracts do, but most of the urinary tract does not. Mucous membranes consist of two and sometimes three elements: always an *epithelium* and an underlying connective tissue layer, the *lamina propria*, which in much of the alimentary tract contains a thin third component of smooth muscle, the *muscularis mucosae*. The whole mucous membrane, often called 'mucosa', usually lies on a further connective tissue layer, the submucous layer or submucosa. The epithelium of a mucous membrane varies according to the site and functional needs, e.g. stratified squamous in the mouth, columnar in the intestine, ciliated in the trachea.

Serous membranes

A serous membrane (serosa) is the lining of a closed body cavity—pericardial, pleural and peritoneal—and consists of connective tissue covered on the surface by a single layer of flattened mesothelial cells (derived from the mesoderm of the coelomic cavity). The part of the serosa that lines the wall of the cavity (the parietal layer of pericardium, pleura or peritoneum) is directly continuous with the same membrane that covers or envelops the mobile viscera within the cavity (the visceral layer). The peritoneal, pericardial and pleural cavities are potential slit-like spaces between the *visceral layer* and the *parietal layer*. The two layers slide readily on each other, lubricated by a film of tissue fluid. There are no glands to produce a lubricating secretion. The serous membranes are usually very adherent to the viscera. The parietal layer is attached to the wall of the containing cavity by loose areolar tissue and in most places can be stripped away easily.

The parietal layer of all serous membranes is supplied segmentally by spinal nerves. The visceral layer possesses no somatic sensory supply.

Blood vessels

Blood vessels are of three types: capillaries; arteries; and veins.

Capillaries are the smallest vessels. Their walls consist only of flattened endothelial cells. Capillaries form an anastomotic network in most tissues. Certain structures, such as the cornea of the eye and hyaline cartilage, are devoid of capillaries.

Arteries conduct blood from the heart to the capillary bed, becoming progressively smaller, and as they do so, give way to arterioles which connect with the capillaries. Arterial walls have three layers. The tunica intima is very thin and comprises the endothelial lining, little collagenous connective tissue and an internal elastic lamina. Surrounding this layer is the tunica media consisting mainly of elastic connective tissue fibres and smooth muscle in varying amounts. The aorta and major arteries have a large proportion of elastic tissue which enables them to regain their original diameter after the expansion that follows cardiac contraction. Smaller arteries have less elastic tissue and more muscle. The tunica media of arterioles is almost entirely composed of smooth muscle. The outermost layer of the arterial wall is the tunica adventitia, which has an external elastic lamina surrounded by collagenous connective tissue.

Veins collect blood from the capillaries. They generally have a thinner wall and a larger diameter than their corresponding arteries. Veins have the same three layers in their walls as arteries, but a distinct internal elastic lamina is absent and there is much less muscle in the media. Peripheral limb veins are often double, as venae comitantes of their arteries. In the proximal parts of limbs venae comitantes unite into a single large vein. Many veins in the limbs and the neck have valves which prevent reflux of blood. These valves usually have two cup-shaped cusps formed by an infolding of the tunica intima. These cusps are apposed to the wall as long as the flow is towards the heart; when blood flow reverses, the valves close by assuming their cup-shaped form. On the cardiac side of a valve the vein wall is expanded to form a sinus. In general, there are no valves in the veins of the thorax and abdomen.

Anastomoses between arteries are either *actual* or *potential*. In the former instance arteries meet end to end, such as the labial branches of the two facial arteries. A potential anastomosis is by terminal arterioles. Given sufficient time these arterioles can dilate to convey adequate blood, but with sudden occlusion of a main vessel the anastomosis is inadequate to immediately nourish the affected part, as in the case of the coronary arteries.

In many cases there is no precapillary anastomosis between adjacent arteries. Such vessels are *end-arteries*, and here interruption of arterial flow necessarily results in gangrene or infarction. Examples are found in the liver, spleen, kidney, lung, medullary branches of the central nervous system, the retina and the straight branches of the mesenteric arteries.

Arteriovenous anastomoses are short-circuiting channels between terminal arterioles and primary venules which occur in many parts of the body. They are plentiful in the skin, where they may have a role in temperature regulation.

Sinusoids are wide capillaries which have a fenestrated or discontinuous endothelium. They are numerous in the liver, spleen, adrenal medulla and bone marrow.

Blood vessels are innervated by efferent autonomic fibres which regulate the contraction of the smooth muscle in their walls. These nerves act on muscular arteries and especially on arterioles. Their main effect is vasoconstriction and increase in vascular tone, mediated by adrenergic sympathetic fibres. In some areas sympathetic cholinergic fibres inhibit muscle activity and cause vasodilatation. On account of the thickness of their walls, large vessels have their own vascular supply through a network of small vessels, the vasa vasorum.

Lymphatics

Not all the blood entering a part returns by way of veins; much of it becomes tissue fluid and returns by way of lymphatic vessels. Lymphatic capillaries are simple endothelial tubes. Larger collecting channels have walls similar to those of veins, but the specific tunics, or layers, are less distinct. They differ from veins in having many more valves. In general superficial lymphatics (i.e. in subcutaneous tissues) follow veins, while deep lymphatics follow arteries.

Clinical spread of disease (e.g. infection, neoplasm) by lymphatics does not necessarily follow strictly anatomical pathways. Lymph nodes may be bypassed by the disease process. If lymphatics become dilated by obstruction their valves may be separated and reversal of lymph flow can then occur. Lymphatics communicate with veins freely in many parts of the body; the termination of the thoracic duct may be ligated with impunity, for the lymph finds its way satisfactorily into more peripheral venous channels.

Lymphoid tissue

The defence mechanisms of the body include **phagocytosis**, which is a non-specific engulfing process, and the **immune response**, which is a specific reaction to micro-organisms and foreign proteins (antigens). The immune response may occur in two ways: (1) by the *humoral antibody response*, with production of antibodies which are protein molecules that circulate in the blood and attach themselves to the foreign protein so that the combination of antigen and antibody can be destroyed by phagocytosis; and (2) by the *cell-mediated immune response*, with the production of specific cells that circulate in the blood and destroy the antigen or stimulate its phagocytosis. Two types of lymphocyte produce these reactions: *T cells* are responsible for cell-mediated immunity and *B cells* for humoral antibody production. The B cells become transformed into plasma cells which produce the antibody molecules (the immunoglobulins: IgG; IgM; IgA; IgE; and IgD).

All lymphocytes arise from common stem cells in bone marrow (in the embryo from yolk sac, liver and spleen). Some of them circulate to and settle in the thymus, where they proliferate. After release into the bloodstream as T cells they colonize the spleen, lymph nodes and other lymphoid follicles by passing through the postcapillary venules of those structures. Other stem cells become B cells and colonize lymphoid follicles without passing through the thymus. The *T* cells are so named because they depend on the thymus for their development; cell-mediated immunity thus depends on this organ. The *B* cells acquire their name from the bursa of Fabricius in birds, for it was in chickens that this organ (a diverticulum of the cloaca) was first found to be the source of humoral antibodies. The main types of T cell are known as T helper, T suppressor, T killer (cytotoxic) and T memory, while B cells can either form plasma cells or become B memory cells.

The **lymphoid organs** consist of the thymus, lymph nodes and spleen. All are encapsulated and have an internal connective tissue framework to support the cellular elements. In all except the thymus the characteristic structural feature is the lymphoid nodule or follicle, which is typically a spherical collection of lymphocytes with a pale central area, the germinal centre. Unencapsulated lymphoid tissue occurs in mucosa-associated lymphoid tissue (MALT) in the mucosa and submucosa of the alimentary, respiratory and genitourinary tracts. Waldeyer's peripharyngeal lymphoid ring of tonsils (palatine, lingual, nasopharyngeal and tubal) and Peyer's patches in the ileum are areas of organized mucosa-associated lymphoid tissue (O-MALT). The overlying epithelium of these sites is able to sample antigens in the lumen and translocate them to the underlying lymphoid aggregation.

In the **thymus** the lymphocytes are not concentrated in rounded follicles but form a continuous dense band of tissue at the outer region or cortex of the lobules into which the organ is divided. The inner (paler) regions of the lobules form the medulla which has fewer lymphocytes and contains the characteristic thymic corpuscles (of Hassall); these are remnants of the epithelium of the third pharyngeal pouches from which the thymus developed.

In a typical **lymph node** the rounded follicles of lymphocytes are concentrated at the periphery (cortex). Lymphocytes, not collected into follicles, are also present in the paracortical areas and medullary region. B lymphocytes are found in the follicles and medulla; T lymphocytes in the paracortical areas and in the cortex between follicles. Several afferent lymph vessels enter through the capsule of the node and open into the subcapsular sinus. From here radial cortical sinuses drain to medullary sinuses which are confluent with the efferent vessel draining the node at the hilum, where blood vessels enter and leave. The thymus, spleen and the O-MALT aggregations, such as the tonsils, do not have afferent lymphatics.

The (palatine and pharyngeal) **tonsils** possess lymphoid follicles similar to those of lymph nodes, but while the nodes have a capsule of connective tissue the tonsils have, on their inner surfaces, a covering of mucous membrane that dips down deeply to form the tonsillar crypts.

The lymphoid follicles of the **spleen** are found in its white pulp, which is scattered in the red pulp that constitutes most of the substance of the spleen and contains large numbers of venous sinuses. In the white pulp T lymphocytes form periarteriolar sheaths, some of which are lymphoid follicles with B lymphocytes in the germinal centres. These follicles are visible to the naked eye on the cut surface of the spleen as whitish nodules up to 1 mm in diameter.

Apart from lymphocytes, all lymphoid organs and organized lymphoid tissue contain macrophages, which are part of the mononuclear phagocyte system of the body.

PART TWO

Nervous system

The nervous system is divided into the **central nervous system**, which consists of the brain and spinal cord, and the **peripheral nervous system** composed of cranial and spinal nerves and their associated ganglia. The central and peripheral parts each have somatic and autonomic components; the somatic are concerned with the innervation of skeletal muscle (along efferent pathways) and the transmission of sensory information (along afferent pathways), and the autonomic are concerned with the control of cardiac muscle, smooth muscle and glands (also involving efferent and afferent pathways). The term **autonomic nervous system** is applied collectively to all autonomic components.

Neurons and nerves

The structural and functional unit of the nervous system is the **nerve cell** or **neuron**. It consists of a part containing the nucleus, the cell body, and a variable number of processes commonly called nerve fibres. A single cytoplasmic process, the **axon** (often very long), conducts nerve impulses away from the cell body, and may give off many collaterals and terminal branches to many different target cells. Other multiple cytoplasmic processes, the **dendrites** (usually very short), expand the surface area of the cell body for the reception of stimuli.

Pathways are established in the nervous system by communications between neurons at **synapses**, which are sites on the cell body or its processes where chemical transmitters enable nerve impulses to be handed on from one neuron to another. Transmission between neurons and cells outside the nervous system, for example muscle cells (neuromuscular junctions), is also effected by neurotransmitters. The small number of 'classic' transmitters such as acetylcholine and noradrenaline (norepinephrine) has been vastly supplemented in recent years by many substances. These include monoamines, amino acids, nitric oxide and neuropeptides.

Cell bodies with similar function show a great tendency to group themselves together, forming **nuclei** within the central nervous system and **ganglia** outside it. Similarly processes from such aggregations of cell bodies tend to run together in bundles, forming **tracts** within the central nervous system and **nerves** outside the brain and spinal cord.

Apart from neurons the nervous system contains other cells collectively known as **neuroglial cells** (neuroglia or glia), which have supporting and other functions but which do not have the property of excitability or conductivity possessed by neurons. The main types of neuroglial cell are *astrocytes* and *oligodendrocytes*, which like neurons are developed from ectoderm of the neural tube. A third type of neuroglial cell is the *microglial cell* (microglia) which is the phagocytic cell of the nervous system, corresponding to the macrophage of connective tissue, and is derived from mesoderm.

Nerve fibres may be **myelinated** or **unmyelinated**. In the central nervous system myelin is formed by oligodendrocytes, and in peripheral nerves by Schwann cells (*neurolemmocytes*). In myelinated fibres, the regions where longitudinally adjacent Schwann cells or oligodendrocyte processes join one another are the *nodes* (of Ranvier). The white matter of the nervous system is essentially a mass of nerve fibres and is so called because of the general pale appearance imparted by the fatty myelin, in contrast to grey matter which is darker and consists essentially of cell bodies.

Peripheral nerve fibres have been classified in relation to their conduction velocity, which is generally proportional to size, and function:

- Group A—Up to 20 μm diameter, subdivided into:
  α: 12–20 μm. Motor and proprioception (Ia and Ib)
  β: 5–12 μm. Touch, pressure and proprioception (II)
  γ: 5–12 μm. Fusimotor to muscle spindles (II)
  δ: 1–15 μm. Touch, pain and temperature (III)
- Group B—Up to 3 μm diameter. Myelinated. Preganglionic autonomic
- Group C—Up to 2 μm diameter. Unmyelinated. Postganglionic autonomic, and touch and pain (IV).

The widest fibres tend to conduct most rapidly. Unfortunately, as can be seen from the above, it is not possible to make a precise prediction of function from mere size. Thus the largest myelinated fibres may be motor or proprioceptive and the smallest, whether myelinated or unmyelinated, are autonomic or sensory.

Spinal nerves

There are 31 pairs of spinal nerves: 8 cervical, 12 thoracic, 5 lumbar, 5 sacral and 1 coccygeal. Each spinal nerve is formed by the union of an **anterior** (ventral) and a **posterior** (dorsal) **root** which are attached to the side of the spinal cord by little rootlets. The union takes place within the intervertebral foramen through which the nerve emerges immediately distal to the swelling on the posterior root, the **posterior root ganglion**; this is also within the foramen. The anterior root of every spinal nerve contains motor (efferent) fibres for skeletal muscle; those from T1 to L2 inclusive and from S2 to S4 also contain autonomic fibres. The anterior root also contains a small number of unmyelinated afferent pain fibres which have 'doubled back' from their cells of origin in the posterior root ganglion to enter the spinal cord by the anterior root instead of by the posterior root. The posterior root of every nerve contains sensory (afferent) fibres whose cell bodies are in the posterior root ganglion. There are no synapses in these ganglia; it is simply the site of the cell bodies.

Immediately after its formation the mixed spinal nerve divides into a larger **anterior** and a smaller **posterior ramus**. The great nerve plexuses—cervical, brachial, lumbar and sacral—are formed from anterior rami; posterior rami do not form plexuses.

Connective tissue binds the fibres of spinal nerves together to form the single nerve. Delicate loose connective tissue, the endoneurium, lies between individual fibres. Rounded bundles of fibres, or fascicles, are surrounded by the perineurium, a condensed layer of collagenous connective tissue. Fascicles are bound together into a single nerve by a layer of loose but thicker connective tissue, the epineurium. In the largest nerve, the sciatic, only about 20% of the cross-sectional area is nerve, so 80% is connective tissue, but in smaller nerves the amount of neural tissue is proportionally greater. The larger nerves have their own nerves, the nervi nervorum, in their connective tissue coverings.

Peripheral nerve trunks in the limbs are supplied by branches from local arteries. The sciatic nerve in the buttock and the median nerve at the elbow each have a large branch from the inferior gluteal and common interosseous arteries respectively. Elsewhere, however, regional arteries supply nerves by a series of longitudinal branches which anastomose freely within the epineurium, so that nerves can be displaced widely from their beds without risk to their blood supply.

General principles of nerve supply

Once the nerve supply to a part is established in the embryo it never alters thereafter, unlike the vascular supply. However far a structure may migrate in the developing fetus it always drags its nerve with it. Conversely, the nerve supply to an adult structure affords visible evidence of its embryonic origin.

Skeletal muscles are innervated from motor neuron 'pools'—groups of motor nerve cell bodies in certain cranial nerve nuclei of the brainstem and anterior horns of the spinal cord. The pool supplying any one muscle overlaps the pools of another, e.g. the anterior horn cells of spinal cord segments C5 and C6 that supply deltoid are intermixed with cells of the same segments supplying subscapularis and other muscles. The only exceptions to the overlapping of neuronal pools are the brainstem nuclei of the fourth and sixth cranial nerves, as they are the only motor nerve cell groups supplying only one muscle (superior oblique and lateral rectus of the eye respectively).

Nerve supply of the body wall

The body wall is supplied segmentally by spinal nerves (Fig. 1.6). The posterior rami pass backwards and supply the extensor muscles of the vertebral column and skull, and to a varying extent the skin that overlies them.

The anterior rami supply all other muscles of the trunk and limbs and the skin at the sides and front of the neck and body.

Posterior rami

In the trunk, all the muscles of the erector spinae and transversospinalis groups that lie deep to the thoraco-lumbar fascia, and the levator costae muscles of the thorax are supplied by the posterior rami of spinal nerves (Fig. 1.7). In the neck, splenius and all muscles deep to it are similarly supplied.

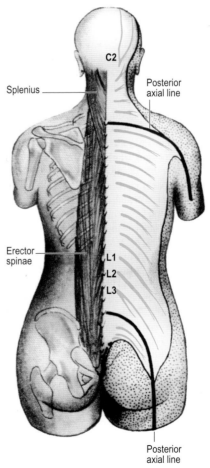

Fig. 1.7   Distribution of posterior rami. On the right, the cutaneous distribution is shown (medial branches down to T6, to clear the scapula, and lateral branches below this); the stippled areas of skin are supplied by anterior rami. On the left, the muscular distribution is shown, to erector spinae and to splenius and the muscles deep to it.

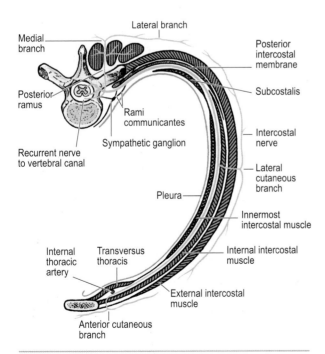

Fig. 1.6   Course of a typical intercostal nerve along the neurovascular plane of the body wall, between the middle and innermost of the three muscle layers.

Each posterior ramus divides into a medial and a lateral branch (Fig. 1.6). Both branches of the posterior rami supply muscle, but only one branch, either medial or lateral, reaches the skin. In the upper part of the body the medial branches, and in the lower part the lateral branches, of the posterior rami provide the cutaneous branches (Fig. 1.7).

C1 has no cutaneous branch, and the posterior rami of the lower two nerves in the cervical and lumbar regions of the cord likewise fail to reach the skin. All 12 thoracic and five sacral nerves reach the skin. No posterior ramus ever supplies skin or muscle of a limb.

Anterior rami

The anterior rami supply the prevertebral flexor muscles segmentally by separate branches from each nerve (e.g. longus capitis and colli, scalene muscles, psoas, quadratus lumborum, piriformis). The anterior rami of the lower four cervical and the first thoracic nerves supply muscles in the upper limb via the brachial plexus. The anterior rami of the 12 thoracic nerves and L1 supply the muscles of the body wall segmentally. Each intercostal nerve supplies the muscles of its intercostal space, and the lower six nerves pass beyond the costal margin to supply the muscles of the anterior abdominal wall. The first lumbar nerve (iliohypogastric and ilioinguinal nerves) is the lowest spinal nerve to supply the anterior abdominal wall. Muscles supplied by anterior rami below L1 are no longer in the body wall; they have migrated into the lower limb.

C1 has no cutaneous branch. C2, 3 and 4 supply skin in the neck by branches of the cervical plexus. C5, 6, 7 and 8 and T1 supply skin of the upper limb via the brachial plexus.

In the trunk the skin is supplied in strips or zones in regular sequence from T2 to L1 inclusive. The intercostal nerves each have a lateral branch to supply the sides and an anterior terminal branch to supply the front of the body wall (Fig. 1.6). The lower six thoracic nerves pass beyond the costal margin obliquely downwards to supply the skin of the abdominal wall (Fig. 1.8).

Neurovascular plane

The nerves of the body wall, accompanied by their segmental arteries and veins, spiral around the walls of the thorax and abdomen in a plane between the middle and deepest of the three muscle layers (see p. 187 and Fig. 1.6). In this neurovascular plane the nerves lie below the arteries as they run around the body wall. But the nerves cross the arteries posteriorly alongside the vertebral column and again anteriorly near the

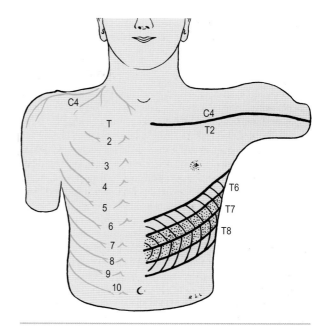

Fig. 1.8 Overlap of dermatomes on the body wall. On the right side, the supraclavicular and thoracic nerves are shown. On the left, the anterior axial line is indicated; this marks the boundary on the chest wall between skin supplied by the cervical plexus and by intercostal nerves. Adjacent dermatomes overlap and thereby, for instance, the dermatomes of T6 and T8 meet each other, completely covering T7, explaining why division of a single intercostal nerve does not give rise to anaesthesia on the trunk.

ventral midline, and at these points of crossing a definite relationship is always maintained between the two. The nerve always lies nearer the skin. The spinal cord lies nearer the surface of the body than the aorta, and as a result the spinal nerve makes a circle that surrounds the smaller arterial circle. The arterial circle is made of the aorta with its intercostal and lumbar arteries, completed in front by the internal thoracic and the superior and inferior epigastric arteries. As a part of the same arterial pattern the vertebral arteries pass up to the cranial cavity. The spinal nerves, as they emerge from the intervertebral foramina, pass laterally behind the vertebral artery in the neck, behind the posterior intercostal arteries in the thorax, behind the lumbar arteries in the abdomen and behind the lateral sacral arteries in the pelvis. The anterior terminal branches of the spinal nerves similarly pass in front of the internal thoracic and the superior and inferior epigastric arteries (Fig. 1.7).

The sympathetic trunk runs vertically within the arterial circle. From the base of the skull to the coccyx the sympathetic trunk lies anterior to the segmental vessels (vertebral, posterior intercostal, lumbar and lateral sacral arteries).

Sympathetic fibres

Every spinal nerve without exception, from C1 to the coccygeal, carries postganglionic (unmyelinated, grey) sympathetic fibres which 'hitch-hike' along the nerves and accompany all their branches. They leave the spinal nerve only at the site of their peripheral destination. They are in the main vasoconstrictor in function, though some go to sweat glands in the skin (sudomotor) and to the arrectores pilorum muscles of the hair roots (pilomotor). In this way the sympathetic system innervates the whole body wall and all four limbs. This is chiefly for the function of temperature regulation. The visceral branches of the sympathetic system have a different manner of distribution (see p. 21).

Nerve supply of limbs

The body wall has been seen to be supplied segmentally by spinal nerves (Fig. 1.6). A longitudinal strip posteriorly is supplied by posterior rami, a lateral strip by the lateral branches of the anterior rami, and a ventral strip by the anterior terminal branches of the anterior rami. In the fetus the limb buds grow out from the lateral strip supplied by the lateral branches of the anterior rami and these lateral branches, by their anterior and posterior divisions, form the plexuses for supply of the muscles and skin of the limbs. The posterior divisions supply extensor muscles and the anterior divisions supply flexor muscles. Both divisions supply skin of the limbs.

Each limb consists of a flexor and an extensor compartment, which meet at the preaxial and postaxial borders of the limb. These borders are marked out approximately by veins. In the upper limb the cephalic vein lies at the preaxial and the basilic vein at the postaxial border. In the lower limb, extension and medial rotation, which replace the early fetal position of flexion, have complicated the picture. The great saphenous vein marks out the preaxial and the small saphenous vein the postaxial borders of the limb.

The spinal nerves entering into a limb plexus come from enlarged parts of the cord, the cervical enlargement for the brachial plexus and the lumbar enlargement for the lumbar and sacral plexuses. The enlargements are produced by the greatly increased number of motor neurons in the anterior horns at these levels (see p. 506).

On account of the way nerve fibres become combined and rearranged in plexuses, any one spinal nerve can contribute to more than one peripheral nerve and peripheral nerves can receive fibres from more than one spinal nerve. It follows that the area of skin supplied by any one spinal nerve or spinal cord segment is not the same as the area supplied by a peripheral spinal nerve. Two kinds of skin maps or charts are therefore required, one showing segmental innervation and the other showing peripheral nerves. The segmental supplies are reviewed below; the peripheral nerves of the upper and lower limbs are summarized on pages 95 and 166.

Segmental innervation of the skin

The area of skin supplied by a single spinal nerve is called a **dermatome**. On the trunk, adjacent dermatomes overlap considerably, so that interruption of a single spinal nerve produces no anaesthesia (Fig. 1.8); the same applies to the limbs, except at the axial lines. The line of junction of two dermatomes supplied from discontinuous spinal levels is demarcated by an **axial line**, and such axial lines extend from the trunk on to the limbs. In the **upper limb** (Fig. 1.9) the anterior axial line runs from the sternal angle across the second costal cartilage and down the front of the limb almost to the wrist. The dermatomes lie in orderly numerical sequence when traced distally down the front and proximally up the back of the anterior axial line (C5, 6, 7, 8 and T1) and these dermatomes are supplied by the nerves of the brachial plexus. In addition, skin has been 'borrowed'

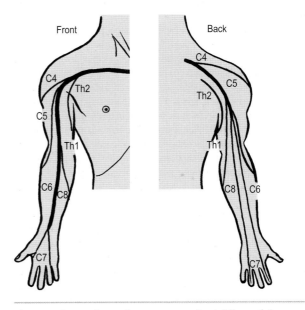

Fig. 1.9   Approximate dermatomes and axial lines of the right upper limb. See text for explanation.

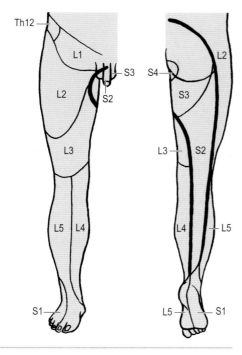

Fig. 1.10 Approximate dermatomes and axial lines of the right lower limb. See text for explanation.

are a compromise between the maximal and minimal segmental areas which experience has shown can occur. Original charts, such as those made by Sherrington, Head and Foerster, are being modified by the continuing accumulation of new information. Thus T1 nerve, for example, is not usually considered to supply any thoracic skin but has sometimes been considered to do so, and L5 and S1 have been reported to extend to buttock skin although this is not usually expected. It is probable that posterior axial lines do not exist, but evidence for anterior axial lines is more convincing. Difficulty in investigation arises in the main from the blurring of patterns due to overlap from adjacent dermatomes. A chart of dermatomes must therefore be interpreted with flexibility. The following summary offers selected guidelines that are clinically useful:

C1 No skin supply
C2 Occipital region, posterior neck and skin over parotid
C3 Neck
C4 Infraclavicular region (to manubriosternal junction), shoulder and above scapular spine
C5 Lateral arm
C6 Lateral forearm and thumb
C7 Middle fingers
C8 Little finger and distal medial forearm
T1 Medial arm above and below elbow
T2 Medial arm, axilla and thorax
T3 Thorax and occasional extension to axilla
T4 Nipple
T7 Subcostal angle
T8 Rib margin
T10 Umbilicus
T12 Lower abdomen, upper buttock
L1 Suprapubic and inguinal regions, penis, anterior scrotum (labia), upper buttock
L2 Anterior thigh, upper buttock
L3 Anterior and medial thigh and knee
L4 Medial leg, medial ankle and side of foot
L5 Lateral leg, dorsum of foot, medial sole
S1 Lateral ankle, lateral side of dorsum and sole
S2 Posterior leg, posterior thigh, buttock, penis
S3 Sitting area of buttock, posterior scrotum (labia)
S4 Perianal
S5 and Co Behind anus and over coccyx.

Segmental innervation of muscles

Most muscles are supplied equally from two adjacent segments of the spinal cord. Muscles sharing a common primary action on a joint irrespective of their anatomical situation are all supplied by the same (usually two) segments. Their opponents, sharing the opposite action,

from the neck and trunk to clothe the proximal part of the limb (C4 over the deltoid muscle, T2 for the axilla).

Considerable distortion occurs to the dermatome pattern of the **lower limb** (Fig. 1.10) for two reasons. Firstly the limb, from the fetal position of flexion, is medially rotated and extended, so that the anterior axial line is caused to spiral from the root of the penis (clitoris) across the front of the scrotum (labium majus) around to the back of the thigh and calf in the midline almost to the heel. Secondly, a good deal of skin is 'borrowed' from the trunk on the cranial side (from T12, L1, 2 and 3). As in the upper limb, the dermatomes can be traced in numerical sequence down in front and up behind the anterior axial line (L1, 2, 3, 4, 5 and S1, 2, 3).

A practical application of the anterior axial line arises in spinal analgesia. A 'low spinal' (caudal) anaesthetic anaesthetizes the skin of the posterior two-thirds of the scrotum or labium majus (S3), but to anaesthetize the anterior one-third of the scrotum or labium L1 must be involved, an additional seven spinal segments higher up.

It must be remembered that a single chart cannot indicate individual variations or the differing findings of several groups of investigators, and that such charts are likewise all supplied by the same (usually two) segments and these segments usually run in numerical sequence with the former. For a joint one segment more distal in the limb the spinal centre lies en bloc one segment lower in the cord.

Thus there are in effect spinal centres for joint movements, and these centres tend to occupy continuous segments in the cord. The upper one or two segments innervate one movement, and the lower one or two innervate the opposite movement (although sometimes the same segment may innervate both movements, but of course from different anterior horn cells). Thus the spinal centre for the elbow is in C5, 6, 7, 8 segments; biceps, brachialis and brachioradialis (the prime flexors of the elbow) are supplied by C5, 6 and triceps (the prime extensor of the elbow) is supplied by C7, 8.

The segments mainly responsible for the various limb joint movements are summarized in Figures 1.11 and 1.12. Flexion/extension at the hip, knee and ankle are the easiest to remember, for each movement involves two segments in logical sequence for each joint, and for each more distal joint the segments concerned are one segment lower:

Hip

$\left.\begin{matrix}2\\3\end{matrix}\right\}$ Flex

$\left.\begin{matrix}4\\5\end{matrix}\right\}$ Extend

Knee

$\left.\begin{matrix}3\\4\end{matrix}\right\}$ Extend

$\left.\begin{matrix}5\\1\end{matrix}\right\}$ Flex

Ankle

$\left.\begin{matrix}4\\5\end{matrix}\right\}$ Dorsiflex

$\left.\begin{matrix}1\\2\end{matrix}\right\}$ Plantarflex

The above pattern enables the segmental innervation of a muscle to be determined, e.g.:

- iliacus (flexes hip) L2, 3
- biceps femoris (flexes knee) L5, S1
- soleus (plantarflexes ankle) S1, 2.

The above are simple flexion–extension movements and, indeed, cover all knee- and ankle-moving muscles. At the hip, however, movements other than flexion and

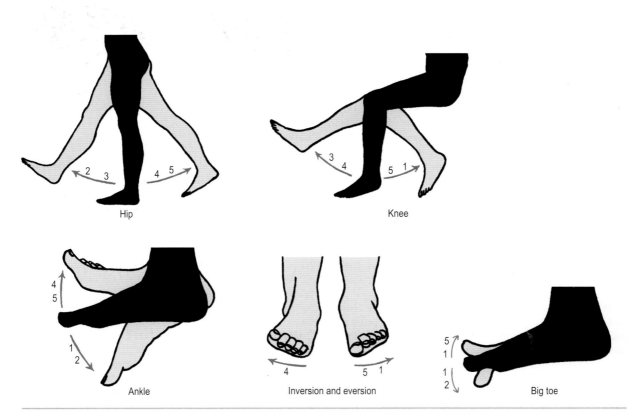

Fig. 1.11 Segmental innervation of movements of the lower limb.

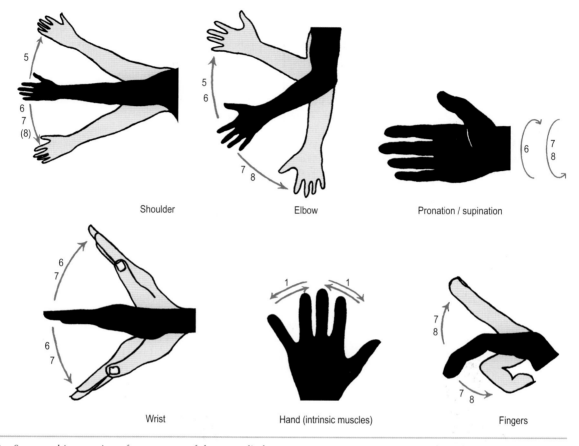

Fig. 1.12 Segmental innervation of movements of the upper limb.

extension are possible, but all are innervated by the same four segments. Thus:

- adduction or medial rotation (same as flexion) L2, 3
- abduction or lateral rotation (same as extension) L4, 5.

For inversion and eversion of the foot the formulae are:

- invert foot L4
- evert foot L5, S1.

Tibialis anterior and tibialis posterior invert the foot and both are innervated by L4 segment. Tibialis anterior is also a dorsiflexor and L4, 5 (from the formula already given for dorsiflexion) is its correct segmental supply. Tibialis posterior, however, lies deep among the plantar flexors of the ankle (S1, 2), but its main action is inversion of the foot (it is the principal invertor) and, although it assists plantar flexion, its segmental innervation is L4, 5.

The upper limb movements, with the segments involved (Fig. 1.12), are as follows:

Shoulder	Abduct and laterally rotate C5
	Adduct and medially rotate C6, 7, 8
Elbow	Flex C5, 6
	Extend C7, 8
Forearm	Pronate C7, 8
	Supinate C6
Wrist only	Flex C6, 7
	Extend C6, 7
Fingers and thumb	Flex C7, 8
(long tendons)	Extend C7, 8
Hand	T1.
(intrinsic muscles)	

In the upper limb the two-and-two segment pattern is not as regular as in the lower limb, probably because in the upper limb much more precise movements are constantly being employed, and the spinal centres have broken up into separate nuclei to control these. Thus, below the elbow the plan does not conform to the basic pattern of four spinal segments for each joint. Flexion and extension share the same two segments; these are C6, 7 for the wrist and C7, 8 for the digits. But the rule holds that the more distal joints are innervated from lower centres in the cord.

As a guide to the level of spinal cord injury it is useful to be aware of a muscle and a movement for which a particular spinal cord segment is mainly responsible:

C4 Diaphragm. Respiration
C5 Deltoid. Abduction of the shoulder
C6 Biceps. Flexion of the elbow. Biceps jerk (see below)
C7 Triceps, Extension of the elbow. Triceps jerk (see below)
C8 Flexor digitorum profundus and extensor digitorum. Finger flexion and extension
T1 Abductor pollicis brevis representing small hand muscles. Abduction of the thumb
T7–12 Anterior abdominal wall muscles. Guarding. Abdominal reflex (see below)
L1 Lowest fibres of internal oblique and transversus abdominis. Guarding
L2 Psoas major. Flexion of the hip
L3 Quadriceps femoris. Extension of the knee. Knee jerk (see below)
L4 Tibialis anterior and posterior. Inversion of the foot
L5 Extensor hallucis longus. Extension of the great toe
S1 Gastrocnemius. Plantarflexion of the foot. Ankle jerk (see below)
S2 Small muscles of the foot
S3 Perineal muscles. Bladder (parasympathetic). Anal reflex (see below).

It is important to note that the term 'root' as used in root injuries may be taken to mean either the nerve root proper, i.e. from the side of the spinal cord to the intervertebral foramen, or the roots of the plexuses, i.e. anterior rami distal to the foramen. In lesions of the nerve roots proper, sweating in the distribution of the appropriate nerves is normal, but in more peripheral lesions sweating is reduced, because the postganglionic sympathetic fibres from the sympathetic trunk join the roots of plexuses distal to the nerve roots proper (Fig. 1.13C).

Spinal reflexes

What is commonly called the 'knee jerk' and similar tendon reflexes are typical examples of spinal myotatic or **stretch reflexes** (deep tendon reflexes). They illustrate the simplest kind of reflex pathway and involve only two neurons with one synapse (monosynaptic reflex arc,

Fig. 1.13A); indeed the tendon reflexes are the only examples of monosynaptic reflex arcs, for all other reflexes involve two or more synapses (multisynaptic, Fig. 1.13B, C).

Tapping the tendon momentarily stretches the spindles within the muscle and this stimulates the afferent (Ia) fibres of the nerve endings surrounding the intrafusal fibres, which pass into the spinal cord by the posterior nerve root. These afferents synapse directly with the α motor neurons of the anterior horn whose axons form the efferent side of the arc, so causing the extrafusal fibres to contract and produce the 'jerk' at the joint.

For most practical purposes the segments mainly concerned with the reflexes most commonly tested may be taken as: biceps jerk—C6; triceps jerk—C7; knee jerk—L3; ankle jerk—S1.

Diminution or absence of the jerk usually indicates some kind of interruption of the arc or muscular defect, but exaggeration of the tendon reflexes is taken as evidence of an *upper motor neuron lesion* due to alterations in the supraspinal control of the anterior horn cells which are rendered unduly excitable. In this case the γ motor neurons of the anterior horn are stimulated by such fibres as the reticulospinal and vestibulospinal. The pathway (Fig. 1.13D) is from the γ motor neuron to the intrafusal muscle fibres of the spindle, then from the afferent fibres of the spindle to the α motor neuron and so to the extrafusal fibres. This is the γ reflex loop or fusimotor neuron loop.

In addition to the above deep tendon reflexes, there are superficial skin reflexes which are multisynaptic. Those most commonly tested are the plantar, abdominal and anal reflexes.

Firm stroking of the lateral surface of the sole of the foot (as with the end of a key) to elicit the **plantar reflex** normally causes plantarflexion of the great toe and probably of the other toes as well. Extension of the great toe—the *extensor response (Babinski's sign)*—indicates an upper motor neuron lesion. In infants under 1 year old the extensor response is the normal response; only with myelination of the corticospinal tracts during the second year does the normal plantar reflex become flexor.

The **abdominal reflex** is elicited by lightly stroking across each quadrant of the anterior abdominal wall. Normally there is contraction of the underlying muscles, but the reflexes are absent in upper motor neuron lesions. Patients with paraplegia who are lying down may exhibit *Beevor's sign*: when trying to lift the shoulders, the umbilicus is displaced upwards, due to weakness of the muscles below the umbilicus.

The **anal reflex** ('anal wink') is a visible contraction of the external anal sphincter following pinprick of the

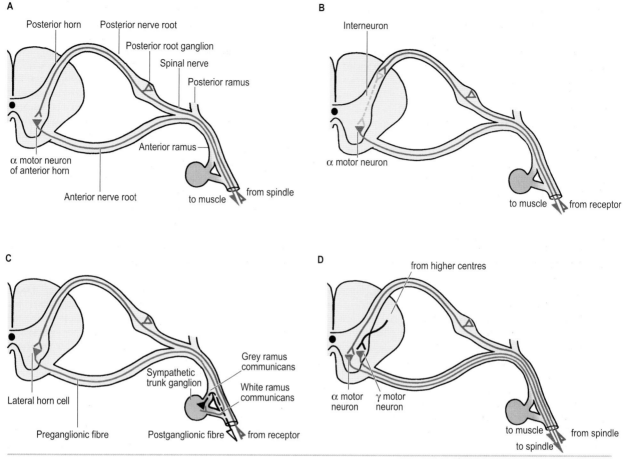

Fig. 1.13 Examples of spinal reflex pathways: **A** the two neurons of a stretch reflex (tendon jerk), which is monosynaptic; **B** a multisynaptic reflex arc; only one interneuron is shown but there may be several; **C** the three neurons of a sympathetic reflex, showing the different positions of cell bodies compared with **B**: that of the preganglionic cell in the lateral grey horn of the spinal cord (instead of the posterior horn), and that of the postganglionic cell in a sympathetic ganglion (instead of the anterior horn). Note that the sympathetic preganglionic fibre runs in the white ramus communicans (which is the more distal connection of the ganglion) and the postganglionic fibre in the grey ramus; **D** the fusimotor neuron loop; the γ efferent neuron, under the influence of higher centres, stimulates the muscle spindle from which afferent fibres pass back to the spinal cord to synapse with the α motor neuron.

perianal skin and depends on intact sacral segments of the cord (mainly S3).

Autonomic nervous system

The motor part of the somatic nervous system is concerned with the innervation of skeletal muscle. The cell bodies are either in the motor nuclei of cranial nerves or the anterior horn cells of the spinal cord, and the nerve fibres which leave the central nervous system run uninterruptedly to the muscles, ending as motor endplates on the muscle fibres. The motor part of the autonomic nervous system is concerned with the innervation of cardiac and smooth muscle and glands, and the great difference between this and the somatic system is that the pathway from nerve cells in the central nervous system to the target organ is interrupted by *synapses in a ganglion*. There are thus two sets of neurons, which are logically called *preganglionic* and *postganglionic*. The preganglionic cell bodies are always within the central nervous system. If sympathetic, they are in the lateral horn cells of all the thoracic and the upper two lumbar segments of the spinal cord; this is the thoracolumbar part of the autonomic nervous system (the 'thoracolumbar outflow'). If parasympathetic, they are in certain cranial nerve nuclei and in lateral horn cells of sacral segments of the spinal cord; this is the craniosacral part of the autonomic nervous system (the 'craniosacral outflow').

The postganglionic cell bodies are in ganglia in the peripheral nervous system. If sympathetic, the ganglia are either in the sympathetic trunk or in autonomic plexuses situated in the abdomen and pelvis (such as the coeliac ganglia). If parasympathetic, the ganglia are usually within the walls of the viscera concerned, while in the head there are four ganglia which are some little distance from the structures innervated.

Sympathetic nervous system

Having reached a sympathetic trunk ganglion, the incoming preganglionic fibres have one of three possible synaptic alternatives. The most common is for them to synapse with cell bodies in a trunk ganglion, either in the one they entered (Fig. 1.14A) or to run up or down the trunk to some other trunk ganglion. The second alternative is to leave the trunk ganglion without synapsing and to pass to a ganglion in an autonomic

plexus for synapse (Fig. 1.14B). The third possibility (which applies only to a small number of fibres) is that they leave the trunk (without synapsing) to pass to the suprarenal gland, where certain cells of the medulla can be regarded as modified ganglion cells.

Because there is no sympathetic outflow from the cervical part of the cord, nor from the lower lumbar and sacral parts, those preganglionic fibres which are destined to synapse with cell bodies whose fibres are going to run with cervical nerves must ascend in the sympathetic trunk to cervical ganglia, and those for lower lumbar and sacral nerves must descend in the trunk to lower lumbar and sacral ganglia.

The segmental levels of the preganglionic cell bodies concerned with the innervation of the different regions of the body (via postganglionic neurons) are indicated in Figure 1.15. In general the body is represented upright from head to perineum but with overlaps and individual variations.

The sympathetic trunk extends alongside the vertebral column from the base of the skull to the coccyx. Theoretically there is a ganglion for each spinal nerve, but fusion occurs, especially in the cervical region where the upper four unite to form the superior cervical ganglion, the fifth and sixth form the middle cervical ganglion,

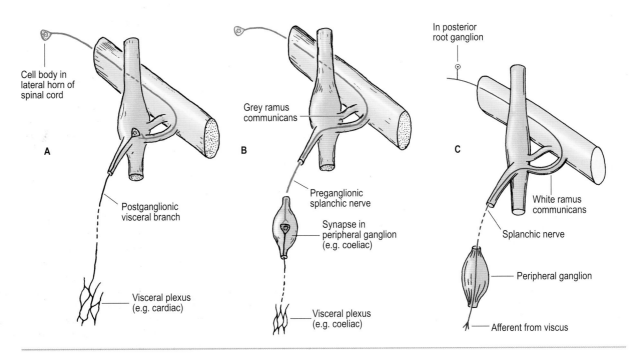

Fig. 1.14   Visceral connections of sympathetic ganglia: **A** efferent pathway with synapse in a sympathetic trunk ganglion; **B** efferent pathway with synapse in a peripheral ganglion; **C** afferent pathway for pain fibres, passing through the trunk ganglion and into the spinal nerve by the white ramus communicans.

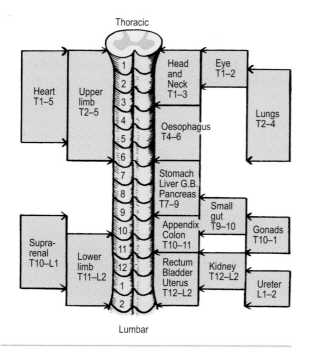

Fig. 1.15 Spinal levels of sympathetic preganglionic cells. There may be considerable individual variations, especially for the upper limb.

and the seventh and eighth fuse as the inferior cervical ganglion (and often with the first thoracic ganglion as well to form the cervicothoracic or stellate ganglion). Elsewhere there is usually one ganglion less than the number of nerves: 11 thoracic; 4 lumbar; and 4 sacral.

The fibres from the lateral horn cells of each segment of the spinal cord leave in the anterior nerve root (with the axons of anterior horn cells) to reach the spinal nerve and its anterior ramus. The connecting links from here to the sympathetic trunk and its ganglia are the *rami communicantes*. There are normally two rami; the *white ramus communicans* is the more distal of the two, and this is the one containing the preganglionic fibres (which are myelinated, hence called white). The other, the *grey ramus communicans*, contains efferent postganglionic fibres (which are unmyelinated, hence grey). The fibres in the grey ramus are those that are distributed via the branches of the spinal nerve to blood vessels, sweat glands and arrector pili muscles (i.e. they are vasomotor, sudomotor and pilomotor). Every spinal nerve receives a grey ramus. All the thoracic and the upper two lumbar nerves have both white and grey rami connecting them to sympathetic ganglia. But the cervical, lower lumbar and sacral nerves do not have white rami; the ganglia

they are connected with receive preganglionic fibres from the thoracolumbar outflow through the chain. Because of the fusion of ganglia, the superior cervical ganglion gives off four grey rami, and the other cervical ganglia two each. Occasionally rami (both grey and white) may be duplicated.

Each sympathetic trunk ganglion has a collateral or *visceral branch*, usually called a *splanchnic nerve* in the thoracic, lumbar and sacral regions, but in the cervical region called a *cardiac branch* because it proceeds to the cardiac plexus. The visceral branches generally arise high up and descend steeply to form plexuses for the viscera (Fig. 1.14). Thus cardiac branches arise from the three cervical ganglia to descend into the mediastinum to the *cardiac plexus*, which is supplemented by fibres from upper thoracic ganglia. From the fifth and lower thoracic ganglia three splanchnic nerves pierce the diaphragm to reach the *coeliac plexus* and other pre-aortic plexuses, which are also joined by lumbar splanchnic nerves from the upper lumbar ganglia. Fibres from these plexuses, and splanchnic nerves from the lower lumbar ganglia, descend to the *superior hypogastric plexus* and thence to the left and right *inferior hypogastric (pelvic) plexuses*. The inferior hypogastric plexuses are joined by visceral branches from all the sacral ganglia (sacral splanchnic nerves).

The sympathetic visceral plexuses thus formed are joined by parasympathetic nerves: vagus to the coeliac plexus; and pelvic splanchnics (S2–4) to the inferior hypogastric plexuses. The mixed visceral plexuses reach the viscera by direct branches and by branches that hitch-hike along the relevant arteries.

In addition to the visceral branches, which supply not only the smooth muscle and glands of viscera but also the blood vessels of those viscera, all trunk ganglia give off *vascular branches* to adjacent large blood vessels. The cervical ganglia give branches to the carotid and vertebral arteries, including (from the superior cervical ganglion) the internal carotid nerve, running upwards on the artery of that name to form the internal carotid plexus on the artery as it enters the skull. The thoracic and lumbar ganglia give filaments to the various aortic plexuses and from there to aortic branches including the common iliac arteries, continued along the internal and external iliac arteries as far as the proximal part of the femoral artery. Branches from the sacral ganglia pass to the lateral sacral arteries. Note that although the head and neck arteries receive direct branches from cervical trunk ganglia, limb vessels get their sympathetic innervation mainly from nerve fibres that run with the adjacent peripheral nerves before passing to the vessels; the fibres do not run long distances along the vessels themselves. Thus the nerve filaments to the vessels of the tip of a finger or toe run not with the digital arteries but with the digital nerves, and only leave the nerves near the actual site of innervation.

Afferent sympathetic fibres

Many afferent fibres hitch-hike along sympathetic efferent pathways. Some form the afferent limb for unconscious reflex activities; others are concerned with visceral pain. All have their cell bodies in the posterior root ganglia of spinal nerves (not in sympathetic ganglia), at approximately the same segmental level as the preganglionic cells (Fig. 1.15). The afferent fibres reach the spinal nerve via the white ramus communicans (Fig. 1.14C) and then join the posterior root ganglion, from which central processes enter the spinal cord by the posterior nerve root (like any other afferent fibres). Visceral pain fibres enter the posterior horn, and thereafter the pain pathway is the same as that for spinal nerve pain fibres. Others concerned with reflex activities may synapse with interneurons in the cord or ascend to the hypothalamus and other higher centres by pathways that are not defined.

Sympathectomy

For the control of excessive sweating and vasoconstriction in the extremities of the limbs, parts of the sympathetic trunk with appropriate ganglia can be removed to abolish the normal sympathetic influence. In upper thoracic ganglionectomy for the upper limb the second and third thoracic ganglia with their rami and the intervening part of the trunk are resected; alternatively, the trunk is divided below the third ganglion and the rami communicantes to the second and third ganglia are severed. The first thoracic ganglion is not removed, as the preganglionic fibres for the upper limb do not usually arise above T2 level (see above), and its removal would result in Horner's syndrome (see p. 423). Upper thoracic ganglionectomy is described further on page 219.

For lumbar sympathectomy the third and fourth lumbar ganglia and the intervening trunk are removed. The first lumbar ganglion should be preserved otherwise ejaculation may be compromised. Lumbar sympathectomy is described further on page 291.

Parasympathetic nervous system

Although all parts of the body receive a sympathetic supply, the distribution of parasympathetic fibres is wholly visceral and not to the trunk or limbs. However, not all viscera are so innervated: the suprarenal glands and the gonads appear to have only a sympathetic supply.

The preganglionic fibres of cranial origin have their cell bodies in the accessory (Edinger–Westphal) oculomotor nucleus, the superior and inferior salivatory nuclei of the seventh and ninth cranial nerves respectively, and the dorsal motor nucleus of the vagus. The postganglionic cells for the first three are in the four parasympathetic ganglia, discussed below; the vagal fibres synapse with postganglionic cell bodies in the walls of the viscera supplied (heart, lungs and gut).

The preganglionic fibres of sacral origin arise from cells in the lateral grey horn of sacral segments 2–4 of the spinal cord, and constitute the *pelvic splanchnic nerves*. Leaving the anterior rami of the appropriate sacral nerves near the anterior sacral foramina, they pass forwards to enter into the formation of the inferior hypogastric plexuses. From there they run to pelvic viscera and to the hindgut as far up as the splenic flexure. Fibres reach the viscera either by running along their blood vessels or making their own way retroperitoneally, and they synapse around postganglionic cell bodies in the walls of these viscera.

Cranial parasympathetic ganglia

The four ganglia—ciliary, pterygopalatine, submandibular and otic—are very similar in plan. Each has parasympathetic, sympathetic and sensory roots, and branches of distribution. The roots and branches are described in general terms below and illustrated in Figure 1.16; the topographical details of each ganglion are dealt with in the regions concerned.

The *parasympathetic root* carries the preganglionic fibres from the cells of origin in a brainstem nucleus. This is the essential functional root of the ganglion; its fibres synapse in it, whereas the fibres of all other roots simply pass through the ganglion without synapse.

The *sympathetic root* contains postganglionic fibres from the superior cervical ganglion, whose preganglionic cell bodies are in the lateral grey horn of cord segments T1–3.

The *sensory root* contains the peripheral processes of cell bodies in the trigeminal ganglion.

The *branches* of each ganglion carry the postganglionic parasympathetic fibres to the particular structure(s) requiring this kind of localized motor innervation: ciliary muscle and sphincter pupillae from the ciliary ganglion, salivary glands from the submandibular and otic ganglia, and lacrimal, nasal and palatal glands from the pterygopalatine ganglion. The other fibres in the branches are sympathetic fibres to the same structures (mainly for their blood vessels) and afferent fibres.

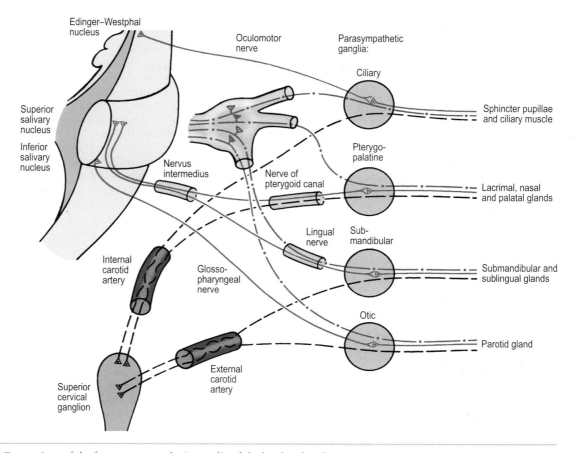

Fig. 1.16   Connections of the four parasympathetic ganglia of the head and neck.

Ciliary ganglion (see p. 418)

Parasympathetic root. From the Edinger–Westphal part of the oculomotor nucleus by a branch from the nerve to the inferior oblique muscle from the inferior division of the oculomotor nerve.

Sympathetic root. From the superior cervical ganglion by branches of the internal carotid nerve.

Sensory root. From a branch of the nasociliary nerve, with cell bodies in the trigeminal ganglion.

Branches. Short ciliary nerves to the eye.

Pterygopalatine ganglion (see p. 384)

Parasympathetic root. From the superior salivary nucleus by the nerve of the pterygoid canal and the greater petrosal nerve from the nervus intermedius part of the facial nerve.

Sympathetic root. From the superior cervical ganglion by the internal carotid nerve, the deep petrosal nerve and the nerve of the pterygoid canal.

Sensory root. From a branch of the maxillary nerve, with cell bodies in the trigeminal ganglion.

Branches. To the lacrimal gland via the zygomatic and lacrimal nerves, and to mucous glands in the nose, nasopharynx and palate via maxillary nerve branches. A few fibres (not shown in Fig. 1.16) are taste fibres from the palate, which run in the greater petrosal nerve and have cell bodies in the geniculate ganglion of the facial nerve.

Submandibular ganglion (see p. 350)

Parasympathetic root. From the superior salivary nucleus by the nervus intermedius part of the facial nerve and the chorda tympani, joining the lingual nerve.

Sympathetic root. From the superior cervical ganglion by fibres running with the facial artery.

Sensory root. From a branch of the lingual nerve, with cell bodies in the trigeminal ganglion.

Branches. To the submandibular and sublingual glands via branches of the lingual nerve.

Otic ganglion (see p. 379)

Parasympathetic root. From the inferior salivary nucleus by the glossopharyngeal nerve and its tympanic branch to the tympanic plexus and then to the lesser petrosal nerve.

Sympathetic root. From the superior cervical ganglion by fibres running with the middle meningeal artery.

Sensory root. From the auriculotemporal nerve with cell bodies in the trigeminal ganglion.

Branches. To the parotid gland via filaments of the auriculotemporal nerve.

Unlike the other three ganglia, the otic ganglion has an additional *somatic motor root*, from the nerve to the medial pterygoid; the fibres pass through (without synapse) to supply the tensor tympani and tensor palati muscles.

Parasympathetic afferent fibres

As in the sympathetic nervous system, afferent fibres often accompany the parasympathetic supply to various structures. Such fibres that run with the glossopharyngeal and vagus nerves have their cell bodies in the inferior ganglia of those nerves, and their central processes pass to the nucleus of the tractus solitarius, through which there are connections with other parts of the brainstem and higher centres for the reflex control of respiration, heart rate, blood pressure and gastrointestinal activity.

The pelvic splanchnic nerves also carry afferent fibres. Their cell bodies are in the posterior root ganglia of the second to fourth sacral nerves and the central processes enter the cord by the posterior nerve roots. Some make local synaptic connections, e.g. for bladder reflexes, but others are pain fibres from pelvic viscera, which often seem to use both sympathetic and parasympathetic pathways for pain transmission, e.g. bladder and rectum.

PART THREE

Embryology

The development of most of the organs and systems is touched upon in the text descriptions of the regions concerned. Here a very brief account of some important features of early development is included, to provide a background for the later notes.

Early development

For the first 8 weeks of the 40-week human gestation period the developing organism is an **embryo**; after that time it is a **fetus**. By the end of the embryonic period most organs have differentiated, and the changes during the fetal period are essentially those of maturation. Many but not all congenital defects are initiated in the embryo rather than the fetus.

The fertilized ovum or **zygote** undergoes repeated cell divisions (cleavage) to produce a mass of cells, the **morula**, which travels along the uterine tube towards the uterus. Further division enlarges the morula and a fluid-filled cavity (the extraembryonic coelom) appears in it; the whole structure is now a **blastocyst**. At this stage implantation into the uterine mucosa takes place, about 6 days after fertilization. The outer layer of cells in the blastocyst, the **trophoblast**, is destined to become placental. The remainder of the cells are concentrated at one end of the blastocyst to form the **inner cell mass** or embryoblast, attached to the inner layer of the trophoblast.

At the beginning of the second week after fertilization, the embryoblast differentiates into two layers, a layer of columnar cells (the epiblast) and a layer of cuboidal cells (the hypoblast). Two cavities then appear, the amniotic cavity, which is related to the epiblast, and the yolk sac, which is related to the hypoblast (Fig. 1.17). The two cavities are surrounded by the extraembryonic coelom, except where the embryoblast is connected to the trophoblast by the connecting stalk.

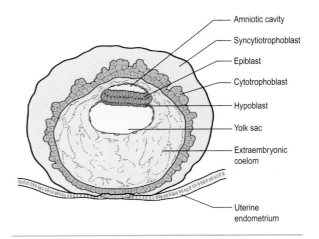

- Amniotic cavity
- Syncytiotrophoblast
- Epiblast
- Cytotrophoblast
- Hypoblast
- Yolk sac
- Extraembryonic coelom
- Uterine endometrium

Fig. 1.17 An embryo at the beginning of the second week. The trophoblast has differentiated into an inner layer of cells with single nuclei (the cytotrophoblast) and an outer layer with multiple nuclei but without distinct cell boundaries (the syncytiotrophoblast).

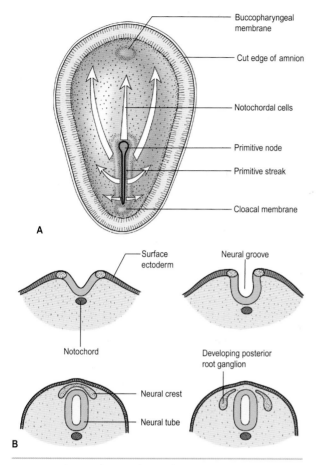

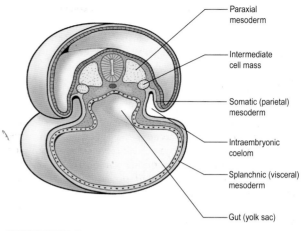

Fig. 1.19   Cross-section through an embryo at the end of the third week.

Fig. 1.18   **A** Dorsal view of an embryo at the beginning of the third week; **B** formation of neural tube and neural crest.

A primitive streak appears on the amniotic aspect of the embryoblast towards what will become the caudal end of the embryo (Fig. 1.18A). The streak indicates the site of a groove at the cephalic end of which is a primitive pit with slightly raised margins; this is the primitive node. In the third week, epiblast cells in the region of the primitive streak invaginate, displacing the hypoblast, and spread bilaterally and cephalad forming two new layers, the **mesoderm** next to the epiblast and the **endoderm** adjacent to the hypoblast. The remaining epiblast cells form the **ectoderm**. From the primitive pit a rod of cells invaginate directly cephalad between ectoderm and endoderm; this is the **notochord**, which extends as far as the buccopharyngeal membrane, where ectoderm and endoderm remain in contact. Similarly at the caudal end of the primitive streak, ectoderm and endoderm are in apposition at the cloacal membrane.

An indentation of the ectoderm overlying the notochord forms the neural groove (Fig. 1.18B). Its edges unite to form the **neural tube**, which becomes depressed below the surface. In due course, the brain and spinal cord develop from the neural tube. Some of the cells derived from the edges of the groove become isolated between the tube and the overlying ectoderm to form the **neural crest**. Its cells are destined to migrate and contribute to the development of several structures, including posterior root ganglia of spinal nerves, corresponding ganglia of cranial nerves, autonomic ganglia, neuroglia, Schwann cells, meninges, bones of the skull and face, sclera and choroid of the eye, dentine and cementum of teeth, parafollicular cells of the thyroid, chromaffin cells of the suprarenal medulla and melanocytes.

Alongside the notochord and neural tube the mesoderm lies in three longitudinal strips (Fig. 1.19). That nearest the midline is the **paraxial mesoderm**; it becomes segmented in cephalocaudal sequence into masses of cells called mesodermal **somites**. The somites produce: (1) the *sclerotome*, medially, which surrounds the neural tube and notochord, producing the vertebrae and ribs; and (2) the *dermomyotome* or muscle plate, laterally, which produces the muscles of the body wall and the dermis of the skin.

The intermediate strip of mesoderm is the **intermediate cell mass**. From its lateral side in cephalocaudal sequence develop successively the pronephros, mesonephros and metanephros and their associated ducts—the progenitors of the urinary and genital systems. Its medial side gives rise to the gonad and the cortex of the suprarenal gland.

The most lateral strip of mesoderm is the **lateral plate**. Very early the embryo begins to curl up, a result of the more rapid growth of the dorsal (ectodermal) surface. The embryo becomes markedly convex towards the amniotic cavity and correspondingly concave towards the yolk sac. As the lateral plate curls around to enclose the yolk sac its mesoderm becomes split into two layers by a space that appears within it. The space is the beginning of the intraembryonic *coelom* or body cavity. The inner layer is the *splanchnic (visceral) mesoderm*. It encloses the yolk sac in an hourglass constriction; the part of the yolk sac outside persists in the umbilical cord as the *vitellointestinal duct*; the part inside the embryo becomes the alimentary canal. The outer layer of the lateral plate is the *somatic (parietal) mesoderm*. Into it the paraxial myotomes migrate in segments to produce the flexor and extensor muscle layers of the body wall. The coelomic cavity at first includes pleural and peritoneal spaces in one continuum; they become separated later. The pleura and peritoneum are thus mesodermal in origin.

The **limb buds** grow from the lateral plate mesoderm and their muscles develop in situ. Although the lateral plate mesoderm is unsegmented, the motor fibres that grow into it from the spinal cord limb plexuses arrange their distribution in a segmental pattern.

The **septum transversum** consists of the mass of mesoderm lying on the cranial aspect of the coelomic cavity. Its cranial part contains the pericardial cavity, the walls of which develop into the pericardium and part of the diaphragm. It is invaded by muscles from cervical myotomes, mainly the fourth; they produce the muscle of the diaphragm. The caudal part of the septum transversum is invaded by the developing liver, which it surrounds as the ventral mesogastrium. The septum transversum later descends, taking the heart with it, to the final position of the diaphragm.

The folding of the embryo is impeded to some extent at the tail end by the presence of the connecting stalk, which later becomes the *umbilical cord*. The greatest amount of folding occurs at the head end of the embryo. By the end of the first fortnight the forebrain capsule is folded down over the pericardium, and a mouth pit, the **stomodeum**, shows as a dimple between the two. Within the body of the embryo the gut cavity extends headwards dorsal to the pericardium, as far forwards as the *buccopharyngeal membrane*, which closes the bottom of the mouth pit. The buccopharyngeal membrane breaks down and disappears in the fourth week and its former site cannot be made out with certainty in the later embryo or adult. Cranial to the site of the membrane the mouth pit is lined with ectoderm; this includes the region of all the mandibular and maxillary

teeth, and the anterior two-thirds of the tongue. *Rathke's pouch* arises from this ectoderm and forms the anterior lobe of the pituitary gland. Caudal to the buccopharyngeal membrane is the pharynx, lined with endoderm and lying dorsal to the pericardium.

Pharyngeal arches and pouches

Mesodermal condensations develop in the side walls of the primitive pharynx to form the **pharyngeal arches** and they grow around towards each other ventrally, where they fuse in the midline. In this way a series of six horseshoe-shaped arches (also called branchial arches) comes to support the pharynx (Fig. 1.20). Deep grooves appear on the surface of the embryo at the intervals between the arches; these are the **pharyngeal** (or branchial) **clefts**. The fifth arch is rudimentary and only four clefts are visible. Outpouchings develop from the lining of the pharynx in between the arches and opposite the clefts: the **pharyngeal** (or branchial) **pouches**. The fourth and fifth pouches share a common opening into the lumen of the pharynx. In each arch a central bar of *cartilage* forms and *muscle* differentiates from the mesoderm around it. An *artery* and cranial *nerve* are allocated to the supply of each arch and its derivatives. Vascular patterns are very changeable during development, but a nerve supply, once established, remains constant and knowledge of the nerve supply of a muscle enables its pharyngeal arch origin to be determined.

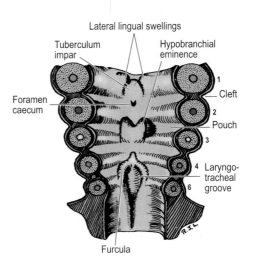

Fig. 1.20   Floor of the developing pharynx. The pharyngeal (branchial) arches are numbered. The foramen caecum lies in the midline between the first and second arches.

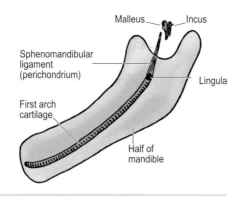

Fig. 1.21 Derivatives of the first arch cartilage.

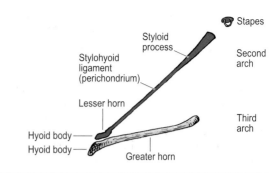

Fig. 1.22 Derivatives of the second and third arch cartilages.

First (mandibular) arch

The right and left halves of the first arch fuse ventrally in the midline. Chondrification in the mesoderm produces *Meckel's cartilage*. The dorsal end of Meckel's cartilage produces the *incus* and *malleus*, and the *anterior ligament of the malleus*. The *sphenomandibular ligament* (Fig. 1.21) is a remnant of the fibrous perichondrium of Meckel's cartilage. The *lingula* at the mandibular foramen develops from the cartilage. The mandible starts ossifying in membrane lateral to Meckel's cartilage, and the rest of the cartilage becomes incorporated in the developing mandible. Some time after birth the cartilage disappears.

Ectodermal and endodermal derivatives of this arch are the mucous membrane and glands (but not the muscle) of the anterior two-thirds of the tongue. The muscles of mastication (masseter, temporal and pterygoids), the mylohyoid and anterior belly of digastric, and the two tensor muscles (tensor palati and tensor tympani) develop from the first arch and are supplied by the mandibular nerve, which is the nerve of this arch. Part of the artery of the first arch persists as the maxillary artery.

Other arches

The skeletal and muscular derivatives of the remaining arches can be summarized as follows.

Second (hyoid) arch

Skeletal derivatives: stapes; styloid process; stylohyoid ligament; lesser horn; and superior part of body of hyoid bone (Fig. 1.22).

Muscular derivatives: muscles of facial expression (including buccinator and platysma); stapedius; stylohyoid; posterior belly of digastric—all supplied by the facial, the nerve of the second arch.

Third arch

Skeletal derivatives: greater horn and inferior part of body of hyoid bone (Fig. 1.22).

Muscular derivatives: stylopharyngeus—supplied by the glossopharyngeal, the nerve of the third arch.

Fourth and sixth arches

Skeletal derivatives: thyroid; cricoid; epiglottic; and arytenoid cartilages.

Muscular derivatives: intrinsic muscles of larynx; muscles of pharynx; levator palati—all supplied by laryngeal and pharyngeal branches of the vagus, the nerve of these arches.

Lateral derivatives of the pharyngeal pouches

Except for the first, each pouch grows laterally into a dorsal and a ventral diverticulum.

First pouch. This is the only pouch in which the endoderm remains in close apposition to the ectoderm of the corresponding cleft, namely at the tympanic membrane, where the mesoderm separating them is minimal. In the other pouches the ectoderm and endoderm are finally widely separated. The endoderm of the first pouch is prolonged laterally, via the auditory tube, to form the middle ear and mastoid antrum (the second pouch gives a contribution to the middle ear; see below). The first pharyngeal cleft becomes deepened to form the external acoustic meatus.

Second pouch. The dorsal part assists the first pouch in the formation of the tympanic cavity, taking what may be its pretrematic nerve (the tympanic branch of the glossopharyngeal) with it; the word 'trema' means a cleft. The ventral part of the pouch develops the tonsillar crypts and the supratonsillar fossa from its endoderm, the surrounding mesoderm contributing the lymphatic tissue of the palatine tonsil. The nerve supply of these derivatives is the glossopharyngeal.

Third pouch. Dorsally the inferior parathyroid gland (termed parathyroid III) and ventrally the thymic rudiment grow from this pouch. The latter progresses caudally and joins with that of the other side to produce the bilobed thymus gland. In its descent the thymic bud draws parathyroid III in a caudal direction, so that ultimately the latter lies inferior to parathyroid IV, which is derived from the fourth pouch. From this thymic bud the medulla of the thymus, including the thymic (Hassall's) corpuscles, is derived; the lymphocytes of the cortex migrate from bone marrow.

Fourth pouch. The superior parathyroid glands (parathyroid IV) are derived from the endodermal lining of this pouch.

Fifth pouch. This forms the *ultimobranchial body*, from which are derived the parafollicular (C) cells of the thyroid gland which produce calcitonin.

Cervical sinus

Concurrently with the growth of the above derivatives from the endoderm of the pouches a change takes place externally in the overlying ectoderm. The only pharyngeal cleft to persist is the first, which forms the external ear. The second arch increases in thickness and grows caudally, over the third, fourth and sixth arches, covering the second, third and fourth clefts and meeting skin caudal to these. During this process a deep groove is formed, which becomes a deep pit, the **cervical sinus**. The lips of the pit then meet and fuse and the imprisoned ectoderm disappears. Persistence of this ectoderm gives rise to a *branchial cyst*. Persistence of the deep pit is termed a branchial sinus. A *branchial fistula* sometimes results from breaking down of the tissues between the floor of the pit and the side wall of the pharynx (endoderm). Usually the track of the fistula runs from the region of the palatine tonsil, between the external and internal carotid arteries, and reaches the skin anterior to the lower end of sternocleidomastoid.

Ventral derivatives of the floor of the pharynx

The tongue, thyroid gland and larynx are derived from the floor of the mouth (Fig. 1.20).

Buds from the first, third and fourth arches form the stroma of the tongue, the epithelium being derived from the ectoderm of the stomodeum and the endoderm of the cranial end of the pharynx. Occipital myotomes migrate

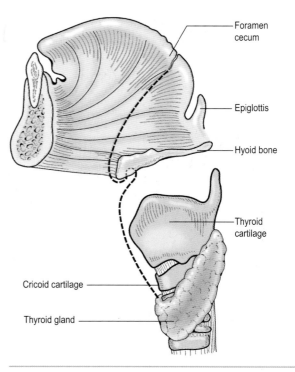

Fig. 1.23   Course of the thyroglossal duct. If a remnant persists it often does so at the kink behind the body of the hyoid bone. The thyroid gland, larynx and trachea have been drawn to a smaller scale than the tongue, mandible and hyoid bone.

Labels: Foramen cecum; Epiglottis; Hyoid bone; Thyroid cartilage; Thyroid gland; Cricoid cartilage

forwards to provide the musculature, carrying their nerve (hypoglossal) supply with them.

The **thyroglossal duct** originates from the endoderm of the floor of the pharynx at the foramen caecum (Fig. 1.20) in the region of the developing tongue, and then passes caudally in front of the hyoid bone, behind which it forms a recurrent loop (Fig. 1.23). The thyroid gland buds from the duct's distal end, which itself may give rise to the pyramidal lobe. Other remnants of the duct may persist as accessory thyroid glands or give rise to thyroglossal cysts (Fig. 1.24). Failure of descent of the thyroglossal duct may result in the development of a lingual thyroid.

In the ventral wall of the pharynx a **laryngotracheal groove** appears. The cephalic end of this gutter is limited by the *furcula*, a ridge in the shape of a wish-bone (Fig. 1.20). The ridges which limit the gutter grow towards each other and, by their fusion, convert the gutter into a tube. This tube, the trachea, then separates from the oesophagus and buds out into the bronchi and lungs at its caudal end. Failure of proper separation

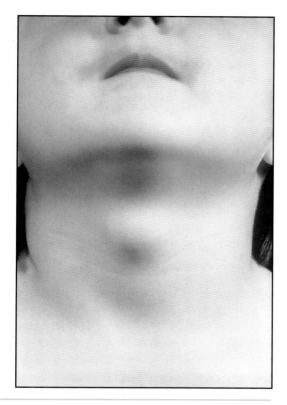

Fig. 1.24 Thyroglossal cyst.

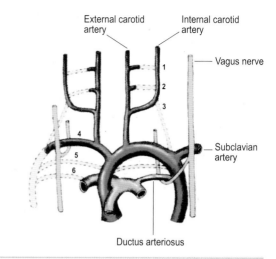

Fig. 1.25 Fate of the arch arteries. The arteries are numbered and the dotted lines indicate the arteries that disappear. The asymmetry of the course of the recurrent laryngeal nerves results from differences in the fate of the lower arch arteries.

of the trachea and oesophagus results in a tracheo-oesophageal fistula. The furcula persists at the aperture of the larynx, whose cartilages, including that of the epiglottis, derive from the underlying fourth and sixth pharyngeal arches.

Branchial arch arteries

From the cephalic end of the primitive heart tube (see p. 31) a *ventral aorta* divides right and left into two branches which curve back caudally as the two *dorsal aortae*. As the branchial arches develop, a vessel in each arch joins the ventral to the dorsal aortae. Thus six aortic arches are to be accounted for. Caudal to this region, the two dorsal aortae fuse to become a single vessel; proximal to the fusion, a part of the right dorsal aorta subsequently disappears.

Parts of the first and second arch arteries form the maxillary and stapedial arteries respectively; the latter does not persist after birth. The third remains as part of the internal carotid artery. The fourth on the right contributes to the subclavian artery, on the left to the

arch of the aorta. The fifth disappears entirely. By the time the sixth artery appears the upper bulbar part of the heart tube has been divided into aorta and pulmonary trunk and it is to the pulmonary trunk that the sixth arch arteries are connected ventrally. Dorsally they communicate with the dorsal aortae. The dorsal part of the sixth arch artery disappears on the right side but persists on the left as the ductus arteriosus, which thus connects the left pulmonary artery to the arch of the aorta (Fig. 1.25). This explains why the recurrent laryngeal (sixth arch) nerve hooks round the ligamentum arteriosum on the left, but migrates up and hooks round the subclavian artery on the right.

Anomalies of the great vessels

The most common anomaly of development is a *patent ductus arteriosus* (persistence of part of the left sixth arch artery), which fails to close in the immediate postnatal period. *Coarctation* of the aorta (narrowing) is due to a defect of the tunica media which forms a shelf-like projection into the lumen, most commonly in the region of the ductus; collateral circulation distal to the obstruction is provided by the internal thoracic and posterior intercostal arteries. An *abnormal origin of the right subclavian artery* is from the arch of the aorta, just distal to the origin of the left one. The abnormal artery passes to the right behind the oesophagus and is a possible cause of dysphagia. With the lack of a normal right subclavian arch, the right recurrent laryngeal nerve is *non-recurrent* and runs down the side of the larynx: a possible hazard in thyroidectomy. The reported incidence of a non-recurrent nerve is around 1%.

Development of mouth and face

The stomodeum (mouth pit) has appeared by the end of the second week and the buccopharyngeal membrane between it and the pharynx breaks down in the fourth week.

The stomodeum is bounded below by the **mandibular prominence** of the first arch (Fig. 1.26), which produces the floor of the mouth, lower jaw and lower lip. From the forebrain capsule the **frontonasal prominence** grows

down towards the stomodeum. This is indented by two **nasal placodes** which develop into **nasal pits**. These are bounded by **medial and lateral nasal prominences** that unite to encircle the nostril. From the cranial aspect of the dorsal region of each mandibular prominence, the **maxillary prominence** grows ventrally above the stomodeum, forming the floor of the orbit and fusing with the lateral nasal prominence along the line of the nasolacrimal duct. The medial nasal prominences merge to form the intermaxillary segment from which develops the philtrum of the upper lip, the part of the upper jaw that carries the four incisor teeth and the adjacent primary palate. The maxillary prominences fuse with the philtrum to form the whole of the upper lip.

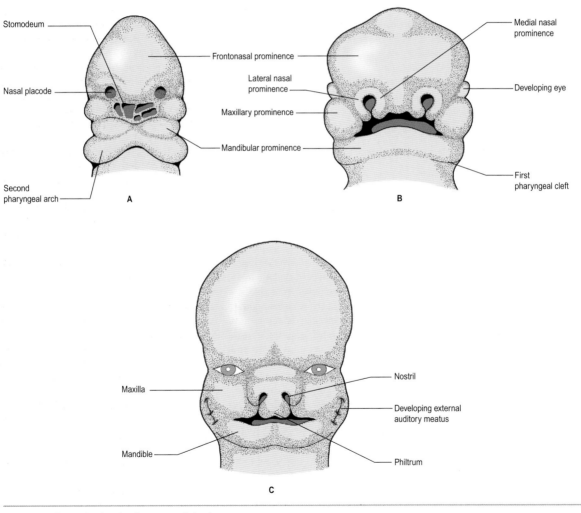

Fig. 1.26   Stages in the development of the face.

At first the developing tongue lies against the floor of the cranium. A midline flange (the nasal septum) grows down from the base of the forebrain capsule (which is the mesenchymal precursor of the skull). From each maxillary process a flange, known as the **palatal shelf**, grows downwards and medially; these shelves are soon elevated to a horizontal position over the dorsum of the tongue. The two palatal shelves meet and unite, forming the secondary palate. They also fuse with the nasal septum and the primary palate, the midline incisive foramen persisting at the site of the latter fusion. These fusions begin anteriorly during the eighth week and extend posteriorly to become complete at the uvula in the tenth week.

The nerve supply of all these structures is derived from the fifth cranial (trigeminal) nerve. The frontonasal prominence and its derivatives are supplied by the ophthalmic division, the maxillary prominence and its derivatives by the maxillary division and the mandibular prominence and its derivatives by the mandibular division.

Defects of development

The most common abnormalities are cleft lip and cleft palate (1 in 1000 and 1 in 2000 births respectively) and there are ethnic variations in these incidences; they may or may not coexist. **Cleft lip** is more frequently lateral. The cleft runs down from the nostril and results from a failure of fusion between the maxillary and medial nasal prominences. Cleft lip may be bilateral and may involve the upper jaw and extend between the primary and secondary palates, the central part being an isolated intermaxillary segment.

Cleft palate may be partial or complete. As the two palatal processes unite with each other progressively from front to back, arrest of union results in a posterior defect that varies from the mildest form of bifid uvula to a complete cleft from uvula to gum. In the latter case the cleft almost always runs between the lateral incisor and canine teeth. Very rarely a midline cleft may separate the two halves of the maxilla. Irregular formations of incisor and canine teeth often accompany these defects of palatal development.

A less common defect arises from the failure of fusion of the lateral nasal process with the maxillary process, producing a groove (*facial cleft*) on the face along the line of the nasolacrimal duct.

Development of the cloaca

At the caudal end of the embryo, the hindgut and the allantois (a diverticulum from the yolk sac) meet in a common cavity, the **cloaca**, bounded distally by the *cloacal membrane* (Fig. 1.27A). From the dorsal wall of the allantois, the *urorectal septum* grows downwards to meet the cloacal membrane, so dividing the cloaca and membrane into two (Fig. 1.27B): at the front are the urogenital sinus and urogenital membrane, and at the back the anorectal canal and the anal membrane, which lies in a small ectodermal depression, the *proctodeum*.

The **urogenital sinus** (endoderm) has three unequally sized parts. The uppermost and largest is the vesical (vesicourethral) part, which forms most of the bladder epithelium (with surrounding mesoderm forming the muscle and connective tissue) and the female urethra (Fig. 1.27D). The lower end of the *mesonephric duct* (see p. 296) opens into this part of the sinus, with the ureter arising as a bud from the duct. The lower ends of the duct and ureter become incorporated into the developing bladder, so forming the trigone and in the male the part of the urethra proximal to the opening of the ejaculatory duct (Fig. 1.27C).

The middle or pelvic part of the sinus forms the rest of the prostatic urethra, the membranous urethra and the prostate (with surrounding mesoderm forming the fibromuscular stroma). In the female it contributes epithelium to the vagina (derived principally from the paramesonephric ducts; see p. 317).

The lowest or phallic part of the sinus becomes the dorsal part of the penis and penile urethra or the lower part of the vagina. At the front of the urogenital membrane (which breaks down) is a midline mesodermal swelling, the *genital tubercle* (Fig. 1.27B), which becomes the glans penis or clitoris. Leading back from the tubercle on either side are the *urogenital folds*, which in the female remain separate as the labia minora. In the male they unite at the back to form the midline raphe of the scrotum, the rest of the scrotum coming from the pair of *genital (labioscrotal) swellings* which develop lateral to the urogenital folds and which in the female become the labia majora. The front parts of the urogenital folds unite from the scrotum forwards as the ventral part of the penis and penile urethra; failure of such fusion results in hypospadias, where the urethra opens on the ventral aspect of a malformed penis.

Cardiac and venous development

Early development of the heart

Primitive blood vessels are laid down by angioblasts on the wall of the yolk sac. Two such vessels fuse together to make a single **heart tube** which develops muscle fibres in its wall and becomes pulsatile. It differentiates into four parts or cavities which in a cephalocaudal direction

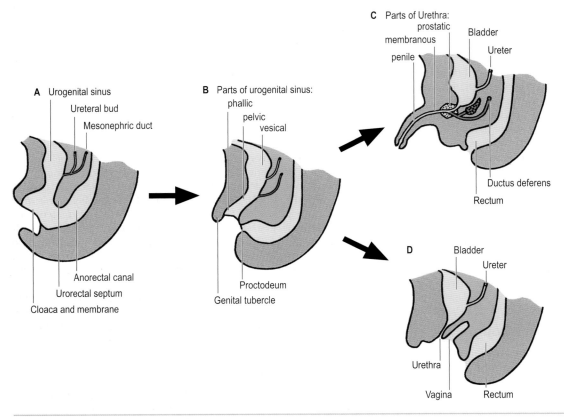

Fig. 1.27   Development of the cloaca: **A** the urorectal septum grows down to divide the cloaca into the urogenital sinus and the anorectal canal; **B** the uppermost (vesicourethral) part of the sinus becomes the bladder and the proximal part of the prostatic urethra, with the pelvic and phallic parts distally; **C** in the male the pelvic part becomes the prostatic urethra distal to the opening of the ejaculatory ducts, and the phallic part becomes the dorsal part of the penile urethra; **D** in the female the bladder and urethra are from the vesicourethral part of the sinus.

are the **bulb, ventricle, atrium** and **sinus venosus**. The tube grows at a greater rate than the cavity (the primitive pericardial cavity) in which it is suspended; it therefore has to bend, and it does so in such a way that the bulb and the ventricle come to lie in front of the atrium and sinus venosus. There is also a slight twisting of the bulb to the right and the ventricle to the left, hence the normal left-sided bulging of the definitive heart.

The upper part of the bulb is the *truncus arteriosus*, which divides to become the aorta and pulmonary trunk. The lower part of the bulb becomes most of the right ventricle, with the original ventricle forming most of the left ventricle. The atrium becomes divided into two, with the sinus venosus becoming mostly absorbed into the right atrium.

Development of veins

From a network of primitive veins, certain longitudinal channels develop to return blood to the sinus venosus. It receives blood from three sources: from the placenta by *umbilical veins*, from the yolk sac (which becomes the alimentary canal) by *vitelline veins*, and from the general tissues of the embryo by *cardinal veins*. In each group there are right and left veins, with anastomosing cross-channels between each pair, and the whole or part of one longitudinal vein of each pair disappears: right umbilical; left vitelline; and left cardinal.

The *vitelline veins*, with their cross-channels, contribute to the formation of the portal vein and the upper end of the inferior vena cava.

The *left umbilical vein* joins the left branch of the portal vein, but its blood short-circuits the liver by passing along a venous shunt, the *ductus venosus*, which joins the inferior vena cava on the cranial side of the liver. After birth the left umbilical vein and its continuation, the ductus venosus, become reduced to fibrous cords, the *ligamentum teres* and *ligamentum venosum*.

On each side, a vein from the head and neck (internal jugular) and from the upper limb (subclavian) unite to form the *anterior cardinal vein*. Similarly, from the lower limb and pelvis, external and internal iliac veins form the *posterior cardinal vein*, into which drain segmental veins (intercostal and lumbar). The anterior and posterior veins unite to form the short *common cardinal vein* which opens into the sinus venosus. The essential features of subsequent changes are the obliteration of the major portions of the left anterior and posterior cardinals, with the persistence of a cross-channel at each end of the body: the left brachiocephalic vein and the left common iliac vein.

In the thorax the right anterior cardinal vein forms the right brachiocephalic and part of the superior vena cava, the rest being derived from the common cardinal. The azygos and hemiazygos veins develop from the right posterior cardinal vein and the supracardinal vein that replaces the left posterior cardinal vein.

In the abdomen other longitudinal channels appear, both medial (subcardinal) and dorsal (supracardinal) to the original posterior cardinal. The end result is the formation of the inferior vena cava and its tributaries from different parts of these vessels and their inter-communications. In the lower abdomen the common iliac veins are behind the corresponding arteries, but higher up the renal veins are in front of the renal arteries, due to their development from dorsal or ventral venous channels.

Fetal circulation

The fetal blood is oxygenated in the placenta not in the lungs. The economy of the fetal circulation is improved by three short-circuiting arrangements, all of which cease to function at the time of birth: the ductus venosus, the foramen ovale and the ductus arteriosus.

Ductus venosus

Oxygenated blood returns from the placenta by the (left) umbilical vein, which joins the left branch of the portal vein in the porta hepatis. This oxygenated blood short-circuits the sinusoids of the liver; it is conveyed directly to the inferior vena cava by the *ductus venosus*.

This channel lies along the inferior surface of the liver, between the attached layers of the lesser omentum. After birth, when blood no longer flows along the thrombosed umbilical vein, the blood in the ductus venosus clots and the ductus venosus becomes converted into a fibrous cord, the *ligamentum venosum*, lying deep in the cleft bounding the caudate lobe of the liver. The intra-abdominal part of the umbilical vein persists as a fibrous cord, the *ligamentum teres*. The two are continuous.

Foramen ovale

The interatrial septum of the fetal heart is patent, being perforated by the *foramen ovale*. Blood brought to the right atrium by the inferior vena cava is directed by its 'valve' through the foramen and so enters the left atrium. The oxygenated placental blood is thus made to bypass the right ventricle and the airless lungs, and is directed into the left ventricle and aorta and so to the carotid arteries.

After birth the foramen ovale is closed by fusion of the primary and secondary septa (see p. 213). After closure all the blood in the right atrium passes into the right ventricle and so to the lungs.

Ductus arteriosus

It has already been noted that oxygenated blood in the umbilical vein passes via the ductus venosus, inferior vena cava and right atrium through the foramen ovale to the left side of the heart and so to the head. Venous blood from the head is returned by way of the brachio-cephalic veins to the superior vena cava. In the right atrium this venous bloodstream crosses the stream of oxygenated blood brought there via the inferior vena cava. The two streams of blood scarcely mix with each other. The deoxygenated blood from the superior vena cava passes through the right atrium into the right ventricle and so into the pulmonary trunk. It now short-circuits the airless lungs by the *ductus arteriosus*. This is a thick-walled artery joining the left branch of the pulmonary trunk to the aorta, distal to the origin of the three branches of the aortic arch. The deoxygenated blood thus passes distally along the aorta and the common and internal iliac arteries, and via the umbilical arteries, to the placenta to be reoxygenated.

After birth the ductus arteriosus is occluded by contraction of its muscular walls. It persists as a fibrous band, the *ligamentum arteriosum*, which connects the commencement of the left pulmonary artery to the concavity of the arch of the aorta. The umbilical arteries close off and become fibrous cords: the medial umbilical ligaments.

PART **FOUR**

Anatomy of the child

The proportions of the newborn child differ markedly from the form of the adult. Some of its organs and structures are well developed and even of full adult size (e.g. the internal ear), while others have yet to develop (e.g. corticospinal tracts to become myelinated, teeth to erupt, secondary sex characters to appear).

General features of the newborn

In comparison with the adult the neonate is much more fully developed at its head end than at its caudal end. The large head and massive shoulders stand out in marked contrast to the smallish abdomen and poorly developed buttocks.

Due to the shortness of the newborn baby's neck, its lower jaw and chin touch its shoulders and thorax. Gradually the neck elongates and the chin loses contact with the chest. The head thus becomes more mobile, both in flexion–extension and in rotation.

The abdomen is not prominent at birth but becomes gradually more and more so. The 'pot-belly' of the young child is due mainly to the large liver and the small pelvis; the pelvic organs lie in the abdominal cavity. In later childhood the pelvic organs and much of the intestinal tract sink into the developing pelvic cavity and the rate of growth of the abdominal walls outpaces that of the liver. In this way, the disposition of the viscera and the contour of the abdominal wall become as in the adult, and the bulging belly flattens.

Some special features of the newborn

Skull

The most striking feature of the neonatal skull is the disproportion between the cranial vault and facial skeleton; the vault is very large in proportion to the face. In Figure 1.28 the photograph of a full-term fetal skull

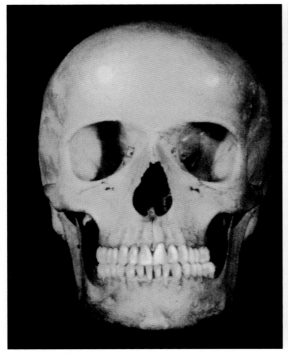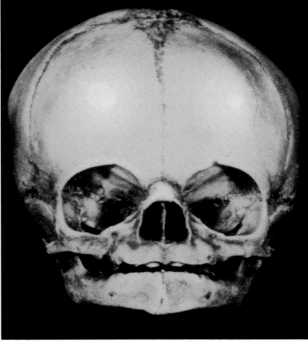

Fig. 1.28   Normal adult and fetal skulls. The fetal skull on the right is projected to the same vertical height as that of the adult. Note the disproportion of the vertical extent of the face. The distance from the lower margin of the orbit to the lower border of the mandible in the adult is three times the diameter of the orbit; in the fetal skull it is equal to the diameter of the orbit.

has been enlarged to the same vertical projection as a normal adult skull and this procedure shows in striking manner the disproportion between the two. In the fetal skull the vertical diameter of the orbit equals the vertical height of maxilla and mandible combined. In the adult skull the growth of the maxillary sinuses and the growth of alveolar bone around the permanent teeth has so elongated the face that the vertical diameter of the orbit is only one-third of the vertical height of maxilla and mandible combined.

Most of the separate skull and face bones are ossified by the time of birth but they are mobile on each other and are fairly readily disarticulated in the macerated skull. The bones of the vault do not interdigitate in sutures, as in the adult, but are separated by linear attachments of fibrous tissue and, at their corners, by larger areas, the fontanelles.

The **anterior fontanelle** lies between four bones. The two parietal bones bound it behind, the two halves of the frontal bone lie in front. It overlies the superior sagittal dural venous sinus. The anterior fontanelle is usually not palpable after the age of 18 months.

The **posterior fontanelle** lies between the apex of the squamous part of the occipital bone and the posterior edges of the two parietal bones. It is closed by the age of 6 months.

At birth the **frontal bone** consists of two halves separated by a median *metopic suture*; this is obliterated by about 7 years. The metopic suture may persist rarely.

The *petromastoid part* of the neonatal temporal bone encloses the internal ear, middle ear and mastoid antrum, all parts of which are full adult size at birth. But the mastoid process is absent and the stylomastoid foramen is near the lateral surface of the skull, covered by the thin fibres of sternocleidomastoid—the issuing facial nerve is thus unprotected and vulnerable at birth. The mastoid process develops with the growth of the sternocleidomastoid muscle and the entry of air cells into it from the mastoid antrum. The process becomes palpable in the second year.

The *tympanic part* is present at birth as the C-shaped *tympanic ring*, applied to the undersurface of the petrous and squamous parts and enclosing the tympanic membrane, which is slotted into it. The external acoustic meatus of the newborn is wholly cartilaginous. The tympanic membrane is almost as big as in the adult, but faces more downwards and less outwards than the adult ear drum; it therefore seems somewhat smaller and lies more obliquely when viewed through the otoscope. The tympanic ring elongates by growth from the lateral rim of its whole circumference, the tympanic plate so produced forming the bony part of the external acoustic meatus and pushing the cartilaginous part of the meatus laterally, further from the ear-drum. The adult bony meatus is twice as long as the cartilaginous part. As the tympanic plate grows laterally from the tympanic ring the tympanic membrane tilts and comes to face rather more laterally and less downwards than in the neonate.

The mandibular fossa (which forms part of the temporomandibular joint) is shallow at birth and facing slightly laterally; with development the fossa deepens and faces directly downwards.

The **maxilla**, between the floor of the orbit and the gum margin, is very limited in height and is full of developing teeth. The maxillary sinus is a narrow slit excavated into its medial wall. Eruption of the deciduous teeth allows room for excavation of the sinus beneath the orbital surface, but the maxilla grows slowly until the permanent teeth begin to erupt at 6 years. At this time it 'puts on a spurt' of growth. The rapid increase in size of the sinus and the growth of the alveolar bone occur simultaneously with increased depth of the mandible. These factors combine to produce a rapid elongation of the face.

The hard palate grows backwards to accommodate the extra teeth; and forward growth of the base of the skull continues at the spheno-occipital synchondrosis (see p. 534) until 18 to 25 years of age.

The **mandible** is in two halves at birth and their cartilaginous anterior ends are separated by fibrous tissue at the symphysis menti. Ossification unites the two halves in the first year. At first the mental foramen lies near its lower border. After eruption of the permanent teeth the foramen lies higher, and is halfway between the upper and lower borders of the bone in adults. In the edentulous jaw of the elderly, absorption of the alveolar margin leaves the mental foramen nearer the upper border of the mandible (Fig. 1.29). Forward growth of the mandible changes the direction of the mental foramen. At birth the mental neurovascular bundle emerges through the foramen in a forward direction. In the adult the mental foramen is directed backwards. At birth the angle is obtuse and the coronoid process lies at a higher level than the condyle. With increase in the length and height of the mandible, to accommodate the erupting teeth, the angle diminishes. In the adult the angle approaches a right angle, and the condyle is at the same level or higher than the coronoid process. In the edentulous mouth of the elderly the angle of the mandible increases again and the neck inclines backwards.

Neck

The newborn baby has a very short neck. The subsequent elongation of the neck is accompanied by positional changes in the covering skin; an incision over the lower neck in an infant usually results in the scar lying over the upper sternum by later childhood.

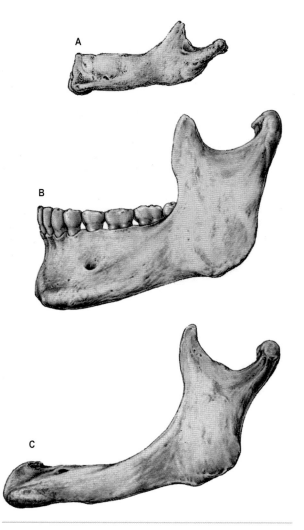

Fig. 1.29   Age changes in the mandible: **A** birth; **B** adult; **C** old age.

larynx and trachea are of small bore at birth. The vocal cords are about 5 mm long by the end of the first year. Laryngitis and tracheitis in infancy thus carry far more risk of respiratory obstruction than they do in later years. Up to the age of puberty there is no difference between the male and female larynx. At puberty the male larynx increases rapidly in size and the vocal cords elongate from 8 to 16 mm within the year, resulting in the characteristic 'breaking' of the voice. Castration or failure of testicular hormone prevents this change taking place.

Thorax

The thoracic cage of the child differs from that of the adult in being more barrel-shaped. A cross-section of the infant thorax is nearly circular; that of the adult is oval, the transverse being thrice the length of the antero-posterior diameter. The large thymus extends from the lower part of the neck through the superior into the anterior mediastinum; it regresses at puberty. The ribs lie more nearly horizontal, so the cage is set at a higher level than in the adult. The high thorax involves a higher level of the diaphragm, with consequent increase of abdominal volume.

Abdomen

At birth the liver is relatively twice as big as in the adult and its inferior border is palpable below the coastal margin. The kidneys are always highly lobulated at birth with very little perinephric fat; grooves on the surface of the adult organ frequently persist as visible signs of the original fetal lobulation. The suprarenal is enormous at birth, nearly as large as the kidney itself. The caecum is conical and the appendix arises from its apex in the fetus; this arrangement is usually still present at birth. During infancy and early childhood the lateral wall of the caecum balloons out and the base of the appendix comes to lie posteriorly on the medial wall. The appendiceal mucous membrane is packed with massed lymphoid follicles in the child. These become much more sparse in later life. The pelvic cavity is very small at birth and the fundus of the bladder lies above the pubic symphysis even when empty.

Upper limb

The upper limb is more fully developed than the lower limb at birth. The grasping reflex of the hand is very pronounced. Growth in length occurs more at the shoulder and wrist than at the elbow. Amputation through the humerus in a young child requires a very

The left brachiocephalic vein crosses the trachea so high in the superior mediastinum that it encroaches above the jugular notch into the neck, especially if it is engorged and the head extended; this should be remembered by the surgeon performing tracheotomy upon the young child.

The shortness of the neck of the newborn involves a higher position of its viscera. The larynx is nearer the base of the tongue and the upper border of the epiglottis is at the level of the second cervical vertebra. From these elevated positions their descent is slow and they reach their adult levels only after the seventh year. The

generous flap of soft tissue lest the growing bone should later protrude through the stump.

Lower limb

At birth the lower limb is not only poorly developed, but occupies the fetal position of flexion, a position which is maintained for 6 months or more. In preparation for standing and walking the limb not only becomes more robust, but undergoes extension and medial rotation that carry the flexor compartment around to the posterior aspect of the limb. The inverted foot of the newborn gradually becomes everted harmoniously with the changes in position of the knee and hip joints. Growth of the limb proceeds more rapidly at the knee than at the hip or ankle. It is not symmetrical across the lower epiphysis of the femur, and 'knock knee' (genu valgum) is normal in the child.

Vertebral column

Until birth the column is C-shaped, concave ventrally. This is imposed by constriction in utero. After birth the column is so flexible that it readily takes on any curvature imposed by gravity. The cervical curve opens up into a ventral convexity when the infant holds up its head, and the lumbar curve opens up into a ventral convexity when the infant walks. The extension of the hip that accompanies walking tilts the inlet of the pelvis forwards, so that the axis of the pelvic cavity is no longer in line with that of the abdominal cavity. This forward tilt of the pelvis necessitates a high degree of forward curvature (lordosis) of the lumbar spine in order to keep the body vertical in the standing position.

The spinal cord extends to the third lumbar vertebra at birth and does not 'rise' to the L1/L2 junction until adult years.

Upper limb 2

General plan

The upper limb of humans is built for prehension. The hand is a grasping mechanism, with four fingers flexing against an opposed thumb. The hand is furthermore the main tactile organ, with a rich nerve supply.

In grasping, the thumb is equal in functional value to the other four fingers; loss of the thumb is as disabling as loss of all four fingers. In order to be able to grasp in any position the forearm is provided with a range of about 140° of pronation and supination, and at the elbow has a range of flexion and extension of like amount. In addition, very free mobility is provided at the shoulder joint, and this mobility is further increased by the mobility of the pectoral girdle through which the upper limb articulates with the axial skeleton.

Although the upper limb is commonly called the arm, this term strictly refers to the upper part of the limb between the shoulder and elbow, while the part between the elbow and wrist is the forearm. Both arm and forearm have anterior or flexor and posterior or extensor compartments. The hand has an anterior (flexor) surface, or palm, and a posterior (extensor) surface, or dorsum.

PART ONE

Pectoral girdle

Limb girdles are defined as the bones that connect the limbs to the axial skeleton. The bones of the pectoral or shoulder girdle are the clavicle and scapula. Only one small joint connects the girdle to the rest of the skeleton—the sternoclavicular joint—and the two bones are joined to one another by an even smaller joint, the acromioclavicular. The remaining attachment to the axial skeleton is mainly muscular, and this helps to account for the mobility of the shoulder girdle. The strong coracoclavicular ligament attaches the clavicle and scapula to each other, and the clavicle is anchored to the first costal cartilage by the costoclavicular ligament. Forces from the upper limb are transmitted by the clavicle to the axial skeleton through these ligaments, and neither end of the clavicle normally transmits much force.

Almost all movement between humerus and glenoid cavity is accompanied by an appropriate movement of the scapula itself. Furthermore, the scapula cannot move without making its supporting strut, the clavicle, move also. Generally speaking the shoulder joint, the acromioclavicular and sternoclavicular joints all move together in harmony, providing a kind of 'thoracohumeral articulation'. Defects in any part of the 'thoracohumeral articulation' must impair the function of the whole.

The bones of the pectoral girdle are described on pages 101–105, the shoulder joint on page 49 and the clavicular joints on pages 45–46.

Muscles of the pectoral girdle

The muscular attachments between pectoral girdle and trunk are direct and indirect.

Direct attachment of the pectoral girdle to the trunk is provided by muscles that are inserted into the clavicle or scapula from the axial skeleton. These muscles are pectoralis minor, subclavius, trapezius, the rhomboids, levator scapulae and serratus anterior. Indirect attachment to the axial skeleton is secured by the great muscles of the axillary folds (pectoralis major and latissimus dorsi); these muscles, by way of the upper end of the humerus, move the pectoral girdle on the trunk.

The muscular attachments between upper limb and pectoral girdle include the deltoid and short scapular muscles, which are inserted about the upper end of the humerus, and the biceps and long head of triceps which, running over the humerus, are inserted beyond the elbow joint into the bones of the forearm. These muscles are important factors in giving stability to the very mobile shoulder joint across which they lie, and are described with the shoulder region (see p. 47).

Pectoralis major

From clavicular and sternocostal heads this large triangular muscle converges on the upper humerus, folding on itself where it forms the anterior axillary wall to become attached to the humerus by means of a bilaminar tendon.

The *clavicular head* arises from the medial half of the anterior surface of the clavicle. Running almost horizontally laterally the fibres of this head lie on the manubrial part of the muscle, from which they are separate. They are inserted by the anterior lamina of the tendon into the lateral lip of the intertubercular (bicipital) sulcus of the humerus.

The *sternocostal head* arises from the lateral half of the anterior surface of the manubrium and body of sternum, the upper six costal cartilages and the aponeurosis of the external oblique muscle over the upper attachment of rectus abdominis. The manubrial fibres are inserted by the anterior lamina of the tendon into the lateral lip of the intertubercular sulcus behind (deep to) the clavicular fibres. The lower sternocostal and abdominal fibres course upwards and laterally to be inserted progressively higher into the posterior lamina of the tendon, producing the rounded appearance of the anterior axillary fold. The fibres which arise lowest of all are thus inserted highest, and by a crescentic fold blend with the capsule of the shoulder joint (Fig. 2.1). The lower medial part of the muscle is thinner and in danger of being perforated when a subpectoral pocket is created for insertion of a prosthesis or muscle flap during *breast reconstruction*. Perforating branches of the internal thoracic artery pierce the deep surface of the muscle at the sternal edge and are at risk of being torn during subpectoral dissection.

Nerve supply. From the brachial plexus via the lateral and medial pectoral nerves, so named because of their origins from the lateral and medial cords of the plexus. The lateral pectoral nerve pierces the clavipectoral fascia medial to the pectoralis minor. Branches of the medial

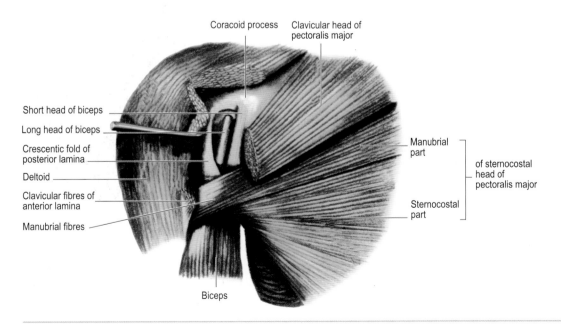

Fig. 2.1   Insertion of the right pectoralis major. Part of the clavicular head has been removed and deltoid incised and retracted to show how the lowest fibres of the sternocostal origin twist upwards deep to the manubrial fibres.

pectoral nerve pierce the pectoralis minor and may pass round its lateral border to reach the pectoralis major. The muscle is the only one in the upper limb to be supplied by all five segments of the brachial plexus; C5, 6 supply the clavicular head and C6–8, T1 the sternocostal part. The degree of paralysis of pectoralis major may be helpful in gauging the extent of a brachial plexus injury (see p. 100).

Action. The muscle is a powerful adductor and a medial rotator of the arm. The sternocostal fibres are the chief adductors. The clavicular head assists in flexion at the shoulder joint. With the upper limb fixed in abduction the muscle is a useful accessory muscle of inspiration, drawing the ribs upwards towards the humerus.

Test. For the clavicular head the arm is abducted to 90° or more and the patient pushes the arm forwards against resistance. For the sternocostal head the arm is abducted to 60° and then adducted against resistance. The contracting heads can be seen and felt.

Pectoralis minor

This small triangular muscle arises from the third, fourth and fifth ribs under cover of pectoralis major (Fig. 2.13). The insertion is by a short thick tendon into the medial border and upper surface of the coracoid process of the scapula (not to the tip of the process, which is fully occupied by biceps and coracobrachialis).

Of no great functional significance, the muscle forms a tight band across the front of the axillary neurovascular and lymphatic contents; division of its tendon facilitates surgical clearance of the axillary lymph nodes (see p. 58).

Nerve supply. By both pectoral nerves (C6–8).

Action. It assists serratus anterior in protraction of the scapula, keeping the anterior (glenoid) angle in apposition with the chest wall as the vertebral border is drawn forwards by serratus anterior. The muscle is elongated when the scapula rotates in full abduction of the arm; its subsequent contraction assists gravity in restoring the scapula to the rest position.

Subclavius

This small and unimportant muscle arises from the costochondral junction of the first rib and is inserted into the subclavian groove on the inferior surface of the clavicle. The muscle thus lies almost horizontally.

Nerve supply. By its own nerve from the upper trunk of the brachial plexus (C5, 6).

Action. It assists in stabilizing the clavicle in movements of the pectoral girdle. It may prevent the jagged ends of a fractured clavicle from damaging the adjacent subclavian vein.

The **pectoral fascia** is a thin lamina of deep fascia that covers the anterior surface of pectoralis major. It is attached medially to the sternum, above to the clavicle and is continuous laterally with the axillary fascia (see p. 53)

The **clavipectoral fascia** is a strong fascial sheet filling in the space between the clavicle and pectoralis minor. Laterally it is attached to the coracoid process and medially it blends with the external intercostal membrane of the upper two spaces. It splits above to enclose subclavius and is attached to the edges of the subclavian groove on the undersurface of the clavicle.

At the lower border of subclavius the two layers fuse and form a well-developed band, the *costocoracoid ligament*, stretching from the knuckle of the coracoid to the first costochondral junction. From this ligament the fascia stretches as a loosely felted membrane to the upper border of pectoralis minor, where it splits to enclose this muscle. Below pectoralis minor the fascia extends downwards as the **suspensory ligament of the axilla**, which is attached to the axillary fascia over the floor of the axilla, and by its tension maintains the concavity of the axilla (Fig. 2.2).

The clavipectoral fascia is pierced by four structures: two passing inwards, two passing outwards. Passing

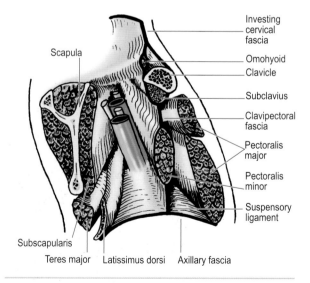

Scapula

Investing cervical fascia

Omohyoid

Clavicle

Subclavius

Clavipectoral fascia

Pectoralis major

Pectoralis minor

Suspensory ligament

Subscapularis

Teres major   Latissimus dorsi   Axillary fascia

Fig. 2.2 Vertical section of the left axilla, looking laterally towards the arm. The clavipectoral fascia encloses subclavius and pectoralis minor, below which it becomes the suspensory ligament of the axilla, joining the axillary fascia which arches upwards between pectoralis major and latissimus dorsi. The neurovascular bundle of the upper limb lies between the anterior and posterior axillary walls.

inwards are lymphatics from the infraclavicular nodes to the apical nodes of the axilla, and the cephalic vein; passing outwards are the lateral pectoral nerve and the thoracoacromial artery, or its branches (pectoral, acromial, deltoid and clavicular); their corresponding veins join the cephalic vein anterior to the fascia.

Trapezius

This large flat muscle, the most superficial of the upper part of the back, arises in the midline from skull to lower thorax and converges on the outer part of the pectoral girdle. Its origin extends from the medial third of the superior nuchal line to the spine of C7 vertebra, finding attachment to the ligamentum nuchae between the external occipital protuberance and the vertebral spine. Below this the origin extends along the spinous processes and supraspinous ligaments of all 12 thoracic vertebrae. Opposite the upper thoracic spines the muscle shows a triangular aponeurotic area, which makes a diamond with that of the opposite side (Fig. 2.5).

The upper fibres are inserted into the posterior border of the lateral third of the clavicle at its posterior border. The middle fibres are inserted along the medial border of the acromion and the superior lip of the crest of the scapular spine. The part of the muscle which arises from the lower six thoracic spines is inserted by a narrow recurved tendon into the medial end of the spine (Fig. 2.5).

Nerve supply. From the spinal part of the accessory nerve (C1–5) and branches from the cervical plexus (C3 and 4); the latter are usually only proprioceptive, although in some cases they contain motor fibres as well (see p. 346). These nerves cross the posterior triangle to enter the deep surface of trapezius. The accessory nerve can be distinguished from the cervical branches by the fact that it emerges from within the substance of sternocleidomastoid; the cervical nerves emerge from behind sternocleidomastoid.

Action. All fibres help to retract the scapula, while the upper and lower fibres are important in scapular rotation, tilting the glenoid cavity upwards, an essential component of abduction of the shoulder. In this action upper fibres elevate the acromion while lower fibres depress the medial end of the spine, like turning a wing nut (Fig. 2.3), and they are strongly assisted by the lowest four digitations of serratus anterior (see p. 44). The upper fibres can elevate the whole scapula (shrug the shoulder) or prevent its depression (as when carrying something heavy). They can also produce lateral flexion of the neck, but acting with the upper fibres of the opposite side they can extend the neck.

Test. The shoulder is shrugged against resistance and the upper border of the muscle is seen and felt.

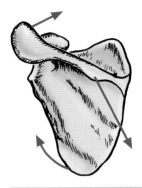

Fig. 2.3 Rotation of the scapula. The upper and lower parts of trapezius pull on the scapular spine in different directions, twisting it like a wing-nut, while serratus anterior pulls on the inferior angle.

Latissimus dorsi

This muscle, covering such a large area of the back, is characterized by its very wide origin and its very narrow insertion. The muscle arises from the spines of the lower six thoracic vertebrae and the posterior layer of the lumbar fascia, by which it is attached to the lumbar and sacral vertebral spines and to the posterior part of the crest of the ilium (Fig. 2.4). Lateral to this it also arises by muscular fibres from the outer lip of the iliac crest. The upper part of the flat sheet of muscle runs horizontally, covered medially by the lower triangular part of trapezius, and passes over the inferior angle of the scapula, from which a few fibres may arise (Fig. 2.5). The lateral part of the muscle runs vertically upwards, being reinforced by four slips from the lowest four ribs, whose fibres of origin interdigitate with those of the external oblique. This lateral border of latissimus dorsi forms a boundary of the lumbar triangle (see p. 231). The muscle converges towards the posterior axillary fold, of which it forms the lower border. The muscle sweeps spirally around the lower border of teres major with some intermingling of their fibres. The muscle is then replaced by a flattened, shiny, white tendon about 3 cm broad which is inserted into the floor of the intertubercular sulcus (Fig. 2.9). As a result of the spiral turn around teres major the surfaces of the muscle, anterior and posterior, are reversed at the tendon; and the fibres that originate lowest at the midline insert highest at the humerus, while those that originate highest insert lowest. This glistening white tendon contrasts with adjacent muscle and is a useful landmark in the lower posterior wall of the axilla.

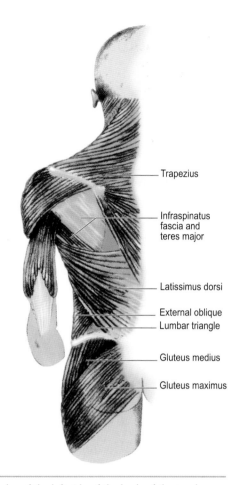

Trapezius

Infraspinatus
fascia and
teres major

Latissimus dorsi

External oblique
Lumbar triangle

Gluteus medius

Gluteus maximus

Fig. 2.4   Muscles of the left side of the back of the trunk.

Nerve supply. By the thoracodorsal nerve (C6–8) from the posterior cord of the brachial plexus. It is vulnerable in operations on the axilla, for in its course down the posterior wall it slopes forwards to enter the medial surface of the muscle just behind its anterior border in front of the thoracodorsal vessels (Fig. 2.15).

Action. It extends the shoulder joint and medially rotates the humerus (e.g. folding the arms behind the back, or scratching the opposite scapula), but in combination with pectoralis major it is a powerful adductor. Especially used in restoring the upper limb from abduction above the shoulder, it is essentially the climbing muscle.

Its costal fibres of origin can assist in deep inspiration, elevating the lower four ribs towards the fixed humerus. But the remainder of the muscle, sweeping from the vertebral column around the convexity of the posterolateral chest wall, compresses the lower thorax in violent expiratory efforts such as coughing or sneezing.

In spinal injury the muscle may move the pelvis and trunk; it is the only muscle of the upper limb to have a pelvic attachment (via the lumbar fascia). The muscle is used in *reconstructive breast surgery*. A part of the muscle is rotated around to the front and positioned in a subpectoral pocket (see p. 40). The thoracodorsal artery is an important source of blood supply to the flap.

Test. The arm is abducted to a right angle and then adducted against resistance; the anterior border of the muscle below the posterior axillary fold can be seen and felt. The muscle can also be felt to contract here when the patient coughs.

Rhomboid major and minor

Rhomboid major arises from four vertebral spines (T2–5), and the intervening supraspinous ligaments. It is inserted into the medial border of the scapula between the root of the spine and the inferior angle (Fig. 2.5).

Rhomboid minor is a narrow ribbon of muscle parallel with the above, arising from two vertebral spines (C7, T1) and inserted into the medial border of the scapula at the root of the spine.

Nerve supplies. By the dorsal scapular nerve (nerve to the rhomboids) from the C5 root of the brachial plexus which passes through scalenus medius, runs down deep (anterior) to levator scapulae (which it supplies) and lies on the serratus posterior superior muscle to the medial side of the descending branch of the transverse cervical artery (Fig. 2.5). It supplies each rhomboid on the deep surface.

Actions. The rhomboids draw the vertebral border of the scapula medially and upwards. With trapezius they contract in squaring the shoulders, i.e. retracting the scapula.

Test. With the hand on the hip or behind the back the patient pushes the elbow backwards against resistance and braces the shoulder back. The muscles are palpated at the vertebral border of the scapula. If the rhomboids of one side are paralysed, the scapula of the affected side remains further from the midline than that of the normal side.

Levator scapulae

This strap-like muscle, which appears in the floor of the posterior triangle, arises from the transverse processus of the atlas and axis and from the posterior tubercles of the third and fourth cervical vertebrae. It is inserted into the medial border of the scapula from the superior angle to the spine.

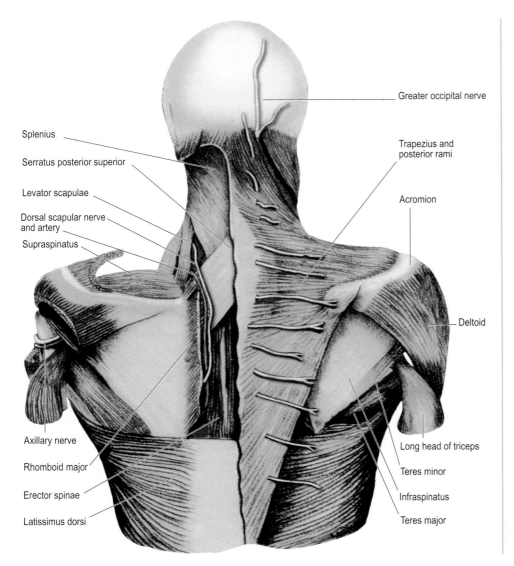

Splenius

Serratus posterior superior

Levator scapulae

Dorsal scapular nerve and artery

Supraspinatus

Axillary nerve

Rhomboid major

Erector spinae

Latissimus dorsi

Greater occipital nerve

Trapezius and posterior rami

Acromion

Deltoid

Long head of triceps

Teres minor

Infraspinatus

Teres major

Fig 2.5 Muscles of the pectoral girdle from behind. On the left most of trapezius, deltoid and the rhomboids have been removed to show the dorsal scapular nerve accompanied by the dorsal scapular artery, and the axillary nerve with the (unlabelled) posterior circumflex humeral artery.

Nerve supply. From the cervical plexus (C3, 4, anterior rami), reinforced by the dorsal scapular nerve (C5).

Action. With the upper part of trapezius, it can elevate the scapula and laterally flex the neck.

Serratus anterior

This is a broad sheet of thick muscle (Fig. 2.15) which clothes the side wall of the thorax and forms the medial wall of the axilla. It arises by a series of digitations from the upper eight ribs. The first digitation arises from the first and second ribs (Fig. 2.6). All the other digitations arise from their corresponding ribs. The muscle is inserted on the costal (inner) surface of the scapula: the first and second digitations at the superior angle, the third and fourth as a thin sheet to the length of the vertebral border, and the lowest four at the inferior angle. The muscle is covered by a strong well-developed fascia.

Nerve supply. By the long thoracic nerve from the C5, 6 and 7 roots of the brachial plexus. The nerve lies behind the midaxillary line (i.e. behind the lateral branches of the intercostal arteries) on the surface of the muscle (Fig. 2.15), deep to the fascia, and is thus usually protected in operations on the axilla.

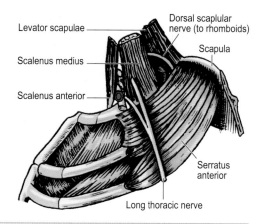

Fig. 2.6 Left long thoracic nerve (to serratus anterior). The branches from C5 and 6 fuse within scalenus medius and emerge as a single trunk which is joined in the axilla over the first digitation of serratus anterior by the branch from C7. The second rib gives origin to half of the first digitation and all the second digitation of the muscle.

Action. The whole muscle contracting en masse protracts the scapula (punching and pushing), thus effectively elongating the upper limb. A further highly important action is that of the lower four digitations, which powerfully assist trapezius in rotating the scapula laterally and upwards in raising the arm above the level of the shoulder. In this action it is a more powerful rotator than trapezius. In all positions the muscle keeps the vertebral border of the scapula in firm apposition with the chest wall.

Test. The outstretched hand is pushed against a wall. Paralysis results in 'winged scapula', where the vertebral border becomes prominently raised off the posterior chest wall.

Joints of the pectoral girdle

Sternoclavicular joint

This is a synovial joint between the bulbous medial end of the clavicle, the superolateral part of the manubrium of the sternum and the adjoining first costal cartilage (Fig. 2.7). The joint is separated into two cavities by an intervening disc of fibrocartilage, which is attached at its periphery to the capsule of the joint. Although synovial, it is atypical as the bony surfaces are covered by fibrocartilage, not the usual hyaline variety. The sternal end of the clavicle projects above the upper margin of the manubrium so that only about the lower half of the clavicular articular surface lies opposite the sternal articular facet.

The **capsule** invests the articular surfaces like a sleeve. The **articular disc** is attached to the capsule. The disc is also firmly attached to the medial end of the clavicle above and behind, and to the first costal cartilage below. The capsule is thickened in front and behind as the **anterior** and **posterior sternoclavicular ligaments**.

The **interclavicular ligament** joins the upper borders of the sternal ends of the two clavicles and is attached to the suprasternal (jugular) notch of the manubrium. The **costoclavicular ligament** binds the clavicle to the first costal cartilage and the adjacent end of the first rib, just lateral to the joint. It is in two laminae. The fibres of the anterior lamina run upwards and laterally, and those of the posterior lamina upwards and medially (these are the same directions as those of the external and internal intercostal muscles). The ligament is very strong and is the major stabilizing factor of the sternoclavicular joint.

Nerve supply. The medial supraclavicular nerves (C3, 4) from the cervical plexus give articular branches to the capsule and ligaments.

Fig. 2.7 Left sternoclavicular joint, sectioned and viewed from the front. The clavicle extends well above the bony socket of the manubrium, and is bound down by the disc and costoclavicular ligament.

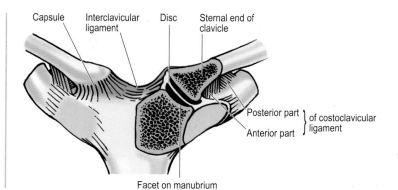

Movements. Elevation (shrugging the shoulder) and depression of the acromial end of the clavicle result in movements downwards and upwards respectively between the sternal end of the clavicle and the disc. Forward and backward (squaring the shoulders) movements of the acromial end likewise cause reciprocal movements at the sternal end; these movements occur between the manubrium and the disc. Similarly, in rotary movements (abduction of the arm above the head) the disc moves with the clavicle. Rotation of the clavicle is passive; there are no rotator muscles. It is produced by rotation of the scapula and transmitted to the clavicle through the coracoclavicular ligaments (see below).

The *stability* of the joint is maintained by the ligaments, especially the costoclavicular ligament. It takes all strain off the joint, transmitting stress from clavicle to first costal cartilage. The latter is itself immovably fixed to the manubrium by a primary cartilaginous joint (see p. 187). Dislocation is unusual; the clavicle breaks in preference.

Acromioclavicular joint

This is a synovial joint between the flat overhanging lateral end of the clavicle and the underlying medial border of the acromion. The articulating surfaces are covered (like those of the sternoclavicular joint) by fibrocartilage (so it is an atypical synovial joint).

A sleeve-like capsule surrounds the articular surfaces; it is not strong, but on top there is a thickening of fibres which constitutes the acromioclavicular ligament. An incomplete disc of fibrocartilage hangs down into the upper part of the joint cavity.

The **coracoclavicular ligament**, extremely strong, is the principal factor in providing stability to the joint. It consists of two parts, conoid and trapezoid (Fig. 2.8). The *conoid ligament*, an inverted cone, extends upwards from the knuckle of the coracoid process to a wider attachment around the conoid tubercle, on the under-surface of the clavicle (Fig. 2.48). The *trapezoid ligament* is attached to the ridge of the same name on the upper surface of the coracoid process and extends laterally, in an almost horizontal plane, to the trapezoid ridge on the undersurface of the clavicle. The two ligaments are connected to each other posteriorly, forming an angle that is open anteriorly.

Nerve supply. By the suprascapular nerve (C5, 6) from the brachial plexus.

Movements. These are passive; muscles which move the scapula cause it to move on the clavicle. Scapular movements on the chest wall fall into three groups: (1) protraction and retraction around the chest wall, (2) rotation, and (3) elevation or depression. These basic

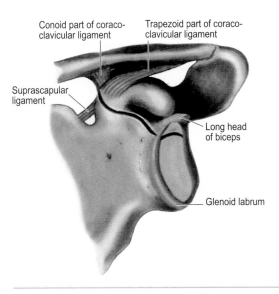

Fig. 2.8   Glenoid cavity of the left scapula and the coracoclavicular ligament. The black line marks the site of the epiphyseal plate between the scapula proper and the coracoid component. The glenoid labrum continues above into the long head of biceps. The trapezoid part of the coracoclavicular ligament lies in front of and lateral to the conoid part.

movements can be combined in varying proportions, and each of these transmits, through ligaments, corresponding movements to the clavicle. All movements of the scapula involve movements in the joint at either end of the clavicle.

Horizontally, in protraction and retraction of the tip of the shoulder, the scapula hugs the thoracic wall, held to it by serratus anterior and pectoralis minor. The acromion glides to and fro on the tip of the clavicle.

In abduction of the arm the total range of scapular rotation on the chest wall is about 60°, but only 20° of this occurs between the scapula and the clavicle. The two parts of the coracoclavicular ligament are then taut, and transmit the rotating force to the clavicle, whose rotation then accounts for the remainder of scapular rotation on the chest wall.

Elevation (shrugging the shoulders) is produced by the upper fibres of trapezius together with levator scapulae and the rhomboids, mutually neutralizing their rotatory effects. Depression of the scapula is produced by gravity, assisted when necessary by serratus anterior and pectoralis minor. Elevation and depression move the medial end of the clavicle (see above), but they scarcely move the acromioclavicular joint.

The *stability* of the joint is provided by the coracoclavicular ligament. The scapula and upper limb hang suspended from the clavicle by the conoid ligament (assisted by the deltoid, biceps and triceps muscles). Forces transmitted medially from the upper limb to the glenoid cavity are transmitted from scapula to clavicle by the trapezoid ligament and from clavicle to first rib by the costoclavicular ligament. Thus a fall on outstretched hand or elbow puts no strain on either end of the clavicle at the joints. If the clavicle fractures as a result, it always does so between these ligaments. Falls on the shoulder may dislocate the acromioclavicular joint, forcing the acromion under the clavicle and tearing the coraco-clavicular ligament.

PART TWO

Shoulder

Muscles of the shoulder

A group of six muscles converge from the scapula on to the humerus and surround the shoulder joint: deltoid, supraspinatus, infraspinatus, teres minor, teres major and subscapularis. Three of them (supraspinatus, infraspinatus and teres minor) extend from the posterior surface of the blade of the scapula to be inserted into the three impressions on the greater tubercle of the humerus. Subscapularis passes from the thoracic surface of the

scapula to the lesser tubercle, and teres major from the inferior angle of the scapula to the shaft of the humerus. All these muscles lie hidden, for the most part, under deltoid and trapezius.

Subscapularis

This arises from the medial two-thirds of the costal surface of the scapula and from the intermuscular septa which raise ridges on the bone. The tendon of the muscle is separated from a bare area at the lateral angle of the scapula by a bursa which communicates with the cavity of the shoulder joint. Lateral to this the tendon fuses with the capsule of the shoulder joint and is inserted into the lesser tubercle of the humerus (Fig. 2.9). The muscle is covered by a dense fascia which is attached to the scapula at the margins of its origin.

Nerve supply. By the upper and lower subscapular nerves (C5, 6) from the posterior cord of the brachial plexus.

Action. With the other short scapular muscles the subscapularis gives stability to the shoulder joint, assisting in fixation of the upper end of the humerus during movements of elbow, wrist, and hand. Acting as a prime mover, it is a medial rotator of the humerus.

There is no satisfactory test for the muscle, as its action is difficult to differentiate from other medial rotators.

Fig. 2.9 Muscles of the posterior wall of the left axilla, from the front. The long head of triceps passes behind teres major, making adjacent to the humerus a quadrangular space (for the axillary nerve) and a triangular space (for the radial nerve). Serratus anterior has been removed, exposing the costal surface of the vertebral border of the scapula, to which it is attached.

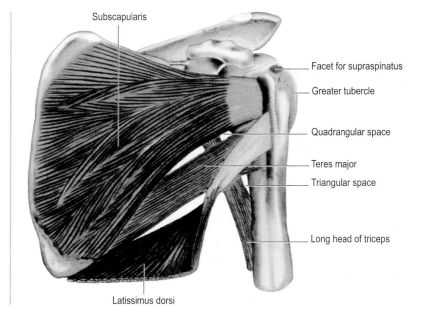

Subscapularis

Facet for supraspinatus

Greater tubercle

Quadrangular space

Teres major

Triangular space

Long head of triceps

Latissimus dorsi

Supraspinatus

The muscle arises from the medial two-thirds of the supraspinous fossa of the scapula. The tendon blends with the capsule of the shoulder joint and passes on to be inserted into the smooth facet on the upper part of the greater tubercle of the humerus (Fig. 2.9).

Nerve supply. By the suprascapular nerve (C5, 6).

Action. The muscle braces the head of the humerus against the glenoid cavity, to give stability during the action of other muscles, especially the deltoid, which it assists in abduction at the shoulder joint.

Test. The arm is abducted against resistance and the muscle palpated (deep to trapezius) above the scapular spine.

Infraspinatus

The muscle arises from the medial two-thirds of the infraspinous fossa and from the deep surface of the infraspinous fascia, which covers the muscle and is attached to the scapula at its margins. A bursa lies between the bare area of the scapula and the muscle; it sometimes communicates with the shoulder joint. The tendon blends with the capsule of the shoulder joint, and is inserted into the smooth area on the central facet of the greater tubercle of the humerus (Fig. 2.52), between supraspinatus above and teres minor below.

Nerve supply. By the suprascapular nerve (C5, 6).

Action. Apart from acting to brace the head of the humerus against the glenoid cavity, giving stability to the joint, the muscle is also a powerful lateral rotator of the humerus.

Test. With the elbow flexed and held into the side, the forearm is moved outwards against resistance and the muscle is palpated (deep to trapezius) below the scapular spine.

Teres minor

The muscle arises from an elongated oval area on the dorsal surface of the axillary border of the scapula. It passes upwards and laterally, edge to edge with the lower border of infraspinatus and behind the long head of triceps. The tendon blends with the capsule of the shoulder joint and attaches to the lowest facet on the greater tubercle of the humerus. The lower part of the lateral border of this muscle lies edge to edge with teres major, but the latter muscle leaves it by passing forward in front of the long head of triceps (Fig. 2.16).

Nerve supply. By a branch from the posterior branch of the axillary nerve (C5, 6).

Action. It assists the other small muscles around the head of the humerus in steadying the shoulder joint. It is a lateral rotator and weak adductor of the humerus. With teres major it holds down the head of the humerus against the upward pull of the deltoid during abduction of the shoulder.

Teres major

This muscle arises from an oval area on the dorsal surface of the inferior angle of the scapula. It is inserted into the medial lip of the intertubercular sulcus of the humerus. The flat tendon of latissimus dorsi winds around its lower border and comes to lie in front of the upper part of the muscle at its insertion (Fig. 2.9).

Nerve supply. By the lower subscapular nerve (C5, 6), which enters the anterior surface of the muscle.

Action. It assists the other short muscles in steadying the upper end of the humerus in movements at the shoulder joint; acting alone it is an adductor and medial rotator of the humerus and helps to extend the flexed arm. With teres minor it holds down the upper end of the humerus as deltoid pulls up the bone into abduction. Its tendon can be transplanted posteriorly to provide lateral rotation when infraspinatus and teres minor are paralysed.

Test. The abducted arm is adducted against resistance, and the muscle is seen and felt from behind the posterior axillary fold.

Infraspinatus fascia

The infraspinatus and teres minor muscles lie deep to a strong membrane which is firmly attached to bone at the margins of these muscles. It is attached above to the lower border of the scapular spine beneath the deltoid muscle. The fascia does not cover teres major (Fig. 2.4). The fascia is a landmark in surgical exposures of this region, and in fracture of the blade of the scapula the resulting haematoma is confined beneath the fascia, producing a characteristic swelling limited to the margins of the bone.

Deltoid

The muscle arises from the anterior border and upper surface of the lateral one-third of the clavicle, from the whole of the lateral border of the acromion and from the inferior lip of the crest of the scapular spine. On the lateral border of the acromion four ridges may be seen; from them four fibrous septa pass down into the muscle. The deltoid tuberosity on the lateral aspect of the humerus is V-shaped, with a central vertical ridge. From the ridge and limbs of the V three fibrous septa pass upwards between the four septa from the acromion. The spaces between the septa are filled with a fleshy mass of muscle fibres which are attached to contiguous septa. The multipennate centre of the deltoid so formed has a diminished range of contraction, but a correspondingly increased force of pull. The anterior and posterior fibres, arising from the clavicle and the scapular spine, are not multipennate. They converge on the anterior and posterior margins of the deltoid tuberosity, and their range of movement is greater but the force of their pull is less.

Nerve supply. By the axillary nerve (C5, 6).

Action. Working with supraspinatus, deltoid abducts the arm by the multipennate acromial fibres. The anterior fibres assist pectoralis major in flexing and medially rotating the arm; the posterior fibres assist latissimus dorsi in extending the arm and act as a lateral rotator.

Test. The arm is abducted against resistance and the muscle is seen and felt.

Intramuscular injection. The site for intramuscular injection into deltoid is on the lateral side of the bulge of the shoulder, no more than 4 cm below the lower border of the acromion; the anterior branch of the axillary nerve curls forwards round the back of the humerus 5 cm below the acromion.

Scapular anastomosis

The *dorsal scapular artery* is a branch of the transverse cervical artery, or arises directly from the third part of the subclavian artery (see p. 362). It accompanies the dorsal scapular nerve and runs down the vertebral border of the scapula to its inferior angle (Fig. 2.10). The transverse cervical artery and the *suprascapular artery* are usually branches of the thyrocervical trunk, which arises from the first part of the subclavian artery. The suprascapular artery crosses over the suprascapular ligament (Fig. 2.8), passes through the supraspinous fossa, turns around the lateral border of the spine of the scapula and supplies the infraspinous fossa as far as the inferior angle. The *subscapular artery*, branching from the third part of the axillary, supplies the subscapularis muscle in the subscapular fossa as far as the inferior angle. Its *circumflex scapular branch* enters the infraspinous fossa on the dorsal surface of the bone, grooving the axillary border as it does so. All these vessels anastomose, thus connecting the first part of the subclavian with the third part of the axillary artery and providing a collateral circulation when the subclavian artery is obstructed, such as by a cervical rib or fibrous band (see p. 439). The companion veins form corresponding anastomoses.

Shoulder joint

The shoulder joint is a multiaxial ball-and-socket synovial joint. There is an approximately 4 to 1 disproportion between the large round head of the humerus and the small shallow glenoid cavity of the scapula (Fig. 2.10). The **glenoid labrum**, a ring of fibrocartilage attached to the margins of the glenoid cavity, deepens slightly but effectively the depression of the glenoid 'fossa' (Fig. 2.8).

The **capsule** of the joint is attached to the scapula beyond the supraglenoid tubercle and the margins of the labrum. It is attached to the humerus around the articular margins of the head (i.e. the anatomical neck) except inferiorly, where its attachment is to the surgical neck of the humerus a finger's breadth below the articular margin (Fig. 2.11A). At the upper end of the intertubercular sulcus the capsule bridges the gap between the greater and lesser tubercles, being here named the **transverse humeral ligament**. A gap in the anterior part of the capsule allows communication between the synovial membrane and the subscapularis bursa (Fig. 2.11). A similar gap is sometimes present posteriorly, allowing

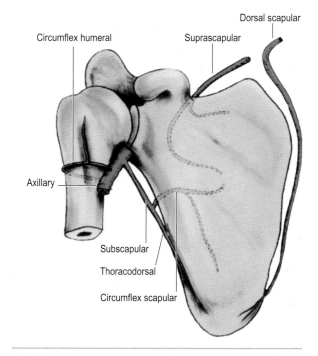

Fig. 2.10 Scapular anastomosis. The dorsal scapular and suprascapular arteries arise from the third and first parts of the subclavian, and the subscapular from the third part of the axillary artery. They and the circumflex scapular anastomose on both surfaces of the scapula.

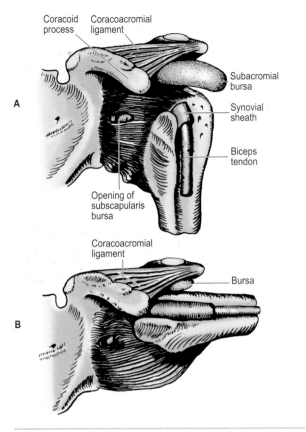

Coracoid process
Coracoacromial ligament
Subacromial bursa
Synovial sheath
Biceps tendon
Opening of subscapularis bursa
Coracoacromial ligament
Bursa

A

B

Fig. 2.11   Left subacromial bursa. In **A** with the arm by the side, the bursa is only half under cover of the acromion, but in **B** with the arm abducted the bursa is withdrawn beneath the acromion.

communication with the infraspinatus bursa. The fibres of the capsule all run horizontally between scapula and humerus. The capsule is thick and strong but it is very lax, a necessity in a joint so mobile as this. Near the humerus the capsule is greatly thickened by fusion of the tendons of the short scapular muscles. The long tendon of biceps is intracapsular.

The **synovial membrane** is attached around the glenoid labrum and lines the capsule. It is attached to the articular margin of the head of the humerus and covers the bare area of the surgical neck that lies within the capsule at the upper end of the shaft. It 'herniates' through the hole in the front of the capsule to communicate with the subscapularis bursa and sometimes it communicates with the infraspinatus bursa. It invests the long head of biceps in a tubular sleeve that is reflected back along the tendon to the transverse ligament and adjoining

floor of the intertubercular sulcus. The synovial sleeve glides to and fro with the long tendon of biceps during abduction–adduction of the shoulder, as shown in Figure 2.11A and B.

The **glenohumeral ligaments** are three thickened bands between the glenoid labrum and humerus which reinforce the anterior part of the capsule. They are visible only from within the joint cavity, which communicates with the subscapularis bursa through an aperture between the superior and middle glenohumeral ligaments.

The **coracohumeral ligament** is quite strong. It runs from the coracoid process to the front of the greater tubercle, blending with the capsule as it does so.

From the medial border of the acromion, in front of the acromioclavicular articulation, a strong flat triangular band, the **coracoacromial ligament**, fans out to the lateral border of the coracoid process (Fig. 2.11). It lies above the head of the humerus and provides support to the head of the humerus. It is separated from the 'rotator cuff' by the subacromial bursa (Fig. 2.11).

The **subacromial (subdeltoid) bursa** is a large bursa which lies under the coracoacromial ligament, to which its upper layer is attached. Its lower layer is attached to the tendon of supraspinatus. It extends beyond the lateral border of the acromion under the deltoid with the arm at the side, but is rolled inwards under the acromion when the arm is abducted. Tenderness over the greater tuberosity of the humerus beneath the deltoid muscle which disappears when the arm is abducted is a feature of subacromial bursitis. Tearing the supraspinatus tendon brings the bursa into communication with the shoulder joint cavity, but in the normal shoulder the bursa does not communicate with the joint.

Nerve supply. By branches from the axillary, musculo-cutaneous and suprascapular nerves.

Stability

The shoulder joint, thus far described, seems to be a very unstable structure. The head of the humerus is much larger than the glenoid cavity (Fig. 2.12), and the joint capsule, though strong, is very lax. These factors suggest that the shoulder joint is an unstable articulation. The factors, however, that contribute to stability are strengthening of the capsule by fusion with it of the tendons of scapular muscles, the glenohumeral and coracohumeral ligaments, the suprahumeral support provided by the coracoacromial arch, the deepening of the glenoid cavity by the labrum and the splinting effect of the tendons of the long heads of biceps and triceps above and below the humeral head.

Upward displacement of the head of the humerus is prevented by the overhanging coracoid and acromion

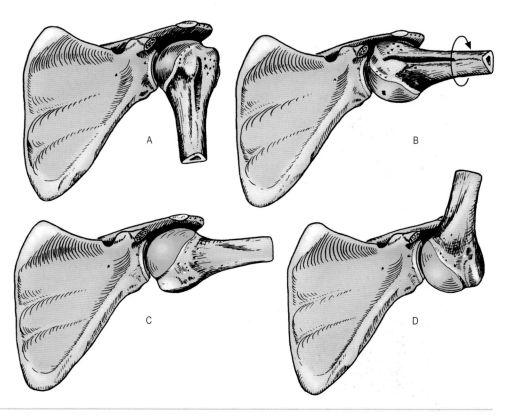

Fig. 2.12 Bony factors in abduction at the shoulder joint. (Anterior view on the left—the coracoid process has been removed.) **A** With the arm by the side; **B** abduction to 90°. Compare with **A** and note that all the available articular surface of the head of the humerus has been used up. **C** With lateral rotation of the humerus from position **B**; more of the articular surface has been made available from below to above the glenoid cavity but such free rotation is limited in the living by the rotator cuff muscles. **D** Full abduction from the rotated position in **C** but note that in the living abduction is limited to about 120°; scapular rotation accounts for the remaining 60°. The movements in **B** to **D** take place in the plane of the paper (the coronal plane of the body) but the final position in **D** can be reached directly by movement at right angles to the paper (flexion in the sagittal plane carried up to full abduction).

processes and the coracoacromial ligament that bridges them. The whole constitutes the coracoacromial arch and the subacromial bursa lies between the arch and the underlying joint capsule and supraspinatus tendon. The arch is very strong. Upward thrust on the humerus will not fracture the arch; the clavicle or the humerus itself will fracture first.

The tendons of subscapularis, supraspinatus, infraspinatus and teres minor fuse with the lateral part of the capsule and are attached to the humerus very near the joint. They are known as the **rotator cuff**, although the supraspinatus is not a rotator of the humerus. There is no cuff inferiorly and here the capsule is least supported.

The shoulder joint is the most frequently dislocated joint in the body. A sudden force applied along the axis of the humerus when it is abducted to more than 90°, extended and laterally rotated, tends to drive the head through the inferior, less supported part of the capsule, frequently tearing the labrum as well. When the arm is returned to the side, the head of the humerus comes to lie in front of the glenoid fossa, below the coracoid process. Dislocation of the shoulder joint in this manner may damage the axillary nerve as it lies directly below the joint capsule (see p. 58). Once the capsule and labrum have been damaged recurrent dislocation tends to occur in a similar manner as above, but with less force being applied. Surgical procedures carried out to prevent redislocation involve repairing the torn labrum, reinforcing the capsule by an overlapping repair and rearrangement of the anterior muscles.

Lesions of the rotator cuff impair movements of the shoulder joint. The supraspinatus tendon is particularly prone to such conditions as it passes over the top of the head of the humerus to its insertion on the greater tubercle. Impingement of the tendon under the coraco-acromial arch and a critical area of diminished vascularity about 1 cm proximal to its humeral insertion are believed to contribute to the occurrence of supraspinatus tendinitis. The inflammatory swelling of the tendon aggravates the impingement. Pain is felt during abduction of the shoulder as the arm traverses an arc between 60° and 120° (the 'painful arc') when impingement is maximal. In advanced cases the tendon may rupture, allowing the subacromial bursa to communicate with the joint cavity, and this can be demonstrated by arthrography as the opaque medium will extend from the joint into the subacromial space.

Movements

As the shoulder joint is of the ball and socket type and as the head of the humerus is four times the area of the glenoid cavity, there is considerable freedom for a variety of movements around many axes. These movements are often associated with movements of the scapula on the thoracic wall and consequential movements of the clavicle.

The movements of the shoulder joint are: flexion and extension; adduction and abduction; and rotation. Circumduction is a rhythmical combination in orderly sequence of flexion, abduction, extension and adduction (or the reverse).

When the arm hangs at rest beside the body, the glenoid fossa faces forwards as well as laterally. *Flexion* at the shoulder joint, without any associated scapular movement, brings the arm forwards and inwards across the front of the body. The clavicular head of pectoralis major and the anterior fibres of deltoid are assisted in this movement by coracobrachialis and the short head of biceps. The opposite movement of *extension* is effected by latissimus dorsi, teres major and the posterior fibres of deltoid. The sternocostal part of pectoralis major is able to extend the fully flexed arm and flex the fully extended arm.

The multipennate acromial fibres of deltoid are the principal abductors at the shoulder joint. But acting alone, deltoid would tend to raise the head of the humerus upwards, as in shrugging the shoulders, rather than abduct it. Supraspinatus initiates *abduction* and holds the head of the humerus against the glenoid fossa, while subscapularis, infraspinatus and teres minor exert a downward pull on the head. At approximately 90° of abduction, the articular surface of the head of the humerus is fully utilized and lies edge to edge with that of the glenoid fossa (Fig. 2.12). Lateral rotation of the humerus is required to bring additional articular surface into play and allow abduction to continue. Not more than 120° of abduction is possible at the glenohumeral articulation. Further abduction, as in bringing the arm vertical beside the head, requires scapular rotation that makes the glenoid fossa face upwards, brought about by trapezius and serratus anterior (Fig. 2.3). Apart from during the initial approximately 30° of abduction, glenohumeral movement and scapular rotation occur simultaneously, their ratio being 2 to 1. Gravity aids *adduction* of the abducted arm; pectoralis major, latissimus dorsi and teres major are powerful adductors.

Rotation is mostly produced by the short scapular muscles: infraspinatus and teres minor for lateral rotation, subscapularis and teres major for medial rotation (assisted by latissimus dorsi and pectoralis major).

Test. The action of placing both hands behind the head is a good test of lateral rotation on the two sides; likewise, actively placing both hands on the back between the scapulae tests medial rotation. With the arm abducted to 90° and the elbow flexed to 90°, moving the hand and forearm upwards and then downwards also tests lateral and medial rotation respectively; the normal range for each is about 90°.

Surgical approach

The joint can be exposed from the front or back. From the front the deltopectoral groove is opened up, ligating tributaries of the cephalic vein, but preserving the vein itself and retracting it medially. The tip of the coracoid process is detached and turned medially with coracobrachialis and the short head of biceps still attached, taking care not to damage the musculocutaneous nerve entering coracobrachialis. Subscapularis is stretched by laterally rotating the humerus and then divided to expose the joint capsule. The anterior circumflex humeral vessels are a guide to the lateral (lower) border of the muscle.

From the back deltoid is detached from the spine of the scapula and acromion and reflected laterally to allow infraspinatus and teres minor to be cut to expose the capsule. The axillary nerve and posterior circumflex humeral vessels must not be damaged when reflecting deltoid.

Injection or *aspiration* of the joint can be carried out from the side below the acromion, from the back below the junction of the acromion with the spine and in the direction of the coracoid process, or from the front with the needle passing through the deltopectoral groove and then below and medial to the tip of the coracoid process through the coracobrachialis-biceps origin and subscapularis.

PART THREE

Axilla

The axilla is the space between the upper arm and the side of the thorax, bounded in front and behind by the axillary folds, communicating above with the posterior triangle of the neck and containing neurovascular structures and lymph nodes, for the upper limb and the side wall of the thorax. Its *floor* is the axillary fascia extending from the anterior to the posterior axillary folds and from the fascia over the serratus anterior to the deep fascia of the arm. The suspensory ligament (Fig. 2.2) from the lower border of pectoralis minor is attached to the fascial floor from above. Its **anterior wall** is formed by pectoralis major, pectoralis minor, subclavius and the clavipectoral fascia; these have been described on pages 40–41. The **posterior wall** extends lower; it is formed by subscapularis and teres major (see pp. 47–48), with the tendon of latissimus dorsi winding around the latter muscle. The **medial wall** is formed by the upper part of serratus anterior, the lower limit of the axilla being defined as the level of the fourth rib. The anterior and posterior walls converge laterally to the lips of the intertubercular groove of the humerus in which lies the tendon of the long head of biceps, overlapped medially by coracobrachialis and the tendon of the short head of biceps (Figs 2.1 and 2.13).

The **apex** is bounded by the clavicle, upper border of the scapula and the outer border of the first rib; it is the channel of communication between axilla and posterior triangle.

Contents of the axilla

Axillary artery

This is the main arterial stem of the upper limb and is a continuation of the third part of the subclavian artery. It commences at the outer border of the first rib and enters the apex of the axilla by passing over the first digitation of serratus anterior, behind the midpoint of the clavicle. At the lower border of teres major it becomes the brachial artery. The axillary artery and the cords of the brachial plexus are enclosed within the axillary sheath, which is projected down from the prevertebral fascia in the neck (see Fig. 6.8, p. 358). The artery is conveniently divided into three parts by pectoralis minor, which crosses in front of it: the part above; the part behind;

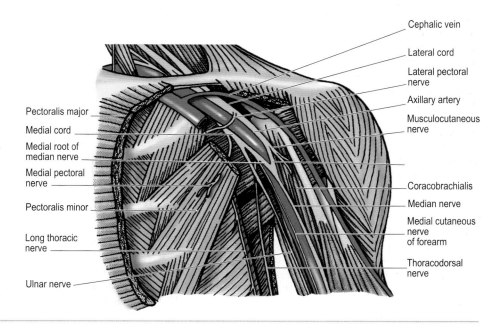

Fig. 2.13   Left axilla and brachial plexus from the front, after removal of much of pectoralis major and minor and the axillary vein. The medial cutaneous nerve of the forearm lies in front of the ulnar nerve medial to the axillary artery. The median nerve is in front of the artery, and laterally the musculocutaneous nerve enters coracobrachialis. (The small medial cutaneous nerve of the arm, which runs distally medial to the axillary vein, is not shown.)

and the part below. The lateral and posterior cords are superolateral, and the medial cord posterior, to the first part of the artery. The second part has the three cords of the plexus lateral, posterior and medial to it, as their names indicate. The third part has the branches from the cords of the brachial plexus, having in general the same relation to the artery as their parent cords. The medial root of the median nerve crosses in front of the artery to join the lateral root and form the nerve lateral to the artery (Fig. 2.13). The axillary vein lies anteromedial to all parts of the artery. The shape of the artery depends upon the position of the arm. With the arm at the side the artery has a bold curve with its convexity lateral. With the arm laterally rotated and abducted, as in operations upon the axilla, the artery pursues a straight course. The *surface marking* of the artery can then be indicated by a line from the middle of the clavicle to the groove behind coracobrachialis.

Surgical approach. The axillary artery can be exposed by a transverse incision below the clavicle or by an incision along the deltopectoral groove. Pectoralis major is split in the line of its fibres in the former and retracted away from deltoid in the latter approaches. The tendon of pectoralis minor is divided. The cords of the brachial plexus and their branches must be safeguarded.

Branches. The first part has one branch, the second part two, and the third part three branches.

The *superior thoracic artery*, from the first part, is a small vessel that runs forwards to supply both pectoral muscles.

The thoracoacromial and lateral thoracic arteries arise from the second part. The *thoracoacromial artery* skirts the upper border of pectoralis minor to pierce the clavipectoral fascia, often separately by its four terminal branches (clavicular, deltoid, acromial and pectoral). These branches radiate away at right angles from each other in the directions indicated by their names.

The *lateral thoracic artery* follows the lower border of pectoralis minor, supplying branches to the pectoralis and serratus anterior muscles and, in the female, being an important contributor of blood to the breast.

The subscapular and the two circumflex humeral arteries arise from the third part. The *subscapular artery*, the largest branch of the axillary, runs down the posterior axillary wall, giving off a dorsal branch, the *circumflex scapular artery*, which passes through the posterior wall of the axilla between subscapularis and teres major, medial to the long head of the triceps and curves backwards round the lateral scapular border. Distal to this large branch, the diminished subscapular artery changes its name to *thoracodorsal*, and runs with the nerve of the same name into latissimus dorsi, having given one to three branches to serratus anterior. These latter branches anastomose with posterior intercostal arteries, providing an alternative source of blood supply to latissimus dorsi (see p. 43) if the subscapular or thoracodorsal arteries have been occluded or divided higher up in the axilla. Although the thoracodorsal nerve arises from the posterior cord of the brachial plexus, it descends to lie in front of the artery in a neurovascular bundle that enters latissimus dorsi close to its anterior edge (Fig. 2.15).

The *anterior circumflex humeral artery* runs deep to coracobrachialis and both heads of biceps (giving here an ascending branch which runs up the intertubercular sulcus and is an important source of blood supply to the head of the humerus), and passes around the surgical neck of the humerus to anastomose with the *posterior circumflex humeral artery*. This, a much larger branch of the axillary artery, passes through the quadrangular space (Fig. 2.9) in the posterior axillary wall between subscapularis and teres major, lateral to the long head of triceps and medial to the humerus. It is accompanied above by the axillary nerve and, like it, supplies the deltoid. It also gives branches to the long and lateral heads of triceps and the shoulder joint, and anastomoses with the profunda brachii artery.

Axillary vein

This large vein commences at the lower border of the teres major as a continuation of the basilic vein. At the outer border of the first rib the axillary vein enters the root of the neck as the subclavian vein in front of scalenus anterior. The venae comitantes of the brachial artery join the axillary vein near its commencement and the cephalic vein drains into it above pectoralis minor. Other tributaries correspond to branches of the axillary artery. The axillary vein has a pair of valves near its distal end and the cephalic and subscapular veins have valves near their terminations. The axillary vein lies medial to the axillary artery, which it partly overlaps anteriorly.

The subscapular veins are multiple and lie on the posterior wall of the axilla; they are encountered during surgical clearance of axillary lymph nodes. The lateral thoracic vein is connected by the thoracoepigastric vein to the superficial epigastric vein, a tributary of the great saphenous vein (see p. 186). This communicating channel becomes prominent on the side of the trunk in cases of inferior vena caval obstruction.

Brachial plexus

Five roots contribute to the formation of the plexus for the upper limb (Fig. 2.14). They are the fibres that

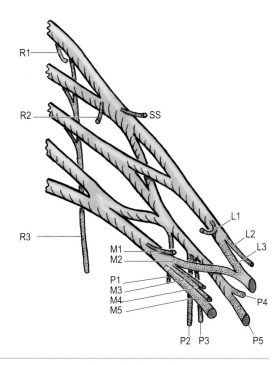

trunks divides into an anterior and a posterior **division** behind the clavicle. Here, at the outer border of the first rib, the upper two anterior divisions unite to form the **lateral cord**, the anterior division of the lower trunk runs on as the **medial cord**, while all three posterior divisions unite to form the **posterior cord**. These three cords enter the axilla above the first part of the artery, approach and embrace its second part, and give off their branches around its third part. Thus the roots are between the scalene muscles, trunks in the (posterior) triangle, divisions behind the clavicle, and cords in the axilla. An extension of the prevertebral fascia in the neck surrounds the axillary artery and cords; local anaesthetics are injected into this axillary sheath to produce a brachial plexus nerve block.

The medial cord frequently receives fibres from the anterior ramus of C7. Rarely there may be a significant contribution to the brachial plexus from the anterior ramus of C4 and a reduction in the contribution from T1 forming a *prefixed plexus*. Alternatively, a *postfixed* plexus receives a substantial contribution from T2 and a diminished input from C5. Other variations may occur in the manner of formation of the trunks, divisions and cords, while the contributions from the spinal cord segments to the branches remain constant.

There are three branches from the roots: one from the upper trunk and 3, 5 and 5 from the lateral, medial and posterior cords, respectively. There are no branches from the divisions (Fig. 2.14).

Branches from the roots

The three branches from the roots are the dorsal scapular nerve, the nerve to subclavius, and the long thoracic nerve; they arise successively from C5, C5, 6 and C5–7, and pass downwards behind, in front of, and behind the roots in that order.

The **dorsal scapular nerve** (nerve to the rhomboids) arises from the posterior aspect of C5, pierces scalenus medius and courses downwards in front of levator scapulae, lying on serratus posterior superior (Fig. 2.5). It is accompanied by the dorsal scapular vessels. It supplies both rhomboids and usually gives a branch to levator scapulae.

The **nerve to subclavius** arises from the roots of C5 and 6. It passes down in front of the trunks and the subclavian vessels to enter the posterior surface of subclavius. It frequently has a branch (accessory phrenic nerve) which connects with the phrenic nerve, providing an alternate pathway for some fibres from the fifth cervical anterior ramus to reach the diaphragm.

The **long thoracic nerve** (nerve to serratus anterior) arises from the posterior aspects of C5, 6 and 7. Branches

Fig. 2.14 Branches of the left brachial plexus.
Branches of roots: R1, dorsal scapular (nerve to rhomboids); R2, nerve to subclavius; R3, long thoracic (nerve to serratus anterior).
Branch of upper trunk: SS, suprascapular nerve.
Branches of lateral cord: L1, lateral pectoral nerve; L2, musculocutaneous nerve; L3, lateral root of median nerve.
Branches of medial cord: M1, medial pectoral nerve; M2, medial root of median nerve; M3, medial cutaneous nerve of arm; M4, medial cutaneous nerve of forearm; M5, ulnar nerve.
Branches of posterior cord: P1, upper subscapular nerve; P2, thoracodorsal nerve (to latissimus dorsi); P3, lower subscapular nerve; P4, axillary nerve; P5, radial nerve.

remain in the anterior rami of C5–8 and T1 after these have given their segmental supply to the prevertebral and scalene muscles. They are to divide into anterior and posterior divisions to supply the flexor and extensor compartments respectively (see p. 14), but before doing so they unite to form three trunks in the following manner. Of the five roots of the plexus the upper two unite to form the upper trunk, the lower two unite to form the lower trunk, and the central root runs on as the middle trunk. The five **roots** lie behind the scalenus anterior muscle and emerge between it and scalenus medius to form the **trunks** which cross the lower part of the posterior triangle of the neck. Each of the three

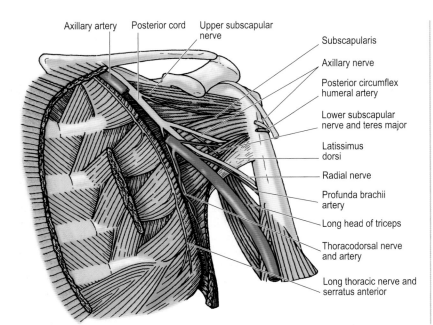

Axillary artery   Posterior cord   Upper subscapular nerve

Subscapularis

Axillary nerve

Posterior circumflex humeral artery

Lower subscapular nerve and teres major

Latissimus dorsi

Radial nerve

Profunda brachii artery

Long head of triceps

Thoracodorsal nerve and artery

Long thoracic nerve and serratus anterior

Fig. 2.15   Posterior wall of the left axilla and posterior cord of the brachial plexus. The radial nerve runs in front of the tendon of latissimus dorsi and then passes back through the triangular space. The axillary nerve passes backwards below subscapularis through the quadrangular space.

of C5 and 6 enter scalenus medius, unite in the muscle, emerge from it as a single trunk and pass down into the axilla. On the surface of serratus anterior (the medial wall of the axilla) this is joined by the branch from C7 which has descended in front of scalenus medius (Fig. 2.6). The nerve passes down posterior to the mid-axillary line, deep to the fascia on serratus anterior, and supplies the muscle segmentally (Fig. 2.15).

Branch from the trunks

The **suprascapular nerve** arises from the upper trunk in the lower part of the posterior triangle and passes back-wards and laterally deep to the border of trapezius. It passes through the suprascapular foramen (beneath the transverse scapular ligament) and supplies supraspinatus, descends lateral to the scapular spine with the supra-scapular vessels and supplies infraspinatus (Fig. 2.16). It supplies the shoulder and acromioclavicular joints.

Branches from the lateral cord

The three branches from the lateral cord are the lateral pectoral, musculocutaneous and lateral root of the median nerve.

The **lateral pectoral nerve** pierces the clavipectoral fascia to supply pectoralis major with fibres from C5, 6 and 7 (Fig. 2.13). It communicates across the front of the first part of the axillary artery with the medial pectoral nerve and through this communication supplies pectoralis minor. It has no cutaneous branch.

The **musculocutaneous nerve** (C5–7) leaves the lateral cord quite high in the axilla, runs obliquely downwards and enters coracobrachialis (Fig. 2.13), giving a twig of supply to it, before passing through the muscle. Lower down in the arm it supplies biceps and brachialis and becomes the *lateral cutaneous nerve of the forearm*. An anaesthetic solution injected through the floor of the axilla to effect a brachial plexus nerve block may not affect the musculocutaneous nerve owing to its high take-off from the lateral cord.

The **lateral root of the median nerve** is the continua-tion of the lateral cord (C5–7). It is joined by the medial root of the median nerve (from the medial cord, C8 and T1); the two roots embrace the artery (Fig. 2.13) and, when the arm is pulled down to depress the shoulder may, in some cases, compress the vessel.

Branches from the medial cord

The five branches from the medial cord are the medial pectoral, medial head of the median nerve, ulnar nerve, and the two cutaneous nerves, to the arm and forearm respectively.

The **medial pectoral nerve** arises from the medial cord (C8, T1) behind the first part of the axillary artery and is joined by a communication from the lateral pectoral nerve. It enters the deep surface of pectoralis minor,

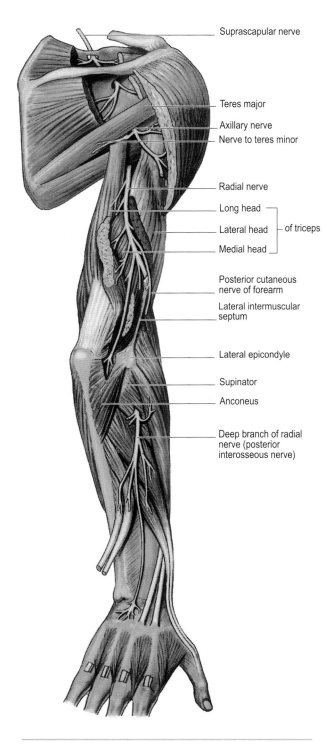

Suprascapular nerve

Teres major

Axillary nerve

Nerve to teres minor

Radial nerve

Long head
Lateral head ⎤ of triceps
Medial head

Posterior cutaneous
nerve of forearm

Lateral intermuscular
septum

Lateral epicondyle

Supinator

Anconeus

Deep branch of radial
nerve (posterior
interosseous nerve)

Fig. 2.16 Suprascapular, axillary and radial nerves on the posterior aspect of the right upper limb.

giving a branch of supply before doing so, perforates the muscle (Fig. 2.13) and enters the pectoralis major, in which it ends by supplying the lower costal fibres. It may give a direct branch to pectoralis major, which passes around the lower margin of pectoralis minor. The medial pectoral nerve has no cutaneous branch. The medial and lateral pectoral nerves are named in accordance with their origins from the medial and lateral cords of the brachial plexus.

The **medial root of the median nerve** is the continuation of the medial cord, with fibres from C8 and T1, and it crosses the axillary artery to join the lateral root (Fig. 2.13).

The **medial cutaneous nerve of the arm** (C8, T1) is the smallest and most medial of all the branches. It runs down on the medial side of the axillary vein and supplies skin over the front and medial side of the arm.

The **medial cutaneous nerve of the forearm** (C8, T1) is a larger nerve that runs down between artery and vein in front of the ulnar nerve (Fig. 2.13) and supplies skin over the lower part of the arm and the medial side of the forearm.

The **ulnar nerve** is the largest branch of the medial cord (C7, 8, T1). It runs down between artery and vein as the most posterior of the structures which run down the medial side of the flexor compartment of the arm. It may receive its C7 fibres as a branch from the lateral cord, if these have not already passed to the medial cord from the anterior ramus of C7.

Branches from the posterior cord

The five branches from the posterior cord are the upper subscapular, thoracodorsal nerve (nerve to latissimus dorsi), lower subscapular, axillary (circumflex) and radial nerves (Fig. 2.15).

The **upper subscapular nerve** is a small nerve (C5, 6) which enters the upper part of subscapularis (Fig. 2.15).

The **thoracodorsal nerve** (nerve to latissimus dorsi C6–8) is a large nerve which runs down the posterior axillary wall, crosses the lower border of teres major and enters the deep surface of latissimus dorsi, well forward near the border of the muscle (Fig. 2.15). It comes from high up behind the subscapular artery, but as it descends to enter the muscle it lies in front of the artery, at this level called the thoracodorsal artery. It is thrown into prominence in the position of lateral rotation and abduction of the humerus and is thus in danger in operations on the lower axilla.

The **lower subscapular nerve** (C5, 6) is larger than the upper subscapular and supplies the lower part of the subscapularis and ends in teres major.

The **axillary nerve** (formerly the circumflex nerve) is one of the two large terminal branches of the posterior cord (the other is the radial nerve). The axillary nerve (C5, 6) supplies nothing in the axilla despite its name having been changed from circumflex to axillary. From its origin, it runs backwards through the *quadrangular space* bounded by subscapularis above, teres major below, long head of triceps medially and the surgical neck of humerus laterally (Fig. 2.9). It then passes just below the capsule of the shoulder joint, with the posterior circumflex humeral vessels below it, and emerges at the back of the axilla below teres minor (Fig. 2.16). Having given a branch to the shoulder joint, it divides into anterior and posterior branches. The *anterior branch* winds round behind the humerus in contact with the periosteum and enters the deep surface of the deltoid to supply it; a few terminal twigs pierce the muscle and reach the skin. The *posterior branch* supplies teres minor and deltoid, then winds around the posterior border of deltoid to become the *upper lateral cutaneous nerve of the arm.*

The **radial nerve** (C5–8, T1) is the continuation of the posterior cord, and is the largest branch of the whole plexus. It crosses the lower border of the posterior axillary wall, lying on the glistening tendon of latissimus dorsi (Fig. 2.15). It passes out of sight through the *triangular space* below the lower border of this tendon as it lies in front of teres major, between the long head of triceps and the humerus (Figs 2.9 and 2.16). Before disappearing it gives nerves of supply to the long head of triceps and the medial head (a nerve which accompanies the ulnar nerve along the medial side of the arm) and a cutaneous branch which supplies the skin along the posterior surface of the upper arm (*posterior cutaneous nerve of the arm*).

Lymph nodes of the axilla

Contained in the fibrofatty tissue of the axilla are many scattered lymph nodes; their number varies between 20 and 30. They are usually described as lying in the following groups:

- An *anterior or pectoral group*, behind pectoralis major along the lateral thoracic artery, at the lower border of pectoralis minor. They receive from the upper half of the trunk anteriorly and from the major part of the breast.
- A *posterior or subscapular group*, on the posterior wall of the axilla along the subscapular artery. They receive from the upper half of the trunk posteriorly, and from the axillary tail of the breast.
- A *lateral group*, along the medial side of the axillary vein. They receive from the upper limb.
- A *central group*, in the fat of the axilla and receiving lymph from the above groups.

- An *apical group*, at the apex of the axilla, receives from all the groups named above. The apical group drains by the subclavian lymph trunk through the apex of the axilla into the thoracic duct or the right lymphatic duct or directly into the jugulosubclavian venous junction in the neck. A few efferents from the apical nodes drain into the supraclavicular (inferior deep cervical) nodes.

Axillary lymph nodes are also described in terms of the levels at which they lie. Level I nodes lie lateral to the lower border of pectoralis minor; level II nodes lie behind the muscle; and level III nodes lie medial to the upper border of the muscle. The lymph node which initially receives lymphatic drainage from an area of the breast, which is the site of a pathological process, is termed a sentinel node; this is usually a level I, occasionally a level II and sometimes an extra-axillary node such as a parasternal node. Its location is confirmed by injecting a dye or radioactive substance into the relevant site in the breast and demonstrating its drainage to the sentinel node visually or by a radioactivity counter.

Surgical approach

The axilla is approached surgically through the axillary skin for the excision of one or more axillary lymph nodes, for the staging and treatment of malignant disease such as cancer of the breast. During such procedures the intercostobrachial (see p. 63), long thoracic (see p. 55) and thoracodorsal (see p. 57) nerves are at risk and need to be safeguarded, unless they are adherent to involved nodes (Fig. 2.17). The thoracodorsal artery accompanies the nerve and its preservation ensures adequate blood supply to latissimus dorsi, which is used in breast reconstruction. The axillary vein must be safeguarded when dividing its subscapular tributaries.

PART FOUR

Breast

The adult **female breast** or mammary gland lies in the subcutaneous tissue (superficial fascia) of the anterior thoracic wall. Despite individual variations in size, the extent of the *base* of the breast is fairly constant: from the sternal edge to near the midaxillary line, and from the second to the sixth ribs. It overlies pectoralis major, overlapping onto serratus anterior and onto a small part of the rectus sheath and external oblique muscle. A small part of the upper outer quadrant may be prolonged

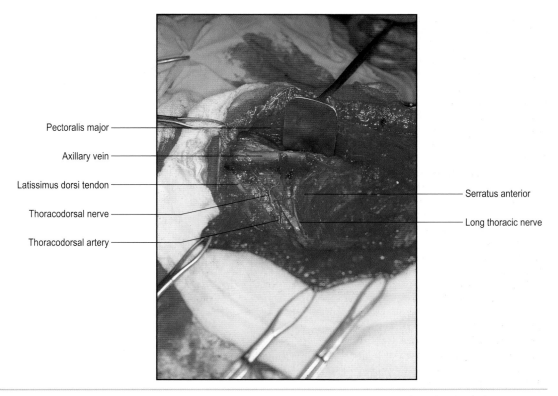

Pectoralis major

Axillary vein

Latissimus dorsi tendon

Thoracodorsal nerve

Thoracodorsal artery

Serratus anterior

Long thoracic nerve

Fig. 2.17   An operative view of the right axilla at the end of surgical clearance of axillary lymph nodes. The pectoralis major is being retracted upwards and medially. The pectoralis minor has been divided to enhance axillary exposure. The long thoracic nerve and the thoracodorsal nerve and artery have been safeguarded. The intercostobrachial nerve has been removed with adherent lymph nodes. The axillary vein has been preserved intact and patent.

towards the axilla. This extension (the *axillary tail*) usually lies in the subcutaneous fat; rarely it may penetrate the deep fascia of the axillary floor and lie adjacent to axillary lymph nodes.

Some 15–20 *lactiferous ducts*, each draining a lobe of the breast, converge in a radial direction to open individually on the tip of the *nipple*, the projection just below the centre of the breast which is surrounded by an area of pigmented skin, the *areola*. Each lactiferous duct has a dilated sinus at its terminal portion in the nipple. Smooth muscle cells are present in the nipple and their contraction causes erection of the nipple. Some large sebaceous and other glands under the areola (*areolar glands*) may form small elevations (tubercles of Montgomery), particularly when they enlarge during pregnancy.

Behind the breast the superficial fascia (the upward continuation of the membranous layer of superficial abdominal fascia of Scarpa) is condensed to form a posterior capsule. Strands of fibrous tissue (forming the *suspensory ligaments* of Cooper) connect the dermis

of the overlying skin to the ducts of the breast and this fascia. They help to maintain the protuberance of the young breast; with the atrophy of age they allow the breast to become pendulous, and when contracted by the fibrosis associated with certain carcinomas of the breast they cause dimpling of the overlying skin. They also cause pitting of the oedematous skin that results from malignant involvement of dermal lymphatics (an appearance often referred to as peau d'orange). Between the capsule and the fascia over pectoralis major is the loose connective tissue of the *retromammary space*.

The *male breast* resembles the rudimentary female breast and has no lobules or alveoli. The small nipple and areola lie over the fourth intercostal space.

Blood supply

This is derived mainly from the *lateral thoracic artery* by branches that curl around the border of pectoralis major and by other branches that pierce the muscle.

The *internal thoracic artery* also sends branches through the intercostal spaces beside the sternum; those of the second and third spaces are the largest. Similar but small perforating branches arise from the *posterior intercostal arteries*. Pectoral branches of the *thoracoacromial artery* supply the upper part of the breast. The various supplying vessels form an anastomosing network. From a circumareolar venous plexus and from glandular tissue venous drainage is mainly by deep veins that run with the main arteries to internal thoracic and axillary veins. Some drainage to posterior intercostal veins provides an important link to the internal vertebral venous plexus veins (see p. 445) and hence a pathway for metastatic spread to bone.

Lymph drainage

Lymphatics within the breast communicate with a subareolar plexus of lymphatics. Around 75% of the lymphatic drainage of the breast passes to axillary lymph nodes, mainly to the anterior nodes, some to the posterior nodes; direct drainage to central or apical nodes is possible. Much of the rest of the lymphatic drainage, originating particularly from the medial part of the breasts, is to parasternal nodes along the internal thoracic artery. A few lymphatics follow the intercostal arteries and drain to posterior intercostal nodes. Occasionally, some lymph from the breast may drain into one or two infraclavicular nodes in the deltopectoral groove or into small inconstant interpectoral nodes between pectoralis major and minor. The superficial lymphatics of the breast have connections with those of the opposite breast and the anterior abdominal wall, from the extraperitoneal tissues of which there is drainage through the diaphragm to posterior mediastinal nodes. Direct drainage from the breast to inferior deep cervical (supraclavicular) nodes is possible. These minor pathways tend to convey lymph from the breast only when the major channels are obstructed by malignant disease.

Development and structure

The breast is a modified sweat gland (see p. 2) and begins to develop as early as the fourth week as a downgrowth from a thickened *mammary ridge* (milk line) of ectoderm along a line from the axilla to the inguinal region. Supernumerary nipples or even glands proper may form at lower levels on this line.

Lobule formation occurs only in the female breast and does so after puberty. Each lactiferous duct is connected to a tree-like system of ducts and lobules, intermingled and enclosed by connective tissue to form a lobe of the gland. The resting (non-lactating) breast, however, consists mostly of fibrous and fatty tissue; variations in size are due to variations in fat content, not glandular tissue which is very sparse. During pregnancy alveoli bud off from the smaller ducts and the organ usually enlarges significantly, and more so in preparation for lactation. When lactation ceases there is involution of secretory tissue. After menopause progressive atrophy of lobes and ducts takes place.

PART FIVE

Anterior compartment of the arm

Coracobrachialis

Functionally unimportant, the muscle arises from the apex of the coracoid process, where it is fused with the medial side of the short head of biceps. The muscle is inserted midway along the medial border of the humerus.

Nerve supply. By the musculocutaneous nerve (C5, 6).

Action. It is a weak flexor and adductor of the shoulder joint.

Biceps

The **long head** of this muscle arises from the supraglenoid tubercle and adjoining part of the glenoid labrum of the scapula (Fig. 2.8). The rounded tendon passes through the synovial cavity of the shoulder joint, surrounded by a sheath of synovial membrane, and emerges beneath the transverse ligament at the upper end of the intertubercular groove. The synovial sheath pouts out below the ligament to an extent which varies with the position of the arm, being greatest in full abduction (Fig. 2.11).

The **short head** arises from the apex of the coracoid process to the lateral side of coracobrachialis. The tendinous origin of each head expands into a fleshy belly; the two bellies lie side by side, loosely connected by areolar tissue, but do not merge until just above the elbow joint, below the main convexity of the muscle bellies. The flattened tendon at the lower end rotates (anterior surface turning laterally) as it passes through the cubital fossa to its insertion into the posterior border of the tuberosity of the radius (Fig. 2.22). A bursa separates the tendon from the anterior part of the tuberosity. At the level of the elbow joint, the tendon has a broad medial expansion, the **bicipital aponeurosis** (Fig. 2.26), which is inserted by way of the deep fascia of the forearm into the subcutaneous border of the upper end of the ulna.

Nerve supply. By the musculocutaneous nerve (C5, 6) with one branch to each belly.

Action. The biceps is a powerful flexor of the elbow and supinator of the forearm. During supination the bicipital aponeurosis draws the distal end of the ulna slightly anteromedially. The biceps is a weak flexor of the shoulder, where the tendon of the long head helps to stabilize the joint as it runs over the top of the head of the humerus.

Test. With the forearm supinated the elbow is flexed against resistance. The contracted muscle in the arm, and the tendon and aponeurosis at the elbow are easily palpable.

Brachialis

The muscle arises from the front of the lower half of the humerus and the medial intermuscular septum. Its upper fibres clasp the deltoid insertion and some fibres arise from the lower part of the radial groove. The broad muscle flattens to cover the anterior part of the elbow joint and is inserted by mixed tendon and muscle fibres into the coronoid process and tuberosity of the ulna (Fig. 2.27).

Nerve supply. By the musculocutaneous nerve (C5, 6). A small lateral part of the muscle is innervated by a branch of the radial nerve (C7).

Action. Brachialis is a flexor of the elbow joint.

Medial intermuscular septum

This fibrous septum is attached along the medial supra-condylar ridge, extends proximally behind the coraco-brachialis insertion and fades out above, between that muscle and the long head of triceps. It gives origin to the most medial fibres of brachialis and the medial head of triceps, and is pierced by the ulnar nerve, the superior ulnar collateral artery and the axillary branch of the radial nerve to the medial head of triceps.

Lateral intermuscular septum

This is attached along the lateral supracondylar ridge and fades out above and behind the insertion of deltoid. Both brachioradialis and extensor carpi radialis longus extend out from the humerus to gain attachment to the septum in front, and posteriorly the medial head of triceps arises from it. It is pierced by the radial nerve and profunda brachii artery (radial collateral branch).

Vessels and nerves of the arm

Brachial artery

This is the continuation of the axillary artery. The axillary vein is formed in the arm from venae comitantes

to the brachial artery, strongly reinforced by the basilic vein, which perforates the deep fascia in the middle of the arm. The brachial artery has the median nerve lateral to it above (Fig. 2.13), but the nerve crosses obliquely in front of the artery at about the middle of the arm and lies on its medial side below. The ulnar nerve, posterior to the artery above, leaves it in the lower part of the arm and slopes backwards through the medial intermuscular septum. The artery is superficial in its course in the arm, lying immediately deep to the deep fascia of the antero-medial aspect of the arm (Fig. 2.18). It passes deeply into the cubital fossa before dividing into the radial and ulnar arteries, usually at the level of the neck of the radius.

The *surface marking* of the brachial artery, with the arm abducted to a right angle, is along a line from the middle of the clavicle to the midpoint between the humeral epicondyles, where it is readily palpable. To palpate the artery in the upper arm, the finger pressure must be directed laterally, not backwards, as the vessel here lies medial to the humerus.

Surgical approach. The artery can be exposed at the medial border of biceps, in the groove between biceps and triceps. The deep fascia is incised and the groove opened up to display the neurovascular bundle embedded in connective tissue.

Branches. Apart from the terminal radial and ulnar arteries, the largest branch is the *profunda brachii artery* (Fig. 2.28). It leaves through the lower triangular space to run in the radial groove with the radial nerve. It supplies triceps, sometimes gives a nutrient artery to the humerus, and divides into two terminal branches which participate in an anastomosis around the elbow; the *middle collateral* descends in the medial head of triceps, while the *radial collateral* continues the course of the artery through the lateral intermuscular septum accompanying the radial nerve.

Other branches are the *superior ulnar collateral*, which accompanies the ulnar nerve, and the *inferior ulnar collateral*, which divides into anterior and posterior branches; all take part in the cubital anastomosis. There are also muscular branches to flexor muscles, and a nutrient artery to the humerus which enters the bone near the coracobrachialis attachment directed distally.

Veins of the arm

Venae comitantes accompany the brachial artery and all its branches. In addition, the **basilic** and **cephalic veins** course upwards through the subcutaneous tissue (Fig. 2.19). The former perforates the deep fascia in the middle of the arm and ascends to become the axillary vein; the latter lies in the groove between deltoid and pectoralis major and ends by piercing the clavipectoral

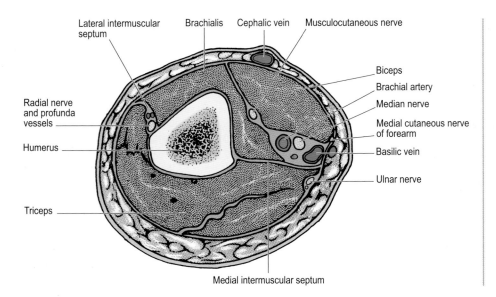

Lateral intermuscular septum
Brachialis
Cephalic vein
Musculocutaneous nerve
Radial nerve and profunda vessels
Humerus
Triceps
Biceps
Brachial artery
Median nerve
Medial cutaneous nerve of forearm
Basilic vein
Ulnar nerve
Medial intermuscular septum

Fig. 2.18 Cross-section of the middle of the right arm, looking towards the shoulder. The brachial artery and the median, ulnar and musculocutaneous nerves are on the medial side, with the radial nerve lateral to the humerus.

fascia to enter the axillary vein. The venae comitantes of the brachial artery join the axillary vein.

Median nerve

The nerve (Fig. 2.13) is formed at the lower border of the axilla by the union of its medial and lateral roots, from the corresponding cords of the brachial plexus. The axillary artery is clasped between the two roots, the medial root crossing in front of the vessel. The commencement of the nerve is lateral to the artery. Passing distally through the arm the nerve lies in front of the brachial artery and at the elbow is found on its medial side. The nerve gives vascular (sympathetic) branches to the brachial artery and may give a branch to pronator teres above the elbow joint.

The *surface marking* of the nerve is along a line from the lateral to the brachial artery in the proximal arm, medial to the artery in the cubital fossa.

Musculocutaneous nerve

The nerve gives a branch to and then pierces coracobrachialis. It comes to lie between biceps and brachialis (Fig. 2.26) and supplies both muscles. The remaining fibres appear at the lateral margin of the biceps tendon as the lateral cutaneous nerve of the forearm. The musculocutaneous is the nerve of the flexor compartment of the arm, supplying all three muscles therein. The branch to brachialis supplies the elbow joint.

Ulnar nerve

Lying posterior to the vessels this nerve inclines backwards away from them and pierces the medial intermuscular septum in the lower third of the arm, accompanied by the superior ulnar collateral artery and a branch of the radial nerve to the medial head of triceps. It gives no branch in the arm; its branch to the elbow joint comes off as it lies in the groove behind the medial epicondyle of the humerus, where it is readily *palpable*.

Medial cutaneous nerve of the arm

Lying medial to the vessels this small nerve pierces the deep fascia in the middle of the arm and supplies the skin on the front and medial side of the arm (Fig. 2.46).

Medial cutaneous nerve of the forearm

Commencing on the medial side of the vessels this large nerve passes anterior to them and pierces the deep fascia with the basilic vein. It divides into anterior and posterior branches which descend to the forearm, the former passing in front of the median cubital vein (Fig. 2.19). The nerve supplies skin over the lower part of the front of the arm and over the medial part of the forearm (Fig. 2.46). The part of the nerve that lies in the upper arm can be used as a graft as this part has a long length without branches.

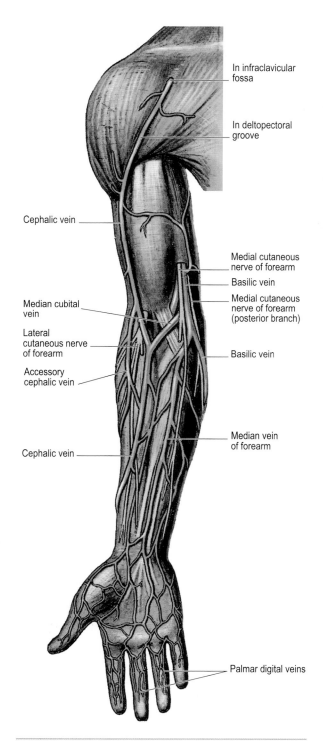

Cephalic vein

Median cubital
vein

Lateral
cutaneous nerve
of forearm

Accessory
cephalic vein

Cephalic vein

In infraclavicular
fossa

In deltopectoral
groove

Medial cutaneous
nerve of forearm

Basilic vein

Medial cutaneous
nerve of forearm
(posterior branch)

Basilic vein

Median vein
of forearm

Palmar digital veins

Fig. 2.19 Superficial veins on the anterior aspect of the right upper limb.

Intercostobrachial nerve

This nerve is the lateral cutaneous branch of the second intercostal nerve. It supplies the skin of the axilla and over a variable extent on the medial side of the upper arm (Fig. 2.46). It may be in contact with level I lymph nodes and be at risk during node excision. The thoraco-epigastric vein (see p. 186) crosses the nerve vertically on its posterior aspect and aids identification. Not infrequently the lateral cutaneous branch of the third intercostal nerve also extends outwards to supply the skin of the axilla.

Lymph nodes

Two groups of one or two lymph nodes each (not part of the axillary group) are found in the arm. The **infraclavicular group** lie along the cephalic vein in the upper part of the deltopectoral groove and drain through the clavipectoral fascia into the apical axillary nodes. They receive afferents from the superficial tissues of the thumb and lateral side of forearm and arm. The **supratrochlear group** lie in the subcutaneous fat just above the medial epicondyle. They drain the superficial tissues of the medial part of the forearm and hand, the afferent lymphatics running with the basilic vein and its tributaries. Their efferent vessels pass to the lateral group of axillary nodes.

PART SIX

Posterior compartment of the arm

The extensor compartment is occupied by the triceps muscle and has the radial nerve and profunda artery running through it. The ulnar nerve passes through the lower part of this compartment.

Triceps

The three heads of this muscle are named long, lateral and medial. The **long head** arises from the infraglenoid tubercle at the upper end of the axillary border of the scapula. The **lateral head** has a linear origin (Fig. 2.16) from the back of the humerus, above the groove for the radial nerve, extending up to the surgical neck. The long and lateral heads converge and fuse to form the superficial lamina of the triceps tendon. The **medial head** arises from the whole of the back of the humerus below the radial groove (Fig. 2.16), and from both intermuscular septa. The medial head is deep to the other two heads and forms the deep lamina of the tendon. Both laminae blend above the elbow and are attached to the upper surface of the olecranon. A few fibres are inserted into the posterior part of the capsule of the elbow joint.

Nerve supply. By the radial nerve (C7, 8). The long and medial heads are supplied by branches given off from the radial nerve in the axilla. In the humeral groove the nerve supplies the lateral head and gives another branch to the medial head, which supplies the anconeus as well. Fractures of the middle of the shaft of the humerus, even though they may damage the radial nerve, are not likely to cause paralysis of triceps because of the high origin of the branches.

Action. The muscle is the extensor of the elbow joint. The long head supports the capsule of the shoulder joint when the arm is abducted, and it aids in extending the shoulder joint.

Test. The flexed forearm is extended against resistance and the muscle seen and felt.

Radial nerve

Leaving the axilla as described on page 58, the nerve passes obliquely across the back of the humerus from medial to lateral in a shallow groove between the long and medial heads of triceps, with the profunda brachii artery. The nerve then pierces the lateral intermuscular septum to enter the anterior compartment and runs towards the elbow between brachialis medially and first brachioradialis and then extensor carpi radialis longus laterally (Fig. 2.26). While in the axilla the nerve gives branches to the long and medial heads of triceps and the posterior cutaneous nerve of the arm. At the back of the humerus the radial nerve supplies the lateral head and the medial head again, the branch to the latter supplying anconeus as well. It also gives the lower lateral cutaneous nerve of the arm and the posterior cutaneous nerve of the forearm, which perforate the lateral head. In the anterior compartment of the arm the radial nerve gives branches to brachioradialis, extensor carpi radialis longus and the lateral part of brachialis. The nerve divides into its terminal superficial branch and the posterior interosseous nerve at the level of the lateral epicondyle. It also supplies the elbow joint.

The *surface marking* of the nerve is from the point where the posterior wall of the axilla and arm meet to a point two-thirds of the way along a line from the acromion to the lateral epicondyle, and thence to the front of the epicondyle.

Ulnar nerve

The nerve courses through the lower part of the extensor compartment and disappears into the forearm by passing between the humeral and ulnar heads of origin of flexor carpi ulnaris (Fig. 2.30). It lies in contact with the bone in the groove behind the medial epicondyle, then lies against the medial ligament of the elbow joint, which it supplies (Fig. 2.22).

Elbow joint

This is a synovial joint of the hinge variety between the lower end of the humerus and the upper ends of radius and ulna (Fig. 2.20). It communicates with the proximal radioulnar joint.

The lower end of the **humerus** has the prominent conjunction of capitulum and trochlea (Fig. 2.21). The *capitulum* is a portion of a sphere which articulates with the upper surface of the head of the radius. It projects forwards and downwards, and is not visible on the posterior aspect of the humerus (Fig. 2.52). In contrast the *trochlea*, which lies medial, is a grooved surface that extends around the lower end of the humerus to the posterior surface of the bone and articulates with the trochlear notch of the ulna. The groove of the trochlea is limited medially by a sharp ridge that extends further distally. Laterally a lower and blunter ridge blends with the articular surface of the capitulum. Thus a tilt is produced at the lower end of the humerus that accounts in part for the carrying angle of the elbow. Fossae immediately above the capitulum and trochlea receive the head of the radius and coronoid process of the ulna, respectively, in full flexion; posteriorly a deep fossa receives the olecranon in full extension.

The upper surface of the cylindrical head of the **radius** is spherically concave to fit the capitulum.

The upper end of the **ulna** shows the deep trochlear notch. A curved ridge joins the prominences of coronoid process and olecranon (Fig. 2.54); the ridge fits the groove in the trochlea of the humerus. The obliquity of the shaft of the ulna to this ridge accounts for most of the carrying angle at the elbow.

The **capsule** is attached to the humerus at the medial and lateral margins of the trochlea and capitulum, respectively, but in front it is attached above the coronoid and radial fossae (Fig. 2.21), and at the back above the olecranon fossa. Distally, the capsule is attached to the margins of the trochlear notch of the ulna, and to the annular ligament of the proximal radioulnar joint (Fig. 2.23). It is not attached to the radius.

The capsule and lower part of the annular ligament are lined with *synovial membrane*, which is attached to the articular margins of all three bones. The synovial membrane thus lines the fossae on the lower end of the humerus. The quadrate ligament, which is attached to the lower margin of the radial notch of the ulna and the

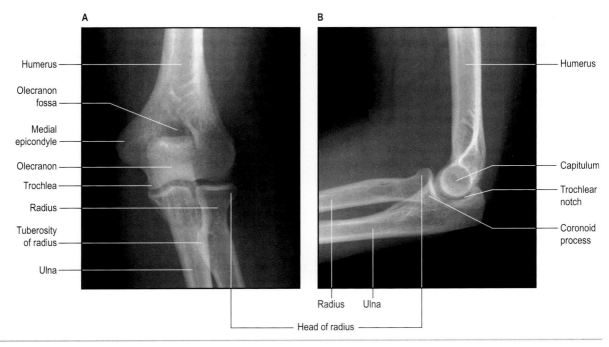

Humerus

Olecranon
fossa

Medial
epicondyle

Olecranon

Trochlea

Radius

Tuberosity
of radius

Ulna

Humerus

Capitulum

Trochlear
notch

Coronoid
process

Radius   Ulna

Head of radius

Fig. 2.20   Radiographs of the elbow joint: **A** anteroposterior projection; **B** lateral projection.
(Provided by Dr R. Sinnatamby, Cambridge University Hospital).

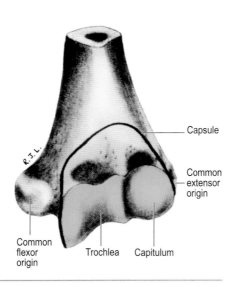

Capsule

Common
extensor
origin

Common
flexor
origin   Trochlea   Capitulum

Fig 2.21   Lower end of the left humerus, showing the line of
attachment of the capsule of the elbow joint.

neck of the radius, prevents herniation of the synovial
membrane between the anterior and posterior free edges
of the annular ligament.

The **ulnar collateral (medial) ligament** of the elbow
joint is triangular and consists of three bands. The
anterior band is the strongest. It passes from the medial
epicondyle of the humerus to a small tubercle (previously
called the sublime tubercle) on the medial border of the
coronoid process. The *posterior band* joins the sublime
tubercle and the medial border of the olecranon. A thin
middle band connects these two and its grooved surface
lodges the ulnar nerve on its way from the arm to the
forearm (Fig. 2.22). The **radial collateral (lateral) ligament** (Fig. 2.23) is a triangular band. Its apex is attached
to the lateral epicondyle and its base fuses with the
annular ligament of the head of the radius. The anterior
and posterior ligaments are merely thickened parts of the
capsule. The **annular ligament** is attached to the anterior
and posterior margins of the radial notch of the ulna,
and clasps the head and neck of the radius in the proximal radioulnar joint. It has no attachment to the radius,
which remains free to rotate in the annular ligament.

Nerve supply. By the musculocutaneous, median,
ulnar and radial nerves.

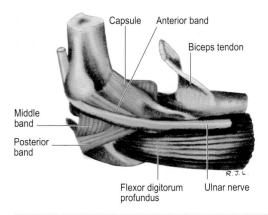

Fig. 2.22   Left elbow joint from the medial side, with the ulnar nerve lying against the ulnar collateral (medial) ligament.

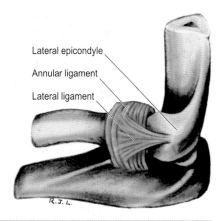

Fig. 2.23   Radial collateral (lateral) ligament of the left elbow joint, passing from the lateral epicondyle to the annular ligament.

Movements

The only appreciable movement possible at the elbow joint is the simple hinge movement of *flexion* and *extension*. From the straight (extended) position the range of flexion is about 140°. This movement does not take place in the line of the humerus, for the axis of the hinge lies obliquely. The extended ulna makes an angle of about 170° with the humerus, the forearm diverging laterally. This so-called '*carrying angle*' fits the elbow into the waist when the arm is at the side, and it is significant that the obliquity of the ulna is more pronounced in women than in men. However, the line of upper arm

and forearm becomes straightened out when the forearm is in the usual working position of almost full pronation (Fig. 2.29). A pathological increase in this 'valgus' angle (e.g. from a fractured lateral epicondyle or damaged epiphysis) may gradually stretch the ulnar nerve behind the medial epicondyle and cause an ulnar nerve palsy. In extension the tip of the olecranon lies in line with the humeral epicondyles, but in full flexion these three bony points make an equilateral triangle.

Surgical approach

The most common approaches are from the sides. Medially the ulnar nerve is displaced backwards and the common flexor origin detached to expose the capsule, while on the lateral side the common extensor origin can be similarly detached. On this side the capsule incision must not extend lower than the level of the head of the radius to avoid damage to the posterior interosseous nerve as it winds round the shaft within the supinator.

For aspiration or injection the needle is inserted on the posterolateral side above the head of the radius, with the elbow at a right angle. The medial side is avoided because of the ulnar nerve.

PART SEVEN

Anterior compartment of the forearm

The flexor muscles in the forearm are arranged in two groups, superficial and deep. The five muscles of the superficial group cross the elbow joint; the three muscles of the deep group do not. The flexor compartment is much more bulky than the extensor compartment, for the necessary power of the grip.

Superficial muscles

These five muscles (Fig. 2.24) are distinguished by the fact that they possess a common origin from the medial epicondyle of the humerus. Three of the group have additional areas of origin. The **common origin** attaches itself to a smooth area on the anterior surface of the medial epicondyle (Fig. 2.21).

With the heel of the hand placed over the opposite medial epicondyle, palm lying on the forearm, the digits point down along the five superficial muscles: thumb for pronator teres; index for flexor carpi radialis; middle finger for flexor digitorum superficialis; ring finger for palmaris longus; and little finger for flexor carpi ulnaris.

Pronator teres

Arising from the common origin and from the lower part of the medial supracondylar ridge, the main superficial belly is joined by the small deep head, which arises from the medial border of the coronoid process of the ulna just distal to the tubercle on it. The median nerve lies between the two heads and the ulnar artery passes deep to the deep head (Fig. 2.26). The muscle, forming the medial border of the cubital fossa (Fig. 2.24), runs distally across the front of the forearm to be inserted by a flat tendon into the middle of the lateral surface of the shaft of the radius at the most prominent part of its outward convexity.

Nerve supply. By the first (highest) muscular branch of the median nerve (C6, 7).

Action. The muscle pronates the forearm and is a weak flexor of the elbow.

Fig 2.24 Superficial muscles of the flexor compartment of the left forearm. Brachioradialis has been retracted laterally to show the radial nerve and its posterior interosseous branch, and the brachial artery and median nerve have been displaced medially to show the insertion of brachialis behind biceps.

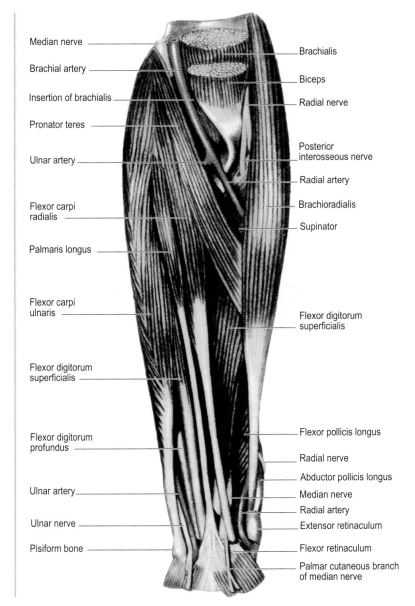

Median nerve

Brachial artery

Insertion of brachialis

Pronator teres

Ulnar artery

Flexor carpi radialis

Palmaris longus

Flexor carpi ulnaris

Flexor digitorum superficialis

Flexor digitorum profundus

Ulnar artery

Ulnar nerve

Pisiform bone

Brachialis

Biceps

Radial nerve

Posterior interosseous nerve

Radial artery

Brachioradialis

Supinator

Flexor digitorum superficialis

Flexor pollicis longus

Radial nerve

Abductor pollicis longus

Median nerve

Radial artery

Extensor retinaculum

Flexor retinaculum

Palmar cutaneous branch of median nerve

Test. From the supine position the forearm is pronated against resistance and the muscle palpated at the medial margin of the cubital fossa.

Flexor carpi radialis

Arising from the common origin the fleshy belly gives way in the middle of the forearm to a long tendon (Fig. 2.24) that runs through its own compartment in the carpal tunnel (see p. 84), lying in the groove of the trapezium, and is inserted into the bases of the second and third metacarpals (symmetrically with extensors longus and brevis). The tendon is a prominent landmark towards the radial side of the front of the wrist. The radial artery lies lateral to the tendon, and the median nerve (with the overlying tendon of palmaris longus) medial to it.

Nerve supply. By the median nerve (C6, 7).

Action. It is a flexor and radial abductor of the wrist. It is an important stabilizer of the wrist in finger and thumb movements.

Test. The wrist is flexed and abducted against resistance and the tendon is easily seen and felt.

Flexor digitorum superficialis

The muscle arises from the common origin, the medial ligament of the elbow joint, and the tubercle on the medial border of the coronoid process of the ulna (humeroulnar head). As this muscle was previously called flexor digitorum sublimis, this tubercle was known as the sublime tubercle. A fibrous arch continues the origin across to the radius, where it arises from the whole length of the anterior oblique line (radial head) (Fig. 2.53). The fleshy belly is partly hidden above by the other superficial flexors, and is therefore frequently described as being in an intermediate layer. Its oblique origin, in continuity from the medial epicondyle to the insertion of pronator teres, forms the upper limit of the space of Parona (see p. 72). Above the wrist the tendons of this muscle appear on each side of the palmaris longus tendon. As the tendons pass beneath the flexor retinaculum, the middle and ring finger tendons lie superficial to those to the index and little finger (Fig. 2.36). Their course in the palm and insertion into the middle phalanges is considered on page 93. In the forearm the muscle has the median nerve plastered to its deep surface by areolar tissue (Fig. 2.25).

Nerve supply. By the median nerve (C7, 8).

Action. It is a flexor of the proximal interphalangeal joints, and secondarily of the metacarpophalangeal and wrist joints. It also assists in flexion of the elbow and wrist.

Test. The fingers are flexed at the proximal interphalangeal joints against resistance applied to the middle phalanges, while the distal interphalangeal joints are kept extended.

Palmaris longus

The muscle arises from the common origin. It is absent in 13% of arms. Its long, flat tendon broadens as it passes in front of the flexor retinaculum, to which it is partly adherent (Fig. 2.24). In the palm it splits to form the longitudinally directed fibres of the palmar aponeurosis (see p. 83). The tendon lies in front of the median nerve just above the wrist.

Nerve supply. By the median nerve (C7, 8).

Action. It is a weak flexor of the wrist, and anchors the skin and fascia of the hand against shearing forces in a distal direction. The tendon can be used in tendon transplant procedures.

Test. The wrist is flexed and the tendon palpated when the pads of the thumb and little finger are pinched together.

Flexor carpi ulnaris

The muscle arises from the common origin and by a wide aponeurosis from the medial border of the olecranon and the upper two-thirds of the subcutaneous border of the ulna (Fig. 2.30). The ulnar nerve passes between the humeral and ulnar heads of this muscle to enter the flexor compartment of the forearm, where the ulnar nerve and artery are overlapped by the muscle (Fig. 2.25). At the wrist the tendon of the muscle is medial to the nerve and artery. The tendon inserts into the pisiform (a sesamoid bone in the tendon) and, by way of the pisohamate and pisometacarpal ligaments, into the hamate and fifth metacarpal bones.

Nerve supply. By the ulnar nerve (C7, 8).

Action. It is a flexor and an ulnar adductor of the wrist. In radial nerve paralysis the tendon can be transplanted to extend the fingers or thumb.

Test. The wrist is flexed and adducted against resistance and the tendon palpated.

Cubital fossa

The cubital fossa is the triangular area between pronator teres, brachioradialis and a line joining the humeral epicondyles (Fig. 2.26). The *roof* is formed by the deep fascia of the forearm, reinforced on the medial side by the bicipital aponeurosis. In front of the bicipital aponeurosis lies the median cubital vein with the medial

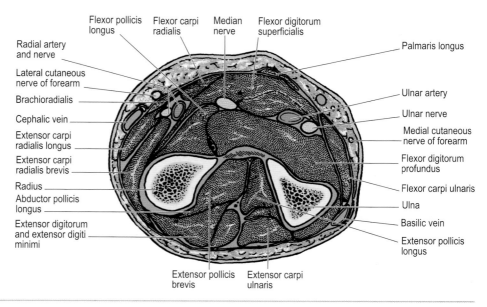

Fig. 2.25 Cross-section through the middle of the right forearm, looking towards the elbow. The median nerve adheres to the deep surface of flexor digitorum superficialis, and the ulnar artery is under cover of the muscle more medially. The ulnar nerve is overlapped by flexor carpi ulnaris. The superficial branch of the radial nerve and the radial artery are under cover of brachioradialis. The deep (posterior interosseous) branch of the radial nerve has divided above this level to supply extensor muscles. The anterior interosseous nerve and vessels lie between flexor pollicis longus and flexor digitorum profundus.

cutaneous nerve of the forearm (Fig. 2.19); the apo-neurosis separates these structures from the underlying median nerve and brachial artery. The *floor* is formed in the main by the brachialis muscle and below by the supinator as it clasps the proximal third of the radius (Fig. 2.27).

The *contents* of the fossa, from medial to lateral side, are the **median nerve, brachial artery, tendon of biceps**, and farther laterally the **radial nerve** and its **posterior interosseous branch**, which are only seen when brachio-radialis is retracted laterally (Fig. 2.26). The artery is palpated here medial to the tendon to define the position for placing the stethoscope when taking the blood pressure. The further courses of the brachial artery and median nerve are discussed below (see pp 72 and 75). The branches of the radial nerve in the cubital fossa have been described on page 64. The posterior interosseous nerve gives branches to extensor carpi radialis brevis and supinator before disappearing from the fossa by passing between the two layers of the supinator muscle (Figs 2.24 and 2.26) into the extensor compartment (see p. 76). The superficial branch of the radial nerve passes down the forearm under cover of the brachioradialis (see p. 77).

Deep muscles

The group consists of flexor digitorum profundus, flexor pollicis longus and pronator quadratus (Fig. 2.27).

Flexor digitorum profundus

The most powerful and the bulkiest of the forearm muscles, it arises by fleshy fibres from the medial surface of the olecranon (Fig. 2.22), from the upper three-quarters of the anterior and medial surfaces of the ulna, including its subcutaneous border, and from the inter-osseous membrane. The tendon for the index separates in the forearm; the three other tendons are still partly attached to each other as they pass across the carpal bones in the flexor tunnel and do not become detached from each other until they reach the palm (Fig. 2.27). At this point of separation the four lumbricals take origin. They are described in the section on the hand (see p. 90).

Nerve supply. By the anterior interosseous branch of the median nerve and by the ulnar nerve (C8, T1). Characteristically, these nerves equally share the bellies, those that merge into the tendons for the index and

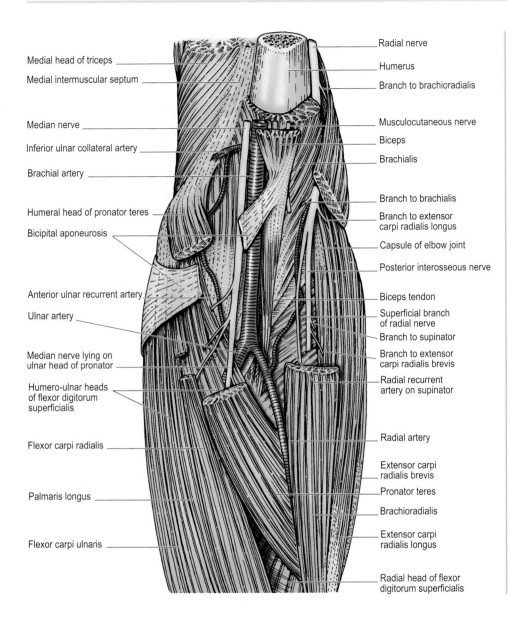

Medial head of triceps

Medial intermuscular septum

Median nerve

Inferior ulnar collateral artery

Brachial artery

Humeral head of pronator teres

Bicipital aponeurosis

Anterior ulnar recurrent artery

Ulnar artery

Median nerve lying on
ulnar head of pronator

Humero-ulnar heads
of flexor digitorum
superficialis

Flexor carpi radialis

Palmaris longus

Flexor carpi ulnaris

Radial nerve

Humerus

Branch to brachioradialis

Musculocutaneous nerve

Biceps

Brachialis

Branch to brachialis

Branch to extensor
carpi radialis longus

Capsule of elbow joint

Posterior interosseous nerve

Biceps tendon

Superficial branch
of radial nerve

Branch to supinator

Branch to extensor
carpi radialis brevis

Radial recurrent
artery on supinator

Radial artery

Extensor carpi
radialis brevis

Pronator teres

Brachioradialis

Extensor carpi
radialis longus

Radial head of flexor
digitorum superficialis

Fig. 2.26 Left cubital fossa. The bicipital aponeurosis has been partly removed. The lateral cutaneous nerve of the forearm is seen emerging from deep to the lateral border of biceps.

middle fingers being supplied from the median, and for the ring and little fingers from the ulnar nerves. The corresponding lumbricals are similarly supplied.

This distribution of 2:2 between median and ulnar nerves occurs in only 60% of individuals. In the remaining 40% the median and ulnar distribution is 3:1 or 1:3 equally (20% each). Whatever the variation, however, the rule is that each lumbrical is supplied by the same nerve which innervates the belly of its parent tendon.

Action. It flexes the terminal interphalangeal joints and, still acting, rolls the fingers and wrist into flexion. It is the great gripping muscle. Extension of the wrist is indispensable to the full power of contraction of the muscle.

Test. With the fingers extended and the hand lying supine on the table, the distal interphalangeal joints are flexed against resistance with the middle phalanx held in extension.

Fig. 2.27 Deep muscles of the flexor compartment of the left forearm. The flexor retinaculum remains in place at the wrist.

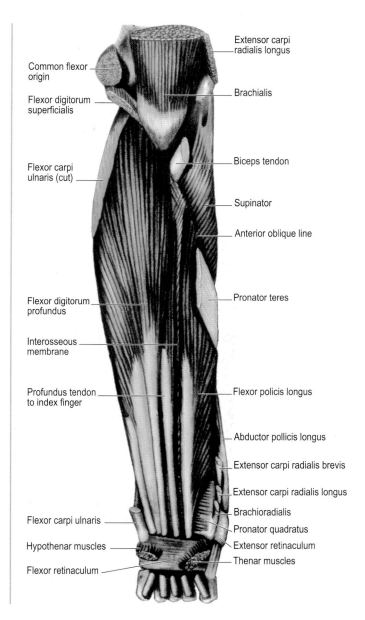

Common flexor origin

Flexor digitorum superficialis

Flexor carpi ulnaris (cut)

Flexor digitorum profundus

Interosseous membrane

Profundus tendon to index finger

Flexor carpi ulnaris

Hypothenar muscles

Flexor retinaculum

Extensor carpi radialis longus

Brachialis

Biceps tendon

Supinator

Anterior oblique line

Pronator teres

Flexor policis longus

Abductor pollicis longus

Extensor carpi radialis brevis

Extensor carpi radialis longus

Brachioradialis

Pronator quadratus

Extensor retinaculum

Thenar muscles

Flexor pollicis longus

This muscle arises from the anterior surface of the radius below the anterior oblique line and above the insertion of pronator quadratus, and from the interosseous membrane. The tendon forms on the ulnar side of this unipennate muscle and receives fleshy fibres into its radial side down to just above the wrist, a distinctive feature which facilitates identification of the tendon (Fig. 2.27). The tendon passes in the carpal tunnel deep to that of the flexor carpi radialis, then spirals around its ulnar side to become superficial. It extends into the thumb to be inserted into the base of the distal phalanx.

Nerve supply. By the anterior interosseous branch of the median nerve (C7, 8).

Action. It is the only flexor of the interphalangeal joint of the thumb, and also flexes the metacarpophalangeal and carpometacarpal joints of the thumb and the wrist joint.

Test. With the proximal phalanx of the thumb held steady, the distal phalanx is flexed against resistance.

Pronator quadratus

Arising from the ridge on the anteromedial aspect of the distal ulna, the muscle is inserted into the anterior surface of the lower fourth of the radius (Fig. 2.53), and into the triangular area above the ulnar notch.

Nerve supply. By the anterior interosseous branch of the median nerve (C7, 8).

Action. The muscle pronates the forearm and helps to hold the lower ends of the radius and ulna together, especially when the hand is weight-bearing. As a pronator it is more powerful than pronator teres.

Space of Parona

In front of pronator quadratus there is a space (of Parona) deep to the long flexor tendons of the fingers and their synovial sheaths. The space is limited proximally by the oblique origin of flexor digitorum superficialis. The space becomes involved in proximal extensions of synovial sheath infections; it can be drained through radial and ulnar incisions to the side of the flexor tendons.

Neurovascular pattern in the forearm

The general arrangement of the deep arteries and nerves of the forearm is that a nerve runs down each border of the forearm (radial and ulnar nerves), and the brachial artery divides into branches (radial and ulnar arteries) that run down to approach these nerves but do not cross them. The radial artery lies medially beside the radial nerve in the middle third, and the ulnar artery lies laterally beside the ulnar nerve in the distal two-thirds of the forearm. The median nerve, on the deep surface of flexor superficialis, crosses the ulnar artery to lie between the two arteries. Radial and ulnar arteries supply the hand; they run down directly into deep and superficial palmar arches. The arterial supply for the forearm comes from the common interosseous branch of the ulnar, which divides into posterior and anterior interosseous arteries. The posterior interosseous artery is rather a failure. Assisted at first by branches of the anterior interosseous that pierce the interosseous membrane, it later fails and is replaced by the anterior interosseous artery, which pierces the membrane to enter the extensor compartment. Anterior (from median) and posterior (from radial) interosseous nerves, on the other hand, remain in their own compartments right down to the wrist, supplying muscles; neither nerve reaches the skin.

Three nerves share in the supply of the muscles of the forearm and each nerve passes between the two heads of a muscle. The median nerve passes between the two heads of pronator teres and the ulnar nerve between the two heads of flexor carpi ulnaris. These two nerves share in the supply of the muscles of the flexor compartment. The muscles of the extensor compartment are supplied by the posterior interosseous nerve, which enters the compartment by passing between the two layers of the supinator muscle.

Vessels of the flexor compartment

The brachial artery enters the forearm by passing into the cubital fossa in the midline; halfway down the fossa (at the level of the neck of the radius) it divides into radial and ulnar arteries (Fig. 2.26). The radial usually appears to be the direct continuation of the brachial artery, whereas the bigger ulnar branches off at an angle (Fig. 2.28). Sometimes the brachial artery divides into its radial and ulnar branches more proximally.

Radial artery

The radial artery passes distally medial to the biceps tendon, across the supinator, over the tendon of insertion of the pronator teres, the radial origin of flexor digitorum superficialis, the origin of the flexor pollicis longus, the insertion of pronator quadratus and the lower end of the radius (against which its pulsation can be readily felt). It disappears deep to the tendons of abductor pollicis longus and extensor pollicis brevis to cross the anatomical snuff box (Fig. 2.32). In the upper part of the forearm it is overlapped anteriorly by brachioradialis (Fig. 2.24). Distally it is covered only by skin and by superficial and deep fascia.

The *surface marking* of the artery is along a line, slightly convex laterally, from medial to the biceps tendon in the cubital fossa to a point medial to the styloid process of the radius. It can be *surgically exposed* at its lower end which is the most common site for arterial cannulation.

Ulnar artery

The ulnar artery disappears from the cubital fossa by passing deep to the deep head of pronator teres and beneath the fibrous arch of the flexor digitorum superficialis and the median nerve (Fig. 2.26). It then runs medially and distally on flexor digitorum profundus

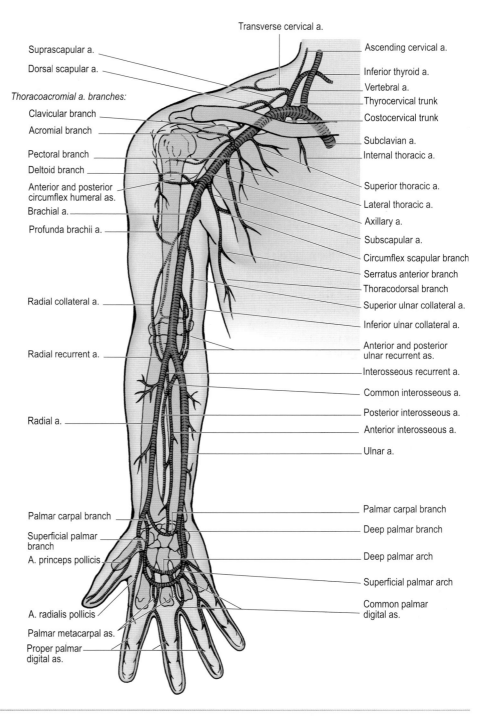

Transverse cervical a.

Suprascapular a.

Dorsal scapular a.

Thoracoacromial a. branches:

Clavicular branch

Acromial branch

Pectoral branch

Deltoid branch

Anterior and posterior circumflex humeral as.

Brachial a.

Profunda brachii a.

Radial collateral a.

Radial recurrent a.

Radial a.

Palmar carpal branch

Superficial palmar branch

A. princeps pollicis

A. radialis pollicis

Palmar metacarpal as.

Proper palmar digital as.

Ascending cervical a.

Inferior thyroid a.

Vertebral a.

Thyrocervical trunk

Costocervical trunk

Subclavian a.

Internal thoracic a.

Superior thoracic a.

Lateral thoracic a.

Axillary a.

Subscapular a.

Circumflex scapular branch

Serratus anterior branch

Thoracodorsal branch

Superior ulnar collateral a.

Inferior ulnar collateral a.

Anterior and posterior ulnar recurrent as.

Interosseous recurrent a.

Common interosseous a.

Posterior interosseous a.

Anterior interosseous a.

Ulnar a.

Palmar carpal branch

Deep palmar branch

Deep palmar arch

Superficial palmar arch

Common palmar digital as.

Fig. 2.28 Arteries of the upper limb.

with the ulnar nerve to its ulnar side and passes down over the front of the wrist into the palm, where it lies in front of the flexor retinaculum and continues as the superficial palmar arch (see p. 85). Ulnar artery pulsation can be felt on the radial side of the tendon of flexor carpi ulnaris just above the pisiform bone.

The *surface marking* is along a line, slightly convex medially, from medial to the biceps tendon in the cubital fossa to the radial side of the pisiform. It can be *surgically exposed* at the lower end and followed upwards by displacing flexor carpi ulnaris. The ulnar nerve on the ulnar side of the artery must be safeguarded.

Its chief branch is the **common interosseous** (Fig. 2.28), which divides into anterior and posterior interosseous branches. The **anterior interosseous artery** lies deeply on the interosseous membrane between flexor digitorum profundus and flexor pollicis longus, supplying each. Perforating branches pierce the interosseous membrane to supply the deep extensor muscles. Nutrient vessels are given to both radius and ulna. The artery passes posteriorly through the interosseous membrane at the level of the upper border of pronator quadratus.

The **posterior interosseous artery** disappears by passing backwards through the interosseous space between the upper end of the interosseous membrane and the oblique cord.

Anastomosis around the elbow joint

Recurrent branches, in some cases double, arise from radial, ulnar and interosseous arteries and run upwards both anterior and posterior to the elbow joint, to anastomose with the radial and middle collateral branches of the profunda brachii, and the superior and inferior ulnar collateral arteries (see p. 61 and Fig. 2.28).

Anastomosis around the wrist joint

Both radial and ulnar arteries give off palmar and dorsal carpal branches. These anatomose with each other deep to the long tendons, forming the palmar and dorsal carpal arches. The **palmar carpal arch** lies transversely across the wrist joint (Fig. 2.28); it supplies the carpal bones and sends branches distally into the hand to anastomose with the deep palmar arch. The **dorsal carpal arch** lies transversely across the distal row of carpal bones. It sends dorsal metacarpal arteries distally into each metacarpal space and these divide to supply the fingers; they anastomose through the interosseous spaces with the deep palmar arch and the digital branches of the superficial palmar arch. Thus a free anastomosis is established between radial and ulnar arteries through the carpal and palmar arches.

Veins of the forearm

The deep veins are plentiful and accompany the arteries, usually by dual venae comitantes which anastomose freely with each other. They drain the forearm but bring relatively little blood from the hand.

Most of the blood from the palm of the hand passes through to a superficial venous network on the dorsum. From the radial side of this arch the **cephalic vein** begins in the roof of the anatomical snuffbox and runs up along the lateral border of the limb (Fig. 2.19). It runs in the upper arm lateral to biceps, to the deltopectoral groove, and perforates the clavipectoral fascia to drain into the axillary vein. From the ulnar side of the dorsal venous arch the **basilic vein** runs up the medial border of the limb. It pierces the deep fascia halfway between elbow and axilla (Fig. 2.19) and becomes the axillary vein at the lower border of teres major.

The **median forearm vein** drains subcutaneous tissue of the front of the wrist and forearm. It ascends to join the median cubital or basilic vein. Commencing distal to the elbow, the **median cubital vein** runs proximomedially from the cephalic to the basilic veins. It lies superficial to the bicipital aponeurosis, but has a communication with the deep veins. There are frequent variations from the standard venous patterns just described.

Lymphatics of the forearm

As elsewhere in the body the superficial lymphatics follow veins, the deep ones follow arteries. From the ulnar side of the hand and forearm the subcutaneous lymphatics run alongside the basilic vein to the supratrochlear nodes. From the radial side the lymphatics run alongside the cephalic vein to the infraclavicular nodes. From the deep parts of the hand and forearm and from the supratrochlear nodes lymphatics pass to the lateral group of axillary nodes (see p. 58).

Nerves of the flexor compartment

The **lateral cutaneous nerve of the forearm**, the cutaneous continuation of the musculocutaneous nerve, pierces the deep fascia above the elbow lateral to the tendon of biceps and supplies the anterolateral surface of the forearm, by anterior and posterior branches, as far distally as the thenar eminence (Fig. 2.46). The **medial cutaneous nerve of the forearm** pierces the deep fascia at the middle of the arm and divides into anterior and posterior branches. It supplies the skin of the front of the lower part of the arm and that of the front and back of the medial part of the forearm (Fig. 2.46).

The superficial terminal branch of the **radial nerve**, the cutaneous continuation of the main nerve, runs from the cubital fossa on the surface of supinator, pronator teres tendon and flexor digitorum superficialis, on the lateral side of the forearm under cover of brachioradialis. In the middle third of the forearm it lies beside and lateral to the radial artery. It then leaves the flexor compartment of the forearm by passing backwards deep to the tendon of brachioradialis and breaks up into two or three branches which can often be rolled on the surface of the tautened tendon of extensor pollicis longus. They are distributed to the radial two-thirds of the dorsum of the hand and the proximal parts of the dorsal surfaces of thumb and lateral two and a half or three and a half fingers (Fig. 2.33), but see page 100 for the effects of nerve injury.

The **median nerve** leaves the cubital fossa between the two heads of pronator teres (Fig. 2.26). It passes deep to the fibrous arch of flexor digitorum superficialis and runs distally adherent to the posterior aspect of this muscle. Above the wrist the nerve comes closer to the surface between the tendons of flexor carpi radialis and flexor digitorum superficialis, lying behind and partly lateral to the tendon of palmaris longus (Fig. 2.24). Near the elbow the median nerve gives muscular branches, first to pronator teres and then to flexor carpi radialis, palmaris longus and flexor digitorum superficialis; the branch to the index finger part of this muscle, however, arises in the middle of the forearm. The nerve supplies the elbow and proximal radioulnar joints.

Deep to flexor digitorum superficialis, the median nerve gives off an **anterior interosseous** branch which runs down with the artery of the same name and supplies flexor digitorum profundus (usually the bellies which move index and middle fingers), flexor pollicis longus, pronator quadratus, and the inferior radioulnar, wrist and carpal joints.

In the distal forearm, above the flexor retinaculum, the median nerve gives off a **palmar branch** to the skin over the thenar muscles.

The *surface marking* of the nerve is along a line from the point in the middle of the cubital fossa medial to the brachial artery to a point at the wrist on the ulnar side of the tendon of flexor carpi radialis.

The **ulnar nerve** enters the forearm from the extensor compartment by passing between the humeral and ulnar heads of origin of flexor carpi ulnaris (Fig. 2.30). It is more easily compressed against the medial surface of the coronoid process than against the humerus, where it lies behind the medial epicondyle (Fig. 2.22). In the forearm the nerve lies under cover of the flattened aponeurosis of flexor carpi ulnaris, with the ulnar artery to its radial side along the distal two-thirds of the forearm. This neurovascular bundle lies on flexor digitorum profundus. Branches of supply are given to flexor carpi ulnaris and the ulnar half (usually) of flexor digitorum profundus. The branch to flexor carpi ulnaris contains C7 fibres brought to the ulnar nerve in the axilla (see p. 57) and C8 fibres; the branch to flexor digitorum profundus contains C8 and T1 fibres.

The ulnar nerve emerges from behind the tendon of flexor carpi ulnaris just proximal to the wrist (Fig. 2.24) and passes across the front of the flexor retinaculum in the hand. Before emerging it gives off a dorsal branch which passes medially between the tendon of flexor carpi ulnaris and the lower end of the ulna. The dorsal branch supplies the dorsum of the hand (Fig. 2.33) and of the ulnar one and a half fingers proximal to their nail beds. The small *palmar cutaneous branch* of the nerve pierces the deep fascia proximal to the flexor retinaculum, and supplies skin of the hypothenar eminence.

The *surface marking* of the nerve is along a line from the medial epicondyle of the humerus to the radial side of the pisiform bone.

Radioulnar joints

The **superior radioulnar joint** is a uniaxial synovial pivot joint between the circumference of the head of the radius and the fibro-osseous ring formed by the annular ligament (see p. 65) and the radial notch of the ulnar (Fig. 2.53). The articular inner aspect of the annular ligament is lined by hyaline cartilage. As has already been noted in connection with the elbow joint (see p. 64), the capsule and lateral ligament of the latter joint are attached to the annular ligament and both joints share the same synovial membrane. The membrane lines the intracapsular part of the radial neck and is supported below by the quadrate ligament.

The **inferior radioulnar joint** is a uniaxial synovial pivot joint between the convex head of the ulnar and the concave ulnar notch of the radius (Fig. 2.54). A triangular, fibrocartilaginous articular disc is attached by its base to the lower margin of the ulnar notch of the radius and by its apex to a fossa at the base of the ulnar styloid. The proximal surface of the disc articulates with the ulnar head. The synovial membrane of the joint projects proximally, as the recessus sacciformis, posterior to the pronator quadratus and anterior to the interosseous membrane.

The **interosseous membrane** connects the interosseous borders of the radius and ulna. Its fibres run from the radius distally to the ulna at an oblique angle.

The *oblique cord* is a flat band whose fibres run in opposite obliquity to those of the interosseous membrane; they slope proximally from just below the radial tuberosity to the side of the ulnar tuberosity. The posterior interosseous vessels pass through the gap between the oblique cord and the upper end of the interosseous membrane.

Nerve supplies. The proximal joint shares the nerve supply of the elbow joint (see p. 65), and the distal joint is supplied by the posterior interosseous and anterior interosseous nerves.

Movements

The movements of pronation and supination occur at the superior and inferior radioulnar joints. In full supination, the anatomical position, the radius lies lateral and parallel to the ulna. During pronation, while the head of the radius rotates within the fibro-osseous ring of the proximal joint, the distal radius rotates in front of and around the head of the ulna, carrying the hand with it; and in full pronation the shaft of the radius lies across the front of the ulna with the distal end of the radius medial to the ulnar head (Fig. 2.29). During supination these movements are reversed. The axis of movement of the radius relative to the ulna passes through the radial head and the ulnar styloid. But the ulnar is not usually entirely stationary during pronation and supination. The distal end of the ulna moves slightly posterolaterally in pronation and anteromedially in supination, these movements being effected by anconeus and the bicipital aponeurosis respectively. Supination is the more powerful action and account is taken of this in the design of screws, which are tightened by supination. Supination is carried out by the biceps and supinator, the former being the stronger provided the elbow is in the flexed position. The muscles producing pronation are principally pronator quadratus and pronator teres. About 140° of rotation occurs at the radioulnar joints during pronation–supination. Synchronous humeral rotation and scapular movement increases the range of rotation to nearly 360°.

PART **EIGHT**

Posterior compartment of the forearm

A dozen muscles occupy the extensor compartment. At the upper part are anconeus (superficial) and supinator (deep). From the lateral part of the humerus arise three muscles that pass along the radial side (brachioradialis, and extensors carpi radialis longus and brevis), and three that pass along the posterior surface of the forearm (extensors digitorum, digiti minimi and carpi ulnaris).

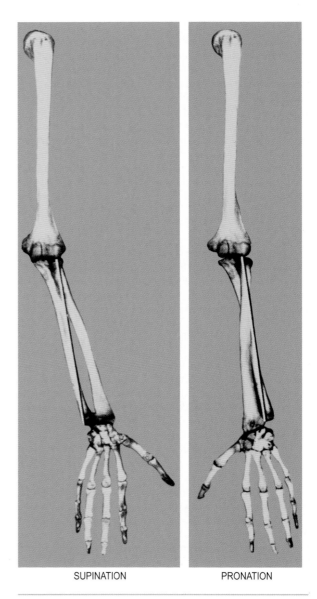

SUPINATION   PRONATION

Fig. 2.29   The limb bones are seen from the front and the axis of pronation–supination is indicated by the black lines.

At the lower end of the forearm these two groups are separated by three muscles that emerge from deeply in between them and go to the thumb (abductor pollicis longus and extensors pollicis longus and brevis). Finally, one muscle for the forefinger runs deeply to reach the back of the hand (extensor indicis).

The nerve of the extensor compartment is the posterior interosseous nerve, which reaches it by passing around the radius (compare the peroneal nerve in the leg); the artery is the posterior interosseous, which gains the extensor compartment by passing between the two bones (compare the anterior tibial artery in the leg). The artery is small and the blood supply of the posterior compartment is reinforced by the anterior interosseous artery.

The six long muscles that come from the lateral side of the humerus have not enough area available at the lateral epicondyle. Two of them arise high above this, from the lateral supracondylar ridge and the lateral intermuscular septum.

Brachioradialis

Arising from the upper two-thirds of the lateral supracondylar ridge, the muscle forms the lateral border of the cubital fossa (Fig. 2.24). At the mid-forearm level the muscle fibres end in a flat tendon, which is inserted into the base of the radial styloid (Fig. 2.27). The muscle and its tendon overlie the radial nerve and the radial artery as they pass down the forearm and deviate posteriorly. The lower part of the tendon is covered by abductor pollicis longus and extensor pollicis brevis as they spiral down to the thumb (Fig. 2.30).

Nerve supply. By the radial nerve (C5, 6) by a branch arising above the elbow joint.

Action. Its action is to flex the elbow joint. It acts most powerfully when the forearm is semipronated.

Test. With the forearm in the midprone position the elbow is flexed against resistance; the muscle can be seen and felt.

Extensor carpi radialis longus

Arising from the lower third of the lateral supracondylar ridge of the humerus the muscle passes down the forearm, behind brachioradialis (Fig. 2.30) and deep to the thumb muscles, to be inserted as a flattened tendon into the base of the second metacarpal.

Nerve supply. By the radial nerve (C6, 7) by a branch arising above the elbow.

Action. It is an extensor and abductor of the wrist. It is indispensable to the action of 'making a fist', acting as a synergist during finger flexion (see p. 94). It assists in flexion of the elbow. In paralysis of forearm flexor muscles it can be transferred into flexor digitorum profundus.

Test. With the forearm pronated the wrist is extended and abducted against resistance and the muscle is palpated below and behind the lateral side of the elbow.

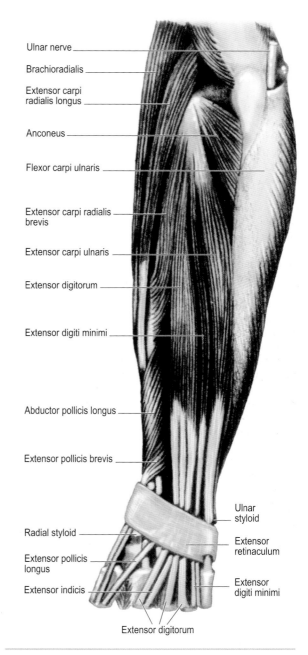

Labels:
Ulnar nerve
Brachioradialis
Extensor carpi radialis longus
Anconeus
Flexor carpi ulnaris
Extensor carpi radialis brevis
Extensor carpi ulnaris
Extensor digitorum
Extensor digiti minimi
Abductor pollicis longus
Extensor pollicis brevis
Radial styloid
Extensor pollicis longus
Extensor indicis
Extensor digitorum
Ulnar styloid
Extensor retinaculum
Extensor digiti minimi

Fig. 2.30 Superficial extensor muscles of the left forearm.

Common extensor origin

The smooth area on the front of the lateral epicondyle is for the attachment of the common extensor origin (Fig. 2.21). From it arise the fused tendons of extensor carpi radialis brevis, extensor digitorum, extensor digiti minimi and extensor carpi ulnaris. All four muscles pass to the posterior surface of the forearm. When the forearm is extended and supinated they spiral around the upper end of the radius; behind this rounded mass of muscle is an elongated pit in which lies the head of the radius. In the working position of the forearm (flexed and half pronated), however, these muscles pass straight from the front of the lateral epicondyle into the forearm.

Extensor carpi radialis brevis

This muscle arises from the common extensor origin on the front of the lateral epicondyle of the humerus, passes down behind and deep to its fellow longus (Fig. 2.30), and is inserted by a flattened tendon into the base of the third metacarpal. It and the longus are inserted into the same metacarpals as flexor carpi radialis. The lower part of both tendons are crossed by abductor pollicis longus and the two extensor muscles of the thumb.

Nerve supply. By a branch in the cubital fossa from the posterior interosseous nerve (C7, 8), before the nerve pierces the supinator muscle.

Action. As a wrist extensor like its longus companion it contracts in making a fist.

Extensor digitorum

Arising from the common extensor origin the muscle expands into a rounded belly in the middle of the forearm, diverging from the three muscles on the radial side and separated from them by the emergence of thumb muscles (Fig. 2.30). Its four tendons pass under the extensor retinaculum crowded together, overlying the tendon of extensor indicis. On the back of the hand the tendons spread out towards the fingers. Commonly the fourth tendon is fused with that to the ring finger, and reaches the little finger only by a tendinous band that passes across near the metacarpophalangeal joint. Other bands join adjacent tendons in a variable manner. The extensor expansions and their insertions into the phalanges are considered with the hand (see p. 93).

Nerve supply. By the posterior interosseous nerve on the back of the forearm (C7, 8).

Action. It is an extensor of the wrist, metacarpophalangeal and interphalangeal joints. Its action is discussed in detail on page 94.

Test. With the forearm in pronation and the fingers extended, the patient tries to keep the fingers extended at the metacarpophalangeal joints while pressure from the examiner on the proximal phalanges tries to flex these joints.

Extensor digiti minimi

Arising in common with the extensor digitorum the belly of the muscle separates after some distance (Fig. 2.30) and then becomes tendinous. Passing beneath the extensor retinaculum on the dorsal aspect of the radioulnar joint the tendon usually splits into two, which lie side by side on the fifth metacarpal bone as they pass to the little finger (Fig. 2.34). The tendon of extensor digitorum to the little finger commonly joins them as a band near the metacarpophalangeal joint and they all form an expansion on the dorsum of the little finger, which behaves as the other extensor expansions (see p. 93).

Nerve supply. By the posterior interosseous nerve (C7, 8).

Action. It assists extensor digitorum in extension of the little finger and wrist joint.

Extensor carpi ulnaris

This muscle arises from the common extensor origin and by an aponeurotic sheet from the subcutaneous border of the ulna (Fig. 2.30). This aponeurosis arises in common with that of flexor carpi ulnaris, the two passing in opposite directions into the extensor and flexor compartments. The tendon of the muscle lies in the groove beside the ulnar styloid as it passes on to be inserted into the base of the fifth metacarpal.

Nerve supply. By the posterior interosseous nerve (C7, 8) at the back of the forearm.

Action. It is an extensor and adductor of the wrist. It acts as a synergist during finger flexion and is indispensable in 'making a fist' (see p. 94).

Test. With the forearm pronated and the fingers extended, the wrist is extended and adducted against resistance. The muscle can be seen and felt in the upper forearm and the tendon palpated proximal to the head of the ulna.

Anconeus

This small muscle arises from the posterior surface of the lateral epicondyle. It fans out to its insertion on the lateral side of the olecranon and adjacent shaft of the ulna (Fig. 2.31).

Nerve supply. By the radial nerve (C7, 8) by a branch that leaves the trunk in the radial groove and passes through triceps, supplying it as well.

Action. The muscle produces the small amount of posterolateral movement of the ulna that occurs during pronation (see p. 76).

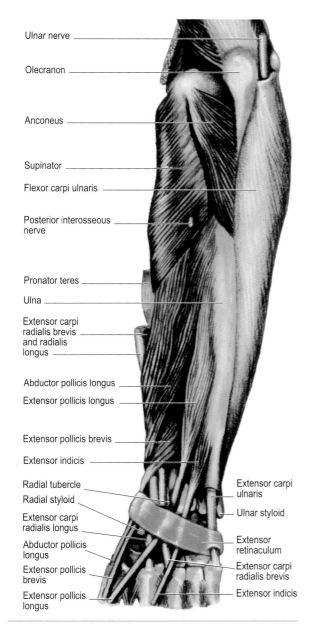

Ulnar nerve

Olecranon

Anconeus

Supinator

Flexor carpi ulnaris

Posterior interosseous
nerve

Pronator teres

Ulna

Extensor carpi
radialis brevis
and radialis
longus

Abductor pollicis longus

Extensor pollicis longus

Extensor pollicis brevis

Extensor indicis

Radial tubercle

Radial styloid

Extensor carpi
radialis longus

Abductor pollicis
longus

Extensor pollicis
brevis

Extensor pollicis
longus

Extensor carpi
ulnaris

Ulnar styloid

Extensor
retinaculum

Extensor carpi
radialis brevis

Extensor indicis

Fig. 2.31   Deep extensor muscles of the left forearm.
Compare with Figure 2.54.

Supinator

This muscle arises from the distal border of the lateral
epicondyle, the lateral ligament of the elbow joint, the
annular ligament of the radius, the supinator crest of
the ulna and the fossa in front of it. The muscle fibres

run behind the radius (Fig. 2.31) and are inserted on its
lateral surface, between the anterior and posterior
oblique lines. It has superficial and deep layers and the
posterior interosseous nerve passes between these two
parts as it leaves the cubital fossa to enter the back of
the forearm. The deep fibres are wrapped around the
proximal third of the radial shaft.

Nerve supply. By the posterior interosseous nerve
in the cubital fossa before the nerve enters the muscle
(C6, 7).

Action. While the biceps is the powerful supinator
of the forearm, supinator fixes the forearm in supination. Only when the elbow is completely extended is the
supinator the prime mover for the action of supination,
which is much weaker in this position.

Abductor pollicis longus

This arises obliquely from the back of both bones of the
forearm and the intervening interosseous membrane,
the ulnar origin being more proximal than the radial
(Figs 2.31 and 2.54). The tendon of the muscle usually
divides into two slips, one being attached to the base of
the first metacarpal, and the other to the trapezium.

Nerve supply. By the posterior interosseous nerve
(C7, 8).

Action. Despite its name this muscle extends the thumb
at the carpometacarpal joint, displacing it laterally in the
plane of the palm (see p. 88). It can assist in abducting
and flexing the wrist, producing a 'trick' flexion when
other flexors are paralysed.

Test. The thumb is extended at the carpometacarpal
joint against resistance. The tendon is seen and felt at
the radial side of the snuffbox and on the radial side of
the adjacent extensor pollicis brevis tendon.

Extensor pollicis brevis

This arises below abductor pollicis longus from the radius
and the adjacent interosseous membrane (Figs 2.31 and
2.54). It spirals from the depths of the forearm around
the radial extensors and brachioradialis, in contact
with abductor pollicis longus, on the radial border of
the snuffbox. Its slender tendon is inserted into the base
of the proximal phalanx.

Nerve supply. By the posterior interosseous nerve
(C7, 8).

Action. It extends the carpometacarpal and metacarpophalangeal joints of the thumb (Fig. 2.32). It prevents flexion of the metacarpophalangeal joint when
flexor pollicis longus is flexing the terminal phalanx, as
in pinching index and thumb pads together (e.g. threading
a needle).

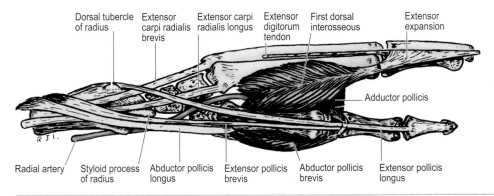

Fig. 2.32   Left anatomical snuffbox. It lies between the extensor tendons of the thumb. In its bony floor are the radial styloid, scaphoid, trapezium and base of the first metacarpal. The floor is crossed by the radial artery.

Test. The thumb is extended at the metacarpophalangeal joint against resistance. The tendon is seen and felt at the radial side of the snuffbox on the ulnar side of the adjacent abductor pollicis longus tendon.

Extensor pollicis longus

This arises from the ulna just distal to abductor pollicis longus (Figs 2.31 and 2.54). Thus it extends higher into the forearm than extensor pollicis brevis. It extends more distally also into the thumb, being inserted into the base of the distal phalanx. Its long tendon changes direction as it hooks around the dorsal tubercle of the radius (Lister's tubercle), whence it forms the ulnar boundary of the snuffbox (Fig. 2.32). In this situation the tendon is supplied with blood by local branches of the anterior interosseous artery. Their occlusion after Colles' fracture may lead to necrosis and spontaneous rupture of the tendon; unopposed action of flexor pollicis longus then produces a flexion deformity of the distal phalanx of the thumb, known as hammer thumb. Such a rupture is not due to wearing through of the tendon as it grates over the fragments.

There is no extensor expansion on the thumb; the tendon of extensor pollicis longus is stabilized on the dorsum of the thumb by receiving expansions from abductor pollicis brevis and adductor pollicis.

Nerve supply. By the posterior interosseous nerve (C7, 8).

Action. It extends the terminal phalanx of the thumb, and draws the thumb back from the opposed position. It assists in extension and abduction of the wrist.

Test. The thumb is extended at the interphalangeal joint against resistance. The tendon is seen and felt on the ulnar side of the snuffbox.

Extensor indicis

This small muscle arises from the ulna distal to the former muscle (Fig. 2.31). Its tendon remains deep and passes across the lower end of the radius covered by the tendons of extensor digitorum, with which it shares a common synovial sheath. From here it passes over the dorsal surface of the metacarpal bone of the index finger lying to the ulnar side of the digitorum tendon (Fig. 2.34). It joins the dorsal expansion of the index finger.

Nerve supply. By the posterior interosseous nerve (C7, 8).

Action. It extends the index finger, as in pointing.

Anatomical snuffbox

If the thumb is fully extended the extensor tendons are drawn up, and a concavity appears between them on the radial side of the wrist. The 'snuffbox' lies between the extensor pollicis longus tendon on the ulnar side and the tendons of extensor pollicis brevis and abductor pollicis longus on the radial side (Fig. 2.32). The cutaneous branches of the radial nerve cross these tendons, and they can be rolled on the tight tendon of extensor pollicis longus. The cephalic vein begins in the roof of the snuffbox, from the radial side of the dorsal venous network. The radial artery, deep to all three tendons, lies on the floor. Bony points readily palpable in the snuffbox from proximal to distal are the radial styloid, scaphoid, trapezium and the base of the thumb metacarpal.

Posterior interosseous nerve

After passing through the supinator muscle between its two layers the nerve appears in the extensor compartment of the forearm (Fig. 2.16) and passes downwards over the abductor pollicis longus origin. It now dips deeply to reach the interosseous membrane on which it passes between the muscles as far as the wrist joint. Here it ends in a small nodule from which branches supply the wrist joint. The nerve supplies the muscles which arise from the common extensor origin and the deep muscles of the extensor compartment.

Posterior interosseous artery

This vessel gains the extensor compartment by passing between the bones of the forearm above the interosseous membrane and below the oblique cord. This small vessel accompanies the posterior interosseous nerve and supplies the deep muscles of the extensor compartment. The arterial supply of the extensor compartment is supplemented by the anterior interosseous artery, which pierces the interosseous membrane just above the upper border of pronator quadratus. The anterior interosseous artery then passes distally to end on the back of the wrist in the dorsal carpal anastomosis.

Extensor retinaculum

The extensor retinaculum is a band-like thickening in the deep fascia of the forearm, about 2.5 cm wide, which lies obliquely across the extensor surface of the wrist (Fig. 2.34). Its proximal attachment is to the antero-lateral border of the radius above the styloid process. It is not attached to the ulna; its distal attachment is to the pisiform and triquetral bones.

From the deep surface of the extensor retinaculum fibrous septa pass to the bones of the forearm, dividing the extensor tunnel into six compartments. The most lateral compartment lies over the lateral surface of the radius at its distal extremity, and through it pass the tendons of abductor pollicis longus and extensor pollicis brevis, each usually lying in a separate synovial sheath. The next compartment extends as far as the dorsal tubercle, and conveys the tendons of the radial extensors of the wrist (longus and brevis), each lying in a separate synovial sheath (Fig. 2.54). The groove on the ulnar side of the radial tubercle lodges the tendon of extensor pollicis longus, which lies within its own compartment invested with a synovial sheath. Between this groove and the ulnar border of the radius is a shallow depression in which all four tendons of extensor digitorum lie, crowded together over the tendon of extensor indicis. All five tendons in this compartment are invested with a common synovial sheath. The next compartment lies over the radioulnar joint and transmits the tendon of extensor digiti minimi in a synovial sheath. Lastly, the groove near the base of the ulnar styloid transmits the tendon of extensor carpi ulnaris in its synovial sheath.

PART **NINE**

Wrist and hand

Wrist joint

The radiocarpal or wrist joint is a biaxial synovial joint. At this joint the concave ellipsoid distal surfaces of the radius and the attached articular disc articulate with the convex proximal surfaces of the scaphoid, lunate and triquetral bones (Fig. 2.55). The fibrocartilaginous disc, which holds the lower ends of the radius and ulna together (see p. 75), separates the radiocarpal joint from the distal radioulnar joint. It does not transmit thrust from the hand. The triangular facet on the lower end of the radius, whose apex is the styloid process, articulates with the scaphoid and the rectangular area next to it with the lunate, which also articulates with the disc. The triquetral articulates with the capsule where it is reinforced by the ulnar collateral ligament; it makes contact with the disc only in full adduction. A capsule surrounds the joint and is thickened to form palmar, dorsal and collateral ligaments.

Nerve supply. By the posterior interosseous (radial) and anterior interosseous (median) nerves.

Movements at the joint are flexion and extension, adduction (ulnar deviation) and abduction (radial deviation). These four movements occurring in sequence produce circumduction. Some of the movement of flexion and extension is always accompanied by similar movement at the midcarpal joint (see p. 95). Of the total range of flexion (about 80°), a greater proportion occurs at the midcarpal joint; in extension (60°), there is a greater proportion at the wrist joint itself. The four movements are carried out by combinations of muscle groups. Thus *flexion* is produced by flexor carpi radialis and flexor carpi ulnaris as prime movers, aided by palmaris longus and the flexors of fingers and thumb and abductor pollicis longus. *Extension* is produced by the radial extensors (longus and brevis) and the ulnar extensor as prime movers assisted by the extensors of fingers and thumb. *Abduction* (limited to about 15° because of the projection of the radial styloid) is carried out by flexor carpi radialis and the two radial extensors acting together, assisted by abductor pollicis longus. Similarly *adduction* (45°) is brought about by simultaneous contraction of flexor and extensor carpi ulnaris. In the resting position, the wrist is in slight adduction and extension.

Surgical approach. The usual approach is on the dorsal surface, on the ulnar side of the tendon of extensor pollicis longus, the tendons of extensor digitorum and extensor indicis being displaced medially to expose the capsule. There are no major vessels or nerves in this region. Needle puncture of the joint is carried out between the tendons of extensor pollicis longus and extensor digitorum; the styloid process of the radius is palpated in the snuffbox to indicate the level of the joint line.

Dorsum of the hand

The skin of the dorsum is thin and can be picked up from the underlying deep fascia and tendons and moved freely over them. There is usually little subcutaneous fat here.

The **cutaneous innervation** of the dorsum is by the terminal branches of the radial nerve and the dorsal branch of the ulnar nerve (Fig. 2.33). They share the hand and its digits 3½ to 1½, though a distribution 2½ to 2½ is not uncommon. The ends of the nerves stop short of the nail beds (which are supplied 3½ to 1½ by the nerves of the flexor skin, the median and the superficial branch of the ulnar nerves).

Large veins forming the **dorsal venous network** lie beneath the skin; they drain from the palm, so that the pressure of gripping does not impede venous return. The network lies superficial to the extensor tendons, proximal to the metacarpal heads, and drains on the radial side into the cephalic vein and on the ulnar side into the basilic vein.

Beyond the extensor retinaculum the extensors of the wrist (two radial and one ulnar) are inserted at the proximal part of the hand, into the bases of their respective metacarpal bones. Lying more superficially, the extensor tendons of the fingers fan out over the dorsum of the hand, attached to the deep fascia of this region and interconnected near the metacarpal heads by a variable arrangement of oblique fibrous bands (intertendinous connections) (Fig. 2.34). The deep fascia and the subjacent extensor tendons roof in a subfascial space that extends across the width of the hand.

The **dorsal carpal arch** is an arterial anastomosis between the radial, ulnar and anterior interosseous arteries. It lies on the back of the carpus and sends *dorsal metacarpal arteries* distally in the intermetacarpal spaces, deep to the long tendons. These split at the webs to supply the dorsal aspects of adjacent fingers. They communicate through the interosseous spaces with the palmar metacarpal branches of the deep palmar arch and the palmar digital branches of the superficial arch. Companion veins bring blood from the palm into the dorsal venous network.

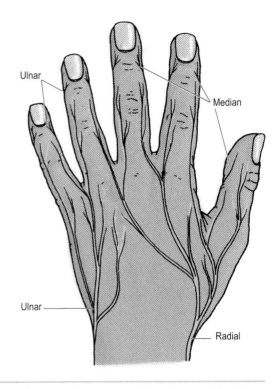

Fig. 2.33   Cutaneous innervation of the dorsum of the left hand.

Palm of the hand

The **skin** of the palm is characterized by flexure creases (the 'lines' of the palm) and papillary ridges, which occupy the whole of the flexor surface, those on the digits being responsible for fingerprints. The ridges serve to improve the grip and they increase the surface area. Sweat glands abound, but there are no sebaceous glands. The little **palmaris brevis** muscle is attached to the dermis. It lies across the base of the hypothenar eminence and is the only muscle supplied by the superficial branch of the ulnar nerve. It may improve the grip by steadying the skin on the ulnar side of the palm.

Elsewhere the skin is steadied by its firm attachment to the palmar aponeurosis. Fibrous bands connect the two and divide the subcutaneous fat into myriads of small loculi, forming a 'water cushion' capable of withstanding considerable pressure. When cut the tension causes some bulging of these fatty loculi.

The *cutaneous innervation* of the palm is mainly by the median nerve and its palmar branch (see pp 75 and

Fig. 2.34 Left extensor retinaculum and synovial sheaths of the extensor tendons. Intertendinous fibrous bands (variable) connect the extensor tendons of the index, middle and ring fingers. The tendon of extensor digiti minimi usually splits into two more distally than seen here; they may have separate synovial sheaths as shown or share a single sheath.

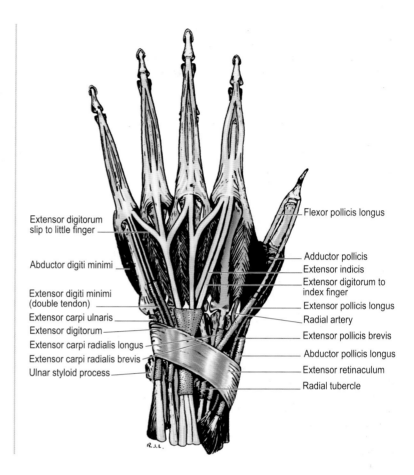

Extensor digitorum slip to little finger

Abductor digiti minimi

Extensor digiti minimi (double tendon)

Extensor carpi ulnaris

Extensor digitorum

Extensor carpi radialis longus

Extensor carpi radialis brevis

Ulnar styloid process

Flexor pollicis longus

Adductor pollicis

Extensor indicis

Extensor digitorum to index finger

Extensor pollicis longus

Radial artery

Extensor pollicis brevis

Abductor pollicis longus

Extensor retinaculum

Radial tubercle

86) and by the superficial and palmar branches of the ulnar nerve (see p. 87)

Palmar aponeurosis

The deep fascia in the central region of the palm is reinforced by a superficial layer of longitudinal fibres continuous with the tendon of the palmaris longus muscle and by deeper transverse fibres (Fig. 2.35). The longitudinal fibres are usually present even when palmaris is absent. This palmar aponeurosis is continuous proximally with the flexor retinaculum and on either side with thinner fascia covering the thenar and hypothenar muscles. The palmar aponeurosis widens distally in the hand and divides into four strips, one for each finger. The most superficial longitudinal fibres insert into the skin of the distal palm and central fibres of the digital strips are attached to the skin at the base of each digit. The main part of each digital slip divides into two diverging bands that are inserted into the deep transverse

metacarpal ligament (see p. 239), the bases of the proximal phalanx and the fibrous flexor sheath (see p. 235). Although a digital slip to the thumb is usually absent, some longitudinal fibres of the palmar aponeurosis curve over and blend with the thenar fascia. A thickening of transversely directed fibres at the level of the heads of the metacarpal bones constitutes the superficial transverse metacarpal ligament (natatory ligament). Contraction of the palmar aponeurosis and its digital strips in Dupuytren's contracture results in fixed flexion of the fingers concerned (usually the ring and little fingers).

Flexor retinaculum

The flexor retinaculum is a strong fibrous band, measuring 2–3 cm transversely and longitudinally, which lies across the front of the carpus at the proximal part of the hand. Its proximal limit lies at the level of the distal, dominant skin crease on the front of the wrist. It is attached to the hook of the hamate and the pisiform

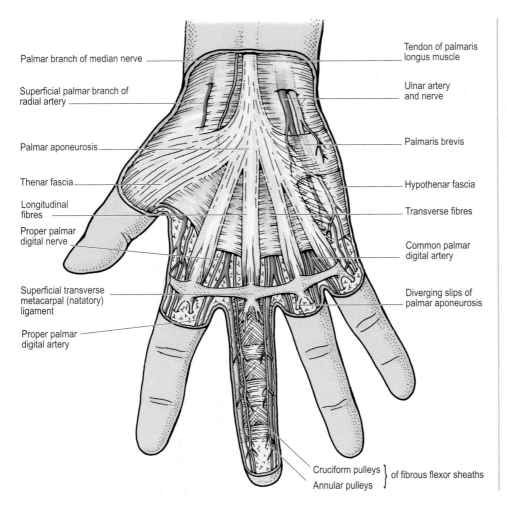

Palmar branch of median nerve

Superficial palmar branch of radial artery

Palmar aponeurosis

Thenar fascia

Longitudinal fibres

Proper palmar digital nerve

Superficial transverse metacarpal (natatory) ligament

Proper palmar digital artery

Tendon of palmaris longus muscle

Ulnar artery and nerve

Palmaris brevis

Hypothenar fascia

Transverse fibres

Common palmar digital artery

Diverging slips of palmar aponeurosis

Cruciform pulleys } of fibrous flexor sheaths
Annular pulleys }

Fig. 2.35 Right palmar aponeurosis and superficial transverse metacarpal ligament. The annular and cruciform pulleys (seen on the middle finger) are conventionally numbered A1 to A5 and C1 to C3. The A1 pulley lies anterior to the metacarpophalangeal joint and the A2 overlies the middle third of the proximal phalanx. (The fascial roof of the canal of Guyon has been removed.)

medially and to the tubercle of the scaphoid and the ridge of the trapezium laterally. The carpus is deeply concave on its anterior aspect, so a fibro-osseous canal, the **carpal tunnel**, lies between the flexor retinaculum and the carpal bones. The median nerve and all the long flexor tendons of the fingers and thumb pass through this tunnel. As they do so, the four tendons of the superficial flexor are separate and lie in two rows, with the middle and ring finger tendons in front of the index and little finger tendons. The tendons of flexor digitorum profundus lie deeply in one plane, with only the tendon to the index finger being separate from the others, which remain attached together till they reach the palm. All eight tendons of the superficial and deep flexors share a common flexor sheath, which does not invest them completely but is reflected from their radial sides, where

arteries of supply gain access. It is as though the tendons had been invaginated into the sheath from the radial side (Fig. 2.36). The tendon of flexor pollicis longus lies in its own synovial sheath as it passes through the fibro-osseous tunnel. At the lateral end of the tunnel a deep lamina from the flexor retinaculum is attached to the medial lip of the groove on the trapezium. The tendon of flexor carpi radialis, enclosed in its own synovial sheath, runs in the groove in this subcompartment of the carpal tunnel. The median nerve passes deep to the flexor retinaculum between the flexor digitorum superficialis tendon to the middle finger and the flexor carpi radialis tendon.

The ulnar nerve lies on the front of the retinaculum lateral to the pisiform bone, with the ulnar artery lateral to the nerve. The ulnar artery and nerve are covered here

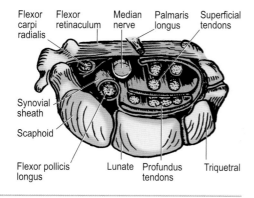

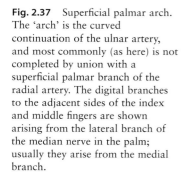

Fig. 2.36 Left carpal tunnel, looking distally towards the palm. For clarity the tendons and median nerve have been separated from each other; in life they are closely packed in the tunnel. The synovial sheath of the finger flexors is open towards the radial side for the access of blood vessels to the tendons.

by a slender band of fascia, forming the *canal of Guyon* in which the nerve may occasionally be compressed. The tendon of palmaris longus is partly adherent to the anterior surface of the retinaculum, which is also crossed superficially by the palmar cutaneous branches of the ulnar and median nerves lying medial and lateral, respectively, to the tendon. The superficial palmar branch of the radial artery lies on the retinaculum further laterally.

Superficial palmar arch

This is an arterial arcade (Fig. 2.37) that lies superficial to everything in the palmar compartment, i.e. in contact with the deep surface of the palmar aponeurosis. It is formed by the direct continuation of the ulnar artery beyond the flexor retinaculum. It is often not a complete arch. If it is complete it becomes continuous with the superficial palmar branch of the radial artery. The arch lies across the centre of the palm, level with the distal border of the outstretched thumb web. From its convexity a *palmar digital artery* passes to the ulnar side of the little finger, and three *common palmar digital arteries* run distally to the webs between the fingers, where each vessel divides into *proper palmar digital arteries* that

Fig. 2.37 Superficial palmar arch. The 'arch' is the curved continuation of the ulnar artery, and most commonly (as here) is not completed by union with a superficial palmar branch of the radial artery. The digital branches to the adjacent sides of the index and middle fingers are shown arising from the lateral branch of the median nerve in the palm; usually they arise from the medial branch.

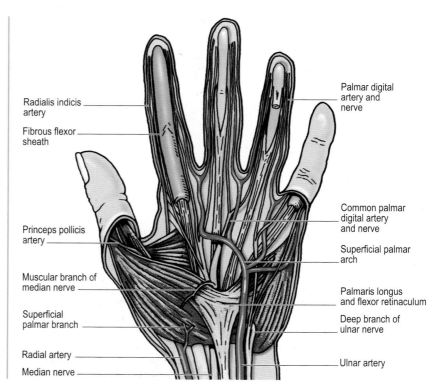

supply adjacent fingers. The thumb side of the index finger and the thumb itself are not supplied from the superficial arch since they receive branches from the radial artery. Palmar digital arteries anastomose with dorsal digital arteries and supply the distal soft parts on the dorsum, including the nail beds.

Digital nerves

Lying immediately deep to the superficial palmar arch are the *common palmar digital nerves* (Fig. 2.37). They pass distally to the webs, between the slips of the palmar aponeurosis, and divide like the arteries (but proximal to the arterial divisions) into *proper palmar digital nerves*, which lie anterior to the arteries in the fingers. Before terminating they each give a dorsal branch and thereby supply all five nail beds (Fig. 2.33). Incisions along the margins of fingers should be sited slightly dorsally to avoid damage to the digital nerves.

The **ulnar nerve** divides into a superficial (cutaneous) and a deep (muscular) branch on the flexor retinaculum. The *superficial branch* divides into two branches: the medial one supplies the ulnar side of the little finger, the lateral the cleft and adjacent sides of little and ring fingers.

The **median nerve** enters the palm beneath the flexor retinaculum. Distal to the retinaculum it enlarges and flattens and gives a *muscular (recurrent) branch* which curls proximally around the distal border of the flexor retinaculum to supply the thenar muscles (see p. 87). Incision of the synovial sheath of the tendon of flexor pollicis longus in the palm will endanger the nerve if the cut is not kept sufficiently distal.

The median nerve then usually divides into two branches. The *medial branch* divides again into two and supplies palmar skin, the cleft and adjacent sides of ring and middle fingers and the cleft and adjacent sides of middle and index fingers. The latter branch supplies the second lumbrical muscle. The *lateral branch* supplies palmar skin, the radial side of the index, the whole of the thumb and its web on the palmar surface and distal part of the dorsal surface. The branch to the index supplies the first lumbrical.

Carpal tunnel syndrome

In the tightly crowded flexor tunnel the median nerve can be compressed by arthritic changes in the wrist joint, synovial sheath thickening or oedema. The symptoms include impaired sensation over three and a half digits on the thumb side of the hand and wasting and weakness of the thenar muscles. There is no sensory loss over the thenar eminence itself, for this area of skin is supplied by the palmar branch of the median nerve, which enters the palm superficial to the retinaculum and so escapes compression. Surgical division of the retinaculum relieves the pressure and the symptoms.

The carpal tunnel syndrome must be distinguished from median nerve damage at a higher level. In the latter case the palmar cutaneous branch will be affected and, in addition, weakness of the relevant flexor muscles in the forearm (e.g. flexor pollicis longus) is a notable feature. In the carpal tunnel syndrome the terminal phalanx of the thumb can be flexed with normal power, but with higher lesions this power is lost.

Radial artery in the hand

The radial artery crosses the anatomical snuffbox over the trapezium and passes to the dorsum of the hand. It then runs deeply between the two heads of the first dorsal interosseous muscle (Fig. 2.32). Lying now between this muscle and adductor pollicis it gives off two large branches. The *arteria radialis indicis* passes distally between the two muscles to emerge on the radial side of the index finger, which it supplies. The *princeps pollicis* artery passes distally along the metacarpal bone of the thumb and divides into its two palmar digital branches at the metacarpal head. The main trunk of the radial artery now passes into the palm between the oblique and transverse heads of adductor pollicis to form the deep palmar arch (Fig. 2.38).

The **deep palmar arch** is an arterial arcade formed by the terminal branch of the radial artery anastomosing with the deep branch of the ulnar artery. Unlike the superficial arch the deep arch is usually complete and runs across the palm at a level about 1 cm proximal to the superficial arch. The deep branch of the ulnar nerve lies within the concavity of the deep arch. From its convexity three *palmar metacarpal arteries* pass distally and in the region of the metacarpal heads they anastomose with the common palmar digital branches of the superficial arch. Branches perforate the interosseous spaces to anastomose with the dorsal metacarpal arteries. Accompanying veins drain most of the blood from the palm into the dorsal venous network (see p. 82). Branches from the anterior carpal arch also anastomose with the deep arch.

For a visual assessment of the contribution of the radial and ulnar arteries to the blood supply of the hand, make a clenched fist and occlude the radial and ulnar arteries. When the fist is released the skin of the palm is seen to be pale, but colour should return rapidly on the release of either one of the arteries. If there is an obvious delay after releasing the ulnar artery compared with the radial, it suggests that the radial supply is dominant and

Fig. 2.38 Left adductor pollicis and the deep palmar arch. The two opponens muscles are also shown.

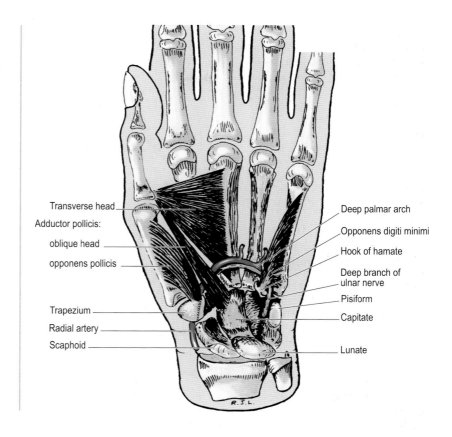

Transverse head

Adductor pollicis:

oblique head

opponens pollicis

Trapezium

Radial artery

Scaphoid

Deep palmar arch

Opponens digiti minimi

Hook of hamate

Deep branch of ulnar nerve

Pisiform

Capitate

Lunate

that procedures that might damage the radial artery (such as cannulation) should be avoided.

Ulnar nerve in the hand

The ulnar nerve leaves the forearm by emerging from deep to the tendon of flexor carpi ulnaris and passes distally on the flexor retinaculum alongside the radial border of the pisiform bone and medial to the ulnar artery. Here it divides into superficial and deep branches (Fig. 2.37). The **superficial branch,** which can be palpated on the hook of the hamate, supplies palmaris brevis and divides into two *digital nerves*; they supply the ulnar one and a half fingers. The small palmar branch, given off by the ulnar nerve in the forearm, supplies skin over the hypothenar muscles. The **deep branch** passes deeply into the palm between the heads of origin of flexor and abductor digiti minimi and through the origin of opponens digiti minimi (Fig. 2.38). Passing down to the interossei, it grooves the distal border of the hook of the hamate and arches deeply in the palm within the concavity of the deep palmar arch. It gives motor branches

to the three hypothenar muscles, the two lumbricals on the ulnar side, all the interossei and both heads of adductor pollicis. Compare the ulnar nerve in the hand with the lateral plantar in the foot (see p. 160): the cutaneous distribution is identical but unlike the ulnar nerve the superficial branch of the lateral plantar nerve supplies three muscles and the deep branch supplies three lumbricals.

Thenar eminence

The thenar eminence is made up of the three short thumb muscles whose origin is essentially from the flexor retinaculum (Fig. 2.39). The most radial of these is **abductor pollicis brevis**. It arises from the flexor retinaculum and the tubercles of the scaphoid and trapezium. It is inserted into the radial side of the base of the proximal phalanx and the tendon of extensor pollicis longus (Fig. 2.32).

Flexor pollicis brevis lies to the ulnar side of the abductor. It arises by a superficial head from the flexor retinaculum and trapezium and by a deep head from

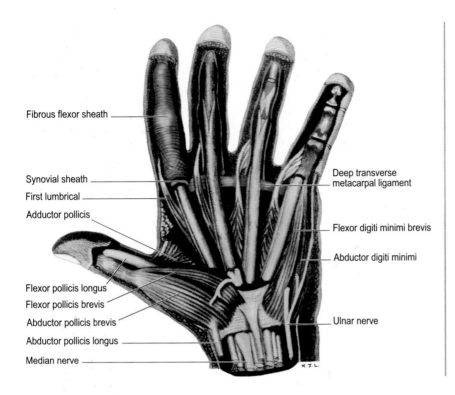

Fibrous flexor sheath

Synovial sheath
First lumbrical
Adductor pollicis

Flexor pollicis longus
Flexor pollicis brevis
Abductor pollicis brevis
Abductor pollicis longus
Median nerve

Deep transverse
metacarpal ligament

Flexor digiti minimi brevis

Abductor digiti minimi

Ulnar nerve

Fig. 2.39 Muscles and tendons of the left palm. The index finger shows the fibrous flexor sheath with the synovial sheath bulging proximally. The middle finger shows the long tendons exposed by incision of the flexor sheath. In the ring finger the profundus tendon has been removed, and in the little finger all is removed down to the phalanges. The first and second lumbricals are unicipital, the third and fourth bicipital. The median nerve passes beneath the flexor retinaculum and immediately gives off the muscular (recurrent) branch to the thenar muscles.

the trapezoid and capitate. It is inserted into the radial sesamoid of the thumb and so to the radial side of the base of the proximal phalanx.

Opponens pollicis lies deep to the former two muscles. It arises from the flexor retinaculum and the trapezium and is inserted into the whole of the radial border of the metacarpal bone of the thumb (Fig. 2.38).

Nerve supplies. All three muscles are supplied by the muscular (recurrent) branch of the median nerve (mainly T1 but with some contribution from C8). However, the nerve supply of flexor pollicis brevis is subject to more variation than that of any other muscle in the body. It may be from the muscular branch of the median nerve or the deep branch of the ulnar nerve, or it may have a double supply from both nerves. The opponens usually has such a double supply.

Actions. The actions of the three muscles are indicated by their names. The abductor abducts the thumb (moving it in a plane at right angles to the palm). By the slip to the tendon of extensor pollicis longus it can assist in extension of the thumb. The flexor flexes the proximal phalanx and draws the thumb across the palm, and the opponens opposes the metacarpal of the thumb (see below).

Tests. For abductor pollicis brevis the thumb is abducted against resistance, at right angles to the palm; the muscle can be seen and felt. For opponens the thumb is brought against resistance towards the base of the little finger and the thumb palpated against the metacarpal. The presence of the long flexor and the variability of the nerve supply makes testing flexor pollicis brevis of doubtful value.

Movements of the thumb

As recommended by the International Federation of Societies for Surgery of the Hand, the terms **flexion** and **extension** of the thumb should be confined to movements at the metacarpophalangeal and interphalangeal joints. Flexion is brought about by flexor pollicis longus and brevis, and extension by extensor pollicis longus and brevis. In **palmar abduction** the thumb moves away from the index finger in a plane at right angles to the palm, and the thumbnail remains in a plane at right angles to that of the four fingernails (Fig. 2.40). This movement is produced by abductor pollicis brevis. In **radial abduction** the thumb is moved away from the index finger in the plane of the palm by abductor pollicis

Fig. 2.40 Movements of the thumb.

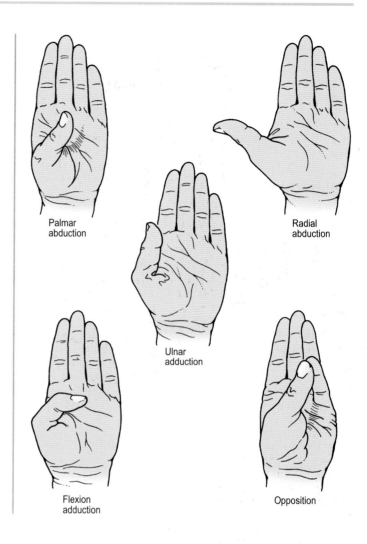

Palmar
abduction

Radial
abduction

Ulnar
adduction

Flexion
adduction

Opposition

longus and extensor pollicis brevis. The opposite movement is (ulnar) **adduction** and is produced by adductor pollicis. Further transpalmar adduction is effected by flexor pollicis brevis. In **opposition** of the thumb adduction is combined with internal rotation of the first metatarsal at its joint with the trapezium, by opponens pollicis, and extension of the thumb at the metacarpophalangeal and interphalangeal joints. This composite movement makes the thumbnail lie parallel with the nail of the opposed finger.

Hypothenar eminence

In name the muscles that form the hypothenar eminence on the ulnar side of the palm are similar to the three thenar muscles. **Abductor digiti minimi** is the most medial of the group (Fig. 2.39). It arises from the pisiform bone and the tendon of flexor carpi ulnaris and is inserted into the ulnar side of the base of the proximal phalanx and into the extensor expansion. **Flexor digiti minimi brevis** (Fig. 2.39) arises from the flexor retinaculum and the hook of the hamate and is inserted into the ulnar side of the base of the proximal phalanx. **Opponens digiti minimi** (Fig. 2.38) also arises from the flexor retinaculum and the hook of the hamate and is inserted into the ulnar border of the fifth metacarpal bone.

Nerve supplies. By the deep branch of the ulnar nerve (mainly T1).

Actions. All three hypothenar muscles help to cup the palm and assist in the grip on a large object.

Long flexor tendons

In the palm the tendons of flexor digitorum superficialis lie anterior to those of flexor digitorum profundus. From the latter tendons the four lumbrical muscles arise. The superficial tendons overlie the profundus tendons as they pass, in pairs, into the fibrous flexor sheaths of the fingers. Their synovial sheaths are considered on page 91.

Lumbrical muscles

Lumbrical muscles arise from the four profundus tendons and pass along the radial sides of the metacarpophalangeal joints on the palmar surface of the deep transverse metacarpal ligament (Fig. 2.39), to be inserted by their tendons into the extensor expansions on the dorsum of the proximal phalanges.

Nerve supply. Characteristically, the two ulnar lumbricals are innervated by the ulnar nerve and the two radial lumbricals by the median nerve (C8, T1). The proportion of ulnar and median distribution to the lumbricals follows that of the parent bellies of the tendons in the forearm (see p. 69). Lumbricals supplied by the ulnar nerve are bicipital, each arising by two heads from adjacent profundus tendons, while those supplied by the median nerve are unicipital and arise from one tendon only.

Actions. See page 94.

Adductor pollicis

This muscle lies deeply in the palm (Figs 2.38 and 2.39) and has two heads of origin. The transverse head arises from the whole length of the palmar border of the third metacarpal from where the muscle converges, fan-shaped, to the ulnar sesamoid of the thumb, the ulnar side of the base of the proximal phalanx and the tendon of extensor pollicis longus. The oblique head arises from the bases of the second and third metacarpals and the capitate and also converges on the ulnar sesamoid.

Nerve supply. By the deep branch of the ulnar nerve (C8, T1).

Action. To approximate the thumb to the index finger, whatever the original position of the thumb.

Interosseous muscles

The interossei are in two groups, palmar and dorsal. The former are small and arise from only one (their own) metacarpal bone; the latter are larger and arise from the adjacent metacarpal bones of the space in which they lie (Fig. 2.41). The palmar interossei are only seen from the palmar aspect of the interosseous spaces, but the dorsal can be seen from both dorsal and palmar aspects. It is easy to recall the attachments of the interossei by appreciating their functional requirements. The formula 'PAD and DAB' indicates that palmar adduct and dorsal abduct the fingers relative to the axis of the palm, which is the third metacarpal bone and middle finger.

The **palmar interossei** adduct the fingers. Thus the thumb requires no palmar interosseous, already possessing its own powerful adductor pollicis muscle. Nevertheless a few fibres are sometimes found passing from the base of the metacarpal of the thumb to the base of its proximal phalanx; when present these fibres represent the first palmar interosseous muscle. The middle finger has no palmar interosseous; it cannot be adducted towards itself. The second, third and fourth palmar interossei arise from the middle finger side of the metacarpal bone of the index, ring and little fingers and are inserted into the same side of the extensor expansion and proximal phalanx of each respective finger.

The **dorsal interossei**, more powerful than the palmar, abduct their own fingers away from the midline of the palm. The thumb and little finger already possess their proper abducting muscles in the thenar and hypothenar eminences. Thus there are dorsal interossei attached only to index, middle and ring fingers. In the case of the index and ring fingers they are inserted into the side of the finger away from the middle finger. The middle finger itself has a dorsal interosseous attached on both sides. All four dorsal interossei arise by two heads, one from each metatarsal bone bounding the interosseous space.

The tendons of palmar and dorsal interossei all pass on the posterior side of the deep transverse metacarpal ligament to reach their distal attachments. They are inserted chiefly into the appropriate side of the extensor expansion, but partly also into the base of the proximal phalanx.

Nerve supply. All the interossei are supplied by the deep branch of the ulnar nerve (C8, T1).

Actions. See page 94.

Fibrous flexor sheaths

From the metacarpal heads to the distal phalanges all five digits are provided with a strong unyielding fibrous sheath in which the flexor tendons lie in a fibro-osseous tunnel (Fig. 2.39). In the thumb the fibrous sheath is occupied by the tendon of flexor pollicis longus alone. In the four fingers the sheaths are occupied by the tendons of the superficial and deep flexors, the superficial splitting to spiral around the deep within the sheath. The proximal ends of the fibrous sheaths of the fingers receive the insertions of the digital slips of the palmar aponeurosis.

Fig. 2.41 Dorsal interossei of the left hand, with the dorsal digital expansions. Compare with Figure 2.34. The tendons occupying the grooves on the radius and ulna are named.

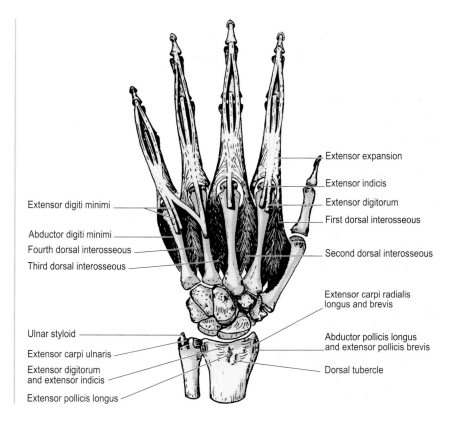

Extensor digiti minimi

Abductor digiti minimi

Fourth dorsal interosseous

Third dorsal interosseous

Ulnar styloid

Extensor carpi ulnaris

Extensor digitorum and extensor indicis

Extensor pollicis longus

Extensor expansion

Extensor indicis

Extensor digitorum

First dorsal interosseous

Second dorsal interosseous

Extensor carpi radialis longus and brevis

Abductor pollicis longus and extensor pollicis brevis

Dorsal tubercle

The sheaths are dense and stiff over the phalanges and the centres of the joints, where they consist of arcuate fibres. In between these *annular pulleys* the sheaths are thin and lax; here the fibres have a cruciate arrangement forming *cruciform pulleys* (Fig. 2.35).

Synovial flexor sheaths

In the carpal tunnel the flexor tendons are invested with synovial sheaths that extend proximally for about 2.5 cm into the lower part of the forearm and proceed distally to a varying extent (Fig. 2.42). On the tendon of flexor pollicis longus the sheath extends from above the flexor retinaculum to the insertion of the tendon into the terminal phalanx of the thumb. The tendons of the superficial and deep flexors are together invested with a common synovial sheath that is incomplete on the radial side. This common sheath extends into the palm and on the little finger it is continued along the whole extent of the flexor tendons to the terminal phalanx. The common flexor sheath ends over the remaining three sets of tendons just distal to the flexor retinaculum. The common flexor sheath communicates at the level of the

wrist with the sheath of flexor pollicis longus in 50% of individuals. In the index, middle and ring fingers, where the common sheath ends beyond the flexor retinaculum, a separate synovial sheath lines the fibrous flexor sheath over the phalanges. The proximal limit of these sheaths is at the level of the distal transverse crease of the palm. There is thus a short distance of bare tendon for index, middle and ring fingers in the middle of the palm. It is from this situation that the lumbrical muscles arise. The fourth lumbrical obliterates the synovial sheath along its origin from the tendon to the little finger.

Palmar spaces

The palmar aponeurosis, fanning out from the distal border of the flexor retinaculum, is triangular in shape. From each of its two sides a septum dips deeply into the palm. That from the ulnar border is attached to the palmar border of the fifth metacarpal bone. Medial to it is the *hypothenar space* that encloses the hypothenar muscles. The remaining part of the palm is divided into two spaces by the septum that dips in from the radial border of the palmar aponeurosis to the palmar surface

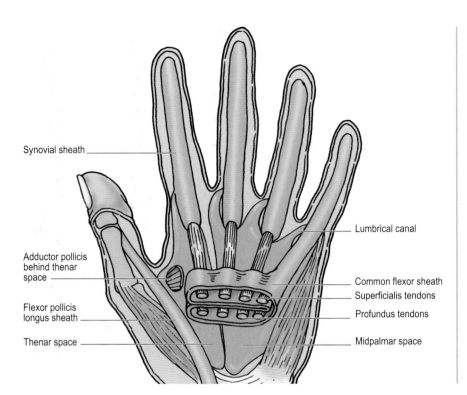

Synovial sheath

Adductor pollicis
behind thenar
space

Flexor pollicis
longus sheath

Thenar space

Lumbrical canal

Common flexor sheath
Superficialis tendons
Profundus tendons

Midpalmar space

Fig. 2.42   Left palmar spaces
and synovial sheaths. Infection in
the thenar or midpalmar spaces
easily breaks through into the
lumbrical canals (connective
tissue sheaths of the lumbrical
muscles), so the canals are
shown in continuity with the
spaces.

of the middle metacarpal bone. This septum lies obliquely and separates the *thenar space* on its radial side from the *midpalmar space* beneath the palmar aponeurosis. The septum usually passes deeply between the flexor tendons of index and middle fingers, i.e. the flexor tendons of the index finger overlie the thenar space. These are potential spaces and their margins are difficult to define. Pus may accumulate in them in infections of the hand and be initially confined within the boundaries described.

Web spaces

Three web spaces lie in the distal part of the palm between the bases of the proximal phalanges of the four fingers. From the skin edge they may be said to extend proximally as far as the metacarpophalangeal joints. Between the palmar and dorsal layers of the skin lie the superficial and deep transverse ligaments of the palm, the digital vessels and nerves, and the tendons of the interossei and lumbricals on their way to the extensor expansions. The web is filled in with a packing of loose fibrofatty tissue.

The **superficial transverse metacarpal ligament**, or natatory ligament, has been described on page 83. It lies just deep to the palmar skin across the free margins

of the webs (Fig. 2.35). The digital vessels and nerves lie immediately deep to the ligament, a point to be remembered in making web incisions for palmar space infections. Here the nerves lie on the palmar side of the arteries. The digital slips of the palmar aponeurosis and the lumbrical tendons lie posterior to the vessels, as they pass distally to their attachments to the fibrous flexor sheaths and extensor expansions respectively.

The **deep transverse metacarpal ligament** lies proximal to the superficial transverse ligament and connects the palmar ligaments of adjacent metacarpophalangeal joints (Fig. 2.39). The digital slips of the palmar aponeurosis are attached to it anteriorly, and transverse bands of the extensor expansion join it posteriorly. The interosseous tendons lie on the dorsal side of the deep transverse ligament; the lumbrical tendons are on the palmar side.

The **web of the thumb** lacks both superficial and deep transverse ligaments, a factor contributing to the mobility of the thumb. The transverse head of adductor pollicis and the first dorsal interosseous muscle lie here and between them emerge the radialis indicis and princeps pollicis arteries. Each hugs its own digit and the central part of the web can be incised without risk to either vessel.

Pulp spaces

The pulp spaces are on the palmar side of the tips of the fingers and thumb. They contain fatty tissue that is divided into numerous compartments by fibrous septa that pass between the distal phalanx and the skin. Terminal branches of the digital vessels course through the spaces and some of them supply the end of the distal phalanx (but not the epiphysis which is supplied by proximal branches); infection of the pulp spaces may occlude these vessels and cause necrosis of the end of the bone. The pulp space is limited proximally by the firm adherence of the skin of the distal flexion crease to the underlying tissue; this prevents pulp infection from spreading proximally along the finger.

Digital attachments of the long tendons

Flexor tendons

The tendon of flexor digitorum superficialis enters the fibrous flexor sheath on the palmar surface of the tendon of flexor digitorum profundus. It divides into two halves, which flatten a little and spiral around the profundus tendon and meet on its deep surface in a chiasma (a partial decussation). This forms a tendinous bed in which lies the profundus tendon. Distal to the chiasma the superficialis tendon is attached to the margins of the front of the middle phalanx (Fig. 2.43).

The profundus tendon enters the fibrous sheath deep to the superficialis tendon, then lies superficial to the partial decussation of the latter, before passing distally to reach the base of the terminal phalanx. In the flexor sheath both tendons are invested by a common synovial sheath that possesses parietal and visceral layers. Each tendon receives blood vessels from the palmar surface of the phalanges. The vessels are invested in synovial membrane. These vascular synovial folds are the **vincula**, and each tendon possesses two, the short and long (Fig. 2.44). The profundus tendon has its short vinculum in the angle close to its insertion. Its long vinculum passes from the tendon between the two halves of the superficialis tendon (proximal to the chiasma) to the palmar surface of the proximal phalanx. The superficialis tendon has a short vinculum near its attachment to the middle phalanx. The long vinculum of the superficialis tendon is double, each half of the tendon possessing a vinculum just distal to its first division, passing to the palmar surface of the proximal phalanx.

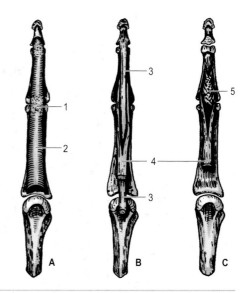

Fig. 2.43 Flexor tendon insertions: **A** fibrous flexor sheath; its fibres are oblique and slender near the interphalangeal (1) joints but transverse and strong across the phalanges (2); **B** tendons exposed after removal of the sheath; the profundus tendon (3) perforates the superficialis tendon (4) to reach the base of the distal phalanx; **C** with the profundus tendon removed to show the gutter-shaped decussation (5) of the superficialis tendon (4) and the insertions into the sides of the palmar surface of the middle phalanx.

Extensor tendons and expansions

The extensor tendons to the four fingers have a characteristic insertion. Passing across the metacarpophalangeal joint, the tendon blends with the central axis of a triangular fibrous expansion on the dorsum of the proximal phalanx. The base of the triangle is proximal and extends around the metacarpophalangeal joint to link with the deep transverse metacarpal ligament. The margins of the expansion are thickened by the attachments of the tendons of the lumbrical and interosseous muscles (the so-called 'wing tendons'), which also contribute transverse fibres to the expansion. As the extensor tendon approaches the proximal interphalangeal joint it splits into a middle slip and two collateral slips. The middle slip is attached to the base of the middle phalanx. The collateral slips are joined by the thickened margins of the expansion and converge to be inserted together into the base of the distal phalanx.

The *retinacular ligaments* are fibrous bands attached to the side of the proximal phalanx, with the fibrous flexor sheath attachment. They extend distally to merge with the margins of the extensor expansion and thereby

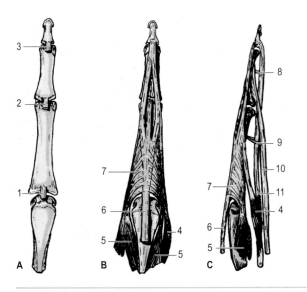

Fig. 2.44 Extensor digitorum tendon and the extensor expansion of the left middle finger: **A** dorsal view showing insertions of the digitorum tendon into the bases of the middle and distal phalanges (2 and 3), with a bursa (1) over the base of the proximal phalanx; **B** dorsal view of the expansion; **C** view of the radial side. The lumbrical (4) is attached to the expansion (7) distal to the interosseous attachment (5). 1, part of bursa; 2 and 3, extensor attachments to middle and distal phalanges; 4, lumbrical muscle; 5, interosseous muscle; 6, extensor digitorum tendon; 7, extensor expansion; 8, long vincula to profundus tendon; 9, long vincula to superficialis tendon; 10, superficialis tendon; 11, profundus tendon.

gain attachment to the base of the distal phalanx. Extension of the proximal joint draws them tight and limits flexion of the distal joint. Flexion of the proximal joint slackens them and permits full flexion of the distal joint. The two joints thus passively tend to assume similar angulations.

Long tendons of the thumb

On the flexor aspect there is only one tendon, that of flexor pollicis longus invested by its synovial sheath as it passes to the distal phalanx. On the extensor surface the tendons of extensor pollicis brevis and longus are each inserted separately (into the proximal and distal phalanx). There is no extensor hood as in the four fingers, but the extensor pollicis longus tendon receives a fibrous expansion from both abductor pollicis brevis and adductor pollicis (Fig. 2.32). These expansions serve to hold the long extensor tendon in place on the dorsum of the thumb.

Grip

Holding a heavy hammer for banging in a nail or holding a needle for delicate sewing (surgical or otherwise!) are but two illustrations of the variety of grips required for different purposes. The *power grip* depends on the long flexors of the fingers, with opposition of the thumb assisting the whole hand to give a tight grip. Synergic contraction of wrist extensors is also essential for a firm grip of this kind; flexion of the wrist weakens the grip. In the *hook grip*, as for carrying a suitcase, the long flexors are in action but wrist extension and opposition may not be necessary accompaniments. The *precision grip* for dealing with small objects requires wrist stability, but opposition of the thumb to finger pads, especially of the index and middle fingers, are the essential features, and here the small hand muscles are of prime importance (see below).

Actions of interossei and lumbricals

The **interossei** are inserted into the proximal phalanges and into the extensor expansions. Contracting as palmar or dorsal groups, respectively, they adduct or abduct the fingers away from the midline of the palm (a longitudinal axis passing through the centre of the middle finger). When palmar and dorsal interossei contract together the adducting and abducting effects cancel out. Flexion of the metacarpophalangeal joints results. The interossei are indispensable for the combined movement of flexion of the metacarpophalangeal joint and simultaneous extension of the interphalangeal joints. The extensor digitorum is, however, indispensable to the action of extending the terminal phalanx with full force. In radial nerve palsy, or if the digitorum tendon is cut on the dorsum of the hand, the distal phalanx cannot be extended with full force even though the interossei are normal.

If the interossei are paralysed, the pull of the digitorum tendon is wholly expended on the metacarpophalangeal joint which is hyperextended and the interphalangeal joints are partially flexed, as in the 'claw hand' of ulnar nerve paralysis (see p. 100).

The **lumbricals** are attached only to the extensor expansions and not to the proximal phalanges as well. Furthermore, their proximal attachments are not to bone but to tendons, and are therefore mobile. The lumbricals thus provide muscular, and hence proprioceptive, bridges between flexor and extensor muscles—a unique occurrence (as also in the foot)—which may have important implications in adjusting the positions of finger joints when using the hand. Acting via the extensor apparatus, the lumbricals extend both interphalangeal joints. Their action at the metacarpophalangeal joint is disputed and any flexor action here is likely to be weak. In the 'claw hand' of ulnar paralysis the index and middle fingers are less flexed at the interphalangeal joints because their lumbrical muscles are intact as they are supplied by the median nerve (Fig. 2.47). Flexion of the ring and little fingers is, however, less pronounced when the level of the ulnar nerve lesion is at, or proximal to, the elbow as the ulnar nerve usually supplies the medial half of flexor digitorum profundus in the forearm (the 'ulnar paradox').

Tests. The first dorsal interosseous can be tested by abducting the index finger against resistance; the muscle can be seen and palpated between the first two metacarpals. The adducting capacity of the palmar interossei can be tested by trying to hold a piece of card between the adjacent extended fingers while an attempt is made to pull the card away. This test carried out between the index and middle fingers provides a reliable assessment of ulnar nerve integrity. The lumbricals can be tested by making a pinching movement between the thumb and each finger successively; if lumbrical function is not intact this results in nail-to-nail contact. The enhancement of distal interphalangeal joint extension by lumbrical action is necessary for firm pulp-to-pulp contact.

Joints of the carpus

An S-shaped **midcarpal joint** forms a continuous synovial space between the two rows of carpal bones, and this extends proximally and distally between adjacent carpal bones, continuous with the *intercarpal joints*. A similar synovial joint lies between the distal row of carpal bones and the metacarpal bones of the four fingers. This **carpometacarpal joint** commonly communicates with the intercarpal joints and with articulations between the bases of the metacarpals. The joint between hamate and fifth metacarpal is the most mobile of the four and the slight flexion possible here aids in 'cupping' the palm. The **first carpometacarpal joint** (of the *thumb*) is a separate synovial cavity between the trapezium and first metacarpal bone. The joint surfaces are reciprocally saddle-shaped, to assist in the vitally important movement of opposition.

The **metacarpophalangeal joints** are synovial joints. They allow of flexion and extension, abduction and adduction. The *palmar ligaments* are strong pads of fibrocartilage, which limit extension at the joint. Those of the index to little fingers are joined together by transverse bands that together constitute the *deep transverse metacarpal ligament* (Fig. 2.39). Bands from the digital slips of the palmar aponeurosis join the palmar surface of this ligament and transverse bands of the extensor

expansions join the dorsal surface. Collateral ligaments flank these joints; they run in a distal and palmar direction from the metacarpal heads to the phalangeal bases. These joints (the 'knuckle joints') lie on the arc of a circle; hence the extended fingers diverge from each other, the flexed fingers crowd together into the palm.

The **interphalangeal joints** are pure hinge joints, no abduction being possible. Extension is limited by palmar and collateral ligaments; the latter have a similar oblique alignment to that in the metacarpophalangeal joints.

PART TEN

Summary of upper limb innervation

Brachial plexus

The *roots* of the plexus (the anterior rami of C5–T1 nerves) are between the scalene muscles, the *trunks* in the posterior triangle, the *divisions* behind the clavicle, and the *cords* arranged round the second part of the axillary artery. About 10% of plexuses are prefixed (from C4–C8) and 10% postfixed (C6–T2).

The preganglionic sympathetic fibres for the upper limb originate mainly from the second to fifth thoracic spinal cord segments, and ascend along the sympathetic trunk. Grey rami communicantes carrying postganglionic fibres from the middle and inferior cervical and the first thoracic sympathetic ganglia join the roots of the brachial plexus. They hitch-hike through the plexus and its branches, remaining in the nerves until very near their area of supply. Thus, the brachial artery receives sympathetic fibres from the median nerve in the arm and arterioles in a finger receive filaments from digital nerves. In the skin, in addition to arterioles, sweat glands and the arrectores pilorum muscles receive sympathetic innervation.

Branches of the roots

C5 Dorsal scapular
C5, 6 Nerve to subclavius
C5–7 Long thoracic.

The **dorsal scapular nerve** (C5) runs down deep to levator scapulae and the two rhomboids, supplying all three muscles. Lying on serratus posterior superior, it forms a neurovascular bundle with the descending scapular vessels alongside the vertebral border of the scapula (Fig. 2.5).

The **nerve to subclavius** (C5, 6) passes down over the trunks of the plexus and in front of the subclavian vein.

It frequently contains accessory phrenic fibres which join the phrenic nerve in the superior mediastinum.

The **long thoracic nerve** (C5, 6, 7) forms on the first digitation of the serratus anterior muscle and runs vertically downwards just behind the midaxillary line, deep to the fascia over the muscle.

Branch of the upper trunk

The **suprascapular nerve** (C5, 6), prominent beneath the fascial floor of the posterior triangle, passes beneath the transverse scapular ligament and round the lateral border of the scapular spine. The nerve supplies supraspinatus, infraspinatus, and the shoulder and acromioclavicular joints.

Branches of the lateral cord

C5–7 Lateral pectoral
C5–7 Musculocutaneous
C5–7 Lateral root of median.

The **lateral pectoral nerve** (C5, 6, 7) passes through the clavipectoral fascia and supplies the upper fibres of pectoralis major. A communicating branch to the medial pectoral nerve crosses in front of the first part of the axillary artery and contributes to the supply of pectoralis minor (Fig. 2.45).

The **musculocutaneous nerve** (C5–7) is muscular to the flexors in the arm and cutaneous in the forearm. It supplies coracobrachialis, then pierces that muscle to slope down between biceps and brachialis, supplying both muscles. Emerging at the lateral border of the biceps tendon, it pierces the deep fascia at the flexure crease of the elbow. Now called the *lateral cutaneous nerve of the forearm*, it supplies skin from elbow to wrist by an anterior and a posterior branch along the radial border of the forearm (Fig. 2.46).

The **lateral root** of the **median nerve** (C5–7) is joined by the medial root at the lateral side of the axillary artery to form the main nerve (see below).

Branches of the medial cord

C8, T1 Medial pectoral
C8, T1 Medial root of median
C8, T1 Medial cutaneous of arm
C8, T1 Medial cutaneous of forearm
C7, 8, T1 Ulnar.

The **medial pectoral nerve** (C8, T1) gives a branch to pectoralis minor and then pierces it to supply the lower (sternocostal) fibres of pectoralis major.

The **medial root** of the **median nerve** (C8, T1) crosses the axillary artery to join its companion and form the median nerve (C5–T1) at the lateral side of the artery.

The **median nerve** (C5–8, T1; Fig. 2.45) supplies most of the flexor muscles of the forearm, but only the three thenar muscles and two lumbricals in the hand. It is cutaneous to the flexor surfaces and nail beds of the three and a half radial digits and a corresponding area of palm.

The **median nerve** leaves the axilla and crosses in front of the brachial artery at the middle of the arm. At the elbow it lies medial to the artery beneath the bicipital aponeurosis. It passes between the two heads of pronator teres and deep to the fibrous arch of flexor digitorum superficialis. Adherent to the deep surface of the muscle, it emerges on the radial side of its tendons, lying deep to the palmaris longus tendon before passing through the carpal tunnel into the hand.

Branches. In the arm the nerve gives sympathetic filaments to the brachial artery, a twig to the elbow joint and may supply pronator teres above the elbow. In the cubital fossa, it supplies pronator teres, palmaris longus, flexor carpi radialis and flexor digitorum superficialis. In the forearm it gives off the *anterior interosseous nerve*, which descends on the interosseous membrane to the wrist. The anterior interosseous is the nerve of the deep flexor compartment; it supplies the radial half (usually) of flexor digitorum profundus, all of flexor pollicis longus and pronator quadratus and is sensory to the wrist and carpal joints. The *palmar cutaneous* branch of the median nerve pierces the deep fascia just above the flexor retinaculum and supplies more than half of the thumb side of the palm.

In the hand the median nerve gives a *muscular recurrent branch*, which recurves around the distal border of the flexor retinaculum to supply the three thenar muscles (abductor and flexor pollicis brevis, and opponens pollicis), and palmar digital branches; these supply both sides of the thumb, index and middle fingers, the radial side of the ring finger and characteristically the two radial lumbricals. The *palmar digital* branches supply the flexor skin of the radial three and a half digits, and the nail beds and distal dorsal skin of these digits.

The **medial cutaneous nerve of the arm** (C8, T1) is the smallest branch of the plexus. It is sometimes replaced entirely by the intercostobrachial nerve. It runs down with the axillary vein to pierce the deep fascia and supply skin on the medial aspect of the arm.

The **medial cutaneous nerve of the forearm** (C8, T1) is a much bigger nerve than the last. It runs down between axillary artery and vein and pierces the deep fascia half way to the elbow, often in common with the basilic vein. It supplies the lower part of the front of

Fig. 2.45 Nerves on the anterior aspect of the left upper limb.

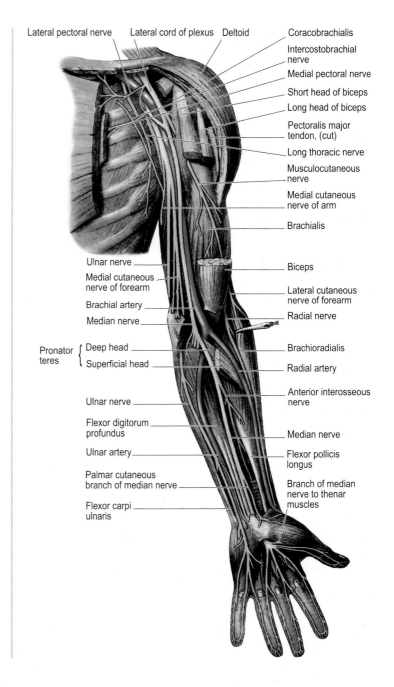

Lateral pectoral nerve
Lateral cord of plexus
Deltoid
Coracobrachialis
Intercostobrachial nerve
Medial pectoral nerve
Short head of biceps
Long head of biceps
Pectoralis major tendon, (cut)
Long thoracic nerve
Musculocutaneous nerve
Medial cutaneous nerve of arm
Brachialis
Ulnar nerve
Medial cutaneous nerve of forearm
Brachial artery
Median nerve
Biceps
Lateral cutaneous nerve of forearm
Radial nerve
Pronator teres { Deep head / Superficial head
Brachioradialis
Radial artery
Anterior interosseous nerve
Ulnar nerve
Flexor digitorum profundus
Ulnar artery
Palmar cutaneous branch of median nerve
Flexor carpi ulnaris
Median nerve
Flexor pollicis longus
Branch of median nerve to thenar muscles

the arm above the elbow and then divides into anterior and posterior branches to supply the skin along the ulnar border of the forearm down to the wrist. In the forearm it is symmetrical with the lateral cutaneous nerve (musculocutaneous) and the two meet without overlap along the anterior axial line. Their territories are

separated posteriorly by the posterior cutaneous branch of the radial nerve.

The **ulnar nerve** (C7, 8, T1) is the direct continuation of the medial cord (C8, T1), with additional C7 fibres picked up in the axilla, usually from the lateral cord. The nerve supplies some flexor muscles on the ulnar side

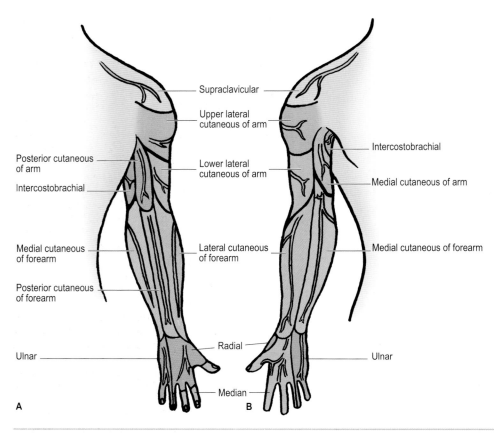

Fig. 2.46   Cutaneous nerves of the right upper limb, **A** from behind, **B** from the front. Compare with the dermatomes on Figure 1.9, page 14.

of the forearm, most of the intrinsic muscles of the hand and the skin of the ulnar one and a half digits.

Running down between the axillary artery and vein, behind the medial cutaneous nerve of the forearm, the ulnar nerve pierces the medial intermuscular septum and descends in the groove on the back of the base of the medial epicondyle. It passes between the two heads of flexor carpi ulnaris and enters the flexor compartment of the forearm. It descends on flexor digitorum profundus, under cover of flexor carpi ulnaris. Here it is joined on its lateral side by the ulnar artery. The two emerge from beneath the tendon of flexor carpi ulnaris just above the wrist and cross the flexor retinaculum lateral to the pisiform bone.

Branches. Articular twigs are given to the elbow joint as the nerve lies on its medial collateral ligament. In the forearm the nerve supplies flexor carpi ulnaris and the ulnar half (usually) of flexor digitorum profundus. It has a *palmar cutaneous* branch which pierces the deep fascia

above the flexor retinaculum to supply skin over the hypothenar muscles. A *dorsal cutaneous* branch winds around the lower end of the ulna deep to the tendon of flexor carpi ulnaris and is distributed to the dorsal skin of one and a half fingers (except that over the distal phalanx of the little finger, and the middle and distal phalanges of the ring finger) and a corresponding area of the back of the hand. Not uncommonly it supplies two and a half instead of one and a half fingers.

The ulnar nerve divides on the flexor retinaculum alongside the pisiform bone. The *superficial branch* runs distally beneath palmaris brevis (which it supplies) and is distributed by two digital branches to the ulnar one and a half fingers, including their nail beds and the skin on the dorsum not supplied by the dorsal branch.

The *deep branch* passes deeply between abductor and flexor digiti minimi then through opponens. It supplies all three hypothenar muscles. It grooves the distal border of the hook of the hamate and crosses the palm in the concavity of the deep palmar arch, supplying the two ulnar lumbricals and all the interossei, both palmar and dorsal. It ends by supplying adductor pollicis.

Branches of the posterior cord

C5, 6 Upper subscapular
C6–8 Thoracodorsal
C5, 6 Lower subscapular
C5, 6 Axillary
C5–8, T1 Radial.

The **upper** and **lower subscapular nerves** (C5, 6) supply the respective parts of subscapularis, with the lower nerve also innervating teres major.

The **thoracodorsal nerve** (nerve to latissimus dorsi) (C6–8) inclines forwards and enters the deep surface of latissimus dorsi just behind the anterior border. Its terminal part lies anterior to the thoracodorsal artery and it is vulnerable in operations on the axillary lymph nodes.

The **axillary nerve** (C5, 6) passes backwards through the quadrangular space (Fig. 2.9), lying above the posterior circumflex humeral vessels and the glistening tendon of latissimus dorsi (as it overlaps teres major) just below the capsule of the shoulder joint, which it supplies. In the quadrangular space it divides. The *posterior branch* supplies teres minor and winds around the posterior border of deltoid, supplying it, and continuing as the *upper lateral cutaneous nerve of the arm* to supply skin over the lower half of deltoid and the upper part of the back of the arm. The *anterior branch* curves round the surgical neck of the humerus, deep to deltoid which it supplies as well as a small area of overlying skin.

The **radial nerve** (C5–8, T1) is the nerve of the extensor compartments of the arm and forearm, supplying skin over them and on the dorsum of the hand. A direct continuation of the posterior cord, the radial nerve passes beyond the posterior wall of the axilla, below the easily identifiable tendon of latissimus dorsi, running dorsally downwards between the long and medial heads of triceps. It spirals across the back of the humerus, between the lateral and medial heads of triceps, lying on the radial groove of the bone, deep to the lateral head. It pierces the lateral intermuscular septum one-third of the way down from the deltoid tuberosity to the lateral epicondyle. In the flexor compartment of the lower arm it descends in the intermuscular slit between brachialis and brachioradialis. After giving off the posterior interosseous branch, the rather slender remnant, purely cutaneous now, retains the name of radial nerve. It runs down the flexor compartment of the forearm, winds around the lower end of the radius deep to the tendon

of brachioradialis and crosses abductor pollicis longus, extensor pollicis brevis and extensor pollicis longus (as one of the contents of the anatomical snuffbox) to reach the back of the hand. Here it supplies the skin of the radial two and a half or three and a half digits (falling short of the nail beds and distal and middle phalanges) and a corresponding area of the dorsum of the hand.

Branches. The *posterior cutaneous nerve of the arm* arises in the axilla and pierces the deep fascia to supply a strip of skin along the extensor surface of the arm down to the elbow. The triceps is supplied by four radial nerve branches. They arise as *nerves to the long, medial, lateral* and *medial heads*, the first two being given off in the axilla and the last two behind the humerus. The first branch to the medial head (the *ulnar collateral nerve*) runs down with the ulnar nerve to enter the lower part of the medial head. The second branch to the medial head continues deep to triceps to supply anconeus.

The *lower lateral cutaneous nerve of the arm* pierces the lateral head of triceps to supply skin over the lateral surface of the arm down to the elbow. In common with it arises the *posterior cutaneous nerve of the forearm* which runs straight down behind the elbow to supply a strip of skin over the extensor surface of the forearm as far as the wrist.

While lying in the flexor compartment of the forearm between brachialis and brachioradialis, the main trunk gives a small branch to the lateral part of brachialis and supplies brachioradialis and extensor carpi radialis longus. At the level of the lateral epicondyle it gives off the posterior interosseous branch, and then continues on as the terminal cutaneous branch already described.

The *posterior interosseous nerve* supplies extensor carpi radialis brevis and supinator in the cubital fossa, and then spirals down around the upper end of the radius between the two layers of supinator to enter the extensor compartment of the forearm. It crosses abductor pollicis longus, dips down to the interosseous membrane and runs to the back of the wrist. In the extensor compartment it supplies seven more muscles; three extensors from the common extensor origin (extensor digitorum, extensor digiti minimi, and extensor carpi ulnaris), the three thumb muscles (abductor pollicis longus, extensor pollicis brevis and extensor pollicis longus) and extensor indicis. It is sensory to the wrist and carpal joints.

PART **ELEVEN**

Summary of upper limb nerve injuries

In order to obtain a quick appraisal of the integrity of a major limb nerve it is not necessary to test every muscle supplied. Usually a key muscle and action can be selected that will indicate whether or not the nerve is intact. The following summary includes notes on selected nerve injuries and methods for exposing nerves if exploration or repair is required.

Brachial plexus

Damage to the *whole plexus* is rare but devastating. The most common cause is a motorbike accident, landing on the shoulder with the neck being forced in the opposite direction, so avulsing the nerve roots. If all the roots are damaged the whole limb is immobile and anaesthetic, and Horner's syndrome (see p. 423) may be present, on account of the connections between nerve roots and the sympathetic trunk. If serratus anterior and the rhomboids are still in action, the damage is distal to the root origins of the dorsal scapular and long thoracic nerves; if supraspinatus and infraspinatus escape, the damage is distal to the upper trunk.

The most common *traction injury* to the plexus is to the upper roots and trunk (C5 and 6—Erb's paralysis) and includes birth injury (Erb–Duchenne paralysis). The abductors and lateral rotators of the shoulder and the supinators are paralysed so that the arm hangs by the side, medially rotated, extended at the elbow and pronated, with loss of sensation on the lateral side of the arm and forearm.

Damage to the *lowest roots* (C8 and T1) is unusual (as with a cervical rib) but includes Klumpke's paralysis due to birth injury during a breech delivery where the arm remains above the head. The small muscles of the hand are those most obviously affected, leading to 'claw hand' with inability to extend the fingers, and sensory loss on the ulnar side of the forearm.

Pectoralis major, being the only muscle supplied by all five segments of the plexus, may be a useful guide to the extent of a plexus injury.

Surgical approach. The supraclavicular part of the plexus can be exposed in the angle between sternocleidomastoid and the clavicle. The inferior belly of omohyoid and the lateral branches of the thyrocervical trunk are divided and the roots of the plexus are identified behind scalenus anterior, which needs to be retracted or severed (carefully avoiding damage to the phrenic nerve) to display the lower trunk. To expose the infraclavicular part, the deltopectoral groove is opened up and pectoralis minor detached from the coracoid process so that the plexus branches around the axillary artery can be dissected out from the axillary sheath. The middle part of the clavicle may have to be removed if a more proximal exposure is needed.

Axillary nerve

The nerve may be damaged in 5% of dislocations of the shoulder, in fractures of the upper end of the humerus or by misplaced injections into deltoid; shoulder abduction is weak and there is a small area of anaesthesia over the lower part of the muscle.

Musculocutaneous nerve

This nerve is rarely injured. Its function may be assessed by testing for elbow flexion by biceps, while palpating the muscle.

Surgical approach. Exposure of the nerve involves opening up the deltopectoral groove and identifying the nerve as it enters coracobrachialis from the lateral cord of the plexus.

Radial nerve

The nerve is most commonly injured high up, by fractures of the shaft of the humerus. The characteristic lesion is 'wrist drop' with inability to extend the wrist and metacarpophalangeal joints (but the interphalangeal joints can still be straightened by the action of the interossei and lumbricals). Sensory loss is minimal and usually confined to a small area overlying the first dorsal interosseous, on account of overlap from the median and ulnar nerves. Transient paralysis may be due to improper use of a crutch pressing on the nerve in the axilla, or 'Saturday night palsy' from draping the arm over a chair when in a state of diminished consciousness. With such high injuries, triceps paralysis can be detected by testing elbow extension. As branches to the long and medial heads of triceps arise in the axilla, elbow extension is not lost after nerve injury following humeral shaft fracture.

Surgical approach. The radial nerve in the arm may be exposed from the back by developing the interval between the long and lateral heads of triceps to reveal the nerve as it crosses the upper part of the medial head before coming to lie in the radial groove (Fig. 2.17). At the elbow brachioradialis and extensor carpi radialis longus are retracted laterally to show the nerve dividing into its superficial and deep (posterior interosseous) branches. The superficial part of supinator can be incised if the deep branch has to be followed downwards.

Ulnar nerve

This is most commonly injured behind the elbow or at the wrist. The classical sign of a low lesion is 'claw hand' (Fig. 2.47), with hyperextension of the

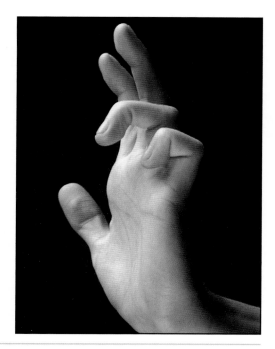

Fig. 2.47 'Claw hand' due to a lesion of the ulnar nerve at the wrist.

metacarpophalangeal joints of the ring and little fingers and flexion of the interphalangeal joints because their interossei and lumbricals are paralysed and so cannot flex the metacarpophalangeal joints or extend the interphalangeal joints. The claw is produced by the unopposed action of the finger extensors and of flexor digitorum profundus. Injury at the elbow or above gives straighter fingers ('ulnar paradox') because the ulnar half of flexor digitorum profundus is now out of action and cannot flex the distal interphalangeal joints of the ring and little fingers. Wasting of interossei eventually becomes obvious on the dorsum of the hand, giving the appearance of 'guttering' between the metacarpals. There is variable sensory loss on the ulnar side of the hand and on the little and ring fingers but often less than might be expected.

Testing for abduction of the index finger by the first dorsal interosseous assesses small muscle function in the hand that is dependent on an intact ulnar nerve supply. Paralysis of the ulnar half of flexor digitorum profundus by a high lesion can be detected by the inability to flex the distal interphalangeal joint of the little finger.

Surgical approach. Exposure of the ulnar nerve in the arm is along the medial border of biceps, where the nerve is medial to the brachial artery. At the elbow it is easily approached behind the medial epicondyle, and in the forearm it can be followed upwards from the

pisiform, where it lies between the bone and ulnar artery, by displacing flexor carpi ulnaris medially.

Median nerve

This is most commonly injured at the wrist—by cuts, or compression in the carpal tunnel. Theoretically there is sensory loss over the radial three fingers and radial side of the palm, but the only autonomous areas of median nerve supply are over the pulp pads of the index and middle fingers. With high lesions of long duration, there is wasting of the front of the forearm because the long flexors (except flexor carpi ulnaris and half of flexor digitorum profundus) and the pronators are paralysed. Typically the hand is held with the index finger straight, in the 'pointing finger' position, often with all other fingers flexed, including the middle finger. Although the part of flexor digitorum profundus to the middle finger tendon usually has a median supply (like the whole of superficialis), its close connection with the part supplied by the ulnar nerve can lead to middle finger flexion, and this part of the muscle may even be supplied by the ulnar nerve. Furthermore the branch to the index finger part of the flexor digitorum superficialis arises near the mid-forearm, rather than in the cubital fossa. For high lesions, test flexor pollicis longus and finger flexors by pinching together the pads of thumb and index finger. Following lesions at wrist level, abduction of the thumb is not possible, and in longstanding cases there is wasting of the thenar eminence (especially abductor pollicis brevis).

Surgical approach. In the mid-arm the median nerve is easily exposed by incision along the medial border of biceps, where the nerve is anterior to the brachial artery, and in the cubital fossa they lie medial to the biceps tendon. In the forearm it is displayed by detaching the radial head of flexor digitorum superficialis from the radius and turning the muscle medially to show the nerve adhering to its deep surface. Relief of compression in the carpal tunnel involves incising the flexor retinaculum longitudinally on the ulnar side of the nerve, to avoid damage to the muscular (recurrent) branch which usually arises immediately distal to the retinaculum and curves radially into the thenar muscles.

PART TWELVE

Osteology of the upper limb

Clavicle

The clavicle is longer and its curvatures are more pronounced in the male. The medial two-thirds is rounded

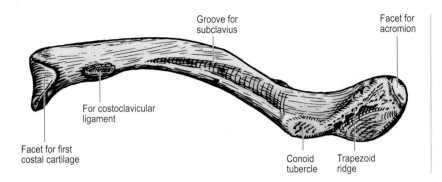

Groove for subclavius

Facet for acromion

Fig. 2.48   Left clavicle, from below.

For costoclavicular ligament

Facet for first costal cartilage

Conoid tubercle

Trapezoid ridge

and convex forwards. The lateral one-third is flat, and curves back to meet the scapula. The upper surface is smoother than the lower. The bone lies horizontally and is subcutaneous, crossed by the supraclavicular nerves.

The bulbous sternal end (Fig. 2.7) has a facet for the sternoclavicular joint. The articular area extends to the under surface, for articulation with the first costal cartilage (Fig. 2.48), and is covered in life by fibrocartilage. The capsule and synovial membrane are attached around the margin of the articular surface. The upper surface receives the interclavicular ligament alongside the capsule attachment.

The clavicular head of sternocleidomastoid arises from the medial third of this surface. Anteriorly, pectoralis major is attached to the medial half and the lateral third gives origin to deltoid. Trapezius is attached to the lateral third posteriorly. Two layers of cervical fascia surround sternocleidomastoid and trapezius and are attached separately to the bone between these muscles, at the base of the posterior triangle (Fig. 2.2).

The lower surface shows a rough area next to the sternal end for attachment of the costoclavicular ligament. A *groove for subclavius* occupies the middle third of this surface and the clavipectoral fascia is attached to the margins of the groove (Fig. 2.2). A nutrient foramen extends laterally in this groove. At the junction of the lateral fourth and the rest of the shaft the *conoid tubercle* marks the attachment of the conoid ligament (Fig. 2.8). From here the rough *trapezoid ridge* extends obliquely to near the lateral articular facet and provides attachment for the trapezoid ligament.

The acromial end has a facet which faces laterally and slightly downwards for articulation with the acromion. The capsule and synovial membrane are attached to the margin of the articular surface, which like that at the sternal end is covered by fibrocartilage.

Fracture of the clavicle is common; when due to indirect violence as in a fall on the outstretched hand, the break is always between the costoclavicular and coracoclavicular ligaments, each of which is stronger than the clavicle itself.

Ossification. The clavicle is the first bone to begin ossifying in the fetus. It does so in membrane from two centres, which ossify at the fifth week and rapidly fuse. A secondary centre appears at the sternal end during the late teens and fuses rapidly.

Scapula

The scapula is a flat triangular bone. The lateral angle is thick to accommodate the glenoid cavity, and projected upwards into the bent coracoid process (Figs 2.49 and 2.50). The lateral border is thick down to the inferior angle. The rest of the blade is composed of thin, translucent bone. From the upper part of the dorsal surface a triangular spine projects back and extends laterally as a curved plate of bone, the acromion, over the shoulder joint (Fig. 2.12).

The *costal surface* is concave, and marked by three or four ridges that converge from the medial border towards the lateral angle. These give attachment to fibrous septa from which the multipennate fibres of subscapularis arise. This muscle is attached to the medial two-thirds of the costal surface. The lateral third is bare and separated from the overlying muscle by the subscapularis bursa. The medial margin of the costal surface receives the insertion of serratus anterior. The first two digitations are attached from the superior angle down to the base of the spine. The next two digitations are thinned out from this level down to the inferior angle, while the last four digitations converge to a roughened area on the costal surface of the inferior angle.

The upper border of the blade slants downwards and laterally to the root of the coracoid process, beside which it dips to form the scapular notch, which lodges the suprascapular nerve. The notch is bridged by the suprascapular ligament. The inferior belly of omohyoid arises from this ligament and the nearby scapular upper

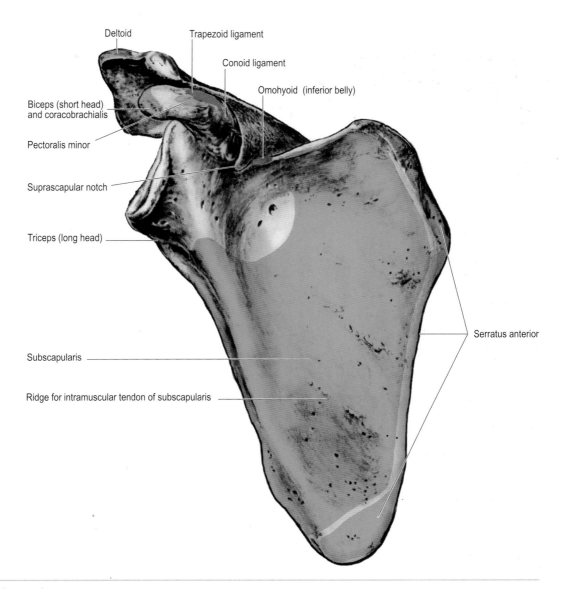

Fig. 2.49 Right scapula: anterior aspect.

border. The medial (vertebral) border, from superior to inferior angle, gives edge to edge attachment to levator scapulae, rhomboid minor and rhomboid major. The lateral (axillary) border extends from the glenoid cavity to the inferior angle. Just below the glenoid fossa is the infraglenoid tubercle (this may be depressed into a fossa), which gives origin to the long head of triceps.

The *dorsal surface* of the blade is divided by the backwardly projecting spine into a small supraspinous and a large infraspinous fossa. The supraspinatus and the infraspinatus arise from the medial two-thirds of their respective fossae and the adjacent area of the spine. Teres major arises from a large oval area at the inferior angle, and teres minor from an elongated narrower area dorsal to the lateral border. This origin of teres minor is commonly bisected by a groove made by the circumflex scapular vessels.

The thick *spine* projects back from a horizontal attachment on the dorsal surface of the blade. It is twisted a little, so its posterior border slopes upwards towards the

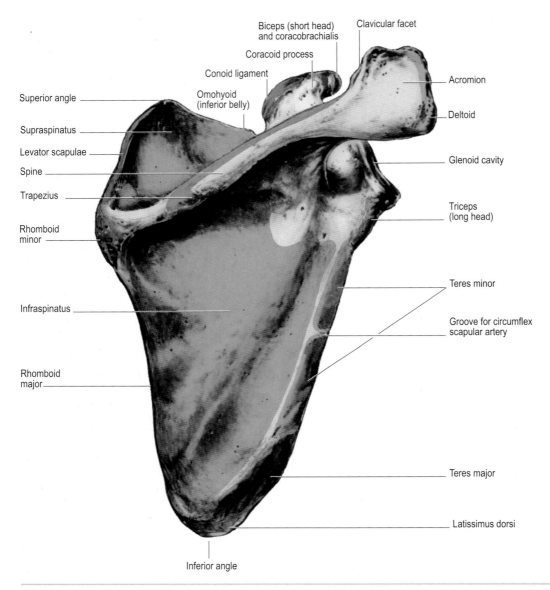

Superior angle

Supraspinatus

Levator scapulae

Spine

Trapezius

Rhomboid minor

Infraspinatus

Rhomboid major

Omohyoid (inferior belly)

Conoid ligament

Coracoid process

Biceps (short head) and coracobrachialis

Clavicular facet

Acromion

Deltoid

Glenoid cavity

Triceps (long head)

Teres minor

Groove for circumflex scapular artery

Teres major

Latissimus dorsi

Inferior angle

Fig. 2.50   Right scapula: posterior aspect.

acromion. Its free lateral border is concave outwards, forming a notch with the back of the lateral angle. The suprascapular vessels and nerve run across this notch to reach the infraspinous fossa. The rectangular *acromion* projects forwards from the lateral end of the spine. The dorsal surface of the spine and acromion are subcutaneous and palpable. Trapezius is attached to the medial border of the acromion and the upper margin of the spine. The attachment curves around a tubercle

just lateral to the medial end of the spine; the lowermost fibres of trapezius converge here. The medial end of the spine is smooth and separated from trapezius by a bursa. Deltoid arises along the inferior margin of the spine and from the posterior, lateral and anterior borders of the acromion. Along its lateral border the acromion shows four or more vertical ridges for attachment of septa in the multipennate central mass of the deltoid. Close to the anterior end of the medial border is the facet for the acromioclavicular joint. In front of the facet the fibres of the coracoacromial ligament converge (Fig. 2.11). Beneath this ligament and the bare bone of the acromion the subacromial (subdeltoid) bursa lubricates the tendon of supraspinatus and the rotator cuff. Above the coracoacromial ligament the deltoid origin continues across the acromion to the lateral part of the clavicle.

The lateral angle of the scapula is wedge-shaped, broadening from the narrow neck out to the prominent margins of the *glenoid cavity*. The upper part of this wedge-shaped bone is projected upwards as the base of the coracoid process. The cavity does not face directly lateral, but peeps forwards a little around the convexity of the chest wall. The margins of the cavity are made more prominent by the attachment of the glenoid labrum. At the upper end of the glenoid rim is the *supraglenoid tubercle*, for attachment of the long head of biceps within the shoulder joint capsule. The capsule is attached to the labrum and to the surrounding bone; The *infraglenoid tubercle* lies below this.

The *coracoid process* rises from its broad base and curves forward and outward like a bent finger. Its tip is palpable by pressing backwards and laterally just below the clavicle, under cover of the anterior margin of deltoid. The process is for muscle and ligament attachments, the ligaments being indispensable to the stability of the pectoral girdle. The conoid ligament is attached by its apex to the knuckle of the coracoid process (Figs 2.49 and 2.50). From here a line runs towards the tip for attachment of the trapezoid ligament. The lateral margin of the process gives attachment to the base of the coracoacromial ligament. The weaker coracohumeral ligament sweeps from the undersurface of the coracoid process to the anatomical neck of the humerus. The pectoralis minor is attached to the medial border and upper surface of the coracoid process. To the tip is attached the short head of biceps and the coracobrachialis.

Ossification. The scapula ossifies in cartilage from several centres. Ossification commences in the eighth week of intrauterine life. Secondary centres for the acromion, coracoid process, glenoid cavity, medial border and inferior angle appear at about puberty, and fuse by about 20 years. The base of the coracoid process and the upper part of the glenoid cavity ossify from the same centre (Fig. 2.8).

Humerus

The shaft of the humerus expands above into an upper end whose articular surface looks up and back (Fig. 2.51). The lower part of the shaft curves gently forwards to a flat lower end projected into medial and lateral epicondyles, between which lie the capitulum and trochlea for articulation at the elbow joint. The medial epicondyle projects in the same direction as the articular surface of the head and is much more prominent than the lateral epicondyle.

The upper end, expanded above the shaft, consists of the convex articular surface and the tubercles (tuberosities) (Fig. 2.51). The articular surface is the head, and the articular margin is the *anatomical neck*. At the junction of the expanded upper end and the shaft is the *surgical neck*; the axillary nerve winds round behind it. Fractures tend to occur here in the elderly.

The *head* (articular surface) forms about one-third of a sphere and is about four times the area of the glenoid cavity of the scapula. It is coated with hyaline cartilage. At rest its lower and anterior quadrant articulates with the glenoid cavity, giving a good range of lateral rotation and abduction from this position. The capsule of the shoulder joint, bridging the bicipital sulcus as the transverse ligament, is attached to the articular margin except medially, where it extends down along the shaft for 2 cm, here enclosing the epiphyseal line.

The *lesser tubercle* (tuberosity) projects prominently forwards, and is continued downwards as the medial lip of the bicipital sulcus. The tendon of subscapularis is inserted on the tubercle and teres major on the medial lip. The *intertubercular sulcus* (formerly the bicipital groove) lies on the anterior surface of the upper end. It is bridged above by the transverse humeral ligament, deep to which the long tendon of biceps leaves the joint. The floor of the sulcus receives the tendon of latissimus dorsi.

The *greater tubercle* (tuberosity) is bare except at its projecting junction with the head, where there are three smooth facets for insertion of the tendons of scapular muscles. Superiorly is the facet for supraspinatus, behind this the facet for infraspinatus, while posteriorly the lowest facet receives teres minor (Fig. 2.52). Below this tendon the bone lies in contact with the axillary nerve and its vessels. The lateral lip of the bicipital sulcus extends down from the anterior margin of the greater tubercle and receives the tendon of pectoralis major.

Much of the *shaft* is triangular in section. The *deltoid tuberosity* is at the middle of the lateral side of the shaft. The tuberosity is a V-shaped prominent ridge, with a smaller ridge between, the three giving attachment to fibrous septa in the multipennate acromial fibres of the deltoid. Below the deltoid tuberosity the lower end of the *radial groove* spirals down. The lower margin of the groove continues as the lateral supracondylar ridge which runs down to the lateral epicondyle. The ridge gives attachment to the lateral intermuscular septum. The less marked medial supracondylar ridge runs down to the prominent medial epicondyle. The ridge gives

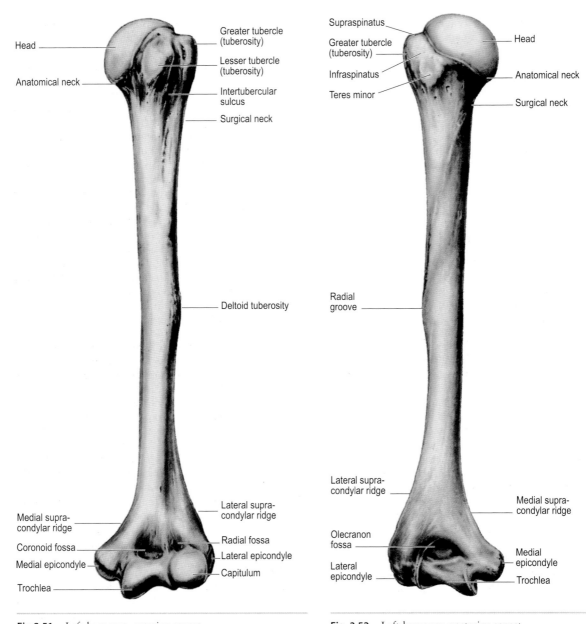

Fig 2.51   Left humerus: anterior aspect.

Fig. 2.52   Left humerus: posterior aspect.

attachment to the medial intermuscular septum. Level with the lower part of the deltoid tuberosity the nutrient foramen, directed down towards the elbow, lies in front of this medial border of the humerus. Above this foramen, opposite the deltoid tuberosity, coracobrachialis is inserted. The flexor surface of the humerus, between the supracondylar ridges, gives origin to brachialis and this

extends upwards to embrace the deltoid tuberosity both in the lower part of the spiral groove and between the tuberosity and the insertion of coracobrachialis.

Viewed from behind the shaft appears twisted due to the radial groove. The lateral (superior) lip of this groove gives attachment to the lateral head of triceps. The medial head of triceps arises from the whole shaft between the supracondylar ridges up to the medial (inferior) lip of the groove. Between the origins of medial and lateral heads the radial nerve and profunda brachii vessels lie in the radial groove.

The lower end of the humerus carries the articular surface for the elbow joint and is projected into medial and lateral epicondyles for attachment of muscles for the flexor and extensor compartments of the forearm. Anterior and posterior appearances are quite different. The articular surface, coated with hyaline cartilage, shows the conjoined capitulum and trochlea. The *capitulum*, for articulation with the head of the radius, is a section of a sphere. It projects forwards and inferiorly from the lateral part and is not visible from the posterior aspect. The *trochlea*, unlike the capitulum, extends also to the posterior surface. Its medial margin is a sharp ridge curving prominently from front to back around the lower end of the humerus. The medial part of the trochlea is at a more distal level than the capitulum, which is a causative factor for the carrying angle at the elbow.

The anterior surface of the shaft of the lower end of the humerus shows a shallow coronoid fossa above the trochlea and a shallow radial fossa above the capitulum. A deep olecranon fossa is seen on the posterior surface. The capsule of the elbow joint is attached to the ridges that form the margins of the capitulum and trochlea and to the shaft of the humerus above the coronoid and radial fossae in front and the olecranon fossa behind.

The *medial epicondyle* has a smooth facet on its anterior surface for the common flexor origin of forearm muscles. Pronator teres arises also from the medial supracondylar ridge just above this. Posteriorly, between the epicondyle and the curving ridge of the trochlea, is a groove which lodges the ulnar nerve. On the distal border of this epicondyle is a small facet for attachment of the ulnar collateral (medial) ligament of the elbow joint.

The *lateral epicondyle* has a smooth facet on its anterior surface for the common extensor origin of forearm muscles. Above this brachioradialis arises from the upper two-thirds and extensor carpi radialis longus from the lower one-third of the lateral supracondylar ridge. At the distal border of the epicondyle the radial collateral (lateral) ligament of the elbow and the superficial fibres of supinator are attached. Anconeus arises from the posterior surface.

Surgical approach. The shaft can be exposed from the front by opening up the deltopectoral groove, and lower down by splitting brachialis vertically. The splitting incision is made anterolaterally and obliquely towards the middle of the front of the shaft, to keep well away from the brachial artery and median nerve. The radial nerve must be remembered when stripping periosteum from the lateral side of the lower part of the shaft.

Exposure of the shaft from behind involves opening up the interval between the long and lateral heads of triceps and splitting the medial head vertically in the midline, avoiding the profunda vessels and the radial nerve with its branches to triceps.

Ossification. A primary centre appears in the centre of the shaft at the eighth week. Upper and lower ends are cartilaginous at birth. Three secondary centres appear at the upper end for the head, greater and lesser tubercles in the first few years after birth. They fuse into a single bony epiphysis. This is the growing end of the bone and fusion occurs with the shaft at about 20 years. Four secondary centres appear at the lower end. The three centres that form the trochlea, capitulum and lateral epicondyle fuse into a single epiphysis, which fuses with the shaft at about 15 years. The medial epicondyle remains as a separate centre, which fuses with a downward projection of the shaft at about 20 years. This late fusion needs to be kept in mind when interpreting radiographs of the elbow region in adolescents.

Radius

The radius has a cylindrical head, which articulates with the capitulum of the humerus, connected by a shaft with a broad distal end, which articulates with the cuboid and the lunate (Fig. 2.53).

The *head* is cylindrical and is covered with hyaline cartilage. It is palpable in the depression behind the lateral side of the extended elbow, where it can be felt rotating in pronation–supination movements. A spherical hollow forms the upper surface, to fit the capitulum. The cylindrical circumference is vertically deepest on the medial side where it articulates with the radial notch of the ulna, while the rest of the circumference articulates with the annular ligament. The narrow *neck* is enclosed by the tapered lower margin of the annular ligament, below which the loose fibres of the quadrate ligament are attached on the medial side.

The *shaft* is characterized at its upper end by an oval prominence, the *radial tuberosity*, projecting towards the ulna. The biceps tendon is attached along the posterior lip, and a bursa lies against the anterior surface of the tuberosity. From the anterior margin of the tuberosity the anterior oblique line forms a ridge that runs down to the point of greatest convexity of the shaft. It is mirrored by a similar, but less prominent, posterior oblique line on the extensor surface of the shaft. Between the two oblique lines the shaft is cylindrical and receives the insertion of supinator. Pronator teres is attached to the greatest convexity of the radius at the middle of its lateral border.

Below the tuberosity the shaft is pinched into a ridge for the interosseous membrane of the forearm. The

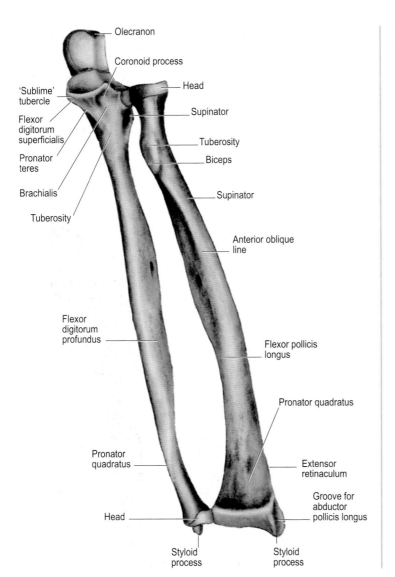

Olecranon

Coronoid process

Head

'Sublime' tubercle

Supinator

Flexor digitorum superficialis

Tuberosity

Pronator teres

Biceps

Brachialis

Supinator

Tuberosity

Anterior oblique line

Flexor digitorum profundus

Flexor pollicis longus

Pronator quadratus

Pronator quadratus

Extensor retinaculum

Groove for abductor pollicis longus

Head

Styloid process

Styloid process

Fig. 2.53 Left radius and ulna, from the front, with sites of muscle attachment indicated.

oblique cord is attached at the upper end and passes up to the ulna; the fibres of the interosseous membrane pass down to the ulna. On the flexor surface the flexor digitorum superficialis is attached to the anterior oblique line, and flexor pollicis longus arises below this down to pronator quadratus. The lower part of the flexor surface is hollowed out above the expanded lower extremity; here pronator quadratus is inserted into the lower one-fifth of the shaft. On the extensor surface below the posterior oblique line is the oblique origin of abductor pollicis longus and distal to this is the origin of extensor pollicis brevis.

The lower end of the bone is expanded and rectangular in transverse section. The ulnar surface shows a notch for articulation with the head of the ulna. Above this is a triangular area which receives pronator quadratus and has the interosseous membrane attached to its posterior edge.

Laterally the lower end is projected into the pyramidal *styloid process*, to the tip of which the radial collateral ligament of the wrist joint is attached and into whose base the tendon of brachioradialis is inserted. The extensor retinaculum is attached to the anterolateral border above the styloid process. This fascial band runs obliquely to its distal attachment on the ulnar side of the carpus. Septa pass from its deep surface to the radius, making compartments for the extensor tendons. Four compartments lie on the posterior surface of the lower end of the radius, and a fifth over the radioulnar joint (Fig. 2.54). The sixth and last compartment lies over the head of the ulna. The tendons of abductor pollicis longus and extensor pollicis brevis lie in a single compartment on the lateral surface. On the posterior surface a broad groove lies lateral to the prominent *dorsal tubercle* (of Lister). It lodges the flat tendons of extensors carpi radialis longus and brevis, sharing a single compartment. On the ulnar side of the dorsal tubercle is a narrow groove that lodges the tendon of extensor pollicis longus in a separate compartment. Between this and the ulnar notch is another broad groove. In the one compartment here lie the four tendons of extensor digitorum with the tendon of extensor indicis deep to them. The tendon of extensor digiti minimi crosses the radioulnar joint in a separate compartment.

Fig. 2.54   Left radius and ulna, from behind, with sites of muscle attachment indicated.

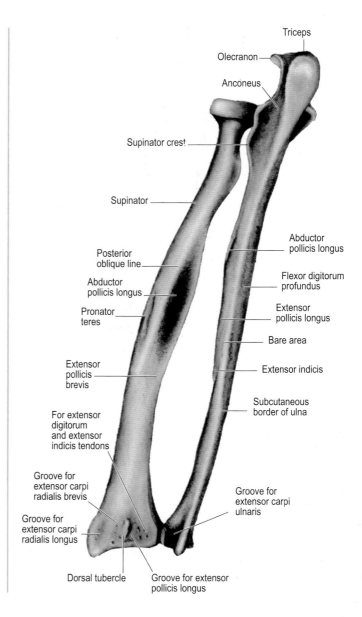

109

Inferiorly the articular surface for the wrist joint has two concave areas covered with hyaline cartilage. The ulnar (medial) surface is square, and articulates with the lunate. To the right-angled border between this surface and the ulnar notch is attached the triangular fibrocartilage which separates the distal radioulnar and wrist joints from each other. The lateral concave area is triangular, with its apex on the styloid process. It articulates with the scaphoid.

This expanded lower end takes the full thrust (via the thenar eminence) of a fall on the outstretched hand, and may lead to Colles' fracture of the lower end. The distal fragment characteristically undergoes lateral and dorsal rotation and displacement, with impaction.

Surgical approach. The head is exposed as for the lateral approach to the elbow joint (see p. 66) by detaching the common extensor origin from the lateral epicondyle of the humerus and incising the capsule. The shaft is exposed from the front. At the upper end brachioradialis and the two radial extensors are mobilized laterally and supinator with its underlying periosteum is detached from the bone, working laterally from the radial tuberosity with the posterior interosseous nerve sandwiched within the muscle. The nerve will not be damaged if the full thickness of the muscle with its periosteum is gently retracted from the bone. Lower down the shaft is exposed between brachioradialis laterally and flexor carpi radialis medially, while the lower end can be approached lateral to flexor carpi radialis by detaching pronator quadratus from the radius and turning it medially. The radial artery lateral to the flexor carpi radialis tendon and the median nerve medial to it need to be safeguarded.

Ossification. The radius starts ossifying in cartilage from a centre in the middle of the shaft at the eighth week. There are secondary centres for the head and the lower end. The lower is the growing end. The upper epiphysis fuses at about 15 years and the lower epiphysis at about 20 years.

Ulna

The ulna tapers in the reverse way to the radius; it is large above and small at its distal extremity, where the head is situated (the head of the radius is at its upper end) (Figs 2.53 and 2.54).

The upper end has two projections, with a saddle-shaped articular surface between them. They are the olecranon and coronoid process, and they grip the trochlear surface of the humerus.

The *olecranon* is the posteriorly situated proximal extension of the shaft, subcutaneous and easily palpable, and in extension of the elbow it is lodged in the olecranon fossa of the humerus. It is bent forwards and has an upper surface that receives the tendon of triceps over a wide area, and has an anterior border that forms a sharp undulating lip at the articular margin; the capsule of the elbow joint is attached just behind this lip. The triangular posterior surface is subcutaneous; the olecranon bursa lies on it. The sides of the triangle are continued below the apex into the sinuous subcutaneous border of the shaft; they give attachment to the deep fascia of the forearm. Flexor digitorum profundus arises from the medial surface of the olecranon. At the upper angle of this area the posterior band of the ulnar collateral (medial) ligament of the elbow is attached. Anconeus is inserted on to the lateral surface of the olecranon.

The *coronoid process* projects forwards from the upper end of the shaft. Its anterior lip is thin and abuts on the articular margin. Medially this lip shows a prominent smooth elevation, the 'sublime' tubercle. Flexor digitorum superficialis is attached here, and deep to this the ulnar collateral (medial) ligament of the elbow. The ulnar nerve lies in contact with the ligament (Fig. 2.22). Distal to the tubercle the deep head of pronator teres is attached to the medial border of the coronoid process. The concave anterior surface of the coronoid process receives the insertion of brachialis, the rough lower part of this surface forming the *ulnar tuberosity*.

The lateral surface of the coronoid process carries a concave facet, the radial notch for the head of the radius, and this surface, covered with hyaline cartilage, continues into that of the trochlear surface. The anterior and posterior margins of the notch give attachment to the annular ligament, while the quadrate ligament is attached to the shaft just below the notch. Just below this the oblique cord is attached.

Between the projections of the olecranon and coronoid process is a deeply saddle-shaped surface, the *trochlear notch*. Convex from side to side, it is concave from top to bottom and fits the trochlea of the humerus. It is covered with hyaline cartilage, which is sometimes constricted in an hour-glass shape or even separated into two surfaces, one on the olecranon and one on the coronoid process. The capsule of the elbow joint is attached around the margins of the trochlear notch and the radial notch; thus the elbow and proximal radioulnar joints form one cavity.

The *shaft* is angled somewhat laterally from the line of the trochlear notch to form the carrying angle (Fig. 2.29). From the posterior margin of the radial notch a vertical ridge runs distally. It is the *supinator crest*. The supinator takes origin from the crest and the concave area in front of it. At the middle of the shaft a prominent ridge, the *interosseous border*, projects laterally; the interosseous membrane is attached here. The narrow extensor surface lies between the interosseous border and the subcutaneous *posterior border*. The broad flexor surface extends around the medial side to the same subcutaneous border; flexor digitorum profundus arises from the flexor surface. Pronator quadratus arises from a ridge on the flexor aspect of the lower shaft. To the subcutaneous border is attached an aponeurosis which is common to flexor digitorum profundus, flexor carpi ulnaris and extensor carpi ulnaris. Abductor pollicis longus, extensor pollicis longus and extensor indicis take origin from the extensor surface in that order from proximal to distal (Fig. 2.31).

The lower end expands into a small rounded prominence, the *head* of the ulna. Its radial and distal surfaces are covered with hyaline cartilage, for articulation with the ulnar notch of the radius and the articular disc of the wrist joint. This triangular fibrocartilage is attached by its apex to the base of the *styloid process*, which projects distally from the medial margin of the lower end. This is smaller than the radial styloid which extends about 1 cm more distally. A groove alongside the process, on the extensor surface, lodges the tendon of extensor carpi ulnaris (Fig. 2.31).

Surgical approach. Being subcutaneous at the back, the bone is easily exposed by incising along the posterior border. The periosteum is elevated and the aponeurotic origins of flexors carpi ulnaris and digitorum profundus retracted medially and that of extensor carpi ulnaris retracted laterally.

Ossification The ulna starts ossifying in cartilage at the eighth week. There is a secondary centre for the head, the growing end, which fuses with the shaft at about 18 years. Two secondary centres contribute to the development of the olecranon; they join the shaft at about 16 years.

Bones of the hand

The articulated bones of the hand are made up of a carpus (eight bones), five metacarpal bones and the phalanges of the five digits.

Carpus

The eight carpal bones articulated together form a semicircle, the convexity of which is proximal and articulates with the forearm. The diameter of the semicircle is distal, and articulates with the metacarpal bases (Fig. 2.55). The flexor surface of the carpus is deeply concave to accommodate the flexor tendons. The extensor surface is gently convex and the extensor tendons pass across it.

The eight carpal bones lie in two rows. In the proximal row are the scaphoid, lunate and triquetral, which

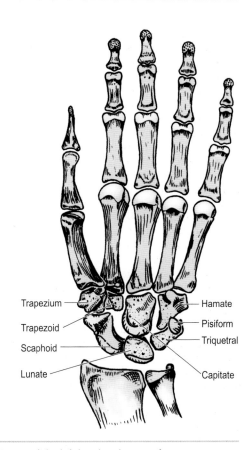

Fig. 2.55 Bones of the left hand: palmar surface.

together form the convexity of the semicircle. The pisiform completes the proximal row by articulating with the front of the triquetral. The four bones of the distal row are the trapezium, trapezoid, capitate and hamate. They articulate with the bones of the proximal row by the midcarpal joint. The bones of each row articulate with each other by intercarpal joints that extend proximally and distally from the S-shaped midcarpal joint.

The **scaphoid** (boat-shaped) bone has a convex, articular proximal surface for the radius that extends on to the dorsal aspect. There is a flat surface medially for the lunate and a concavity distomedially for the capitate. The distal convex surface articulates with trapezium and trapezoid. The *tubercle* is a blunt prominence to the thumb side of the distal surface, and is palpable. The narrow non-articular *waist* of the bone is palpable in the snuffbox distal to the radial styloid (Fig. 2.32). It is perforated, especially on its dorsal surface, by vascular foramina. These are more numerous distally, so that fracture across the waist sometimes results in avascular necrosis of the proximal fragment. The scaphoid is the carpal bone most commonly fractured. If it needs to be approached *surgically* the route is from the front between the flexor carpi radialis tendon medially and the radial artery laterally, so exposing the wrist joint capsule, which is incised to reach the bone.

The **lunate** (semilunar) bone shows a convex proximal facet for the radius and the articular disc of the wrist joint, which extends on to the dorsal aspect. To each side there is a facet for the adjoining bones (scaphoid and triquetral) of the proximal row, and there is a concavity distally for the capitate. The palmar surface is broader than the dorsal surface. The lunate is the carpal bone most commonly dislocated and is displaced anteriorly when this occurs.

The **triquetral** bone has an oval facet on the distal palmar surface for the pisiform. The proximal surface is smooth for the capsule and disc of the wrist joint. Distally the triquetral articulates with the hamate, and laterally with the lunate.

The **pisiform** has a flat surface for articulation with the triquetral, and the convexity of the remainder of the bone leans somewhat towards the radial side, over the concavity of the carpus.

The **trapezium** articulates with the adjacent trapezoid, and these together by concave facets fit the distal convexity of the scaphoid. A distal articular surface, saddle-shaped, is for the thumb metacarpal, and this is a separate synovial joint. The trapezium articulates narrowly with the tubercle on the base of the index-finger metacarpal. There is a prominent ridge (tubercle) with a groove on its medial side lying obliquely on the palmar surface. The tendon of flexor carpi radialis runs in the groove. The radial artery is related to the dorsal surface.

The **trapezoid** is a small bone that lies wedged between trapezium and capitate, articulating proximally with the scaphoid and distally with the index-finger metacarpal.

The **capitate** is the largest of the carpal bones. It lies between the hamate medially and the trapezoid and scaphoid laterally. Proximally its convex surface fits the distal concavity of the lunate. Distally it articulates with the base of the middle and a tiny part of the ring-finger metacarpals.

The **hamate** is wedge-shaped. Proximally the thin edge of the wedge articulates with the lunate, while distally the base articulates with the fourth and fifth metacarpals. The lateral surface articulates with the capitate and the medial surface with the triquetral. The palmar surface is projected as a hook-like flange that overhangs the anterior concavity of the carpus distal to the pisiform. A slight groove on the distal surface of the base of the

hook makes contact with the deep branch of the ulnar nerve.

Metacarpus

The thumb metacarpal is shorter and thicker than the others. Its base has a saddle-shaped facet for the trapezium. The convex facet on its head is not so prominently rounded as those of the other four metacarpals (Fig. 2.55); the flexor margin of the facet is grooved for the sesamoids of the thenar muscles. The shaft is set at right angles to the plane of the other four, so that its flexor surface faces across the palm.

The remaining four metacarpals show expanded bases by which they articulate with the distal row of carpal bones and with each other. The middle metacarpal shows a prominent styloid process that projects dorsally into the angle between capitate and trapezoid (Fig. 2.56). The heads carry boldly rounded articular facets which extend further on the flexor than the extensor surface. The four metacarpal bones together form a gentle concavity for the palm. Their heads form the knuckles of the fist.

Phalanges

Two phalanges form the thumb, three form each finger. Each of the five proximal phalanges has a concave facet on the base, for the head of its own metacarpal. Middle

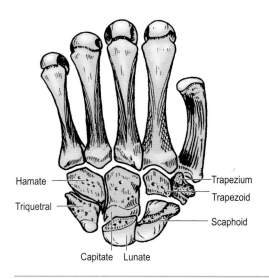

Fig. 2.56   Bones of the left carpus and metacarpus: dorsal surface.

and distal phalanges carry a facet on each base that is divided by a central ridge into two concavities. The heads of the proximal and middle phalanges are correspondingly trochlea-shaped, with their facets on the distal and flexor surfaces, not on the extensor surface. Each distal or terminal phalanx expands distally into a tuberosity, roughened on the flexor surface for attachment of the digital fibrofatty pad.

Sesamoid bones

The pisiform is a sesamoid bone in the tendon of flexor carpi ulnaris, but it is included in the carpus as a functional constituent of its bony skeleton. In the thumb a pair of sesamoid bones articulate with the flexor surface of the metacarpal head. That on the radial side lies in the tendon of flexor pollicis brevis, and that on the ulnar side in the tendon of adductor pollicis. Sesamoid bones are commonly found also at the other metacarpal heads, especially the fifth and second, lodged in the palmar capsule of the metacarpophalangeal joints, and occasionally at the interphalangeal joints. Fibrocartilaginous at first, they ossify generally soon after puberty.

Ossification

The carpus is all cartilaginous at birth. The largest carpal bone, the capitate, ossifies first (first year) and the smallest, the pisiform, ossifies last (tenth year). The others ossify in sequence, according to their size, and the whole carpus, except the sesamoid pisiform bone, is ossified by the seventh year. The shafts of all the metacarpals and phalanges ossify in utero. Secondary centres of ossification develop at the bases of all the phalanges and the thumb metacarpal. The metacarpals of the second, third, fourth and fifth digits develop secondary centres at their heads.

Surface features

On the flexor surface the tubercle of the scaphoid and the pisiform are palpable in the distal skin crease of the wrist, which marks the proximal extent of the flexor retinaculum. The proximal skin crease (or the middle crease if three are present) marks the wrist joint (Fig. 2.57). The ridge of the trapezium and the hook of the hamate are each palpable deep to their overlying muscles; pressure on the overlying digital branches of the ulnar nerve may cause pain when palpating the latter. The prominence of the metacarpal heads can be felt in the palm; they lie along the distal skin crease of the palm. In the snuffbox, distal to the radial styloid, the scaphoid, trapezium and base of the thumb metacarpal can be felt. The lunate, too deep to be readily felt on the flexor surface, is easily palpable midway between radial and ulnar styloids on the extensor surface; it rolls prominently under the palpating fingertip during full flexion of the wrist.

Fig. 2.57 Surface projections of some bony features of the left wrist and hand and skin creases. The proximal wrist crease indicates the level of the wrist joint. The metacarpophalangeal joints are far proximal to the interdigital webs.

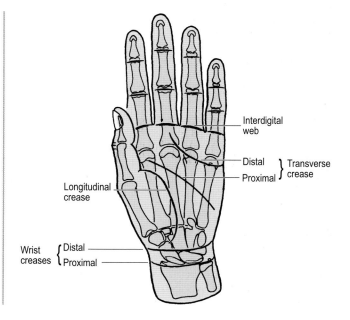

Lower limb 3

General plan

The human lower limb is built for support and propulsion. The two hip bones articulate with one another in front at the pubic symphysis, and each is firmly fixed to the lateral part of the sacrum by the relatively immobile sacroiliac joint. The rigid bony pelvis thus produced transmits the body weight through the acetabulum of the hip bone to the lower limb and likewise transmits the propulsive thrust of the lower limb to the hip bone. In sitting, body weight is transmitted to the ischial tuberosities and the legs are free to rest.

The fixation of the hip bones restricts movements in the hip region compared with the shoulder, but a wide range of flexion–extension movements and a lesser degree of abduction–adduction are still possible. At the knee and ankle flexion and extension are the essential movements (although some rotation occurs at the knee), while in the foot there are limited movements at small joints.

Although the lower limb is commonly called the leg, this term strictly refers to the region between knee and foot. Above the knee is the thigh, which can be divided into three compartments: anterior or extensor; medial or adductor; and posterior or flexor. (The limb rotates medially during development and the original dorsal or extensor surface becomes anterior, and the ventral or flexor surface becomes posterior.) The gluteal region or buttock lies behind the pelvis and hip, above the posterior compartment of the thigh. The leg proper also has three compartments: anterior or extensor; lateral or peroneal; and posterior or flexor (calf). The foot has a dorsum or upper surface and a sole or plantar surface.

PART ONE

Anterior compartment of the thigh

Subcutaneous tissue

The fat of the front of the thigh contains cutaneous nerves, lymphatic vessels and nodes, the termination and tributaries of the great saphenous vein and cutaneous branches of the femoral artery.

Superficial nerves

The cutaneous branches of the lumbar plexus that supply the thigh are derived from the first three lumbar nerves. They are the ilioinguinal, femoral branch of the genitofemoral, medial, intermediate and lateral femoral cutaneous nerves, and the anterior branch of the obturator nerve (Fig. 3.43). All these nerves supply fascia lata as well as skin. The dermatomes of the lower limb are illustrated on page 15.

The **ilioinguinal nerve** is the collateral branch of the iliohypogastric, both being derived from the first lumbar nerve. It has no lateral but only a terminal cutaneous distribution. In the anterior abdominal wall it lies in the neurovascular plane between the internal oblique and transversus abdominis muscles, pierces internal oblique and supplies its lower fibres, and passes down deep to the external oblique (see Fig. 5.7, p. 235) to emerge on the front of the cord through the superficial inguinal ring. Piercing the external spermatic fascia its chief distribution is to the skin of the root of the penis and the anterior one-third of the scrotum, but it supplies also

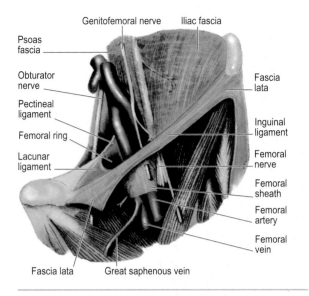

Psoas fascia

Obturator nerve

Pectineal ligament

Femoral ring

Lacunar ligament

Genitofemoral nerve   Iliac fascia

Fascia lata

Inguinal ligament

Femoral nerve

Femoral sheath

Femoral artery

Femoral vein

Fascia lata   Great saphenous vein

Fig. 3.1   Left femoral ring and sheath. The femoral canal, vein and artery are within the sheath; the nerve is outside it.

a small area of thigh below the medial end of the inguinal ligament.

The **genitofemoral nerve** is derived from the first and second lumbar nerves, but fibres from only L1 pass into the femoral branch. This branch is given off from the nerve as it lies on psoas major. It runs down on the external iliac artery and passes beneath the inguinal ligament into the femoral sheath. It pierces the anterior wall of the sheath and the overlying fascia lata below the middle of the inguinal ligament (Fig. 3.1) to supply skin over the femoral triangle. The genital branch passes through the deep ring with the other constituents of the spermatic cord (see p. 236).

The **medial femoral cutaneous nerve** is a branch of the femoral nerve (L2, 3). Inclining medially across the femoral vessels it pierces the fascia lata at the mid-thigh and supplies the medial side of the thigh; its terminal twigs join the patellar plexus (see below).

The **intermediate femoral cutaneous nerve** (L2, 3) is also a branch of the femoral nerve. It passes vertically downwards, usually pierces sartorius, and then pierces the fascia lata at a higher level than the medial cutaneous nerve to supply the front of the thigh as far down as the knee, where its terminal twigs join the patellar plexus.

The **lateral femoral cutaneous nerve** is a branch of the lumbar plexus (L2, 3). Passing from the lateral border of psoas major across the iliac fossa it lies at first behind the fascia iliaca; but approaching the inguinal ligament

it inclines forwards and is incorporated within the substance of the iliac fascia, which is here a thick tough membrane (Fig. 3.1). The nerve now passes behind or pierces the inguinal ligament a centimetre to the medial side of the anterior superior iliac spine (Fig. 3.2).

The nerve enters the thigh deep to the fascia lata, and divides into anterior and posterior branches which pierce the fascia lata separately. The anterior branch is distributed along the anterolateral surface of the thigh, and its terminal twigs enter the patellar plexus. The posterior branch supplies the skin on the posterolateral aspect from the level of the greater trochanter to the mid-thigh.

The nerve is sometimes compressed as it passes through the inguinal ligament, causing pain and altered sensation in the lateral side of the thigh (*meralgia paraesthetica*). Less commonly the nerve may be compressed as it passes through the iliac fascia. Surgical treatment of this condition requires division of the inguinal ligament and freeing the nerve of any fascial compression.

The **obturator nerve** (L2–4) sends a twig from its anterior division into the subsartorial plexus, whence cutaneous branches pass to skin over the medial side of the thigh (Figs 3.43 and 3.44).

Patellar plexus

This is a fine network of communicating twigs in the subcutaneous tissue over and around the patella and patellar ligament. It is formed by the terminal branches of the medial and intermediate femoral cutaneous nerves, anterior branch of the lateral femoral cutaneous nerve and infrapatellar branch of the saphenous nerve.

Superficial arteries

Four cutaneous branches of the femoral artery are found in the subcutaneous tissue below the inguinal ligament.

The **superficial circumflex iliac artery** pierces the fascia lata lateral to the saphenous opening and passes up below the inguinal ligament to the anastomosis at the anterior superior iliac spine.

The **superficial epigastric artery** emerges through the saphenous opening. It crosses the inguinal ligament and runs towards the umbilicus.

The **superficial external pudendal artery** emerges from the saphenous opening and passes medially, in front of the spermatic cord (round ligament) to the penis and scrotum (labium majus).

The **deep external pudendal artery** pierces the fascia lata and passes behind the spermatic cord (round ligament) to supply the skin of the scrotum (labium majus).

Fig. 3.2 Left femoral triangle and adductor canal. Part of sartorius has been removed to show the contents of the canal.

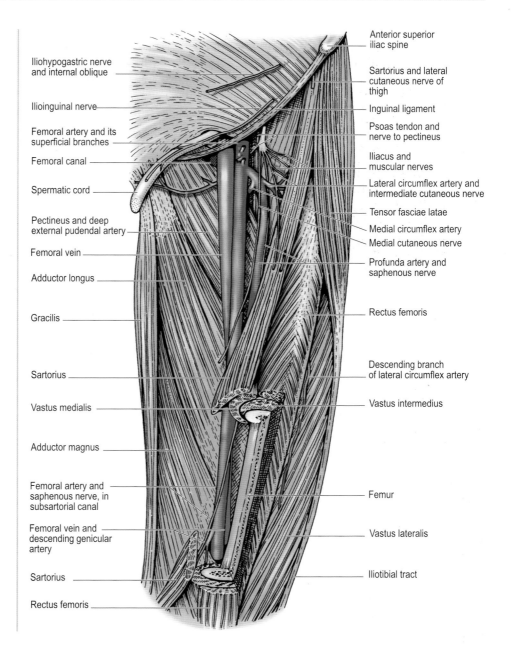

Iliohypogastric nerve and internal oblique

Ilioinguinal nerve

Femoral artery and its superficial branches

Femoral canal

Spermatic cord

Pectineus and deep external pudendal artery

Femoral vein

Adductor longus

Gracilis

Sartorius

Vastus medialis

Adductor magnus

Femoral artery and saphenous nerve, in subsartorial canal

Femoral vein and descending genicular artery

Sartorius

Rectus femoris

Anterior superior iliac spine

Sartorius and lateral cutaneous nerve of thigh

Inguinal ligament

Psoas tendon and nerve to pectineus

Iliacus and muscular nerves

Lateral circumflex artery and intermediate cutaneous nerve

Tensor fasciae latae

Medial circumflex artery

Medial cutaneous nerve

Profunda artery and saphenous nerve

Rectus femoris

Descending branch of lateral circumflex artery

Vastus intermedius

Femur

Vastus lateralis

Iliotibial tract

Superficial veins

These are essentially tributaries of the great (long) saphenous vein, one of the most important veins in the body in view of its tendency to become dilated (varicose), and its use as a conduit in vascular surgery.

The **great (long) saphenous vein,** the longest vein in the body, begins as the upward continuation of the medial marginal vein of the foot (p. 149). It courses upwards in front of the medial malleolus (Fig. 3.28), crosses the lower quarter of the medial surface of the tibia obliquely and runs up behind the medial border of the tibia towards the knee, where it lies a hand's breadth behind the medial border of the patella. It spirals forwards round the medial convexity of the thigh and ends by passing through the cribriform fascia covering the saphenous opening (Fig. 3.3), which lies about 3 cm below and lateral to the pubic tubercle. Here it joins the femoral vein. It contains up to 20 valves, more of them below knee level than above. Incompetence of valves is a cause of varicosity of the vein.

A number of tributaries may be expected to join the great saphenous vein in the region of the saphenous opening; like venous patterns elsewhere the exact number is variable since some may unite with others to form common trunks or may be missing. There are usually four veins that correspond to the four cutaneous branches of the femoral artery (superficial circumflex iliac, superficial epigastric, and superficial and deep external pudendal). The superficial external pudendal artery runs horizontally between the superficial and deep external pudendal veins. The deep external pudendal artery runs medially behind the saphenous vein near its termination. Anterolateral and posteromedial veins of

the thigh frequently join the great saphenous vein a little below the saphenous opening.

The superficial epigastric vein may form the lower end of the thoracoepigastric vein which serves as a communication between the superior and inferior venae cavae (see p. 186).

The deep connections of the lower end of the great saphenous vein in the leg are described on page 145.

Lymph nodes and vessels

Large lymphatic vessels accompany the great saphenous vein from the foot, leg and thigh, and numerous large vessels spiral around the outer side of the thigh to converge on the **superficial inguinal nodes** (Fig. 3.4). These consist of about 10 nodes. A proximal group lies just distal to the inguinal ligament and a distal group lies vertically along the terminal great saphenous vein. The lateral nodes of the proximal group receive lymph from the buttock, flank and back below the waist. The medial nodes of this group receive lymph from the umbilicus and anterior abdominal wall below it, the external genitalia of both sexes (excluding the testis, but including the lower vagina), the lower anal canal and perineum, and a small proportion of the drainage from the uterus via lymphatics accompanying the round ligament. The distal group receives all the superficial lymphatics of the lower limb, except for those from the posterolateral part of the calf. The superficial inguinal nodes drain mainly to the external iliac nodes by efferent lymphatics, some of which pierce the cribriform fascia.

Three of four **deep inguinal nodes** lie deep to the fascia lata, medial to the femoral vein, one or two being in the femoral canal. They receive the deep lymphatics that accompany the femoral vessels from the popliteal fossa, lymphatics from the glans penis (or clitoris) and a few efferent lymphatics from the superficial inguinal nodes. The deep inguinal nodes drain to the external iliac nodes through the femoral canal.

Superficial fascia

The membranous layer of the superficial fascia of the abdominal wall (see Scarpa's fascia, p. 185) extends into the thigh and fuses with the fascia lata (Fig. 3.5) at the flexure skin crease of the hip joint (Fig. 4.1A, B, p. 185). The attachment extends laterally from the pubic tubercle below the inguinal ligament. The saphenous opening lies below this line, so a femoral hernia, emerging from the saphenous opening, can never come to lie in the space deep to Scarpa's fascia. The hernia emerges into ordinary subcutaneous fat and therefore does not become very large.

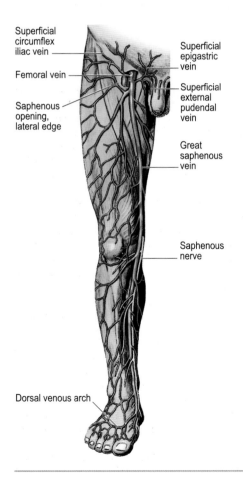

Superficial circumflex iliac vein

Femoral vein

Saphenous opening, lateral edge

Superficial epigastric vein

Superficial external pudendal vein

Great saphenous vein

Saphenous nerve

Dorsal venous arch

Fig. 3.3 Right great saphenous vein and its tributaries.

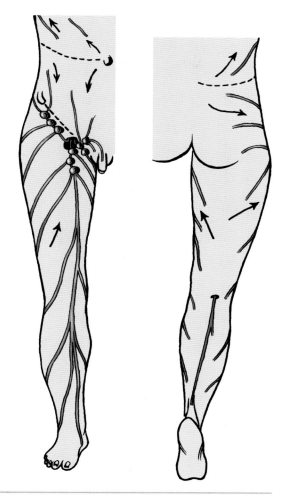

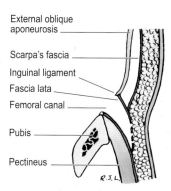

Fig. 3.5 Sagittal section through the femoral canal. The membranous layer of superficial fascia of the abdomen is attached to the fascia lata below the inguinal ligament but above the saphenous opening, so that a femoral hernia passing through the cribriform fascia at the opening is directed into the subcutaneous fat and not into the potential space deep to the abdominal fascia.

Fig. 3.4 Superficial lymph drainage of the right lower limb (front and back). The superficial inguinal nodes also receive all the lymph from the subcutaneous tissues of the trunk below the waist.

Fascia lata

The deep fascia, the fascia lata, encloses the thighs like a stocking but one whose top is too large. A vertical slit has been cut at the top of the stocking, so to speak, and the cut edges overlapped to fit the bony pelvis, so forming the margin of the saphenous opening, as described below.

The upper end of the lateral part of the cut fascial stocking (Fig. 3.6A) is attached to the inguinal ligament, which it draws into a downward convexity when the thigh is extended. The line of fascial attachment extends posteriorly from the anterior superior iliac spine along the external lip of the iliac crest, splitting to enclose the tensor fasciae latae and gluteus maximus muscles. The two layers that enclose the gluteus maximus are very thin. Posterior to gluteus maximus the fascia lata is attached to the sacrum and the sacrotuberous ligament. The attachment of the fascia lata extends along the convexity of the ischial tuberosity and the ischiopubic ramus around the medial side of the limb to the body of the pubic bone.

The medial part of the cut fascial stocking (Fig. 3.6B) passes deep to the lateral part (A) over pectineus, posterior to the femoral sheath, and is attached to the pectineal line of the pubic bone. To change the simile, the edges of A and B of the slit in Figure 3.6 are overlapped like lapels of a double-breasted jacket and the great saphenous vein passes through the gap like a hand reaching into the inside pocket. The cut edge of A forms a crescentic or falciform margin to the **saphenous opening**, which is merely the oblique space lying between the cut edges as they overlap each other. The saphenous opening is covered in by a loose fascia attached laterally to the falciform edge and medially to the fascia lata where it lies over adductor longus. This fascia is pierced by the great saphenous vein and its tributaries and by efferent lymphatics from the superficial inguinal lymph nodes, giving it a sieve-like appearance, whence it derives the name of *cribriform fascia*.

The fascia lata is attached below to the tibial condyles and to the head of the fibula. Anteriorly it is reinforced by expansions from the quadriceps femoris. Over the

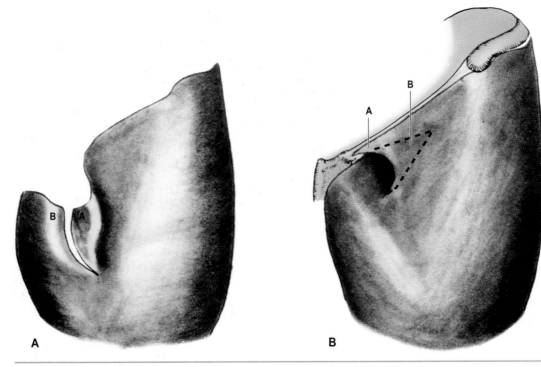

Fig. 3.6 Fascia lata and the formation of the left saphenous opening. The lateral margin of the slit in the fascia **A** becomes attached to the pubic tubercle and inguinal ligament, while the medial edge **B** is tucked deep to **A** and attached to the pectineal line, so forming the saphenous opening.

popliteal fossa it is strengthened by transverse fibres and continues below into the deep fascia of the calf.

Tensor fasciae latae

This arises from a 5-cm length of the external lip of the iliac crest between the anterior superior iliac spine and the tubercle of the crest. It is a thin sheet of muscle at its origin and becomes thicker at its insertion into the iliotibial tract.

Nerve supply. By the superior gluteal nerve (L4, 5, S1).

Action. Its action is to pull upon the iliotibial tract, so assisting gluteus maximus in extending the knee joint. The muscle is also active in helping to stabilize the pelvis during walking, when it assists gluteus medius and minimus in resisting adduction at the hip (see p. 129).

Iliotibial tract

This is a thickening of the fascia lata on the lateral side of the thigh. The upper end of the tract splits to enclose tensor fasciae latae and the superficial layer is attached to the iliac crest. Three-quarters of gluteus maximus is inserted into it. The tract passes vertically down and is inserted into a smooth circular facet on the lateral condyle of the tibia (Fig. 3.48A). When the knee is straight the tract passes in front of the axis of flexion. Thus it maintains the knee in the hyperextended position while the quadriceps is relaxed and the patella freely mobile.

The **lateral intermuscular septum** is a strong layer extending from the deep surface of the iliotibial tract to the linea aspera of the femur. Vastus lateralis lies in front and the short head of biceps femoris behind it (Fig. 3.7).

Femoral triangle

When the fascia lata is removed from the front of the thigh the underlying muscles are exposed (Fig. 3.2). The most superficial of all is sartorius, a parallel-sided ribbon of muscle that swings obliquely across the thigh. The adductor longus is prominent on the medial side, and the two muscles enclose, with the inguinal ligament, the femoral triangle.

Fig. 3.7 Cross-section of the left upper thigh, looking towards the hip. The vasti embrace the femur, and the lateral intermuscular septum lies between vastus lateralis and biceps, so attaching the iliotibial tract to the linea aspera of the femur. The sciatic nerve is surrounded by the hamstrings, and the femoral vessels are in the triangular adductor canal in front of adductor longus, with the profunda vessels behind adductor longus adjacent to the femur.

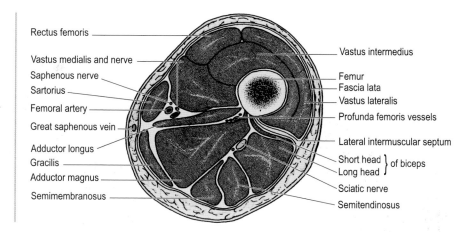

The femoral triangle is defined as the triangle that lies between the inguinal ligament, the medial border of sartorius, and the medial border of adductor longus. The floor of the triangle is gutter-shaped and the hollow can be seen when the thigh is flexed. The femoral nerve and vessels lie in the gutter. The muscles lying in the floor of the femoral triangle are the iliacus, psoas, pectineus and adductor longus.

Sartorius

This muscle, the longest in the body, arises from the anterior superior iliac spine and the notch below it. Its parallel fibres extend for the whole length of the muscle. It crosses the thigh obliquely along the medial border of the femoral triangle (Fig. 3.2) and on the fascial roof of the adductor canal, and then descends more vertically to the upper part of the medial surface of the tibia. It is inserted here in front of gracilis and semitendinosus by an aponeurosis, the upper end of which arches backwards over the top of the gracilis tendon.

Nerve supply. By a branch from the anterior division of the femoral nerve (L2–4).

Action. Sartorius draws the lower limb into the sitting tailor's position (thigh flexed, laterally rotated and abducted, knee flexed).

Adductor longus is described with the other adductors on page 126.

Iliacus

This muscle arises from the iliac fossa (see p. 283). Entering the thigh beneath the lateral part of the inguinal ligament, it curves backwards behind the femoral vessels to be inserted into the front of the psoas tendon

(Fig. 3.8) and a small area of femoral shaft just below the lesser trochanter. The lower part of the iliac fossa is occupied by a bursa, the iliac (psoas) bursa, which lies deep to iliacus and psoas and extends with them into the upper thigh.

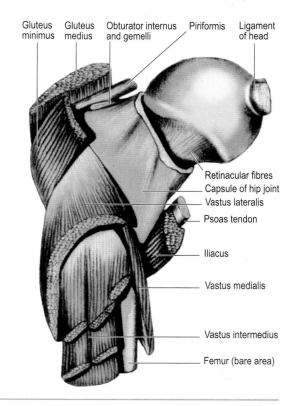

Fig. 3.8 Attachments at the upper end of the right femur, from the front.

Nerve supply. By the femoral nerve (L2, 3) in the iliac fossa.

Action. With psoas, it is a powerful flexor of the hip joint (see p. 133).

Psoas major

This arises from the lumbar spine (see p. 283). It passes into the thigh deep to the middle of the inguinal ligament. Its rounded tendon is inserted into the lesser trochanter (Fig. 3.8). Both iliacus and psoas pass across the front of the capsule of the hip joint, with the bursa intervening. The bursa may communicate with the hip joint through a gap in the capsule that lies between the iliofemoral and pubofemoral ligaments.

Nerve supply. By the first three lumbar nerves (mainly L2).

Action. With iliacus it is a powerful flexor of the hip. The action of psoas on the lumbar spine is described on page 283.

Pectineus

This is a quadrilateral muscle that arises from the pectineal line of the pubis and from a narrow area of bone below (Fig. 3.11). It slopes backwards down to the upper end of the femoral shaft, where it is inserted into a vertical line below the lesser trochanter (Fig. 3.12). The muscle is covered anteriorly by an infolding of fascia lata that passes deep to the falciform margin of the saphenous opening (Fig. 3.6B). The femoral vein and femoral canal lie on the surface of the muscle, while adductor brevis and the anterior division of the obturator nerve lie behind it.

Nerve supply. By the anterior division of the femoral nerve (L2, 3) by a branch that passes behind the femoral sheath. Occasionally it receives a twig from the obturator nerve (L2, 3).

Action. Pectineus flexes and adducts the thigh.

Femoral sheath

The femoral vessels, passing beneath the inguinal ligament, draw around themselves a funnel-shaped prolongation of the transversalis fascia in front and the psoas fascia behind (Fig. 3.1). This prolongation of fascia, the femoral sheath, fuses with the adventitia of the artery and vein about 3 cm distal to the inguinal ligament.

The femoral nerve in the iliac fossa lies in the gutter between psoas and iliacus, behind the iliac fascia. Lateral to the femoral sheath the transversalis fascia and iliac fascia fuse with the inguinal ligament, and the

femoral nerve thus enters the thigh outside the femoral sheath. Within the sheath there is a space on the medial side of the femoral vein, the **femoral canal** (Fig. 3.2). The femoral canal is widest at its abdominal end, where its opening, the **femoral ring**, has four boundaries. Anteriorly lies the medial part of the inguinal ligament, medially the crescentic edge of the lacunar ligament, posteriorly the pectineal ligament and laterally the femoral vein (Fig. 3.1). A femoral hernia enters the femoral canal through this ring. The lacunar ligament may have to be incised to release a strangulated hernia, and here an accessory (abnormal) obturator artery is at risk (see p. 320). The canal contains a lymph node (of Cloquet) which in the female drains directly from the clitoris, and in the male from the glans penis.

Femoral artery

The artery enters the thigh at a point midway between the anterior superior iliac spine and the pubic symphysis (midinguinal point). Here it lies on the psoas major tendon, which separates the artery from the capsule of the hip joint. This is the position where its pulsation can be felt and where it can be entered for arterial catheterization. It emerges from the femoral sheath, courses downwards and enters the adductor canal deep to sartorius. It has four small branches below the inguinal ligament (see p. 116) and just below the termination of the femoral sheath gives off a large branch, the profunda femoris, the chief artery of the thigh.

The *surface marking* of the femoral artery, with the hip slightly flexed and laterally rotated, is from the midpoint between the pubic symphysis and the anterior superior iliac spine, along the upper two-thirds of a line towards the adductor tubercle. The *surgical approach* to the artery in the adductor canal is through an incision on the medial aspect of the lower thigh; sartorius is retracted medially and the fascial roof of the canal divided.

Cannulation. The femoral artery is second only to the radial (see p. 72) as the site of choice for the placement of an arterial line. Its superficial position below the inguinal ligament makes it easily accessible. The most common complications include retroperitoneal haemorrhage and perforation of the gut (by entering the abdominal cavity), and arteriovenous fistula (with the femoral or external iliac vein).

The **profunda femoris artery** is normally the vessel of supply for all thigh muscles (unless its circumflex branches come directly from the femoral). It arises from the lateral side of the femoral artery about 3–4 cm distal to the inguinal ligament and then spirals down deep to it, passing between pectineus and adductor longus, whose upper border separates the femoral and profunda arteries (Fig. 3.2). The profunda vein lies in front of the profunda artery, which continues down on adductor brevis and magnus and ends as the fourth perforating artery. Apart from the perforating arteries and muscular branches, it gives off large lateral and medial circumflex femoral arteries.

The **lateral circumflex femoral artery** arises from the lateral side of the profunda artery (Fig. 3.2) or occasionally from the femoral artery. It passes laterally between the branches of the femoral nerve, and disappears from the femoral triangle beneath sartorius to lie deep to rectus femoris. Here it breaks up into three branches.

The *ascending branch* runs up on the vastus lateralis, under cover of sartorius and tensor fasciae latae. It gives a branch to the trochanteric anastomosis (see p. 131) and passes on towards the anterior superior iliac spine, where it ends by anastomosing with the superficial and deep circumflex iliac, an iliac branch of the iliolumbar and the superior branch of the superior gluteal artery. This ascending branch is a large vessel and in the anterior approach to the hip joint between sartorius and tensor fasciae latae, it and its venae comitantes must be secured when separating the muscles.

The *transverse branch* passes across the vastus lateralis and winds around the femur to form one limb of the cruciate anastomosis (see p. 131).

The *descending branch* slopes steeply downwards, with the nerve to vastus lateralis, in a groove between the anterior edge of the vastus lateralis and the vastus intermedius. It supplies both muscles and ends by sending twigs to the anastomosis around the knee.

The **medial circumflex femoral artery** arises from the medial side of the profunda (occasionally from the femoral), often above its lateral companion, and immediately passes backwards between pectineus and the psoas tendon. Running above adductor brevis and below obturator externus, it passes between quadratus femoris and adductor magnus to enter the gluteal region. It gives an *ascending branch* to the trochanteric anastomosis, and a *horizontal branch* to the cruciate anastomosis.

The four **perforating arteries** pass backwards through adductor magnus, the first having passed above, the second through and the third and fourth below adductor brevis. They supply the adductor muscles and the hamstrings and make a series of anastomoses with one another, with the cruciate anastomosis above and with the popliteal artery below.

In the vascular surgical literature, the femoral artery above the origin of the profunda branch (deep femoral artery) is termed the common femoral artery, and the vessel below this branch is the superficial femoral artery.

Femoral vein

The vein enters the lower angle of the femoral triangle, where it lies posterior to the artery. It ascends through the femoral triangle and comes to lie on the medial side of the artery. It receives a tributary corresponding to the profunda femoris artery and just below the femoral sheath the great saphenous vein joins its anteromedial side (Fig. 3.1). Within the sheath it passes under the inguinal ligament and runs along the brim of the pelvis as the external iliac vein. It has four or five valves, the most constant ones being just above the junctions with the profunda and great saphenous veins.

In the living body the position of the femoral vein below the inguinal ligament is found by feeling the pulsations of the femoral artery, which is immediately lateral to the vein. In thin people the femoral vein may be surprisingly near the surface even though it is within the femoral sheath.

Femoral nerve

This is the nerve of the extensor compartment of the thigh, and is formed from the *posterior* divisions of the anterior rami of the lumbar nerves 2, 3 and 4. The obturator nerve, which supplies the adductor muscles derived from the flexor muscles of the thigh, is formed by the *anterior* divisions of the same rami (see p. 14). The femoral nerve *supplies iliacus* in the abdomen. Lying in the iliac fossa between psoas and iliacus the femoral nerve enters the thigh by passing deep to the inguinal ligament at the lateral edge of the femoral sheath, which separates it from the femoral artery (Fig. 3.1).

As it enters the femoral triangle it gives a *branch to pectineus*; this branch passes behind the femoral sheath to reach the muscle (Fig. 3.2). Just distal to the inguinal ligament the femoral nerve divides into several branches. The intermediate and medial femoral cutaneous nerves have already been described (see p. 115).

There are two **nerves to sartorius**, one of which usually pierces the muscle and continues as the intermediate cutaneous nerve. The **nerve to rectus femoris** is usually double; the upper nerve gives a branch to the hip joint. The **nerve to vastus medialis**, the largest of the muscular branches, passes down on the lateral side of the femoral artery into the adductor canal, where it gives branches to and enters vastus medialis, and continues downwards to the capsule of the knee joint. The **nerve to vastus lateralis** runs downwards with the descending branch of the lateral femoral circumflex artery to supply the muscle and the knee joint. The **nerve to vastus intermedius** enters the anterior surface of the muscle and also supplies the knee joint. The **saphenous nerve** leaves the femoral triangle at its lower angle and in the subsartorial canal passes across the front of the femoral artery to reach its medial side (Fig. 3.2). It gives twigs to the subsartorial plexus and leaves the canal at its distal end by passing between sartorius and gracilis.

Quadriceps femoris

This muscle is the main extensor of the knee joint and has four parts: rectus femoris and the three vastus muscles: lateralis; intermedius; and medialis. All converge to form the quadriceps tendon which contains the patella and which continues down as the patellar ligament to be inserted into the tuberosity of the tibia.

Rectus femoris arises from the ilium by two heads (Fig. 3.45). The *reflected head* arises from a groove above the acetabulum, the *straight head* from the upper half of the anterior inferior spine, above the iliofemoral ligament. The two heads unite to form the anterior lamina of the quadriceps tendon. The posterior surface of the muscle is clad in a glistening aponeurosis that glides on the anterior surface of vastus intermedius. The anterior surface is covered with a similar aponeurosis on its upper part.

Vastus lateralis has an extensive linear origin from the upper part of the intertrochanteric line, the greater trochanter (Fig. 3.8) and the lateral lip of the linea aspera of the femur. It also arises from the lateral intermuscular septum. Inferiorly the muscle is incorporated in the quadriceps tendon (Fig. 3.10). The anterior edge of the muscle lies free on vastus intermedius; the descending branch of the lateral circumflex artery and the nerve to vastus lateralis lie in the shallow gutter between the two.

Vastus intermedius arises from the anterior and lateral surfaces of the upper two-thirds of the shaft of the femur. The anterior surface of the muscle is covered by an aponeurosis which is continued down into the quadriceps tendon.

Articularis genu is a small muscle which arises from the anterior surface of the lower femoral shaft, deep to vastus intermedius, and is inserted into the upper convexity of the suprapatellar bursa (see p. 143).

Vastus medialis arises from the lower part of the intertrochanteric line and the medial lip of the linea aspera and from the tendon of adductor magnus below the hiatus for the femoral vessels. The muscle slopes around the medial surface of the femur, merging with vastus intermedius, and is continuous below with the quadriceps tendon, while the lowest fibres, lying nearly horizontal, are inserted directly into the medial border of the patella. These fibres are indispensable to the stability of the patella.

The **quadriceps tendon** is attached to the base and sides of the patella. A thin sheet passes across the front of the patella into the patellar ligament and the retinacula.

The **patellar ligament** connects the lower border of the patella with the smooth convexity on the tuberosity of the tibia (Fig. 3.48). The *patellar retinacula* are fibrous expansions from the quadriceps tendon and patellar ligament, which connect the sides of the patella with the condyles of the tibia and the collateral ligaments.

Nerve supplies. Each muscle is supplied by its own branch from the femoral nerve (L3, 4).

Actions. The muscle is the main extensor of the knee joint. Rectus femoris can assist iliopsoas to flex the hip.

Test. While lying on the back with the knee partly flexed, the patient extends the knee against resistance. Rectus femoris can be seen and felt contracting.

Stability of the patella

The patella is a sesamoid bone in the quadriceps tendon. It is mobile from side to side. The patellar ligament is vertical, but the pull of the quadriceps is oblique, in the line of the shaft of the femur, and when the muscle contracts it tends to draw the patella laterally. Three factors discourage this lateral dislocation; they are the usual bony, ligamentous and muscular factors that control the stability of any bone. The bony factor consists in the forward prominence of the lateral condyle of the femur (Fig. 3.9), the ligamentous factor is the tension of the medial patellar retinaculum, but they are in themselves incapable of preventing lateral displacement of the patella. The lowest fibres of vastus medialis, inserted into the border of the bone, hold the patella medially when the quadriceps contracts (Fig. 3.10). These fibres of vastus medialis are indispensable to the stability of the patella.

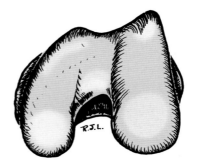

Fig. 3.9 Lower end of the left femur, from below. The prominence of the lateral condyle discourages lateral displacement of the patella.

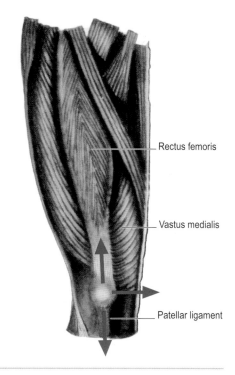

Rectus femoris

Vastus medialis

Patellar ligament

Fig. 3.10 Stabilization of the right patella. The slightly oblique pull of rectus femoris is counteracted by the lowest fibres of vastus medialis.

Adductor canal

This canal (also known as the subsartorial or Hunter's canal) is a gutter-shaped groove between vastus medialis and the front of the adductor muscles, below the apex of the femoral triangle. The gutter is roofed in by a fascia which contains in its meshes the subsartorial plexus. The canal so formed contains the femoral artery and vein, the saphenous nerve and, in the upper part, the nerve to vastus medialis (Fig. 3.7). Sartorius lies on the fascial roof. The adductors in the floor of the canal are the adductor longus above and the adductor magnus below. The subsartorial plexus receives small branches from the medial cutaneous nerve of the thigh, the saphenous nerve and the anterior division of the obturator nerve. The plexus supplies the overlying fascia lata and an area of skin above the medial side of the knee. The femoral artery leaves the canal by passing into the popliteal fossa through the hiatus between the hamstring and adductor parts of the adductor magnus muscle. In the distal part of the canal the femoral vein is postero-lateral to the artery. The vein ascends posteriorly until

in the femoral triangle it lies medial to the artery. This is in keeping with the rotation medially of the lower limb from the fetal position, and is further reflected in the spiral manner in which the saphenous nerve passes across the femoral artery. At all levels in the thigh the artery lies between saphenous nerve and femoral vein. Below the opening in the adductor magnus the saphenous nerve continues to descend in the canal. The *descending genicular artery* arises from the femoral artery just above the adductor hiatus and, passing downwards, divides into a superficial saphenous artery that accompanies the saphenous nerve and a deep muscular branch that enters the vastus medialis and joins the arterial anastomosis around the knee.

The **saphenous nerve** passes out of the canal by escaping from behind the posterior border of sartorius (in front of gracilis). It pierces the fascia lata here and passes downwards behind the great saphenous vein. Just before leaving the canal the *infrapatellar branch* is given off; this nerve pierces sartorius, joins the patellar plexus and supplies prepatellar skin.

PART TWO

Medial compartment of the thigh

The contents of this (adductor) compartment of the thigh are separated from the anterior (extensor) compartment by the medial intermuscular septum, but there is no septum dividing them from the posterior (flexor or hamstring) compartment. The muscles consist of gracilis and the three adductors, longus, brevis and magnus, while deeply lies obturator externus. The nerve of the compartment is the obturator, and the artery is the profunda femoris, assisted proximally by the obturator artery.

The **medial intermuscular septum** is a thin fascia that lies between vastus medialis and the adductors and pectineus. It is attached to the fascia lata and the linea aspera of the femur, and is continuous above with the fascia on pectineus (see p. 119).

Gracilis

This, the most superficial muscle of the medial side of the thigh, arises as a flat sheet from the edge of the inferior ramus of the pubis and the adjoining ischial ramus (Fig. 3.45). The muscle narrows in triangular fashion and is replaced by a cylindrical tendon which is inserted into the upper part of the medial surface of the shaft of the tibia just behind sartorius.

Adductor longus

This, the most superficial of the three adductors, arises from a circular area on the body of the pubis, in the angle between the pubic crest and symphysis (Fig. 3.45), by a strong round tendon, sometimes ossified ('rider's bone'). The muscle rapidly becomes fleshy and flattens out to be inserted by an aponeurotic flat tendon into the middle third of the linea aspera of the femur (Fig. 3.11).

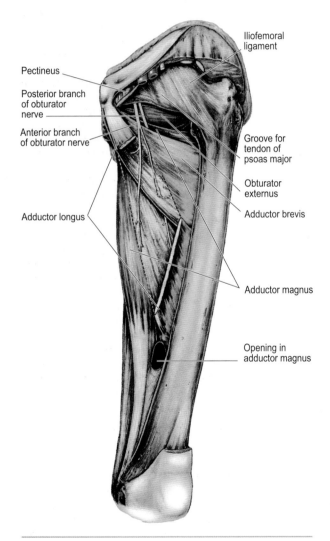

Iliofemoral
ligament

Pectineus

Posterior branch
of obturator
nerve

Anterior branch
of obturator nerve

Groove for
tendon of
psoas major

Obturator
externus

Adductor brevis

Adductor longus

Adductor magnus

Opening in
adductor magnus

Fig. 3.11 Adductor muscles and anterior and posterior divisions of obturator nerve of the left thigh: anterior aspect.

Adductor brevis

This muscle arises from the body and inferior ramus of the pubic bone, deep to pectineus and adductor longus (Fig. 3.45). It widens in triangular fashion to be inserted into the upper part of the linea aspera immediately behind the insertion of pectineus and adductor longus. The anterior division of the obturator nerve passes vertically downwards on its anterior surface (Fig. 3.11); the posterior division passes down behind it. The upper border of adductor brevis thus lies between the two divisions of the obturator nerve in the same way as the upper border of adductor longus lies between the femoral and the profunda femoris vessels.

Adductor magnus

This is a composite muscle formed by the fusion of adductor and hamstring muscle masses, each with their own nerve supply.

The *hamstring part* arises from the ischial tuberosity (Fig. 3.45), and the fibres pass vertically downwards to a tendinous attachment to the adductor tubercle of the femur, with an expansion to the medial supracondylar line. In continuity with the ischial origin, the *adductor part* arises from the ischiopubic ramus. These fibres are inserted progressively higher along the medial supracondylar line, the linea aspera and up to the gluteal tuberosity (Fig. 3.47). The upper border of the muscle is horizontal, lying edge to edge with the lower border of quadratus femoris, and the medial circumflex femoral artery passes between the two muscles from front to back to reach the cruciate anastomosis (Fig. 3.13). Near the top of the medial supracondylar line there is a gap in the muscle attachment through which the femoral vessels pass, changing their name to popliteal as they do so. Along the linea aspera attachment there are four small openings, the lowest for the end of the profunda femoris vessels, and the others for their perforating branches.

Nerve supplies of adductors. Gracilis and adductor longus and brevis are supplied by the anterior division of the obturator nerve, the hamstring part of magnus by the tibial part of the sciatic nerve and the rest of magnus by the posterior division of the obturator (L2, 3 for all muscles).

Actions of adductors. The adductor mass of muscles, though large, is less important in the prime movement of adduction than in synergic activities associated with posture and gait.

Tests for adductors. While lying on the back with the knee straight, the patient adducts the thigh against resistance, and the upper ends of gracilis and adductor longus are palpated.

Obturator externus

This muscle arises from the whole of the obturator membrane and from the anterior bony margin of the obturator foramen. Both membrane and muscle fall short of the obturator notch above, thereby forming a canal for the passage of the obturator nerve and vessels (Fig. 3.11). The muscle passes laterally and posteriorly beneath the neck of the femur where it narrows into a tendon that spirals in contact with the back of the femoral neck to be inserted on the medial surface of the greater trochanter into a deep pit, the trochanteric fossa. The capsule of the hip joint encloses the back of the neck of the femur only as far as the place where obturator externus tendon is in contact with periosteum, namely half the neck of the femur (Fig. 3.12), whereas in front the capsule of the hip joint includes the whole of the neck of the femur (Fig. 3.8).

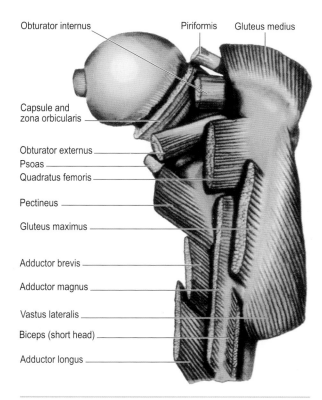

Obturator internus Piriformis Gluteus medius

Capsule and zona orbicularis

Obturator externus
Psoas
Quadratus femoris

Pectineus

Gluteus maximus

Adductor brevis

Adductor magnus

Vastus lateralis

Biceps (short head)

Adductor longus

Fig. 3.12 Attachment at the upper end of the right femur, from behind.

Nerve supply. By the posterior division of the obturator nerve (L3, 4).

Action. With the other short muscles around the hip joint, it stabilizes and supports the proximal part of the limb. As its line of pull passes behind the hip joint, it is a lateral rotator of the femur.

Obturator artery and nerve

The **obturator artery**, on emerging from the obturator foramen with the nerve, divides into anterior and posterior branches that encircle the foramen between the obturator externus and the membrane. They anastomose with each other and with the medial circumflex artery. From the posterior branch the *articular* twig to the hip joint arises; it enters the acetabular notch and runs in the ligament of the head of the femur to supply a small scale of bone in the region of the pit for the attachment of the ligament (see p. 133).

The **obturator nerve** divides in the obturator notch into anterior and posterior divisions; the anterior passes above obturator externus, the posterior passes through the muscle, giving off a branch to supply it before doing so.

The *anterior division*, giving an articular branch to the hip joint, descends in the thigh behind the adductor longus, which it supplies. Passing over the anterior surface of adductor brevis (Fig. 3.11), which it usually supplies, it goes on to supply gracilis and end in the subsartorial plexus, whence branches supply the skin over the medial side of the thigh. Direct branches to the skin are often given off at a level above the subsartorial plexus.

The *posterior division* emerges through obturator externus (having already supplied that muscle), and passes vertically downwards on adductor magnus deep to the other adductor muscles. It supplies adductor magnus and gives a terminal branch which runs with the femoral artery through the hiatus in the muscle to the popliteal fossa and supplies the capsule of the knee joint by passing in with the middle genicular artery.

PART THREE

Gluteal region and hip joint

The gluteal region or buttock lies behind the pelvis, and extends from the iliac crest to the gluteal fold (fold of the buttock). Various muscles, nerves and vessels emerge from the pelvis to enter the lower limb in this region. The muscles of the region are the three gluteal—gluteus maximus, medius and minimus—and the deeply placed piriformis, obturator internus, superior and inferior gemellus, and quadratus femoris (Fig. 3.13). Bony and ligamentous features of the region include the back of the sacrum and hip bone, the upper end of the femur,

and the sacrotuberous and sacrospinous ligaments. The greater sciatic foramen is formed above and in front by the greater sciatic notch of the hip bone, behind by the sacrotuberous ligament, and below by the sacrospinous ligament (see Figs 5.72 and 5.73, pp 334 and 335).

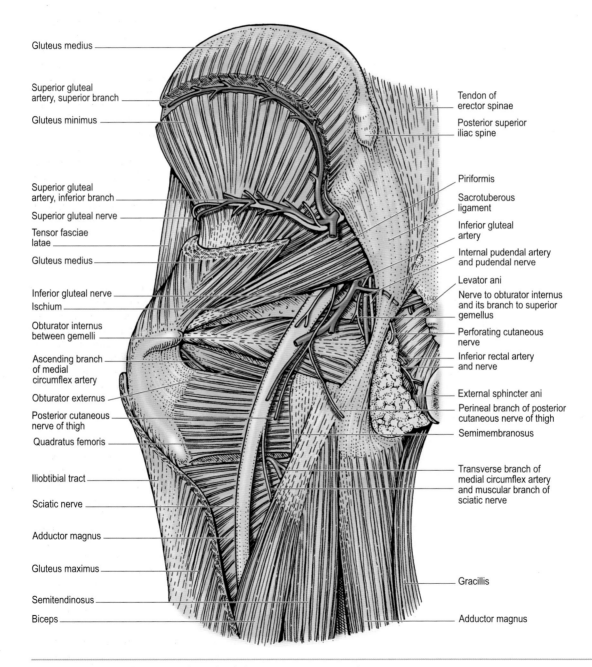

Gluteus medius

Superior gluteal artery, superior branch

Gluteus minimus

Superior gluteal artery, inferior branch

Superior gluteal nerve

Tensor fasciae latae

Gluteus medius

Inferior gluteal nerve

Ischium

Obturator internus between gemelli

Ascending branch of medial circumflex artery

Obturator externus

Posterior cutaneous nerve of thigh

Quadratus femoris

Ilioabtibial tract

Sciatic nerve

Adductor magnus

Gluteus maximus

Semitendinosus

Biceps

Tendon of erector spinae

Posterior superior iliac spine

Piriformis

Sacrotuberous ligament

Inferior gluteal artery

Internal pudendal artery and pudendal nerve

Levator ani

Nerve to obturator internus and its branch to superior gemellus

Perforating cutaneous nerve

Inferior rectal artery and nerve

External sphincter ani

Perineal branch of posterior cutaneous nerve of thigh

Semimembranosus

Transverse branch of medial circumflex artery and muscular branch of sciatic nerve

Gracillis

Adductor magnus

Fig. 3.13   Left gluteal region, with much of gluteus maximus removed.

The lesser sciatic foramen is formed by the lesser sciatic notch of the hip bone, and the same two ligaments. The ligaments cross each other and so convert the two sciatic notches into foramina.

Subcutaneous tissue

The subcutaneous fat is well developed in the gluteal region and gives the buttock its characteristic convexity. The fold of the buttock is the transverse skin crease for the hip joint and is not caused by the lower border of the gluteus maximus, which crosses the line of the fold obliquely. The blood supply of the skin and fat is derived from branches of the superior and inferior gluteal arteries, and the lymphatic drainage is into the lateral group of the superficial inguinal lymph nodes.

The **cutaneous nerves** of the buttock (Fig. 3.44) are derived from posterior and anterior rami. The posterior rami of the upper three lumbar nerves slope downwards over the iliac crest to supply the upper skin of the buttock. The posterior rami of all five sacral nerves are cutaneous. The upper three supply the skin of the natal cleft, the lower two, with the coccygeal nerve, supply skin over the coccyx.

The anterior rami are derived from widely separated segments. The upper part of the lateral skin is supplied by lateral cutaneous branches of the subcostal and ilio-hypogastric nerves (T12 and L1), the lower part by branches of the lateral femoral cutaneous nerve (L2). The perforating cutaneous nerve (S2, 3) and branches of the posterior femoral cutaneous nerve (S2, 3) supply the lower central part of the buttock. Thus the segments between L2 and S2 are not represented in the skin of the buttock; their dermatomes lie peripherally, in the skin of the limb (see Fig. 1.10, p. 15). The posterior axial line lies between these discontinuous dermatomes.

Gluteus maximus

This is the largest and the most superficial of the gluteal muscles, and it is characterized by its large fibre bundles. A thick flat sheet of muscle, it slopes from the pelvis down across the buttock at 45° (see Fig. 2.4, p. 43). It arises from the gluteal surface of the ilium behind the posterior gluteal line, from the lumbar fascia, from the lateral mass of the sacrum below the auricular surface, and from the sacrotuberous ligament. The deep half of its lower half is inserted into the gluteal tuberosity of the femur (Fig. 3.12). The remaining three-quarters of the muscle is inserted into the upper end of the iliotibial tract (Fig. 3.13).

There are usually three *bursae* beneath the muscle: one over the ischial tuberosity, one over the greater trochanter, and another over vastus lateralis.

The blood supply comes from both the superior and inferior gluteal arteries, and the veins form a plexus beneath the muscle.

Nerve supply. By the inferior gluteal nerve (L5, S1, 2), the only muscle supplied by this nerve.

Action. Its action on the femur is a combination of lateral rotation and extension at the hip joint, while through the iliotibial tract its contraction supports the extended knee. In paralysis of quadriceps femoris it can become an active but weak extensor of the knee. It can be felt in contraction in standing with hip and knee each slightly flexed, in which case it is a powerful antigravity muscle. It comes into play as an extensor of the hip joint chiefly at the extremes of hip movement, as in running, climbing stairs, etc., and it is called into play little if at all in the mid-position of the hip joint, as in quiet walking, when the main extensors of the hip are the hamstrings. It is the chief antigravity muscle of the hip during the act of sitting down from standing, controlling flexion of the hip joint.

Test. While lying face down with the leg straight, if the patient tightens the buttock and extends the hip, the contracting muscle can be observed and palpated.

Gluteus medius

This muscle arises from the gluteal surface of the ilium between the middle and posterior gluteal lines (Fig. 3.45). Its posterior third is covered by the gluteus maximus (see Fig. 2.4, p. 43) and its anterior two-thirds by thick deep fascia. The muscle converges to a flat tendon which is attached to the lateral surface of the greater trochanter (Fig. 3.12). A bursa separates the tendon from the upper part of the lateral surface of the greater trochanter.

Gluteus minimus

This muscle arises under cover of gluteus medius (Fig. 3.13) from the gluteal surface of the ilium between the middle and inferior lines, whence its fibres converge to a tendon which is attached to the anterior surface of the greater trochanter (Fig. 3.8). Its anterior border lies edge to edge with that of gluteus medius from origin to insertion. A bursa separates the tendon from the medial part of the anterior surface of the greater trochanter.

Nerve supplies. Gluteus medius and minimus are supplied by the superior gluteal nerve (L4, 5, S1).

Actions. These two muscles abduct the hip joint and their anterior fibres rotate the thigh medially. The two muscles are constantly called into play as the foot on one side is raised during walking and running, when the muscles on the opposite (supporting) side contract to prevent the pelvis from sagging on the unsupported side. In this they are assisted by tensor fasciae latae (see p. 120). If they are paralysed the gait is markedly affected, the trunk swaying from side to side towards the weight-bearing limb to prevent downward tilting of the pelvis on the unsupported side.

Test. While lying face down with the leg flexed to a right angle, the patient turns the foot outwards against resistance. Gluteus medius is palpated below the iliac crest behind tensor fasciae latae, which can also be felt contracting. In the *Trendelenburg test* with the patient standing on one leg, the pelvis on the opposite side should rise slightly; if it falls due to loss of abductor power on the supporting side, the test is positive.

Piriformis

This is an important muscle in that its relations provide the key to the arrangement of the structures in the gluteal region (Fig. 3.13). The muscle arises from the front of the middle three pieces of the sacrum, within the pelvis, and passes laterally behind the sacral plexus to emerge through the greater sciatic foramen, which it almost completely fills. Some additional fibres arise from the upper margin of the notch (Fig. 3.45). In the buttock its upper border lies alongside gluteus medius, its lower border alongside the superior gemellus. It converges into a rounded tendon which is inserted into the medial surface of the upper border of the greater trochanter (Fig. 3.12).

The *surface marking* of the lower border of piriformis is from the midpoint of a line between the posterior superior iliac spine (indicated by an overlying dimple on the surface of the back) and the tip of the coccyx to the tip of the greater trochanter.

Nerve supply. By the anterior rami of S1 and S2.

Obturator internus and gemelli

Obturator internus arises from the internal surface of the lateral wall of the pelvis (see p. 299) and makes a right-angled bend around the lesser sciatic notch of the ischium to enter the gluteal region (Fig. 3.13). Its deep tendinous surface is separated by a bursa from the lesser sciatic notch, which is covered here by hyaline cartilage. As the muscle emerges into the buttock it is reinforced by additional muscle fibres arising from the margins of the lesser sciatic notch. These are the superior and inferior gemelli. They blend with the tendon of obturator internus, which is inserted into the medial surface of the greater trochanter above the trochanteric fossa (Fig. 3.12).

Nerve supply. By its own nerve (L5, S1, 2).

The **superior gemellus** arises from the spine of the ischium and is supplied by the nerve to obturator internus, while the **inferior gemellus** arises from the ischial tuberosity at the margin of the lesser sciatic notch and is supplied by the nerve to quadratus femoris (Fig. 3.45).

The tendon of obturator internus and the gemelli lie horizontal in the buttock, the superior gemellus below piriformis and the inferior gemellus above quadratus femoris. The sciatic nerve passes down on their posterior surface.

Quadratus femoris

This rectangular muscle (Fig. 3.13) arises from the ischial tuberosity and is inserted into the quadrate tubercle of the femur. It is separated from the back of the neck of the femur by the tendon of obturator externus. The upper and lower borders of this horizontal muscle lie edge to edge with the inferior gemellus above and the upper border of adductor magnus below.

Nerve supply. By its own nerve (L4, 5, S1).

Actions. Pyriformis, obturator internus, the gemelli and quadratus femoris act together to adjust and stabilize the joint. Acting as prime movers they are lateral rotators of the extended thigh and abductors of the flexed thigh.

A number of structures emerge from the pelvis through the greater sciatic foramen into the gluteal region; to do so they pass above or below the piriformis muscle. Above the upper border emerge the superior gluteal nerve and vessels. Below the lower border emerge the inferior gluteal nerve and vessels, the pudendal nerve and vessels, the nerve to obturator internus, and the sciatic nerve with the posterior femoral cutaneous nerve on its surface and the nerve to quadratus femoris deep to it.

The **superior gluteal nerve** (L4, 5, S1) emerges from the greater sciatic notch above the upper border of piriformis and immediately disappears beneath the posterior border of gluteus medius and runs forwards between gluteus medius and minimus (Fig. 3.13). It supplies both muscles and ends in tensor fasciae latae. It has no cutaneous distribution.

The **superior gluteal artery** emerges from the pelvis above the upper border of piriformis and divides into superficial and deep branches. The superficial branch enters the deep surface of gluteus maximus to supply it and the overlying skin. The deep branch passes laterally between gluteus medius and minimus and divides into an upper and a lower branch. The upper reaches the anastomosis at the anterior superior iliac spine; the lower supplies the two glutei and joins the trochanteric anastomosis.

The **inferior gluteal nerve** (L5, S1, 2) leaves the pelvis beneath the lower border of piriformis and sinks into the deep surface of gluteus maximus (Fig. 3.13). It has no cutaneous distribution.

The **inferior gluteal artery** appears in the buttock between piriformis and the superior gemellus. It breaks up into muscular branches which supply piriformis, obturator internus, and gluteus maximus. It sends anastomotic branches to the trochanteric and cruciate anastomoses. One branch, the artery to the sciatic nerve, runs down on the sciatic nerve which it supplies. Cutaneous branches supply the buttock and back of thigh.

Trochanteric anastomosis

This provides the main source of blood for the supply of the head of the femur. The anastomosis lies near the trochanteric fossa. It is formed by anastomosis of the descending branch of the superior gluteal artery with the ascending branches of both lateral and medial circumflex femoral arteries. The inferior gluteal artery usually joins the anastomosis. Branches from the anastomosis pass along the femoral neck with the retinacular fibres of the capsule (see p. 132).

Cruciate anastomosis

At the level of the middle of the lesser trochanter the transverse branch of the medial circumflex femoral artery meets the transverse branch of the lateral circumflex femoral at the lower border of the insertion of quadratus femoris. They are joined by an ascending branch of the first perforating artery and the cross is completed above by a descending branch of the inferior gluteal artery.

The **pudendal nerve** (S2–4) makes a brief appearance in the buttock (Fig. 3.13). On emerging from beneath piriformis the nerve turns forward around the back of the sacrospinous ligament, on which it lies just medial to the spine of the ischium. It leaves the buttock by passing forward through the space between the sacrotuberous and sacrospinous ligaments (the lesser sciatic foramen) to enter the pudendal canal (see Fig. 5.69, p. 327).

The **internal pudendal artery** follows a similar course to that of the nerve, lying on its lateral side. It crosses the tip of the ischial spine, against which it can be compressed to control arterial haemorrhage in the perineum. A companion vein lies on each side of the artery.

The **nerve to obturator internus** (L5, S1, 2) lies still more laterally and loops around the base of the ischial spine as it passes forward to sink into the muscle, deep to its fascia, in the side wall of the ischioanal fossa (see Fig. 5.69, p. 327). It also supplies the superior gemellus.

The **sciatic nerve** (L4, 5, S1–3) emerges from below the piriformis muscle more laterally than the inferior gluteal and pudendal nerves and vessels (Fig. 3.13). It lies upon the ischium over the posterior part of the acetabulum. It is in contact with bone at a point one-third of the way up from the ischial tuberosity to the posterior superior iliac spine; this point is the surface marking for the entry of the nerve into the gluteal region. It passes vertically down over the posterior surface of obturator internus and quadratus femoris to the hamstring compartment of the thigh, where it is crossed posteriorly by the long head of biceps femoris. In the buttock it lies under cover of gluteus maximus just to the medial side of the midpoint between the greater trochanter and the ischial tuberosity, which is the *surface marking* of the nerve at the top of the thigh.

Its tibial and common peroneal (fibular) components usually separate in the upper part of the popliteal fossa but occasionally there is a high division and the two components may leave the pelvis separately, in which case the common peroneal nerve (L4, 5, S1, 2) usually pierces the piriformis while the tibial nerve (L4, 5, S1–3) emerges from beneath the muscle in the ordinary way.

The **posterior femoral cutaneous nerve** (S1–3) emerges from beneath piriformis and in its course in the buttock it lies on the sciatic nerve under cover of gluteus maximus. Below the buttock the nerve passes vertically down the midline of the back of the thigh and leg as low as the mid-calf. It lies beneath the fascia lata, superficial to the hamstrings, which separate it from the sciatic nerve, and supplies the fascia and overlying skin by a series of branches. Gluteal branches curl around the lower border of gluteus maximus to supply skin over the convexity of the buttock (Fig. 3.44). The long *perineal branch* winds medially and forward between gracilis and the fascia lata at the root of the limb to supply the posterior part of the scrotum or labium majus.

It is significant that the segments (S2, 3) of this nerve are also those of the pelvic parasympathetic nerves which supply pelvic viscera. Pain from pelvic disease is often referred over the distribution of the posterior femoral cutaneous nerve, and such pain along the back of the thigh and calf must be distinguished from sciatica.

The **nerve to quadratus femoris** (L4, 5, S1) lies on the ischium deep (anterior) to the sciatic nerve. It passes over the back of the hip joint, to which it gives an articular branch, and continues downwards deep to obturator internus and the gemelli, to sink into the anterior surface of quadratus femoris. It also supplies the inferior gemellus.

Gluteal intramuscular injection

The upper outer quadrant of the gluteal region is a common site for intramuscular injections. To avoid damage to the sciatic nerve it must be noted that the gluteal region extends from the iliac crest to the gluteal fold. In the above quadrant the needle may enter gluteus medius or gluteus maximus, depending on the exact position chosen.

Hip joint

The hip joint is a multiaxial synovial joint of the ball-and-socket variety, between the acetabulum of the innominate (hip) bone (Fig. 3.45) and the head of the femur (Fig. 3.47). In general it can be said that in all joints stability and range of movement are in inverse proportion to each other; the hip joint provides a remarkable example of a high degree of both. Its stability is largely the result of the adaptation of the acetabulum and femoral head to each other, and its great range of mobility results from the femur having a long neck that is much narrower than the head.

The cup-shaped acetabulum is formed by fusion of the three components of the hip bone: ilium, ischium, and pubis. The articular surface, covered with hyaline cartilage, does not occupy the whole of the acetabular fossa, but is a C-shaped concavity that is broadest above, where the body weight is transmitted in the erect posture. Its peripheral edge is deepened by a rim of fibrocartilage—the **acetabular labrum**—which encloses the femoral head beyond its equator, thus increasing the stability of the joint. The labrum is triangular in section, with its base attached to the acetabular rim. It is continued across the acetabular notch at the inferior margin of the acetabulum as the **transverse ligament**. The central non-articular part of the acetabulum is occupied by a pad of fat (the Haversian pad).

The spherical head of the femur is covered with hyaline cartilage. The non-articulating summit of the head is excavated into a pit (*fovea*) for attachment of the **ligament of the head of the femur** (ligamentum teres), whose other end is attached to the transverse ligament and the margins of the acetabular notch.

The **capsule** of the joint is attached circumferentially around the labrum and transverse ligament, whence it passes laterally, like a sleeve, to be attached to the neck of the femur. In front it is attached to the inter-trochanteric line, but at the back it extends for only half this distance, being attached halfway along the femoral neck (Fig. 3.12). The capsule is loose but extremely strong.

From these attachments the fibres of the capsule are reflected back along the neck of the femur to the articular margin of the femoral head. This reflected part constitutes the **retinacular fibres**, which bind down the nutrient arteries that pass, chiefly from the trochanteric anastomosis, along the neck of the femur to supply the major part of the head. Fracture of the femoral neck

within the capsular attachment ruptures the retinacular fibres and the vessels, causing avascular necrosis of the head.

The fibrous capsule is strengthened by three ligaments, which arise one from each constituent bone of the hip bone.

The **iliofemoral ligament** (of Bigelow) is the strongest of the three, and has a triangular shape (Fig. 3.14A). The apex is attached to the lower half of the anterior inferior iliac spine and the base is attached to the inter-trochanteric line. The margins are thick and the ligament has the appearance of an inverted V (though often being referred to as the Y-shaped ligament). The ligament limits extension at the hip joint.

The **pubofemoral ligament** is attached to the superior ramus and obturator crest of the pubic bone. It passes distally deep to the iliofemoral ligament, and blends with the capsule (Fig. 3.14A).

The **ischiofemoral ligament** is the weakest of the three. It arises from the posteroinferior margin of the acetabulum, and its fibres, passing laterally to the capsule, spiral upwards and blend with circular fibres of the capsule, the *zona orbicularis* (Fig. 3.14B). The zona is responsible for the hourglass constriction of a normal arthrogram.

As in all synovial joints, the **synovial membrane** is attached to the articular margins. From its attachment around the labrum and transverse ligament it lines all the capsule and is reflected back along the neck of the femur, where it invests the retinacular fibres up to the articular margin of the head of the femur. The Haversian fat pad and the ligament of the head are likewise invested in a sleeve of synovial membrane that is attached to the articular margins of the concavity of the acetabulum and of the fovea on the femoral head. Occasionally (10%) a perforation in the anterior part of the capsule, between the iliofemoral and pubofemoral ligaments, permits communication between the synovial cavity and the iliac bursa.

Relations

Anteriorly the psoas major tendon separates the capsule from the femoral artery and more medially pectineus intervenes between the capsule and the femoral vein. The femoral nerve lies lateral to the artery in a groove between iliacus and the psoas tendon. Iliacus is partly separated from the capsule by the bursa. *Superiorly* the reflected head of rectus femoris (medially) and gluteus minimus (laterally) are in contact with the capsule. *Inferiorly* obturator externus spirals below the capsule to the back of the femoral neck. *Posteriorly* lies piriformis, and below it the obturator internus tendon and the

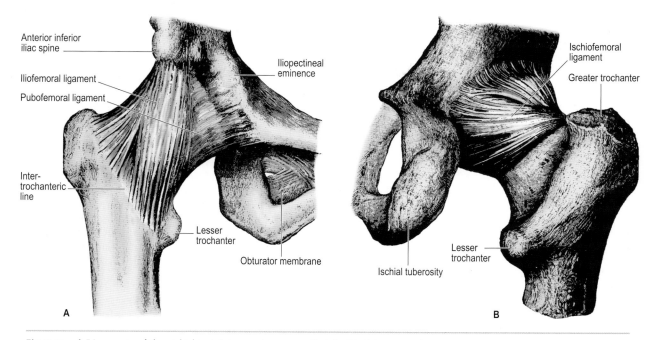

Fig. 3.14 **A** Ligaments of the right hip joint: anterior aspect; **B** right hip joint: posterior aspect.

gemelli separate the sciatic nerve from the capsule. *Laterally* the capsule blends with the iliotibial tract. *Medially* the acetabular fossa forms part of the lateral wall of the pelvis, and in the female the ovary lies adjacent, separated only by obturator internus, the obturator nerve and vessels and the peritoneum.

Blood supply

The capsule and synovial membrane are supplied from nearby vessels. The head and intracapsular part of the neck receive their blood from the trochanteric anastomosis (see p. 131), mainly through branches of the medial circumflex femoral artery. Although the artery in the ligament of the head of the femur (from the obturator artery) is important in the young child, it is usually considered to have atrophied by the age of about 7 years (but bleeding from it at adult hip operations suggests that it may often remain patent for much longer).

Nerve supply

The femoral nerve via the nerve to rectus femoris, the obturator nerve directly from its anterior division, the nerve to quadratus femoris and articular twigs from the sciatic nerve all supply the hip joint. The femoral, obturator and sciatic nerves also supply the knee joint

(see p. 144), and pain arising in the hip joint may be referred to the knee.

Movements

As in any ball and socket joint, movement is possible in all directions. Flexion, extension, adduction and abduction are free; a combination of all four produces circumduction. In addition, medial and lateral rotation of the femur occur.

In **flexion** of the hip the head of the femur rotates about a transverse axis that passes through both acetabula (Fig. 3.15) and the thigh is flexed upon the trunk. The muscles responsible for flexion are psoas major and iliacus, assisted by rectus femoris, sartorius and pectineus. Flexion is limited by the thigh touching the abdomen, or by tension of the hamstrings if the knee is extended; the normal range is about 120°, with the knee flexed.

Extension of the thigh, the reverse of the above movement, is performed by gluteus maximus at the extremes of the movement and by the hamstrings in the intermediate stage. The movement is limited by tension in the iliofemoral ligament, and amounts to about 20°.

In **adduction** and **abduction** of the thigh the femoral head rotates in the acetabulum about an anteroposterior axis. Adduction of about 30° is produced by contraction of the pectineus, adductors longus, brevis and magnus

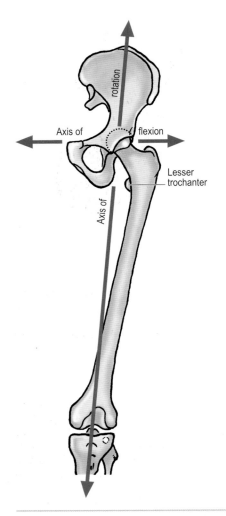

Axis of rotation

Axis of flexion

Lesser trochanter

Axis of

Fig. 3.15   Axes of rotation at the hip joint.

femoral head (Fig. 3.15). On account of the angulation of the neck of the femur, this axis does not coincide with the axis of the femoral shaft. Consequently the femoral neck and greater trochanter move forwards during medial rotation, and backwards during lateral rotation.

Medial rotation is produced by the anterior fibres of gluteus medius and minimus assisted by tensor fasciae latae. It is restricted by tension in the lateral rotators and the ischiofemoral ligament. Pyriformis, obturator internus and the gemelli, quadratus femoris and obturator externus are lateral rotators, assisted by gluteus maximus and sartorius. Lateral rotation is restricted by tension in the medial rotators and the iliofemoral ligament. Rotation in either direction amounts to about 40°.

If the neck of the femur is fractured, the shaft is free to rotate about its own axis, and psoas and iliacus produce the lateral rotation of the limb that is the characteristic feature of a fractured femoral neck.

Stability

The snug fit of the femoral head into the acetabulum, deepened by the labrum, makes the hip a very stable joint, further reinforced by the ligaments on the outside of the capsule, especially the iliofemoral. The short muscles of the gluteal region are important muscular stabilizers. The joint is least stable when flexed and adducted; dislocation requires considerable force but may occur, for example, in serious car accidents; the head of the femur is typically displaced posteriorly and there is often an associated fracture at the back of the acetabulum.

Surgical approach

The hip joint can be approached from the front, side or back. From the front and side the routes lie in front of, through or behind tensor fasciae latae. The anterior approach is through the interval between sartorius and tensor fasciae latae, detaching the tensor, rectus femoris and the anterior part of gluteus minimus from the hip bone so that the upper and anterior parts of the joint capsule can be reached. The anterolateral approach is between tensor fasciae latae and gluteus medius, exposing the capsule by retracting the anterior borders of gluteus medius and minimus or by detaching them from the greater trochanter. The ascending branches of the lateral circumflex femoral vessels are a source of bleeding during this approach, and the superior gluteal nerve is at risk at the upper end of the exposure. The posterior approach involves splitting the middle of gluteus maximus in the line of its fibres. Piriformis, obturator internus and the gemelli are divided at their

and the gracilis. It is limited by contact with the other leg or, if the latter is abducted out of the way, by the tension of gluteus medius and minimus. Abduction is produced by contraction of gluteus medius and minimus, assisted by tensor fasciae latae and sartorius. It is limited by tension in the adductors and in the pubofemoral ligament, and amounts to about 60°. Contraction of the abductors is essential in normal one-legged stance and in walking and running (see p. 129). In the sitting position, piriformis and the gemelli and obturator muscles act as abductors, e.g. helping to move the leading leg when getting out of a car.

In **rotation** the femoral head rotates in the acetabulum about a vertical axis that passes through the centre of the

femoral attachments to display the capsule. The sciatic nerve is retracted medially and is protected by turning the cut ends of obturator internus and the gemelli backwards over the nerve.

Injection or *aspiration* of the joint can be carried out from the front or side. At the front the needle is inserted 5 cm below the anterior inferior iliac spine and directed upwards, backwards and medially. For the lateral approach the needle passes in front of the greater trochanter and parallel with the femoral neck, entering the capsule through the lower ends of gluteus medius and minimus.

PART FOUR

Posterior compartment of the thigh

The posterior or hamstring compartment of the thigh extends from the buttock to the back of the knee. It is separated from the anterior compartment by the lateral intermuscular septum, but there is no septum dividing it from the medial or adductor compartment, for the adductor magnus is a muscle consisting of fused adductor and hamstring components.

The **cutaneous nerve supply** is by the posterior femoral cutaneous nerve, which runs vertically downwards deep to the fascia lata, pierces it behind the knee, and ends halfway down the calf. It sends branches through the fascia lata to supply the overlying skin.

Hamstring muscles

The hamstring muscles all arise from the ischial tuberosity and are inserted into the tibia or fibula; they thus span both the hip and knee joints. They are the semimembranosus, semitendinosus and biceps femoris (long head). The short head of biceps arises from the back of the femur.

Semimembranosus

This extends from the ischial tuberosity to the medial condyle of the tibia. It arises from the lateral part of the ischial tuberosity (Fig. 3.16), above the part that bears weight in sitting. This origin is a long flat tendon, from which muscle fibres commence about mid-thigh. The distal attachment of the muscle is by a rounded tendon into the horizontal concavity on the back of the medial condyle of the tibia (Figs 3.17 and 3.48B). From this insertion three expansions diverge. One passes forwards along the medial surface of the condyle deep to the tibial collateral ligament of the knee, separated

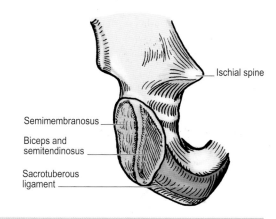

Fig. 3.16 Left ischial tuberosity, from behind.

from it by a bursa. A second expansion passes obliquely upwards to the lateral femoral condyle as the oblique popliteal ligament (see p. 142), while the third forms a strong fascia overlying popliteus and reaches the soleal line of the tibia.

Semitendinosus

This arises, in common with the long head of biceps, from the medial part of the ischial tuberosity (Fig. 3.16). The fleshy belly diminishes in size from above downwards to a cord-like tendon that lies on the posterior surface of the muscular belly of semimembranosus (Fig. 3.17). The tendon of semitendinosus passes behind the medial condyle of the femur and then curves forwards to be inserted behind gracilis into the upper part of the subcutaneous surface of the tibia.

Biceps femoris

This muscle has two heads of origin. The *long head* arises, in common with semitendinosus, from the ischial tuberosity (Fig. 3.16). It passes downwards and laterally, crossing the sciatic nerve on its posterior aspect, and joins the *short head* which has a long origin, from the whole length of the linea aspera and the upper part of the lateral supracondylar line of the femur (Fig. 3.47B). Distally the single tendon of the muscle is folded or split around the fibular collateral ligament of the knee joint and is inserted into the head of the fibula (Fig. 3.21).

Blood supply of the hamstrings. The hamstring compartment receives its blood supply mainly from the profunda femoris artery and its perforating branches. These pierce the adductor magnus and give off large

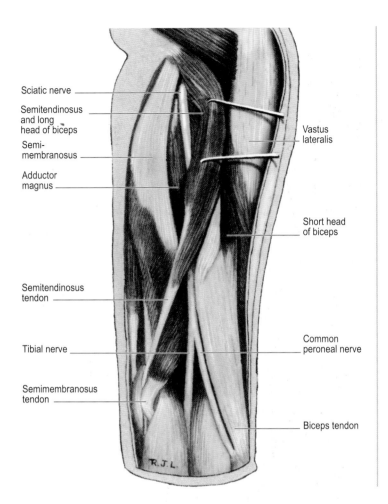

Sciatic nerve

Semitendinosus and long head of biceps

Semi-membranosus

Adductor magnus

Semitendinosus tendon

Tibial nerve

Semimembranosus tendon

Vastus lateralis

Short head of biceps

Common peroneal nerve

Biceps tendon

R.J.L.

Fig. 3.17 Right hamstring muscles. Semitendinosus and long head of biceps are retracted laterally to show the sciatic nerve lying on adductor magnus lateral to the tendinous upper end of semimembranosus.

branches to the hamstrings and the overlying fat and skin. The blood supply of the upper part of the hamstrings is derived from the inferior gluteal artery and that of the lower part from the popliteal artery. These and the perforating branches of the profunda femoris form a series of anastomoses along the back of the thigh. The highest is the cruciate anastomosis.

Nerve supplies. The three muscles are supplied, with the ischial part of adductor mangus, by the tibial component of the sciatic nerve (L5, S1), with the exception of the short head of biceps, which is supplied by the common peroneal (fibular) part of the sciatic nerve.

Actions. Acting from above the hamstrings flex the knee joint, and acting from below they extend the hip joint. With the knee semiflexed, biceps femoris is a lateral rotator, while semimembranosus and semitendinosus are medial rotators of the leg.

Test. While lying face downwards with the limb straight, the knee is flexed against resistance, and the tendons of biceps and semitendinosus palpated above the knee on the lateral and medial sides respectively.

Sciatic nerve

The sciatic nerve runs vertically through the hamstring compartment, lying deep to the long head of biceps, between it and the underlying adductor magnus (Fig. 3.17). At the apex of the popliteal fossa, a hand's breadth or more above the knee joint, it divides into its tibial and common peroneal (fibular) components; but the division may occur at a higher level (see p. 131).

The *surface marking* of the nerve is from the midpoint between the ischial tuberosity and greater trochanter to the apex of the popliteal fossa.

Fig. 3.18 Right popliteal fossa. Semitendinosus, semimembranosus and the two heads of gastrocnemius have been retracted to expose the contents of the fossa more fully.

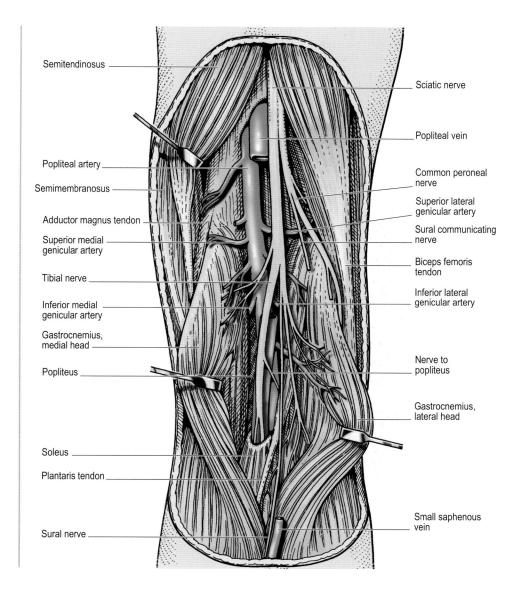

Semitendinosus

Sciatic nerve

Popliteal vein

Popliteal artery

Common peroneal nerve

Semimembranosus

Superior lateral genicular artery

Adductor magnus tendon

Sural communicating nerve

Superior medial genicular artery

Biceps femoris tendon

Tibial nerve

Inferior lateral genicular artery

Inferior medial genicular artery

Gastrocnemius, medial head

Nerve to popliteus

Popliteus

Gastrocnemius, lateral head

Soleus

Plantaris tendon

Small saphenous vein

Sural nerve

PART FIVE

Popliteal fossa and knee joint

The **popliteal fossa** is a diamond-shaped space behind the knee (Fig. 3.18). It is limited above by the semimembranosus and the semitendinosus on the medial side and the biceps femoris on the lateral side, diverging from the apex. In the living, the back of the flexed knee is hollow between the ridges made by the tensed hamstring tendons. In the extended knee the hamstring tendons lie against the femoral condyles and the fat of the popliteal space bulges the roof of the fossa. The lower part of the 'diamond' is occupied by the heads of the gastrocnemius and is opened up only when they are artificially separated (Fig. 3.18).

The *roof* of the fossa is formed by the fascia lata, which is here strongly reinforced by transverse fibres. It is pierced by the small saphenous vein and the posterior femoral cutaneous nerve. The *floor* is provided, from above downwards, by the popliteal surface of the femur, the capsule of the knee joint, reinforced by the oblique popliteal ligament, and the popliteus muscle covered by its fascia. The popliteal artery and vein and the tibial and common peroneal nerves pass through the fossa. A small group of popliteal lymph nodes lie alongside the popliteal vein.

The **common peroneal nerve** (*common fibular* nerve) runs downwards and laterally, medial to the biceps tendon, and disappears into the substance of peroneus longus to lie on the neck of the fibula, against which it can be rolled in the living. It gives off the following branches:

1. The *sural communicating nerve*, which pierces the roof of the fossa and runs downwards in the subcutaneous fat to join the sural nerve below the bellies of gastrocnemius.
2. The *lateral cutaneous nerve* of the calf, which pierces the roof of the fossa over the lateral head of gastrocnemius and supplies the skin over the upper part of the peroneal and extensor compartments of the leg.
3. The superior and inferior *genicular nerves*, which travel with the arteries of the same name and supply the capsule of the knee joint and the lateral ligament.
4. The *recurrent genicular nerve*, which arises in the substance of peroneus longus, perforates tibialis anterior and supplies the capsules of the superior tibiofibular and knee joints.

The common peroneal nerve ends by dividing, in the substance of peroneus longus, into the deep and superficial peroneal nerves.

The **tibial nerve** runs vertically down along the middle of the fossa and disappears by passing deeply between the heads of gastrocnemius (Fig. 3.17). If the latter are separated the nerve is seen passing, with the popliteal vessels, beneath the fibrous arch in the origin of soleus (Fig. 3.18). Below this fibrous arch it enters the calf. The nerve gives *motor branches* to all the muscles that arise in the popliteal fossa, namely to plantaris, both heads of the gastrocnemius, soleus and popliteus. The last branch hooks around the lower border of popliteus to enter its deep (tibial) surface.

The tibial nerve here has only one cutaneous branch, the *sural nerve*. It runs vertically down in the narrow interval between the two heads of gastrocnemius and pierces the deep fascia halfway down the calf, where it replaces the posterior cutaneous nerve of the thigh. Passing down in the subcutaneous fat it joins the sural communicating nerve below the bellies of gastrocnemius where it is always close to the small saphenous vein which is the guide to the nerve (it can be used for grafts); the nerve is usually lateral to the vein.

Articular branches, the *genicular nerves*, are three in number. They accompany the superior and inferior medial genicular arteries to supply the medial ligament and the capsule of the knee joint, and the middle genicular artery to pierce the oblique popliteal ligament, supplying it and the cruciate ligaments.

Popliteal vessels

Throughout the whole of its course the **popliteal artery** is the deepest of the large neurovascular structures in the fossa (Fig. 3.18). It extends from the hiatus in adductor magnus (a hand's breadth above the knee) to the fibrous arch in soleus (a hand's breadth below the knee). It enters the fossa on the medial side of the femur; there it lies not only deep but medial to the sciatic nerve and its vertical continuation the tibial nerve. As it passes downwards it is convex laterally, coming to lie lateral to the tibial nerve. Below the fibrous arch in soleus, as the posterior tibial artery, it returns to the medial side of the nerve. At all levels the popliteal vein lies between the artery and the nerve. The artery lies successively on the popliteal surface of the femur, separated from it by a little fat, on the oblique popliteal ligament and on the fascia over the popliteus muscle. It passes under the fibrous arch in soleus and immediately divides into anterior and posterior tibial arteries. Rarely the popliteal artery may divide proximal to popliteus, the anterior tibial artery then descending anterior to the muscle.

The popliteal artery may be compressed by the medial head of gastrocnemius (popliteal artery entrapment syndrome) when the artery takes a variant course, deviating medially behind the muscle and passing distally deep to the muscle. The artery may also be compressed by an accessory slip of the muscle arising more laterally from the femur, separating the artery and vein or passing behind both.

Palpation of popliteal pulsation against the back of the femur, with the fingertips of both hands pressing into the centre of the fossa, must be accompanied by flexion of the knee to relax the overlying popliteal fascia.

Muscular branches are given to the muscles in the popliteal fossa including two large *sural arteries* that supply the two heads of gastrocnemius. The **genicular arteries** are five in number, upper and lower lateral and medial, and a middle. The medial and lateral superior genicular arteries encircle the lower end of the femur proximal to the attachment of the gastrocnemius muscles. The medial and lateral inferior arteries encircle the upper end of the tibia. The *middle genicular artery* pierces the oblique popliteal ligament to supply the cruciate ligaments; it is accompanied by the genicular branch of the posterior division of the obturator nerve (see p. 127).

The *medial superior genicular artery* lies deep to semitendinosus, semimembranosus and the tendon of adductor magnus.

The *lateral superior genicular artery* is deep to the tendon of biceps femoris.

The *medial inferior genicular artery* courses obliquely downwards deep to the medial head of gastrocnemius and the medial ligament of the knee. The *lateral inferior genicular artery* runs horizontally deep to the lateral head of gastrocnemius, crosses the popliteus tendon and passes deep to the lateral ligament of the knee.

The genicular branches of the popliteal artery form an anastomosis, around the patella and the femoral and tibial condyles, with the descending genicular branch of the femoral artery, the descending branch of the lateral circumflex femoral artery, the circumflex fibular branch of the posterior tibial artery and the anterior and posterior recurrent branches of the anterior tibial artery.

Surgical approach. Various surgical approaches to the popliteal artery are possible: from behind or from either side with the knee partly flexed. The posterior approach opens up the interval between the heads of the gastrocnemei, retracting these muscles apart, and carefully avoiding the nerves and the popliteal vein. The lateral approach passes behind the iliotibial tract and the lateral intermuscular septum, displacing biceps backwards. The medial approach gives superior access. The above-knee popliteal artery is accessed along the anterior border of sartorius with division of the adductor magnus tendon. Below-knee access to the artery requires medial retraction of the tendons of sartorius, gracilis and semitendinosus, and posterior retraction of the medial head of gastrocnemius. These musculotendinous structures may be divided for greater access. The great saphenous vein needs to be safeguarded.

The **popliteal vein** lies, at all levels, between the artery and the tibial nerve (Fig. 3.18). It is formed by the union of the venae comitantes of the anterior and posterior tibial arteries; ascending through the aperture in the adductor magnus it becomes the femoral vein. It receives tributaries that accompany the branches of the popliteal artery and the *small saphenous vein* (see p. 150). The popliteal vein may take the form of venae comitantes on either side of the artery.

The **popliteal lymph nodes** consist of a few scattered nodes lying about the termination of the small saphenous vein, beneath the deep fascia. They receive from a small area of skin just above the heel by a few superficial afferents which run with the small saphenous vein and pierce the roof of the fossa, and from the deep structures of the calf by afferents that accompany the posterior tibial vessels. They send their efferents alongside the popliteal and femoral vessels to the deep inguinal nodes.

Popliteus

This muscle (Fig. 3.19) is attached to a triangular area on the posterior surface of the tibia above the soleal line. The muscle slopes upwards and laterally towards a cord-like tendon, which is attached to a pit at the anterior end of a groove on the lateral surface of the lateral condyle of the femur (Fig. 3.23); the tendon runs along the groove when the knee is fully flexed. The tendon lies within the capsule of the knee joint, entering it beneath the *arcuate popliteal ligament*, to which superficial fibres of the muscle are attached (Fig. 3.19). The muscle also has some attachment to the capsule and the posterior convexity of the lateral meniscus (Fig. 3.22). A pouch of synovial membrane from the knee joint lies between the tendon and the superior tibiofibular joint, with which it may communicate.

Nerve supply. By a branch of the tibial nerve which winds around its lower border and sinks into its deep (anterior) surface. This nerve also supplies the superior tibiofibular joint.

Action. In the fully extended knee the femur has rotated medially on the tibia to 'lock' the joint (see p. 144). The femur is rotated laterally to unlock the joint at the commencement of flexion by the popliteus, acting from below with the tibia fixed as in the erect position. The attachment to the lateral meniscus suggests that the posterior horn of the meniscus may be retracted during this movement. In the supine or seated position, popliteus medially rotates the mobile tibia at the commencement of flexion.

Knee joint

The knee joint is a synovial joint, the largest in the body. It is a modified hinge joint; in addition to flexion and extension a small amount of rotation of the leg is possible in the flexed position of the knee. It is a compound joint that includes two condylar joints between the femur and the tibia (Fig. 3.21A) and a sellar (saddle) joint between the patella and the femur (Fig. 3.20), the former being partly divided by menisci. The lateral and medial articular surfaces of the femur and tibia are asymmetrical. The distal surface of the medial condyle of the femur is narrower and more curved than that of the lateral condyle. The lateral tibial articular surface is almost circular, the medial is oval with a longer anteroposterior axis, and these differences are reflected in the shapes of the menisci. The articular surface of the patella is

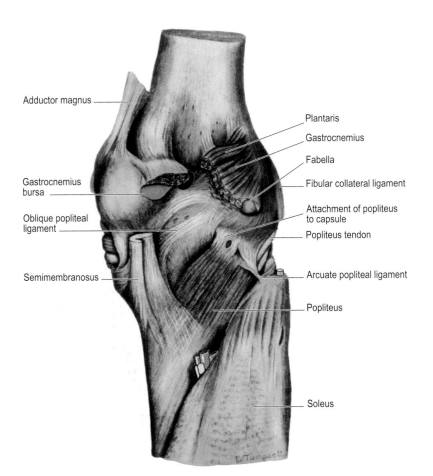

Adductor magnus

Gastrocnemius bursa

Oblique popliteal ligament

Semimembranosus

Plantaris

Gastrocnemius

Fabella

Fibular collateral ligament

Attachment of popliteus to capsule

Popliteus tendon

Arcuate popliteal ligament

Popliteus

Soleus

Fig. 3.19   Right knee joint from behind, showing the reinforcement of the capsule by the oblique popliteal ligament, and popliteus emerging from the capsule. The fabella is a sesamoid bone sometimes present in the lateral head of gastrocnemius.

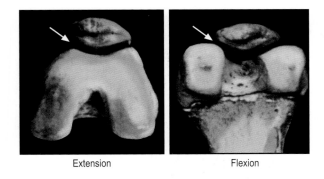

Extension   Flexion

Fig. 3.20   Left femur and patella, as seen when looking upwards from the tibia with the knee in extension and flexion. The medial facet of the patella (arrow) is free in extension but in flexion it articulates with the medial condyle of the femur.

divided by a vertical ridge into a large lateral and a small medial surface; the latter is further subdivided by a vertical ridge into two smaller areas. The large lateral area articulates with the lateral condyle of the femur in extension and flexion. In extension the area next to it is in contact with the medial femoral condyle and the most medial area does not articulate with the femur (Fig. 3.20). In flexion this surface is in contact with the medial condyle and the middle area is opposite the intercondylar notch of the femur.

The **capsule** of the knee joint is attached posteriorly to the proximal margins of the femoral condyles and the intercondylar fossa. Medially the capsule is attached to the articular margin of the femur, but laterally the attachment is proximal to the groove for the popliteus tendon (Fig. 3.23). Anteriorly the capsular attachment on the femur is deficient above the level of the patella, permitting the suprapatellar bursa to be in full communication with the joint. The capsule blends with the patellar retinacula, thereby gaining attachment to the sides of the patella and patellar ligament. Posteriorly on the tibia the capsule is attached to the margins of the tibial condyles, and in the intercondylar area to the distal edge of the groove for the posterior cruciate ligament (Fig. 3.48B); the attachment to the lateral condyle is interrupted by an aperture for the passage of the popliteus tendon. On the sides, the capsule is attached to the margins of the tibial condyles, and laterally to the head of the fibula as well. A thickening of the capsule on the medial side is a deep component of the tibial collateral ligament and is firmly attached to the medial meniscus. On its deep aspect the capsule has weak attachments to the rims of both menisci, the coronary ligaments, which connect them to the tibia. Anteriorly the line of attachment on the tibia of the fused capsule and patellar retinacula inclines distally from the medial and lateral condyles to the tibial tuberosity.

The **tibial collateral ligament** (medial ligament) (Figs 3.21 and 3.22) is a flat, triangular band attached

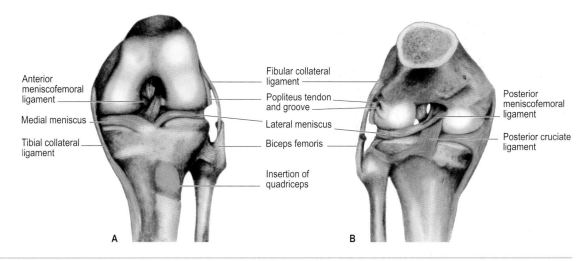

Anterior meniscofemoral ligament

Medial meniscus

Tibial collateral ligament

Fibular collateral ligament

Popliteus tendon and groove

Lateral meniscus

Biceps femoris

Insertion of quadriceps

Posterior meniscofemoral ligament

Posterior cruciate ligament

A   B

Fig. 3.21 Ligaments of the left knee joint, with the knee partially flexed: **A** from the front; **B** from behind.

Fig. 3.22 Menisci of the left knee joint, from behind.

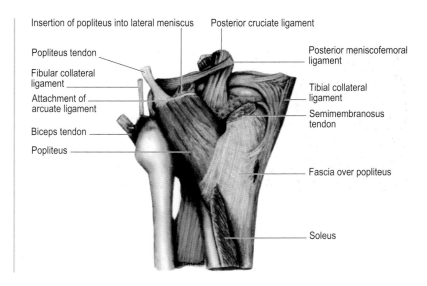

Insertion of popliteus into lateral meniscus   Posterior cruciate ligament

Popliteus tendon

Fibular collateral ligament

Attachment of arcuate ligament

Biceps tendon

Popliteus

Posterior meniscofemoral ligament

Tibial collateral ligament

Semimembranosus tendon

Fascia over popliteus

Soleus

above to the medial femoral epicondyle, just distal to the adductor tubercle, and attached below to the upper part of the medial surface of the tibia. Its anterior margin, which forms the vertical base of the triangle, is free except at its attached extremities. The posterior apex of the triangular ligament blends with the capsule and is thereby attached to the medial meniscus. Above its distal attachment the ligament is crossed by the tendons of sartorius, gracilis and semitendinosus with a bursa interposed. The medial inferior genicular vessels and nerve and the anterior expansion of the semimembranosus tendon are deep to the distal part of the ligament with another bursa intervening.

The **fibular collateral ligament** (lateral ligament) (Figs 3.21 and 3.22) is cord-like and is attached proximally to the lateral epicondyle, below the attachment of the lateral head of gastrocnemius and above that of the tendon of popliteus (Fig. 3.23). Its distal attachment is to the head of the fibula overlapped by the tendon of biceps femoris, a bursa intervening between them. The ligament is not attached to the capsule and has no connection with the lateral meniscus. A bursa lies between the ligament and the capsule, and the tendon of popliteus lies deep to the capsule here. The lateral inferior genicular vessels and nerve run deep to the distal part of the ligament.

The **oblique popliteal ligament** (Fig. 3.19) is an expansion from the tendon of semimembranosus that blends with the capsule at the back of the joint and ascends laterally to the intercondylar fossa and lateral femoral condyle. The popliteal artery lies on it, and genicular vessels and nerves penetrate it.

The **arcuate popliteal ligament** (Fig. 3.19) is a Y-shaped thickening of posterior capsular fibres. The stem of the Y is attached to the head of the fibula. The medial limb arches over the tendon of popliteus to the posterior edge of the tibial intercondylar area. Some popliteus muscle fibres are attached to it. The lateral limb ascends to the lateral femoral condyle.

The **cruciate ligaments** are a pair of very strong ligaments connecting tibia to femur (Figs 3.21 and 3.24). They lie within the capsule of the knee joint, but not within the synovial membrane. It is as though they had been herniated into the synovial membrane from behind, so that they are covered by synovial membrane on their front and sides but not posteriorly. The **anterior cruciate ligament** is attached to the anterior part of the tibial plateau between the attachments of the anterior horns of the medial and lateral menisci. The ligament ascends posterolaterally, twisting on itself, and is attached to the posteromedial aspect of the lateral femoral condyle. The **posterior cruciate ligament** is stronger, shorter and broader, and less oblique. It is attached to a smooth impression on the posterior part of the tibial intercondylar area which extends to the uppermost part of the posterior surface of the tibia (Fig. 3.48B). The ligament ascends anteromedially and is attached to the antero-lateral aspect of the medial femoral condyle. The cruciate ligaments cross each other like the limbs of the letter X, the anterior ligament lying mainly anterolateral to the posterior ligament.

The **menisci**—formerly called semilunar cartilages—are crescentic discs of fibrocartilage comprising mainly collagenous fibrous tissue that lie on and are attached to the tibial plateau (Fig. 3.24). They are triangular in cross-section, being thicker at their convex periphery. Their distal surfaces are flat, while their proximal surfaces are concave and articulate with the convex femoral condyles. The menisci are mainly avascular but their peripheral zone is vascularized by capillaries from the capsule. The **medial meniscus** is almost a semicircle

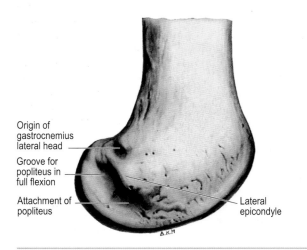

Origin of gastrocnemius lateral head

Groove for popliteus in full flexion

Attachment of popliteus

Lateral epicondyle

Fig. 3.23 Distal end of the right femur: lateral aspect.

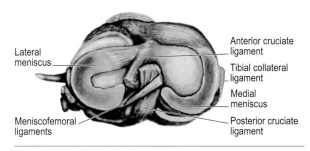

Lateral meniscus

Meniscofemoral ligaments

Anterior cruciate ligament

Tibial collateral ligament

Medial meniscus

Posterior cruciate ligament

Fig. 3.24 Menisci of the left knee joint, from above.

and is broader posteriorly. Its anterior horn is attached to the intercondylar area in front of the anterior cruciate ligament, while the posterior horn is similarly attached in front of the posterior cruciate ligament. As mentioned above, the medial meniscus is firmly attached to the capsule and the tibial collateral ligament.

The **lateral meniscus** is about four-fifths of a circle and is of uniform width. Its anterior horn is attached in front of the intercondylar eminence of the tibia, behind the anterior cruciate ligament with which it partly blends. The posterior horn is attached behind the intercondylar eminence, in front of the posterior horn of the medial meniscus. From the posterior convexity of the lateral meniscus fibrous bands pass upwards and medially to the medial femoral condyle, in front of and behind the posterior cruciate ligament (Figs 3.21 and 3.24). These are the **anterior** and **posterior meniscofemoral ligaments** (of Humphry and Wrisberg). More medially some fibres of the popliteus muscle are attached to the posterior convexity of the lateral meniscus. The **transverse ligament** is a variable band that connects the anterior convexity of the lateral meniscus to the anterior horn of the medial meniscus.

The **synovial membrane** is the most extensive in the body but the amount of synovial fluid in a normal joint is only 0.5 ml—a mere capillary film. It is attached to the articular margins of the femur, tibia and patella and lines the deep aspect of the capsule, but it is separated from the capsule by the popliteus tendon and the cruciate ligaments, which are thereby excluded from the synovial cavity. Anteriorly the membrane is separated from the patellar ligament by the *infrapatellar fat pad*, which herniates the membrane into the joint cavity as a pair of folds, the *alar folds*; these converge in the midline into a single fold, the *infrapatellar fold*, which extends posteriorly and is attached to the femoral intercondylar fossa (Fig. 3.25). The synovial membrane does not cover the surfaces of the menisci. It is continuous with the lining of the suprapatellar bursa. Posteriorly a small pouch of membrane projects distally between the tendon of popliteus and the upper ends of the tibia and fibula; it may communicate with the superior tibiofibular joint. The synovial cavity of the knee joint often communicates with the bursa deep to the medial head of gastrocnemius, and sometimes communicates with the bursa deep to the lateral head of gastrocnemius.

There are a dozen **bursae** related to the knee joint: four on the anterior aspect; two on either side; and four at the back. The suprapatellar bursa lies between the femur and the quadriceps femoris; the articularis genu muscle is attached to it (see p. 124). The subcutaneous prepatellar bursa lies between the skin and the patella and the subcutaneous infrapatellar bursa between the

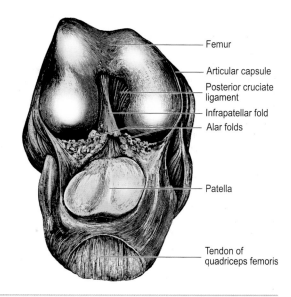

Femur

Articular capsule

Posterior cruciate ligament

Infrapatellar fold

Alar folds

Patella

Tendon of quadriceps femoris

Fig. 3.25 Right knee joint in flexion: anterior aspect. The quadriceps tendon has been divided and reflected downwards.

skin and the tibial tuberosity. The deep infrapatellar bursa is situated between the patellar ligament and the upper part of the tibia. Laterally there is a bursa between the fibular collateral ligament and the biceps femoris tendon, and another bursa between the ligament and the capsule where it overlies the popliteus tendon. Medially there is a bursa between the tibial collateral ligament and the tendons of sartorius, gracilis and semitendinosus; a bursa deep to the ligament partly separates it from the tibia, the capsule and an expansion from the semimembranosus tendon. Two bursae are situated deeply between the posterior aspect of the capsule and the medial and lateral heads of gastrocnemius. The semimembranosus bursa lies between that muscle and the medial head of gastrocnemius; it may communicate with the bursa deep to the latter muscle and thereby with the joint cavity. The bursa between the popliteus tendon and the back of the upper tibia and fibula is an extension of the synovial membrane of the knee joint.

Blood supply

The capsule and joint structures are supplied from the anastomoses around the knee (see p. 139). The chief contributors are the five genicular branches of the popliteal artery, of which the middle genicular supplies the cruciate ligaments.

Nerve supply

The joint is supplied from the femoral nerve through its branches to the three vasti, from the sciatic nerve by the genicular branches of its tibial and common peroneal components, and from the obturator nerve by the twig from its posterior division, which accompanies the femoral artery through the gap in the adductor magnus into the popliteal fossa. During arthroscopy it must be remembered that, although local anaesthesia affects the overlying skin, the cruciate ligaments remain sensitive (tibial nerve). The horns of the menisci are innervated but their central parts are devoid of sensory fibres.

Movements

The movements of the knee joint are flexion, extension and rotation.

Flexion is performed primarily by the hamstrings—semimembranosus, semitendinosus and biceps femoris—assisted by gracilis, sartorius, popliteus, gastrocnemius and plantaris. It is limited to about 150° by compression of the soft parts behind the knee.

Extension is performed by the quadriceps femoris, assisted by tensor fasciae latae. As the knee extends, the shorter and more rounded lateral femoral condyle completes its extension excursion about 30° short of full extension. The lateral condyle then rotates forwards around a taut anterior cruciate ligament, and allows the longer and more oval medial condyle to glide backwards into its own full extension. This passive medial rotation of the femur is part of a 'locking' mechanism which secures the joint in 5–10° of hyperextension, when both cruciate ligaments, the tibial and fibular collateral ligaments and the oblique popliteal ligament are all taut. The femur rotates as described when extension occurs with the foot on the ground. When the foot is free to move, passive lateral rotation of the tibia occurs instead at the terminal phase of extension. From the locked position lateral rotation of the femur must precede flexion. This lateral rotation is produced by the popliteus muscle; when flexion occurs with the foot free, popliteus medially rotates the tibia instead. The unlocked knee can now be flexed by the hamstrings.

When the knee flexes, the fibular collateral ligaments and the posterior part of the tibial collateral ligaments are relaxed and a smaller femoral surface articulates with the menisci. In this position about 10° of active *rotation* is possible. Lateral rotation is produced by biceps femoris and medial rotation by semimembranosus and semitendinosus. Passive rotation in the flexed position amounts to about 60°, such as when a clinician takes hold of a subject's leg and rotates it.

Flexion and extension take place above the menisci, in the upper compartment of the joint. The menisci are passively opened up in extension when a broader area of femoral condyle is in contact with them, separating their anterior and posterior convexities. Rotation takes place below the menisci, in the lower compartment.

Stability

The bony contours contribute little to the stability of the joint, but the intercondylar eminence of the tibia prevents sideways slipping of femur on tibia. Nevertheless, ligaments and muscles make it a very stable joint which rarely dislocates. The cruciate ligaments are indispensable to anteroposterior stability in flexion. Forward displacement of the tibia on the femur is prevented by the anterior cruciate ligament and backward displacement of the tibia on the femur is prevented by the posterior cruciate ligament. The integrity of the posterior cruciate ligament is therefore important when walking downstairs or downhill (Fig. 3.26).

The menisci are liable to injury resulting from twisting strains applied to the flexed weight-bearing knee. The medial meniscus is more prone to damage, probably because it is firmly attached to the capsule and the collateral ligament. Likewise the flat medial ligament, which is attached to the posteromedial capsule, is more likely to be torn than the cord-like lateral ligament, which is unattached to the capsule. A combined rotation

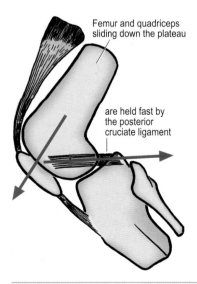

Femur and quadriceps sliding down the plateau

are held fast by the posterior cruciate ligament

Fig. 3.26   Weight-bearing on the flexed knee. The body weight is suspended on the posterior cruciate ligament. This is the position of the upper knee during progression downhill.

and impact injury to the flexed knee, as in sports injuries, may cause rupture of the anterior cruciate ligament. The stronger posterior cruciate ligament is less likely to be damaged, but it may be torn when the tibia is violently thrust backwards in relation to the femur.

Surgical approach

The knee joint can be exposed from the front on either side of the patella by incisions through the vasti and alongside the patella and its ligament; incisions lateral to the patella avoid damage to the infrapatellar branch of the saphenous nerve. A limited approach to the medial meniscus with the knee flexed is along the medial side of the patella but with the incision extending no more than 1 cm below the upper margin of the tibia, to avoid damage to this branch, which curves forwards below that level. Exposure of the back of the joint capsule through the popliteal fossa involves opening up the interval between the tibial nerve and semimembranosus, then displacing the nerve and popliteal vessels laterally and detaching the medial head of gastrocnemius from its origin. This head is also displaced laterally, so revealing the capsule and helping to protect the vessels and nerve. The middle genicular artery will require ligation.

Aspiration is usually carried out from the side at the upper lateral margin of the patella, the needle entering the suprapatellar bursa. For injection the joint is entered at the lower border of the patella on either side of the patellar ligament. The needle tip must not damage the menisci or joint surfaces. For arthroscopy the approach is usually on the lateral side of the patellar ligament.

PART SIX

Anterior compartment of the leg

The front of the leg includes the subcutaneous surface of the tibia on the medial side and the extensor muscular compartment on the anterolateral side.

The **cutaneous nerves** are derived from the femoral nerve over the tibia and from the common peroneal nerve over the extensor compartment (Fig. 3.43). The *saphenous nerve* gives off its infrapatellar branch, to supply the subcutaneous periosteum of the upper end of the tibia and the overlying skin, and then descends just behind the great saphenous vein with which it passes in front of the medial malleolus. It usually bifurcates above the malleolus, and the branches run in front of and behind the vein. The main nerve (anterior branch) often extends on the medial side of the foot as far as the bunion region: the metatarsophalangeal joint. The

lateral cutaneous nerve of the calf, a branch of the common peroneal, supplies deep fascia and skin over the upper parts of the extensor and peroneal compartments and the *superficial peroneal nerve* replaces it over the rest of these surfaces.

The subcutaneous surface of the tibia has subcutaneous fat in direct contact with the periosteum; the deep fascia here is blended with the periosteum. The great saphenous vein and the saphenous nerve lie in the fat, accompanied by numerous lymphatic vessels which pass up from the foot to the vertical group of superficial inguinal nodes. This is an important part of the course of the **great saphenous vein** (see p. 117) for here it has most of its deep connections. Along the medial side of the calf behind the medial border of the tibia a variable number of perforating (anastomotic) veins connect the great saphenous with deep veins of the calf (Fig. 3.27). Their location is variable but there is usually one just below and one about 10 cm above the medial malleolus, and another one a little below the middle of the leg. Higher up, there is a perforator just distal to the knee, and a rather long perforator in the lower thigh joining the great saphenous or one of its tributaries to the femoral vein in the adductor canal. The perforators in the leg may connect instead with a superficial longitudinal trunk, the **posterior arch vein** (Fig. 3.27), which usually joins the great saphenous some way below the knee. When traced deeply through the deep fascia, some of the perforating veins in the leg are seen to join the venae

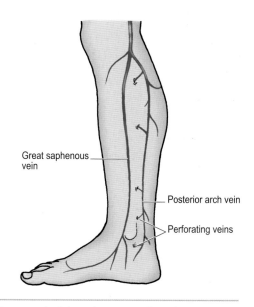

Great saphenous vein

Posterior arch vein

Perforating veins

Fig. 3.27 Lower end of the right great saphenous vein, passing upwards in front of the medial malleolus.

comitantes of the posterior tibial artery, while others join the venous plexus in soleus. The valves in the perforating veins are directed inwards and are found where the veins pierce the deep fascia and also where they join the deep veins. Much of the saphenous blood passes from superficial to deep through the perforators, to be pumped upwards in the deep veins by the contractions of soleus and other calf muscles. If the valves in the perforators become incompetent, the direction of blood flow is reversed and the veins become varicose (Fig. 3.28).

The upper end of the subcutaneous surface of the shaft of the tibia receives the tendons of *three muscles* that converge from the three constituent parts of the hip bone (Fig. 3.45). They are sartorius (supplied by the femoral, the nerve of the ilium), gracilis (supplied by the obturator, the nerve of the pubis) and semitendinosus (supplied by the sciatic, the nerve of the ischium) in that order from before backwards. The three tendons are separated by a bursa which lies deep to the flattened sartorius tendon.

The **deep fascia** of the leg covers only muscles, being attached to periosteum at all places where bone is subcutaneous; these include the medial surface of the tibial shaft and malleolus, and the lateral surface of the fibular

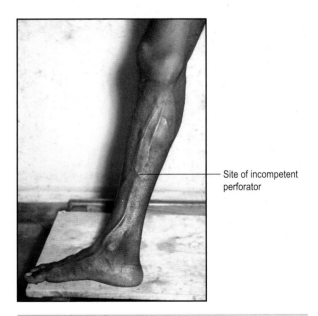

Fig. 3.28 The great saphenous and posterior arch veins are dilated (varicose). A small subcutaneous bulge (clinically called a blow-out) at the middle of the leg marks the site of an incompetent perforator.

— Site of incompetent perforator

malleolus and the triangular area above it. The deep fascia thus extends from the anterior border of the tibia around the lateral aspect of the leg to the posterior border of the tibia, enclosing the muscles of the leg. Two intermuscular septa pass from its deep surface to become attached to the fibula. They enclose the peroneal compartment. Between the anterior intermuscular septum and the tibia lies the extensor compartment, while between the posterior intermuscular septum and the tibia posteriorly lies the much more bulky flexor compartment or calf of the leg.

Extensor compartment

The compartment comprises the space between the deep fascia and the interosseous membrane, bounded medially by the extensor surface of the tibia and laterally by the extensor surface of the fibula and the anterior intermuscular septum. Its contents are muscles: tibialis anterior, extensor hallucis longus, extensor digitorum longus, and peroneus tertius, together with the deep peroneal nerve and anterior tibial vessels. This is a tight space and any further increase of its contents, by for instance a haematoma or muscle oedema, could cause compression and ischaemia of neurovascular and muscular structures in the compartment (compartment syndrome).

In its lower extent the deep fascia is thickened to form the **superior extensor retinaculum** (Fig. 3.29), which is attached to the anterior borders of the tibia and fibula. Deep to the retinaculum lie the tendons of tibialis anterior, extensor hallucis longus, extensor digitorum longus and peroneus tertius, in that order from medial to lateral, in front of the lower end of the tibia. Only the tibialis anterior tendon has a synovial sheath here. The anterior tibial vessels and deep peroneal nerve are also deep to the retinaculum, lying between extensor hallucis longus and extensor digitorum longus, with the vessels medial to the nerve (Fig. 3.29).

Tibialis anterior

This muscle, which is readily palpable lateral to the tibia, arises from the upper two-thirds of the extensor surface of the tibia, from the interosseous membrane and from the deep fascia overlying it. The muscle descends as a tendon, enclosed in a synovial sheath, through the medial compartments of the superior and inferior extensor retinacula, and is inserted into the medial and inferior surfaces of the medial cuneiform and the adjacent part of the first metatarsal bone (Fig. 3.29).

Nerve supply. By the deep peroneal and recurrent genicular nerves (L4).

Fig. 3.29 Left lower leg and dorsum of the foot.

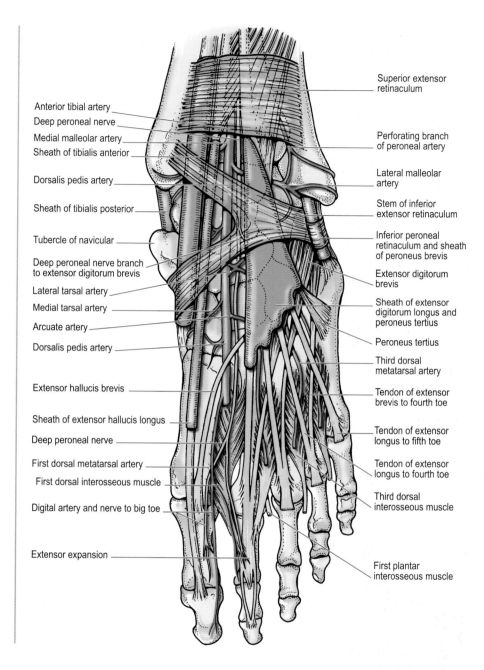

Anterior tibial artery

Deep peroneal nerve

Medial malleolar artery

Sheath of tibialis anterior

Dorsalis pedis artery

Sheath of tibialis posterior

Tubercle of navicular

Deep peroneal nerve branch to extensor digitorum brevis

Lateral tarsal artery

Medial tarsal artery

Arcuate artery

Dorsalis pedis artery

Extensor hallucis brevis

Sheath of extensor hallucis longus

Deep peroneal nerve

First dorsal metatarsal artery

First dorsal interosseous muscle

Digital artery and nerve to big toe

Extensor expansion

Superior extensor retinaculum

Perforating branch of peroneal artery

Lateral malleolar artery

Stem of inferior extensor retinaculum

Inferior peroneal retinaculum and sheath of peroneus brevis

Extensor digitorum brevis

Sheath of extensor digitorum longus and peroneus tertius

Peroneus tertius

Third dorsal metatarsal artery

Tendon of extensor brevis to fourth toe

Tendon of extensor longus to fifth toe

Tendon of extensor longus to fourth toe

Third dorsal interosseous muscle

First plantar interosseous muscle

Action. Combined dorsiflexion of the ankle joint and inversion of the foot. Tibialis anterior helps to maintain the medial longitudinal arch of the foot (see p. 165).

Test. The foot is dorsiflexed against resistance; the tendon can be seen and felt.

Extensor hallucis longus

This muscle arises from the middle half of the fibula and the adjacent interosseous membrane. (Flexor hallucis longus, too, arises from the fibula.) The muscle lies deep at its origin, but emerges between tibialis anterior and extensor digitorum longus in the lower part of the leg, where its tendon crosses in front of the anterior tibial vessels and deep peroneal nerve from their lateral to medial sides. It passes deep to the superior and is slung by the inferior extensor retinacula and proceeds along the medial side of the dorsum of the foot to be inserted into the base of the terminal phalanx of the great toe. It has a separate synovial sheath on the foot (Fig. 3.29).

Nerve supply. By the deep peroneal nerve (L5).

Action. To dorsiflex (anatomically this is to extend) the great toe. Secondarily it is a dorsiflexor of the ankle.

Test. The big toe is dorsiflexed against resistance; the tendon can be seen and felt. This test is a useful index of the L5 anterior ramus and spinal nerve.

Extensor digitorum longus

This muscle arises from the upper three-quarters of the extensor surface of the fibula, a small area on the lateral condyle of the tibia and the interosseous membrane. Its tendon passes deep to the superior extensor retinaculum and then acquires a synovial sheath, which it shares with the tendon of peroneus tertius, and is enclosed in a loop of the interior extensor retinaculum. It divides into four tendons which diverge superficial to extensor digitorum brevis and are inserted into the lateral four toes (Fig. 3.29). Their mode of insertion is the same as that of the extensor digitorum tendons in the hand. A dorsal extensor expansion over the proximal phalanx divides into three slips, the central (middle) slip being inserted into the base of the middle phalanx. The two side slips reunite after being joined by the tendons of the interossei and lumbricals and are inserted into the base of the distal phalanx.

Nerve supply. By the deep peroneal nerve (L5, S1).

Action. To dorsiflex the lateral four toes.

Test. The four lateral toes are dorsiflexed against resistance; the tendons can be seen and felt.

Peronius tertius

This muscle arises from the lower third of the fibula. The tendon passes deep to the superior extensor retinaculum and through the stem of the inferior retinaculum, where it shares the synovial sheath of extensor digitorum longus, and is inserted into the dorsum of the base of the fifth metatarsal bone and by an extension into the superior surface of that bone (Fig. 3.29).

Nerve supply. By the deep peroneal nerve (L5, S1).

Action. To dorsiflex and evert the foot.

The **deep peroneal (deep fibular) nerve** arises within peroneus longus, over the neck of the fibula, at the bifurcation of the common peroneal nerve. It spirals around the neck of the fibula deep to the fibres of extensor digitorum longus, and so reaches the interosseous membrane, on the lateral side of the anterior tibial vessels. With them it lies between extensor digitorum longus and tibialis anterior. In the middle of the leg the neurovascular bundle lies on the interosseous membrane between tibialis anterior and extensor hallucis longus. The latter muscle then crosses in front of the bundle, and lies on its medial side. The deep peroneal nerve supplies the four muscles of the extensor compartment of the leg.

The **anterior tibial artery**, formed at the bifurcation of the popliteal artery in the calf, passes forwards through the upper part of the interosseous membrane near the neck of the fibula, with a companion vein on each side. The artery with its companion veins runs vertically downwards on the interosseous membrane and crosses the lower end of the tibia at the front of the ankle joint, midway between the malleoli, where it changes its name to the dorsalis pedis artery. It gives off an anterior recurrent branch, which pierces tibialis anterior, to the arterial anastomosis around the upper end of the tibia. (An inconstant posterior recurrent branch arises in the popliteal fossa.) The anterior tibial artery supplies the muscles of the extensor compartment and gives malleolar branches to both malleolar regions. The deep peroneal nerve reaches it from the lateral side, runs in front of it in the crowded space of the middle of the leg and returns to its lateral side below. The accompanying *anterior tibial veins* run, one on each side of the artery, in close contact with it and anastomose by cross channels at frequent intervals.

Tibiofibular joints

The **superior tibiofibular joint** is a synovial joint between the lateral tibial condyle and the fibular head. The articulating surfaces are almost flat. The capsule is reinforced by anterior and posterior ligaments. The joint cavity may occasionally communicate posteriorly with the bursa deep to the popliteus tendon and thence with the knee joint.

The **interosseous membrane** consists of strong fibres that slope steeply from the tibia down to the fibula, and are continuous distally with the interosseous tibiofibular ligament.

The **inferior tibiofibular joint** is a fibrous joint (syndesmosis) between the convex medial surface of the distal end of the fibula and the concave fibular notch of the distal tibia. The bones are held together by anterior and posterior tibiofibular ligaments and are strongly bound by the interosseous tibiofibular ligament, whose fibres occupy the triangular area on each bone at the lower end of the interosseous border (Fig. 3.51).

Only slight movements occur at the tibiofibular joints, the fibula rotating laterally a little during dorsiflexion at the ankle.

PART **SEVEN**

Dorsum of the foot

The skin of the dorsum of the foot is supplied mainly by the superficial peroneal nerve, assisted by the deep peroneal, saphenous, and sural nerves (Fig. 3.43). The large veins form a **dorsal venous arch** which receives most of its blood by marginal and interosseous tributaries from the sole of the foot. The dorsal venous arch, lying over the heads of the metatarsals, drains from its medial and lateral ends into the great and small saphenous veins respectively.

The **superficial peroneal (superficial fibular) nerve** surfaces in the distal third of the leg and divides into medial and lateral branches which supply the skin of the dorsum of the foot. The medial branch further divides to supply the medial side of the dorsum of the great toe and the sides of the second cleft. The lateral branch divides to supply the third and fourth clefts. The lateral side of the foot and lateral side of the little toe are supplied by the sural nerve, while the first cleft is supplied by the deep peroneal nerve. The skin over the terminal phalanges is supplied by the medial and lateral plantar nerves. The medial side of the foot, usually as far forward as the metatarsophalangeal joint, is supplied by the termination of the saphenous nerve.

The subcutaneous layer of the dorsum of the foot, as of the hand, contains but little fat in most people, and the veins are consequently easily seen when distended.

The **deep fascia** on the dorsum of the foot binds down the underlying tendons. A Y-shaped thickening of the fascia, the inferior extensor retinaculum, prevents bowstringing of the extensor tendons as they pass across the front of the ankle joint.

The **inferior extensor retinaculum** arises by a stem from the anterior part of the upper surface of the calcaneus, on the lateral border of the dorsum of the foot (Fig. 3.29). From the stem two limbs diverge. The upper limb is attached to the medial malleolus, the lower limb arches across the tendons on the dorsum and blends with the plantar aponeurosis under the medial longitudinal arch of the foot. Most of the inferior retinacular fibres, however, sling around the tendons and return to be attached to the calcaneus, and only the superficial fibres pass across to the medial malleolus and plantar

aponeurosis. All the extensor tendons are enclosed in synovial sheaths where they are slung in the inferior extensor retinaculum.

Extensor digitorum brevis

This is a muscle whose fleshy belly can be seen in most feet and felt in all. It arises from the upper surface of the calcaneus and from the deep surface of the stem of the Y-shaped inferior extensor retinaculum. It passes obliquely across the dorsum of the foot and gives off four tendons to the medial four toes. The tendon to the great toe is different from the others and is named **extensor hallucis brevis**. Its belly usually separates early from the main muscle mass and the tendon is inserted separately into the base of the proximal phalanx of the great toe. As in the thumb, so in the great toe there is no dorsal extensor expansion. The remaining three tendons are inserted into the dorsal extensor expansions of the second, third and fourth toes. All four tendons of the muscle pass deep to the tendons of extensor digitorum longus.

Nerve supply. By the deep peroneal nerve (S1, 2).

Action. To extend the medial four toes. It is particularly of value when the long extensor is out of action, in the fully dorsiflexed ankle.

Test. The toes are dorsiflexed and the muscle belly towards the lateral side of the dorsum of the foot is observed and palpated.

The anterior tibial artery, lying over the lower end of the tibia midway between the malleoli, extends forwards as the **dorsalis pedis artery** (Fig. 3.29). This runs to the base of the first intermetatarsal space and passes down into the sole, where it joins the lateral plantar artery to complete the plantar arch. It lies between the tendon of extensor hallucis longus medially and the digital branch of the deep peroneal nerve laterally, and it is crossed by the tendon of extensor hallucis brevis. Its pulsation can be *palpated* lateral to the extensor hallucis longus tendon on a line from the midpoint between the two malleoli towards the first toe cleft on the underlying navicular and intermediate cuneiform bone. Occasionally the vessel is replaced by an enlarged perforating peroneal artery in front of the lateral malleolus. It has three named branches. The **lateral tarsal artery** runs laterally beneath extensor digitorum brevis to supply that muscle and the underlying tarsal bones. The **arcuate artery** runs laterally beneath the tendons of extensor digitorum brevis over the bases of the metatarsal bones. It gives off dorsal metatarsal arteries to supply the lateral three clefts. Each metatarsal artery gives off a perforating branch at the posterior and anterior end of its intermetatarsal space to communicate with the plantar arch and its metatarsal branches. It is the accompanying perforating veins that are responsible for bringing much of the blood from the sole of the foot through the intermetatarsal spaces to the dorsal venous arch. The *first dorsal metatarsal artery*, given off just before the dorsalis pedis enters the sole, supplies the first cleft and the medial side of the dorsum of the great toe.

The **deep peroneal (deep fibular) nerve** crosses the tibia lateral to the artery, midway between the malleoli. It passes forward, deep to the tendons, on the lateral side of the dorsalis pedis artery, to pierce the deep fascia and supply the first cleft. It gives off a branch which curves laterally beneath the muscle belly of extensor digitorum brevis and supplies this muscle and the underlying periosteum and joint capsules. It also gives a branch as an additional supply to the first dorsal interosseous muscle.

PART EIGHT

Lateral compartment of the leg

This muscular compartment lies between the peroneal surface of the fibula and deep fascia of the leg and is bounded in front and behind by the anterior and posterior intermuscular septa. It contains the peroneus longus and brevis muscles and the superficial peroneal nerve. Its blood supply is derived from branches of the peroneal artery which pierce flexor hallucis longus and the posterior intermuscular septum. Its veins drain, for the most part, into the small saphenous vein.

Peroneus longus and peroneus brevis

Peroneus longus arises from the head and the upper two-thirds of the peroneal surface of the fibula and from the intermuscular septa. **Peroneus brevis** arises from the lower two-thirds of the fibula; in the middle third of the bone its origin lies in front of that of peroneus longus and the two muscles, and their tendons maintain this relationship.

The broad tendon of peroneus brevis lies behind (and grooves) the lateral malleolus. The narrower tendon of peroneus longus lies on that of brevis and does not come into contact with the malleolus. The two tendons pass forwards to the peroneal trochlea on the lateral surface of the calcaneus, which separates them. The tendon of brevis passes above the peroneal trochlea to be inserted into the tubercle at the base of the fifth metatarsal bone. The tendon of peroneus longus passes below the peroneal trochlea and enters the sole of the foot, lying against the posterior ridge of the groove on the cuboid bone. Here

the tendon possesses a sesamoid fibrocartilage which often ossifies. The tendon crosses the sole obliquely to be inserted into the lateral side of the base of the first metatarsal and the adjoining part of the medial cuneiform (Fig. 3.35).

The tendons are bound down at the lateral malleolus by the **superior peroneal retinaculum**, a band of deep fascia that extends from the back of the malleolus to the lateral surface of the calcaneus; and at the peroneal trochlea by the **inferior peroneal retinaculum**, a band of fascia attached to the peroneal trochlea and to the calcaneus above and below the peroneal tendons. Its upper part is continuous with the stem of the Y-shaped inferior extensor retinaculum. The two tendons are enclosed in a common synovial sheath from above the lateral malleolus to the peroneal trochlea, where the sheath divides to accompany each tendon separately to its insertion.

Nerve supplies. Both muscles are supplied by the superficial peroneal nerve (L5, S1).

Action. Both muscles evert, and weakly plantarflex, the foot; they are the plantarflexors when the tibial nerve is paralysed. In addition, peroneus longus is a factor in maintaining the lateral longitudinal and transverse arches of the foot (see p. 165).

Test. The foot is everted and the tendons can be seen and felt below the lateral malleolus.

The **superficial peroneal (superficial fibular) nerve** begins in the substance of peroneus longus at the division of the common peroneal nerve. It passes downwards in the muscle and emerges at its anterior border behind the anterior intermuscular septum. It supplies both peronei, pierces the deep fascia between the middle and lower third of the leg, and divides into medial and lateral branches. (The distribution on the dorsum of the foot has been described on page 149.) It also supplies the skin of the anterolateral aspect of the lower leg (Fig. 3.43).

PART NINE

Posterior compartment of the leg

This is commonly called the **calf**. The skin of the upper half of the calf is supplied by the termination of the posterior femoral cutaneous nerve. Below this level the sural and sural communicating nerves, from tibial and common peroneal nerves, supply the back and lateral side of the calf, and the saphenous nerve supplies the medial side (Fig. 3.44).

The **small (short) saphenous vein**, draining the lateral side of the dorsal venous arch and the lateral margin of the foot, lies with the sural nerve behind the lateral malleolus. It passes upwards in the subcutaneous fat to the midline of the calf and pierces the deep fascia anywhere from midcalf to the roof of the popliteal fossa. It usually runs within and then beneath the deep fascia for some distance before it enters the popliteal vein. It communicates by several channels with the great saphenous vein.

The deep fascia is thickened above the heel, where it is attached to the tibia and fibula, across the back of the tendo calcaneus (Achilles' tendon), forming a 'pulley' for the tendon and separated from it by a bursa. A further thickening of fascia, the **flexor retinaculum**, bridges the deep flexor tendons and neurovascular bundle; it extends posteriorly from the tip of the medial malleolus to the medial process of the calcaneus.

The muscles of the calf, the posterior compartment of the leg, fall into superficial and deep groups, with the *deep transverse fascia* of the leg between them. This fibrous septum extends transversely from the soleal line and posterior border of the tibia to the posterior border of the fibula; it is continuous above with the fascia covering the popliteus. The superficial muscles consist of gastrocnemius, plantaris and soleus which all converge on a thick tendon at the back of the heel, the tendo calcaneus or Achilles' tendon. They are the main plantarflexors of the ankle joint. The deep group includes popliteus (see p. 139), and three muscles—flexor digitorum longus, flexor hallucis longus and tibialis posterior—whose tendons pass under the flexor retinaculum into the sole of the foot. The nerve of the posterior compartment is the tibial part of the sciatic, and the arteries are the posterior tibial (from the popliteal) and its peroneal branch.

Superficial muscles of the calf

Gastrocnemius and plantaris

The **lateral head** of **gastrocnemius** arises on the lateral surface of the lateral femoral condyle, from a smooth pit above that of popliteus; the pits are separated by the epicondyle (Fig. 3.23). The **medial head** of gastrocnemius arises from the back of the medial condyle and the popliteal surface of the shaft of the femur (Fig. 3.19). There is a bursa between each head and the capsule of the knee joint. They may communicate with the joint cavity and the medial bursa may also communicate with the semimembranosus bursa.

The two heads converge to lie side by side (Fig. 3.30), and the larger medial head extends to a lower level than the lateral head. The broad bellies of the muscle insert into a dense aponeurosis on their anterior surfaces, bearing on the soleus muscle. The aponeurosis blends with that of soleus to form the tendo calcaneus, which is inserted into a smooth transverse area on the middle third of the posterior surface of the calcaneus. A bursa lies between it and the upper part of the calcaneus. A second bursa lies between it and the thickened deep fascia 5 cm above its insertion.

Plantaris arises from the lower part of the lateral supracondylar line of the femur. Its slender tendon runs

Fig. 3.30 Cross-section of the middle of the right upper leg, looking towards the knee. Tibialis posterior is the deepest calf muscle, immediately behind the interosseous membrane. Note the many veins associated with soleus—a potential site of dangerous deep venous thrombosis.

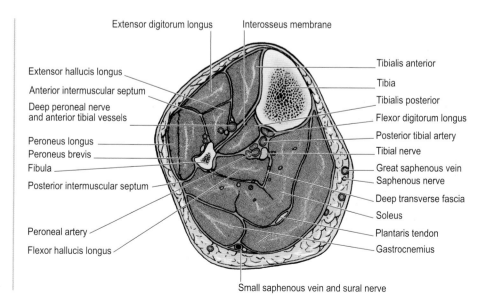

Extensor digitorum longus
Interosseus membrane
Extensor hallucis longus
Anterior intermuscular septum
Deep peroneal nerve and anterior tibial vessels
Peroneus longus
Peroneus brevis
Fibula
Posterior intermuscular septum
Peroneal artery
Flexor hallucis longus
Tibialis anterior
Tibia
Tibialis posterior
Flexor digitorum longus
Posterior tibial artery
Tibial nerve
Great saphenous vein
Saphenous nerve
Deep transverse fascia
Soleus
Plantaris tendon
Gastrocnemius
Small saphenous vein and sural nerve

151

distally deep to the medial head of gastrocnemius (Fig. 3.18), and continues along the medial border of the tendo calcaneus with which it fuses. It can be harvested for use as a tendon graft but is absent unilaterally or bilaterally in about 10–20% of subjects.

Soleus

The muscle arises from the upper quarter of the back of the fibula, including the head of the bone, whence a fibrous arch (which bridges over the popliteal vessels and tibial nerve) carries it in continuity to the soleal line of the tibia and the middle third of the posterior border of the tibia (Fig. 3.31). The muscle has a dense aponeurosis upon either surface and muscle fibres that slope downwards from the anterior to the posterior lamella; these fleshy fibres are visible at the medial and lateral borders of the muscle. The posterior (superficial) lamella is continued at its lower end into the tendo calcaneus, and the muscle fibres of soleus are received into its deep surface down to within a short distance of the calcaneus.

Perforating veins from the great saphenous vein enter the substance of soleus. The muscle contains a rich plexus of veins (Fig. 3.30), and these are pumped empty by contraction of the muscle, thus aiding venous return. Stagnation in these veins predisposes to deep venous thrombosis and the danger of pulmonary embolism. The 'soleal pump' is aided by the 'sole pump' (see p. 160).

Nerve supply. All three muscles are supplied by the tibial nerve (S1, 2). Each head of gastrocnemius receives a branch from the nerve in the popliteal fossa, and the lateral branch usually supplies plantaris as well. Soleus receives two branches, one from above the muscle in the popliteal fossa and one on its deep surface in the calf. In cases of intractable intermittent claudication both branches must be cut if soleus is to be completely denervated.

Actions. Soleus and gastrocnemius are the chief plantar flexors of the foot, and gastrocnemius is also a flexor of the knee. The powerful multipennate soleus is an antigravity muscle. In standing it contracts alternately with the extensor muscles of the leg to maintain balance. It is a very strong but relatively slow plantar flexor of the ankle joint, a necessary mechanical result of the obliquity of its multipennate fibres. The gastrocnemius bellies provide the necessary rapid contraction required for propulsion in walking, running and leaping. One strolls along quietly mainly with soleus; one wins the long jump mainly with gastrocnemius.

Test. The foot is plantarflexed against resistance; the tendo calcaneus and muscles above it can be seen contracting and can be palpated.

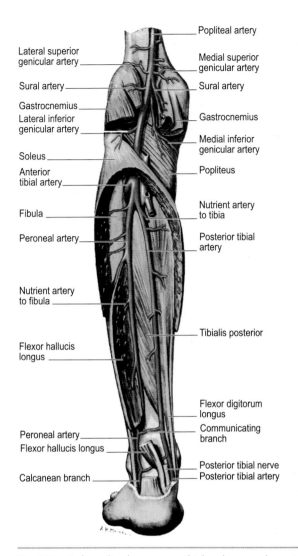

Fig. 3.31 Left popliteal, posterior tibial and peroneal arteries: posterior aspect. The high origin of the peroneal artery from the posterior tibial artery makes the popliteal artery to appear in arteriograms as though it ends by trifurcating.

Deep muscles

The deep muscles of the calf consist of flexor digitorum longus, flexor hallucis longus and tibialis posterior. Their three tendons pass under the flexor retinaculum into the sole of the foot. Those of tibialis posterior and flexor hallucis longus are parallel throughout their course, the tibialis medial to the hallucis. The tendon of flexor digitorum longus takes an oblique course superficial to both. In the calf it lies medially, crosses tibialis posterior to lie under the flexor retinaculum between the two, and in the sole it crosses flexor hallucis longus to pass to the lateral four toes.

Flexor digitorum longus

This muscle arises from the posterior surface of the tibia below the soleal line. The tendon of the muscle slopes downwards across the posterior surface of the tendon of tibialis posterior in the lower part of the leg. Enclosed in a synovial sheath it passes deep to the flexor retinaculum. It passes along the medial side of the sustentaculum tali of the calcaneum and enters the sole of the foot, where it crosses the inferior surface of the tendon of flexor hallucis longus (Fig. 3.34). At this point it divides into four tendons, the medial two of which receive a strong slip from the tendon of flexor hallucis longus. The four tendons at their commencement receive the insertion of the flexor accessorius muscle. More distally each gives origin to a lumbrical muscle. The tendons pass into the fibrous flexor sheaths of the lateral four toes, perforate the tendons of flexor digitorum brevis, and are inserted into the bases of the distal phalanges.

Nerve supply. By the tibial nerve (S1, 2).

Action. Its principal action is to plantarflex the lateral four toes and, secondarily, to plantarflex the ankle joint. Its tonus, with that of the other deep calf muscles, assists in maintaining the longitudinal arch of the foot (see p. 165).

Flexor hallucis longus

This is the bulkiest and most powerful of the three deep muscles of the calf. It arises from the flexor surface of the fibula and from the interosseous membrane (Fig. 3.48).

The fibres spiral down to be inserted into a central tendon which escapes from the muscle just at the lower end of the tibia, hence 'beef to the heel' describes the flexor hallucis longus (Fig. 3.31). The tendon passes deep to the flexor retinaculum, enclosed in a synovial sheath. It grooves the posterior surface of the talus and the undersurface of the sustentaculum tali (Figs 3.41 and 3.54), from where it passes directly forwards like a bowstring beneath the arched medial border of the foot to be inserted into the base of the distal phalanx of the great toe.

It is crossed in the sole by the tendons of flexor digitorum longus and gives a strong slip to the medial two of these (those for the second and third toes). In the calf the peroneal artery runs down deep to the muscle on the tibialis posterior.

Nerve supply. By the tibial nerve (S1, 2).

Action. Its principal action is to flex the great toe, and it is significant that this is the 'take-off' point, the last part to leave the ground in propulsion (see p. 166). It plantarflexes the ankle joint simultaneously. The pull of this powerful muscle is an important factor in maintaining the medial longitudinal arch of the foot.

Tests. The terminal phalanges of the great toe (for flexor hallucis longus) and of other toes (for flexor digitorum longus) are flexed against resistance.

Tibialis posterior

Tibialis posterior is the most deeply placed muscle in the calf. It arises from the interosseous membrane and the adjoining surface of both bones of the leg below the origin of soleus. Enclosed in a synovial sheath, the tendon passes deep to the flexor retinaculum and grooves the back of the medial malleolus (Fig. 3.32). It passes forward above the medial side of the sustentaculum tali, superficial to the deltoid ligament (see p. 161) and is inserted mainly into the tuberosity of the navicular. Tendinous slips also pass to the sustentaculum tali, all three cuneiforms, the cuboid and the second, third and fourth metatarsals. The proximal attachment of the muscle consists of two pointed processes, between which the anterior tibial vessels pass.

Nerve supply. By the tibial nerve (L4).

Action. It inverts and adducts the forefoot and, since it passes behind the medial malleolus, it plantarflexes the ankle joint. It contributes to maintaining the medial longitudinal arch of the foot.

Test. With the foot in slight plantarflexion, it is inverted against resistance; the tendon can be felt behind the medial malleolus.

The **posterior tibial artery** arises at the lower border of the popliteus, where the popliteal artery divides into anterior and posterior tibial branches. It passes under the fibrous arch in the origin of soleus and runs down on tibialis posterior, between flexor digitorum longus and flexor hallucis longus. It ends under the flexor retinaculum by dividing into medial and lateral plantar arteries. It is accompanied throughout its course by a pair of venae comitantes which frequently communicate with each other around the artery.

The pulsation of the artery can be *palpated* behind the medial malleolus, 2.5 cm in front of the medial border of the tendo calcaneus. It can be exposed here, e.g. for making an arteriovenous shunt with the great saphenous vein for haemodialysis.

Branches. The *peroneal (fibular) artery* arises 2.5 cm distal to popliteus. Its proximal course is in line with the

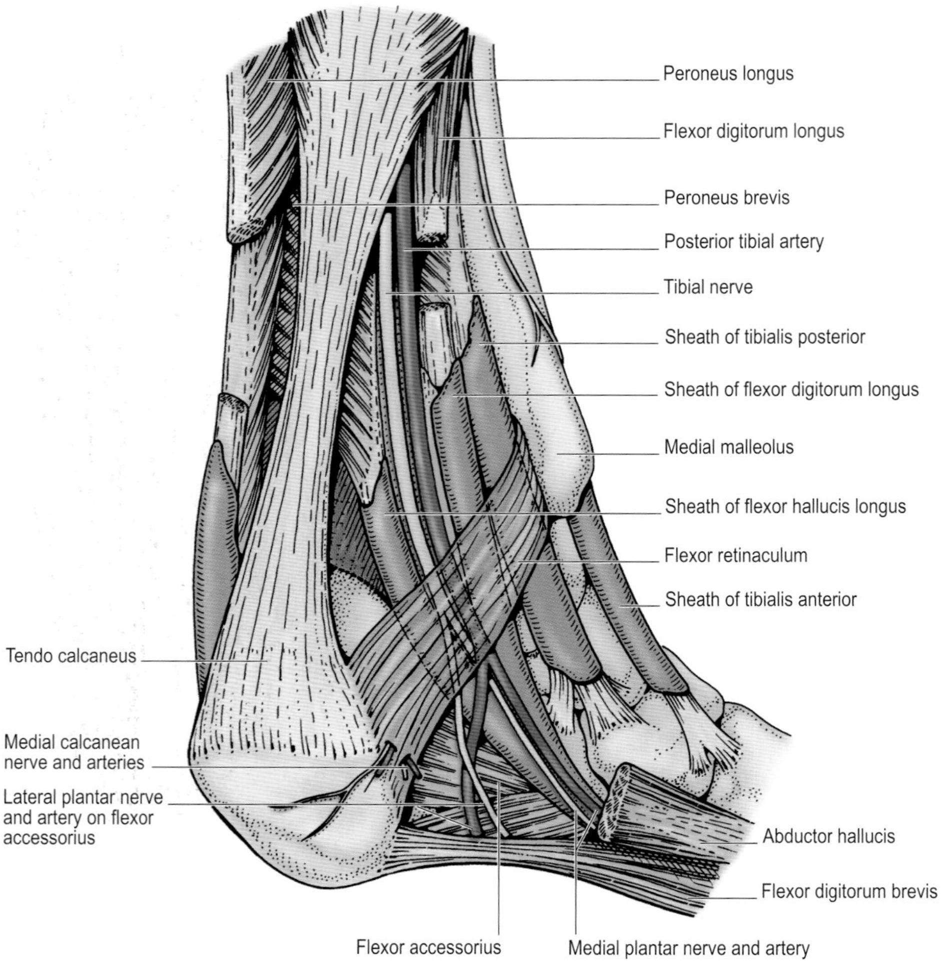

Fig. 3.32 Left ankle region: medial aspect.

Peroneus longus

Flexor digitorum longus

Peroneus brevis

Posterior tibial artery

Tibial nerve

Sheath of tibialis posterior

Sheath of flexor digitorum longus

Medial malleolus

Sheath of flexor hallucis longus

Flexor retinaculum

Sheath of tibialis anterior

Tendo calcaneus

Medial calcanean nerve and arteries

Lateral plantar nerve and artery on flexor accessorius

Abductor hallucis

Flexor digitorum brevis

Flexor accessorius

Medial plantar nerve and artery

popliteal artery (Fig. 3.31), and in some arteriograms the latter may appear to have trifurcated into anterior and posterior tibial and peroneal arteries. It runs distally in a fibrous canal between flexor hallucis longus and tibialis posterior, giving branches to the calf muscles and others that wind around the fibula to supply peroneus longus and brevis. It gives a nutrient artery to the fibula. It ends by dividing into a perforating branch which pierces the interosseous membrane to enter the extensor compartment and a lateral calcanean branch to the lateral side of the heel. The perforating branch may replace or supplement the dorsalis pedis artery.

The *circumflex fibular artery* passes laterally around the fibular neck to join the arterial anastomosis around the knee. The large *nutrient artery to the tibia* pierces tibialis posterior and runs downwards to enter the bone

just distal to the soleal line. Muscular branches supply soleus and the deep flexors. Medial calcanean branches pierce the flexor retinaculum and supply the medial side of the heel.

The **tibial nerve** runs straight down the midline of the calf, deep to soleus. The posterior tibial artery is at first lateral to it, but passes anterior to it and continues downwards on its medial side. The nerve ends under the middle of the flexor retinaculum by dividing into the medial and lateral plantar nerves (Fig. 3.32); its *surface marking* is from the middle of the popliteal fossa to midway between the medial malleolus and the tendo calcaneus.

It is the nerve of the flexor compartment, giving branches to soleus, flexors digitorum longus, hallucis longus and tibialis posterior. It gives *medial calcanean nerves* which pierce the flexor retinaculum to supply the skin of the heel, including the weight-bearing surface (Fig. 3.32).

PART TEN

Sole of the foot

The **skin** of the sole is supplied from the medial and lateral plantar nerves by branches that perforate the plantar aponeurosis along each edge of the strong central portion. Blood vessels accompany all the cutaneous nerves of the sole. The plantar surfaces of the toes are supplied by digital branches of the medial (three and a half toes) and lateral (one and a half toes) plantar nerves. The plantar digital nerves also supply the nail bed and surrounding skin. The median and ulnar nerve distributions to the fingers are identical.

The **subcutaneous tissue** in the sole, as in the palm, differs from that of the rest of the body in being more fibrous. Fibrous septa divide the tissue into small loculi which are filled with a rather fluid fat under tension, so that the cut tissue bulges. This makes a shock-absorbing pad, especially over the heel. The septa anchor the skin to the underlying plantar aponeurosis and limit the mobility of the skin.

The **plantar aponeurosis** is composed of dense collagen fibres arranged mainly longitudinally. It arises posteriorly from the medial process of the calcaneus and fans out over the sole (Fig. 3.33). It divides into five bands, one for each toe. Just distal to the metatarsal heads, these are connected by transverse fibres, the superficial transverse metatarsal ligament. The digital slips bifurcate for the passage of the flexor tendons and are inserted around the edges of the fibrous flexor sheaths and into the deep transverse metatarsal ligaments that unite the plantar ligaments of adjacent metatarsophalangeal joints. From each edge of the plantar aponeurosis a septum penetrates the sole, separating the flexor digitorum brevis from the abductors of big and little toes. The septa are attached to the first and fifth metatarsal bones. The abductors of the big and little toes, lying along the margins of the sole, are covered by deep fascia that is much thinner than the central plantar aponeurosis.

The muscles of the sole are arranged in four layers. The superficial layer consists of three short muscles that cover the sole, beneath the plantar aponeurosis. The second layer consists of long tendons to the digits, and their connections. The third layer consists of the short muscles of the great and little toes; it is confined to the metatarsal region of the foot. The fourth layer

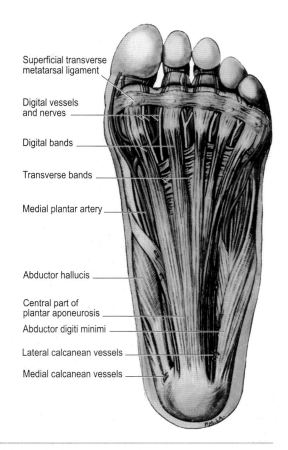

Fig. 3.33 Left plantar aponeurosis.

consists of both plantar and dorsal interossei and it includes also the tendons of peroneus longus and tibialis posterior. The segmental nerve supply of all the muscles is essentially S2.

First layer

Three short muscles lie side by side along the sole of the foot. The central of these, flexor digitorum brevis, is the counterpart of flexor superficialis in the upper limb, and is represented in the palm by the four tendons of that muscle.

Flexor digitorum brevis arises from the medial process of the calcaneus and the deep surface of the central part of the plantar aponeurosis. It divides into four tendons which pass to the lateral four toes. Each tendon enters the fibrous flexor sheath on the plantar aspect of its digit, divides and spirals around the long flexor tendon, and partially reunites in a chiasma before dividing again to be inserted into the sides of the middle phalanx.

This is an identical arrangement with that of the flexor digitorum superficialis.

Nerve supply. By the medial plantar nerve.

Action. To flex the toes with equal effect in any position of the ankle joint.

Abductor hallucis arises from the medial process of the calcaneus and from the flexor retinaculum. It runs along the medial margin of the foot (Fig. 3.33) to be inserted into the medial side of the base of the proximal phalanx of the great toe.

Nerve supply. By the medial plantar nerve.

Action. It abducts the great toe.

Abductor digiti minimi arises from both *medial and lateral* processes of the calcaneus, deep to the origin of flexor digitorum brevis. It lies along the lateral margin of the foot (Fig. 3.33). Its tendon is inserted into the lateral side of the base of the proximal phalanx of the fifth toe and the tubercle of the fifth metatarsal bone.

Nerve supply. By a branch from the main trunk of the lateral plantar nerve.

Action. It abducts the little toe.

Second layer

This consists of the long flexor tendons and their connections in the sole.

The **tendon of flexor hallucis longus** passes forward like a bowstring beneath the medial longitudinal arch of the foot (Fig. 3.41). It is crossed inferiorly by the tendon of flexor digitorum longus, to the medial two of whose divisions it gives off a strong slip. It next lies in a groove between the two sesamoids beneath the head of the first metatarsal bone, and finally is inserted into the base of the distal phalanx of the big toe (Fig. 3.34). It is invested by a synovial sheath throughout its whole course in the foot.

The **tendon of flexor digitorum longus** enters the sole on the medial side of the tendon of flexor hallucis longus. At its point of division into its four tendons of insertion it crosses superficial to the tendon of flexor hallucis longus, which gives a strong slip to the tendons for the second and third toes. It also receives the insertion of flexor accessorius (Fig. 3.34). The four tendons pass forwards in the sole deep to those of flexor digitorum brevis and after giving off the lumbricals they enter the fibrous sheaths of the lateral four toes. Each tendon perforates the tendon of flexor digitorum brevis and passes on to be inserted into the base of the distal phalanx.

Flexor accessorius arises by a large medial head from the medial surface of the calcaneus and by a small lateral head that arises from the lateral border of the plantar surface of the calcaneus; they converge on the muscle belly. The posterior part of the long plantar ligament is visible in the triangular interval between the two heads. The muscle belly is inserted into the tendon of flexor digitorum longus as it subdivides into tendons for the digits.

Nerve supply. By the main trunk of the lateral plantar nerve.

Action. By pulling on the tendons of flexor digitorum longus, it provides a means of flexing the lateral four toes in any position of the ankle joint. It also straightens the pull of the long flexor tendons on the toes.

The **lumbrical muscles** arise from the tendons of flexor digitorum longus, and pass forward on the medial (big toe) sides of the metatarsophalangeal joints of the lateral four toes (Fig. 3.34). (In the hand the lumbricals are on the thumb side of the corresponding joints.) Their tendons lie on the plantar surfaces of the deep transverse ligament of the metatarsal heads and pass dorsally to be inserted into the extensor expansions.

Nerve supply. As in the hand, a lumbrical supplied by the medial plantar (cf. median) nerve is unicipital; one supplied by the lateral plantar (cf. ulnar) nerve is bicipital. In the foot only the first lumbrical is supplied by the medial plantar nerve; it arises by a single head from its own tendon. The lateral three lumbricals are supplied by the lateral plantar nerve (deep branch) and each arises by two heads from the adjoining sides of the tendons.

Action. The lumbricals maintain extension of the digits at the interphalangeal joints while the flexor digitorum longus tendons are flexing the toes, so that in walking and running the toes do not buckle under.

Third layer

This consists, like the first layer, of three muscles but they are shorter and confined to the metatarsal region of the foot. Two act on the big toe, one on the little toe.

Flexor hallucis brevis lies against the undersurface of the metatarsal bone of the first toe. It arises from the cuboid, the lateral cuneiform and the tendon of tibialis posterior. The belly of the muscle splits into two parts which are inserted, each by way of a sesamoid bone, into the medial and lateral sides of the base of the plantar surface of the proximal phalanx of the great toe. The medial insertion blends with that of abductor hallucis, the lateral with that of adductor hallucis.

Nerve supply. By the medial plantar nerve.

Action. To flex the proximal phalanx of the big toe.

Fig. 3.34 Plantar muscles of left foot: second and third layers.

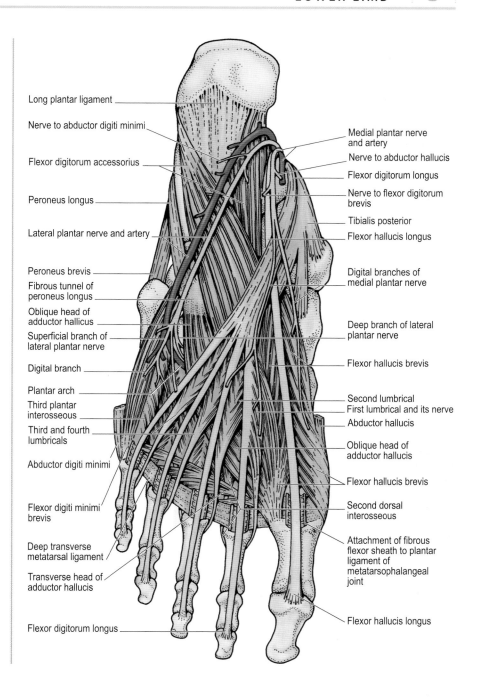

Long plantar ligament

Nerve to abductor digiti minimi

Flexor digitorum accessorius

Peroneus longus

Lateral plantar nerve and artery

Peroneus brevis

Fibrous tunnel of peroneus longus

Oblique head of adductor hallucis

Superficial branch of lateral plantar nerve

Digital branch

Plantar arch

Third plantar interosseous

Third and fourth lumbricals

Abductor digiti minimi

Flexor digiti minimi brevis

Deep transverse metatarsal ligament

Transverse head of adductor hallucis

Flexor digitorum longus

Medial plantar nerve and artery

Nerve to abductor hallucis

Flexor digitorum longus

Nerve to flexor digitorum brevis

Tibialis posterior

Flexor hallucis longus

Digital branches of medial plantar nerve

Deep branch of lateral plantar nerve

Flexor hallucis brevis

Second lumbrical

First lumbrical and its nerve

Abductor hallucis

Oblique head of adductor hallucis

Flexor hallucis brevis

Second dorsal interosseous

Attachment of fibrous flexor sheath to plantar ligament of metatarsophalangeal joint

Flexor hallucis longus

Adductor hallucis has two heads. The large oblique head arises anterior to flexor hallucis brevis, from the long plantar ligament where it roofs over the peroneus longus tendon, and from the bases of the second, third and fourth metatarsal bones. The slender transverse head has no bony origin; it arises from the deep transverse ligament and from the plantar ligaments of the lateral four metatarsophalangeal joints. The two heads unite in a short tendon which is inserted, with the lateral insertion of flexor hallucis brevis, into the lateral side of the plantar surface of the base of the proximal phalanx of the big toe (Fig. 3.34).

Nerve supply. By the deep branch of the lateral plantar nerve.

Action. The muscle draws the big toe towards the axis of the metatarsus and assists in maintaining the transverse arch.

Flexor digiti minimi brevis arises from the base of the fifth metatarsal bone and the adjoining fibrous sheath of peroneus longus. The muscle belly lies along the undersurface of the fifth metatarsal bone. Its tendon is inserted into the base of the proximal phalanx medial to the insertion of abductor digiti minimi (Fig. 3.34).

Nerve supply. By the superficial branch of the lateral plantar nerve.

Action. To assist in flexing the little toe.

Fourth layer

The fourth layer of muscles consists of the interossei in the intermetatarsal spaces. The tendons of tibialis posterior and peroneus longus, lying deeply against the undersurface of the tarsus, are conveniently included in this layer.

Interosseous muscles

The actions of the interossei of the foot (Fig. 3.35), as of the hand, are indicated by the mnemonic 'PAD and DAB': the plantar adduct and the dorsal abduct, but with the important difference that the longitudinal axis of the foot has shifted medially, and lies along the second metatarsal bone and the phalanges of the second toe (which is usually the longest toe). As in the hand, a **plantar interosseous** arises from the metatarsal bone of its own toe, while the bulkier **dorsal interosseous** arises by two heads from the two metatarsals between which it lies.

The three plantar adducting muscles adduct towards the second toe. The first toe has its own adductor mechanism (oblique and transverse heads of adductor hallucis) so that only the lateral three toes require adducting interossei. The first, second and third plantar interossei, each arising from the metatarsal bone of its own digit, are inserted by tendons into the medial sides of the third, fourth and fifth digits. The three tendons pass dorsal to the deep transverse ligament of the metatarsal heads and are inserted chiefly into the bases of the proximal phalanges, and also into the dorsal extensor expansion.

The four dorsal abducting muscles abduct away from the line of the second toe. The big and little toes each possess an abductor muscle. The second requires an abducting muscle on each side while the third and fourth require a single muscle each to abduct the digit laterally, away from the second toe. Each arises from both bones of its own intermetatarsal space. The first is inserted on the big toe side of the second toe, the second, third and fourth on the little toe side of the second, third and fourth toes. The tendons are inserted chiefly into the bases of the proximal phalanges, and each also gives an extension to the dorsal extensor expansion.

Nerve supplies. All interossei are supplied by the lateral plantar nerve. Those of the fourth space are supplied by the superficial branch, all the remainder by the deep branch.

Action. The adducting and abducting actions of the interossei are of little significance in the human foot. It is more important that they assist the lumbricals in extending the interphalangeal joints (through the extensor expansions), and they flex the metatarsophalangeal joints (by their attachments to the proximal phalanges).

The **tendon of peroneus longus** crosses the sole obliquely (Fig. 3.35). It lies against the posterior ridge of the groove, under the cuboid. At the lateral margin of the foot it contains a sesamoid fibrocartilage which may be ossified. As it crosses the groove of the cuboid it is held in position by the long plantar ligament, which is attached to the anterior and posterior ridges as it bridges the groove. Emerging from this tunnel the tendon proceeds to its insertion at the base of the first metatarsal and adjoining area on the lateral surface of the medial cuneiform. A synovial sheath accompanies it throughout its course.

The **tendon of tibialis posterior** lies above the sustentaculum tali and spring ligament and is inserted mainly into the tuberosity of the navicular (Fig. 3.41). From its insertion many bands of fibres are traceable to other parts of the foot; usually described as insertions of the muscle, they are rather in the nature of ligaments. They pass to the sustentaculum tali, all three cuneiforms, the floor of the groove in the cuboid and the bases of the second, third and fourth metatarsals (Fig. 3.35).

Vessels and nerves

These are derived from the posterior tibial neurovascular bundle in the calf. The posterior tibial artery and tibial nerve divide, each into medial and lateral plantar branches, under cover of the flexor retinaculum. On the medial and lateral borders of the sole the artery is more marginal than the nerve and each artery is accompanied by a pair of venae comitantes. Where they cross, the nerve is nearer the skin. The plantar arteries and nerves lie between the first and second layers, inferior to the long tendons.

Fig. 3.35 Plantar muscles and tendons of left foot: fourth layer.

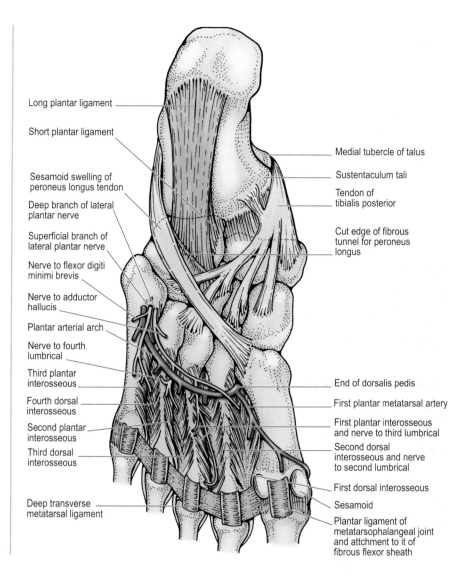

Long plantar ligament

Short plantar ligament

Sesamoid swelling of peroneus longus tendon

Deep branch of lateral plantar nerve

Superficial branch of lateral plantar nerve

Nerve to flexor digiti minimi brevis

Nerve to adductor hallucis

Plantar arterial arch

Nerve to fourth lumbrical

Third plantar interosseous

Fourth dorsal interosseous

Second plantar interosseous

Third dorsal interosseous

Deep transverse metatarsal ligament

Medial tubercle of talus

Sustentaculum tali

Tendon of tibialis posterior

Cut edge of fibrous tunnel for peroneus longus

End of dorsalis pedis

First plantar metatarsal artery

First plantar interosseous and nerve to third lumbrical

Second dorsal interosseous and nerve to second lumbrical

First dorsal interosseous

Sesamoid

Plantar ligament of metatarsophalangeal joint and attchment to it of fibrous flexor sheath

The **medial plantar artery** is smaller than its fellow; it gives rise to no plantar arch and its digital supply is restricted practically to the big toe. In the hand there are two palmar arches, a superficial from the ulnar artery, and a deep from the radial artery; but in the foot there is only one plantar arch, derived from the lateral plantar artery.

The **medial plantar nerve** (Fig. 3.34) supplies abductor hallucis, flexor digitorum brevis, flexor hallucis brevis and the first lumbrical; in addition it gives off digital cutaneous branches that supply the medial three and a half toes. Its most lateral cutaneous branch communicates with the neighbouring lateral plantar digital

branch across the plantar surface of the fourth metatarsophalangeal joint, where pressure on the nerve may give rise to the painful condition known as metatarsalgia.

The **lateral plantar artery** crosses the sole obliquely deep to the first layer of the sole, towards the base of the fifth metatarsal bone. It gives off a branch that accompanies the superficial branch of the lateral plantar nerve, but its main trunk accompanies the deep branch of the nerve to form the plantar arch. The **plantar arch** curves convexly forwards, across the bases of the fourth, third and second metatarsals and is joined in the proximal part of the first intermetatarsal space by the dorsalis pedis artery.

From the convexity of the plantar arch plantar metatarsal arteries run forwards and bifurcate to supply the four webs and digits. Perforating arteries from the plantar arch and its metatarsal arteries reinforce the dorsal metatarsal arteries.

The **veins** accompanying the perforating arteries take most of the blood from the sole and from the interosseous muscles to the dorsal venous arch. The veins among the plantar muscles act as a 'sole pump' which aids the 'soleal pump' of the posterior compartment of the calf (see p. 152).

The **lateral plantar nerve** crosses the sole obliquely medial to the lateral plantar artery (Fig. 3.34). Its course and distribution have similarities with those of the ulnar nerve in the hand. It supplies flexor accessorius and abductor digiti minimi and sends perforating branches through the plantar aponeurosis to supply skin on the lateral side of the sole. Near the base of the fifth metatarsal bone it divides into superficial and deep branches. The *superficial branch* supplies the fourth cleft and communicates with the medial plantar nerve and, by a lateral branch, supplies the skin of the lateral side and distal dorsum of the little toe. Unlike the superficial branch of the ulnar nerve, this branch supplies three muscles, namely flexor digiti minimi brevis and the two interossei of the fourth space (third plantar and fourth dorsal). The *deep branch* lies within the concavity of the plantar arch and ends by sinking into the deep surface of the oblique head of adductor hallucis. It gives off

branches to the remaining interossei, to the transverse head of adductor hallucis and to the three lateral (bicipital) lumbricals.

PART **ELEVEN**

Ankle and foot joints

Ankle joint

The ankle joint, or *talocrural joint*, is a synovial joint of the modified hinge variety. The axis of rotation is not fixed but changes between the extremes of plantarflexion and dorsiflexion. The articulating surfaces are covered with hyaline cartilage. The weight-bearing surfaces are the upper facet of the talus and the inferior facet of the tibia (Fig. 3.36). Stabilizing surfaces are those of the medial and lateral malleoli, which grip the sides of the talus. The joint is enclosed in a capsule lined with synovial membrane. The **capsule** is attached to the articular margins of all three bones except the anterior part of the talus, where it is fixed some distance in front of the articular margin, on the neck of the bone. Posteriorly the capsule, on its way up to the tibia, is attached also to the posterior tibiofibular ligament.

The **synovial membrane** is attached to the articular margin of the talus and clothes the intracapsular part of

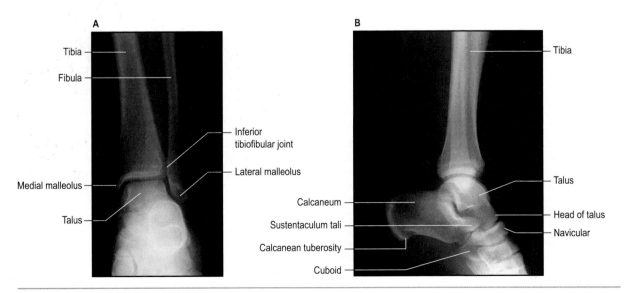

Fig. 3.36   Radiographs of the ankle joint: **A** anteroposterior projection; **B** lateral projection.
(Courtesy of Dr R. Sinnatamby, Cambridge University Hospital.)

Fig. 3.37   Left ankle and heel from behind.

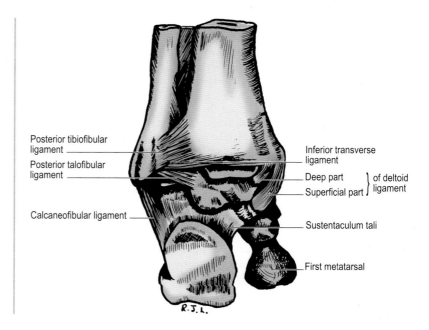

Posterior tibiofibular ligament

Posterior talofibular ligament

Calcaneofibular ligament

Inferior transverse ligament

Deep part } of deltoid
Superficial part } ligament

Sustentaculum tali

First metatarsal

the neck. Elsewhere it is attached to all articular margins and lines the inside of the capsule.

Strong medial and lateral ligaments strengthen the joint. The **deltoid ligament**, on the medial side, is in two layers. The *deep part* (Fig. 3.37) is a narrow band extending from the tibial malleolus to the side of the talus. The *superficial part* is triangular, like a delta. It fans downwards from the borders of the tibial malleolus and its lower margin has a continuous attachment from the medial tubercle of the talus along the edge of the sustentaculum tali and spring ligament to the tuberosity of the navicular (Fig. 3.40).

On the lateral side there are three separate bands, radiating from the lateral malleolus, which are collectively commonly called the *lateral ligament*. Anterior and posterior bands pass to the talus, the intermediate band to the calcaneus. The **anterior talofibular ligament** (Fig. 3.38) joins the anterior border of the lateral malleolus to the neck of the talus. The **calcaneofibular ligament** (Fig. 3.38) extends from the tip of the malleolus down and back to the lateral surface of the calcaneus. The **posterior talofibular ligament** (Fig. 3.37) lies horizontally between the malleolar fossa of the fibula and the lateral tubercle of the talus. Above it lies the **posterior tibiofibular ligament**, whose lower part (also called the *inferior transverse ligament*) is covered by hyaline cartilage and articulates with the talus. In plantarflexion these two ligaments lie edge to edge, but in dorsiflexion they diverge like the blades of an opening pair of scissors.

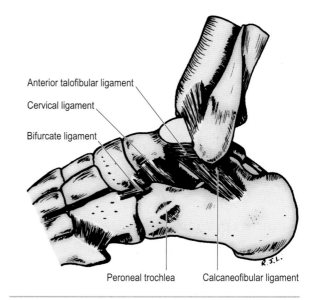

Anterior talofibular ligament

Cervical ligament

Bifurcate ligament

Peroneal trochlea   Calcaneofibular ligament

Fig. 3.38   Left ankle from the lateral side.

The blood supply of the capsule and ligaments is derived from anterior and posterior tibial arteries and the peroneal artery, and the nerve supply is by the deep peroneal and tibial nerves.

Movements

The upper facet of the talus, slightly concave from side to side, is convex anteroposteriorly. It is broad in front and narrow behind. In full dorsiflexion the broad anterior articular area of the talus is grasped by the mortice formed by the malleoli and the inferior surface of the tibia. This requires widening of the malleolar gap through slight lateral rotation of the fibula by stretching at the inferior tibiofibular syndesmosis and gliding at the superior tibiofibular joint. In full plantar-flexion the smallest area of the talus is in contact with the malleoli and distal tibia, but even in this position inversion and eversion are not possible at the ankle. For all practical purposes the ankle may be regarded as a true hinge joint.

The axis of rotation is not horizontal, but slopes downwards and laterally. It passes through the lateral surface of the talus just below the apex of the triangular articular area and through the medial surface at a higher level, just below the concavity of the comma-shaped articular area. It passes through the malleoli just above their apices. The axis changes during movement, for the upper convexity of the talus is not the arc of a circle, but rather of an ellipse. The obliquity of the axis involves a slight movement resembling inversion in full plantar-flexion, and the reverse, resembling slight eversion, in full dorsiflexion, but these apparent movements are not of true inversion and eversion.

From the upright position, with the foot at right angles to the leg, active plantar flexion of about 20° is produced by gastrocnemius and soleus, assisted by the long flexor tendons and the long and short peronei. Active dorsiflexion of about 10° is produced by tibialis anterior, the long toe extensors and peroneus tertius. The degree of passive movements possible is approximately double the above.

Surgical approach

The ankle joint can be exposed from the front between the tendons of extensor hallucis and digitorum longus, avoiding damage to the intervening deep peroneal nerve and anterior tibial vessels. For an approach behind the medial malleolus the tendons of tibialis posterior and flexor digitorum longus are displaced forwards, while on the lateral side the peroneus longus and brevis can be displaced forwards to reach the capsule behind the lateral malleolus. For *aspiration* the joint can be entered in front of the lateral malleolus and lateral to the tendon of peroneus tertius, or in front of the medial malleolus medial to tibialis anterior. The joint line should be defined by moving the foot.

Tarsal joints

The most important joints in the tarsus are those between the talus, calcaneus and navicular and between the calcaneus and cuboid.

On the undersurface of the talus there are two separate joints. At the back is the talocalcanean joint, where the upper surface of the calcaneus articulates with the undersurface of the talus. In front of this is a more complicated joint, with part of the undersurface of the head of the talus articulating with the upper surface of the sustentaculum tali and body of the calcaneus and the spring ligament, and the front of the head of the talus articulating with the navicular (Fig. 3.39). The whole joint with its single synovial cavity is called talocalcaneonavicular.

The **talocalcaneonavicular joint** is a synovial joint of the ball and socket variety. The ball is the head of the talus (Fig. 3.39) and the socket comprises the navicular and calcaneus and the spring ligament. The posterior surface of the navicular has an articular surface which is concave reciprocally with the anterior convexity of the head of the talus. The anterior end of the upper surface of the calcaneus has a concave facet, and the sustentaculum tali a similar one for articulation with the inferior convexity of the head of the talus. Between these navicular and calcanean surfaces the head of the talus

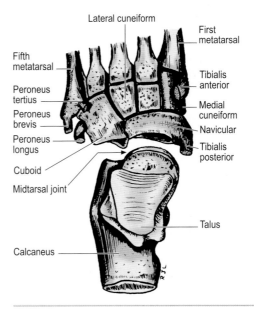

Fig. 3.39   Bones of the left foot from above, separated at the midtarsal joint. The insertions of all tendons producing inversion and eversion of the foot are in front of this joint.

articulates with the fibrocartilaginous upper surface of the spring ligament. All these structures are enclosed in a single capsule.

The **talocalcanean joint** lies behind the talocalcaneonavicular joint. It is a synovial joint between the concave facet on the undersurface of the talus and the convex facet on the upper surface of the calcaneus (Fig. 3.52).

The **calcaneocuboid joint** is a separate synovial joint between the front of the calcaneus and the back of the cuboid; this and the talonavicular part of the talocalcaneonavicular joint form what is usually called the **midtarsal joint** (Fig. 3.39). The calcaneocuboid joint is surrounded by a capsule, thickened above and below. The long and short plantar ligaments are accessory ligaments on its plantar surface. Simple gliding movement takes place at this joint during inversion and eversion of the foot.

The **short plantar ligament** (properly called the plantar calcaneocuboid) is a thick bundle which fills in the adjacent hollows in front of the anterior tubercle of the calcaneus and behind the posterior ridge of the cuboid (Figs 3.40 and 3.54). It is covered over by the long plantar ligament.

The **long plantar ligament** (Fig. 3.40) is attached to the plantar surface of the calcaneus anterior to its tuberosity, and to the anterior tubercle of that bone. From here it extends forwards to cover the short plantar ligament, and its deeper fibres are attached to the posterior ridge of the cuboid. Its superficial fibres bridge the groove of the cuboid, making a fibrous roof over the peroneus longus tendon, and are attached to the anterior ridge of the cuboid and extend forwards to the bases of the central three metatarsal bones. It is covered by flexor accessorius, and its posterior part is visible in the gap between the medial fleshy and lateral tendinous heads of that muscle.

Various other smaller but stronger interosseous plantar ligaments unite adjacent bones and help to support the arches of the foot.

The **plantar calcaneonavicular (spring) ligament** is a very strong band that connects the anterior edge of the sustentaculum tali to the plantar surface of the navicular (Fig. 3.40). Its upper surface articulates with the head of the talus, and bears a fibrocartilaginous facet for this purpose. Its lower fibres extend well under the sustentaculum tali and lie almost transversely across the foot. Like ligaments in general, it consists of collagenous tissue and, despite its common name 'spring ligament', it is not elastic.

The *bifurcate ligament* (Fig. 3.38) arises from the upper surface of the calcaneus, under cover of the extensor digitorum brevis muscle at the front of the tarsal sinus. From this origin two limbs diverge from each

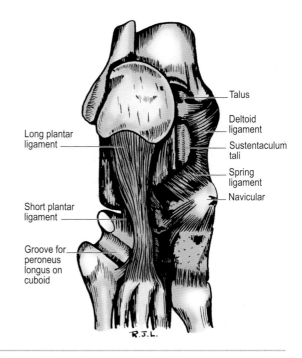

Long plantar ligament

Short plantar ligament

Groove for peroneus longus on cuboid

Talus

Deltoid ligament

Sustentaculum tali

Spring ligament

Navicular

R.J.L.

Fig. 3.40   Plantar ligaments of the left foot. On the medial side the deltoid ligament of the ankle joint fuses with the spring ligament.

other. The medial limb is attached to the navicular and the lateral limb is attached to the cuboid.

The *tarsal sinus* lies obliquely between the talocalcaneonavicular joint and the talocalcanean joint. It is a cylindrical canal that opens anteriorly at its lateral end like the broad end of a funnel. The sinus is occupied by a strong, flat bilaminar *interosseous talocalcanean ligament*. The central portion of each bony gutter is perforated by vascular foramina. At the lateral end of the sinus is the *cervical ligament* between the neck of the talus and the upper surface of the calcaneus (Fig. 3.38).

Inversion and eversion of the foot

Inversion and eversion of the foot occur at the subtalar and midtarsal joints, more movement occurring at the former joint. (Adduction and supination of the forefoot accompany inversion; abduction and pronation of the forefoot accompany eversion.) The range of inversion is increased in plantarflexion, and the fully inverted foot is also plantarflexed. The more restricted movement of eversion is linked in an allied manner with dorsiflexion.

The movement of **inversion** (raising the medial border of the foot) is produced by any muscle that is attached

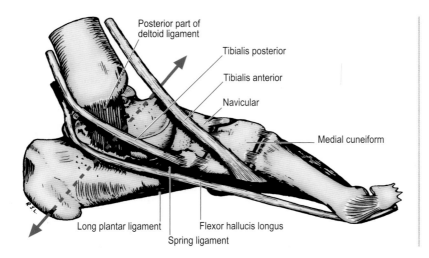

Posterior part of
deltoid ligament

Tibialis posterior

Tibialis anterior

Navicular

Medial cuneiform

Long plantar ligament

Flexor hallucis longus

Spring ligament

Fig. 3.41   Left foot from the medial side, with the axis of inversion and eversion indicated by the interrupted arrow. The inverting tendons pull at right angles around the axis. The everting peroneal tendons act in a similar way on the lateral side.

to the medial side of the foot. Tibialis anterior and tibialis posterior are responsible, assisted by extensor and flexor hallucis longus on occasion.

The movement of **eversion** (raising the lateral border of the foot) is produced by any muscle that is attached to, or pulls upwards upon, the lateral side of the foot. Peroneus longus, brevis, and tertius are responsible.

All the muscles producing inversion and eversion are attached to the fore part of the foot, anterior to the midtarsal joint (Fig. 3.39). The calcaneus and cuboid are firmly connected by the long and short plantar ligaments, which limit the range of mobility at the midtarsal joint; when they and the spring ligament are taut they transmit the rotatory force to the calcaneus. This bone then rotates (i.e. inverts or everts) under the talus, which is firmly wedged against the tibia between the malleoli and cannot therefore be inverted or everted.

The axis of inversion–eversion movement is along an oblique line (Fig. 3.41) passing from the lateral tubercle of the calcaneus upwards, forwards and medially through the neck of the talus and the medial part of the tarsal sinus. The lines of pull of the muscles lie at right angles to this oblique axis. The balanced actions of these muscles combine in different patterns to produce ordered movements of the ankle and tarsal joints.

Forefoot joints

The metatarsus is much more rigid than the metacarpus. The **first tarsometatarsal joint** possesses its own capsule and synovial membrane and is capable of some movement in a vertical plane to conform with movements in the medial longitudinal arch of the foot, and it becomes hyperextended in flat foot; but the joint movements in no way compare with those of the carpometacarpal joint of the thumb and no opposition of the big toe is possible. The **second tarsometatarsal joint** is immobile, the base of the metatarsal being firmly fixed between the anterior ends of the medial and lateral cuneiforms. This is a result of the shifting of the axis of the foot towards its medial side, and the second toe forms the line for adduction and abduction of the digits. The immobility of the second metatarsal and the slenderness of its shaft are contributory factors in 'spontaneous' fracture ('march fracture') of this bone.

The **first metatarsophalangeal joint** is the site of hallux valgus. The big toe has no dorsal extensor expansion nor fibrous flexor sheath; its long tendons are held in position by strands of deep fascia. If the phalanges become displaced laterally and the fibrous bands give way, the pull of extensor hallucis longus, like that of extensor hallucis brevis, becomes oblique to the long axis of the toe and tends to increase the deformity.

The **interphalangeal joints** are similar to those of the hand, with capsules and collateral ligaments (see p. 95).

Supporting mechanisms of the foot

In the erect position the heel, lateral margin of the foot, the ball of the foot (the part underneath the metatarsal heads) and the pads of the distal phalanges touch the ground. The medial margin of the foot arches up between the heel and the ball of the big toe, forming a visible and obvious medial longitudinal arch. The lateral margin of the foot is in contact with the ground, but its constituent bones do not bear with equal pressure on the ground. As on the medial side, so, on the lateral side, there is a bony longitudinal arch extending from the heel to the heads of the metatarsal bones, but the lateral longitudinal arch is much flatter than the medial.

The bones that form the *medial longitudinal arch* are calcaneus, talus, navicular, the three cuneiform bones and their three metatarsal bones. The pillars of the arch are the tuberosity of the calcaneus posteriorly and the heads of the medial three metatarsal bones anteriorly. The *lateral longitudinal arch* consists of calcaneus, cuboid and the lateral two metatarsal bones.

The *transverse arch* is, in reality, only half an arch, being completed as an arch by that of the other foot. It consists of the bases of the five metatarsal bones and the adjacent cuboid and cuneiforms. The heads of the five metatarsal bones lie flat upon the ground, though the first and fifth heads bear more weight than the others.

The factors maintaining the integrity of the arches of the foot are identical with those responsible in any joint of the body, namely, bony, ligamentous and muscular, but their relative importance is different in the three arches.

Medial longitudinal arch

Bony factors do not play a significant role in maintaining the stability of this arch. The head of the talus is supported on the sustentaculum tali, but this is a negligible factor. Ligaments are important, but are unable to maintain the arch entirely on their own. The most important ligament is the plantar aponeurosis, stretching like a tie beam or bowstring between the supporting pillars of the arch. If it is shortened by extension of the toes, especially the big toe, it draws the pillars together and so heightens the arch. Next in importance is the spring ligament, for it supports the head of the talus. If it stretches it allows the navicular and calcaneus to separate and so the head of the talus, the highest point of the arch, sinks lower between them. All the other interosseous ligaments also contribute towards maintaining the arch.

Muscles are indispensable to the maintenance of the medial longitudinal arch. The most important muscular supporting structure is the tendon of flexor hallucis longus (Fig. 3.41). It is assisted by the tendons of flexor digitorum longus to the second and third toes, which receive a slip from the tendon of flexor hallucis longus. These tendons act as bowstrings along the medial longitudinal arch from the sustentaculum tali to the medial three digits and draw the pillars of the arch towards each other. They are not called into play during short periods of standing, for generally the weight is borne well back on the heel and the pads of the toes are not pressed on the ground. Meanwhile the ligaments support the arch.

But during prolonged standing the ligaments 'tire', and relief is obtained by pressing the pads of the toes to the ground. During movements of propulsion and during landing on the feet the inertia and momentum of the body weight throw a vastly greater strain on the arch, and this strain is taken up especially by the contraction of the flexor hallucis longus muscle and the tension of its tendon.

The short muscles in the first layer that are inserted into the medial three toes (abductor hallucis, and the medial half of flexor digitorum brevis) likewise assist in maintaining the arch.

The tendons of tibialis anterior and peroneus longus are inserted into the same two bones (medial cuneiform and first metatarsal bone), but they exert opposite effects upon the medial longitudinal arch. Peroneus longus tends to evert the foot and lower the medial side of the foot, as is so well seen in the everted *flat* foot of peroneal spasm in children. On the other hand, tibialis anterior and tibialis posterior have a significant beneficial effect on the arch by their tendency to invert the foot, in other words to raise the medial border from the ground.

Lateral longitudinal arch

No bony factor contributes to the stability of this arch, but ligaments play a relatively more important part than in the case of the medial arch. The plantar aponeurosis in its lateral part and the plantar ligaments act as bowstrings beneath the arch.

The peroneus longus tendon, as it enters the groove on the undersurface of the cuboid, pulls upwards on the lateral longitudinal arch through its sesamoid fibrocartilage and is the most important single factor in maintaining its integrity. The tendons of flexor digitorum longus to the fourth and fifth toes (assisted by flexor accessorius) and the muscles of the first layer of the sole (lateral half of flexor digitorum brevis and abductor digiti minimi) also assist by preventing separation of the pillars of the arch.

Transverse arch

The intermediate and lateral cuneiforms are wedge-shaped, and in this single respect the bones are adapted to the maintenance of the transverse arch of the foot. The lateral cuneiform overhangs the cuboid and thus rests on it to some extent. The medial cuneiform is wedge-shaped the wrong way for an arch. Thus bony factors play a mixed role in maintaining the transverse arch.

The ligaments that bind together the cuneiforms and bases of the five metatarsal bones are more important, and the most important factor of all is the tendon of peroneus longus, the pull of which tends to approximate medial and lateral borders of the foot across the sole.

Propulsive and shock-absorbing mechanisms of the foot

If the foot were entirely rigid it would serve as a propulsive member by plantarflexion at the ankle joint and, indeed, the contraction of soleus and gastrocnemius is the chief factor responsible for propulsion in walking, running and jumping. But the propulsive action of these great muscles of the calf is enhanced by arching of the foot and flexion of the toes. Thus the tendo calcaneus plantarflexes a very mobile, not a rigid, foot. The sequence of events in walking is usually described as four phases: heel-strike, support (stance or weight-bearing), toe-off (push off) and swing (Fig. 3.42). The weight of the foot is taken successively on the heel, lateral border, and the ball of the foot, and the last part to leave the ground is the anterior pillar of the medial longitudinal arch and the medial three digits. In running the heel remains off the ground, the toes and the forefoot taking the thrust of the weight; but the take-off point is still the anterior pillar of the medial longitudinal arch.

At the moment of heel-strike, the extensors of the foot and toes contract and then gradually relax to prevent the toes from slapping on the ground. While the heel is rising from the ground the medial toes are gradually extended. The extended toes elongate the flexor hallucis longus and flexor digitorum longus muscles, and this increases the force of their subsequent contraction.

Contraction of the toe flexors, long and short, heightens the medial longitudinal arch and increases the force of the take-off by the pressure of the toes on the ground. Meanwhile, the lumbricals prevent the toes from buckling under when pulled upon by flexor digitorum longus. Contraction of the long flexors also aids plantarflexion at the ankle joint.

PART TWELVE

Summary of lower limb innervation

Cutaneous innervation

The segmental supply (dermatomes) of the lower limb has been considered on page 15. The cutaneous nerves have been described in the preceding pages but for convenience are summarized here (Figs 3.43 and 3.44).

The skin of the buttock receives fibres that run down from the subcostal and iliohypogastric nerves, the posterior rami of the first three lumbar and first three sacral nerves, and the perforating cutaneous nerve, with an upward contribution from the posterior femoral cutaneous nerve. The latter supplies a long strip down the back of the limb to the midcalf, with lateral and medial femoral cutaneous nerves on either side and a small contribution from the obturator nerve on the medial side. On the front of the thigh, the subcostal, femoral branch of genitofemoral and ilioinguinal nerves supply skin below the inguinal ligament, while the lateral,

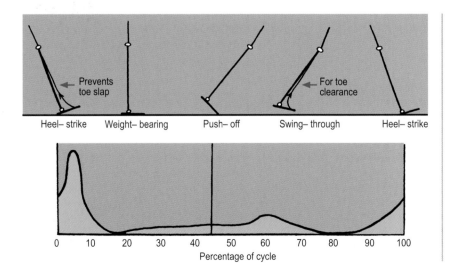

Heel– strike   Weight– bearing   Push– off   Swing– through   Heel– strike

0   10   20   30   40   50   60   70   80   90   100
Percentage of cycle

Fig. 3.42 Phasic action of the pretibial muscle group during walking. The contraction during heel-strike (shock-absorbing) is much greater than that needed for toe clearance during the swing-through phase.

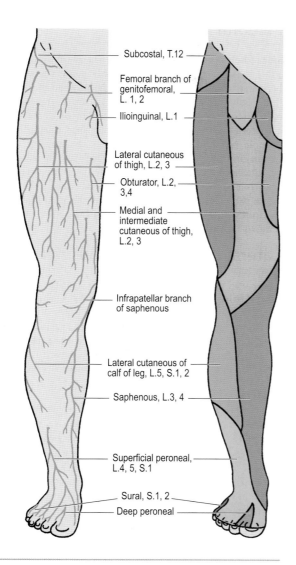

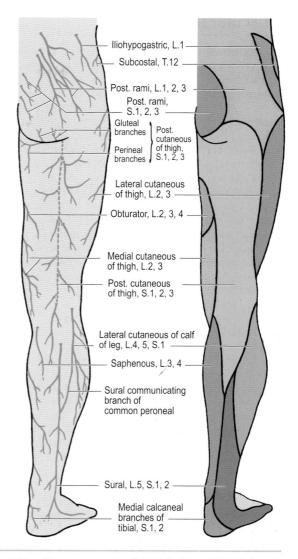

Fig. 3.43 Cutaneous nerves of the right lower limb, their areas of distribution and segmental origins: anterior aspect.

Fig. 3.44 Cutaneous nerves of the right lower limb, their areas of distribution and segmental origins: posterior aspect.

intermediate and medial femoral cutaneous nerves supply the skin of the rest of the thigh, with the obturator nerve contributing to the supply of the medial side.

The skin of the front of the knee receives branches from the medial femoral cutaneous nerve, the lateral cutaneous nerve of the calf and the saphenous nerve, the last reaching as far as the level of the metatarsophalangeal joint of the great toe. The superficial peroneal extends over the front of the lower leg and dorsum of

the foot, with the deep peroneal supplying the first toe cleft. The sural nerve takes over from the lateral cutaneous nerve of the calf on the lateral side of the back of the leg and extends along the lateral side of the foot to the little toe. Medial calcanean branches of the tibial nerve supply the heel, and medial and lateral plantar nerves the sole. The medial plantar, like the median nerve in the hand, usually supplies three and a half and the lateral plantar the rest of the digits.

Muscular innervation

The segmental innervation of lower limb muscles has been considered on page 16. In the thigh the anterior compartment is supplied by the femoral nerve and the adductor group by the obturator nerve. The tibial part of the sciatic nerve is the nerve of the posterior compartment, with only the short head of biceps supplied by the common peroneal part. In the gluteal region, the inferior gluteal nerve innervates gluteus maximus with the other two glutei receiving their supply from the superior gluteal which also supplies tensor fasciae latae. The short lateral rotator muscles behind the hip have their own nerves, with the obturator externus supplied by the obturator nerve. The tibial nerve is the nerve of the flexor compartment of the leg and its plantar branches supply the muscles of the sole. The common peroneal nerve divides into the superficial peroneal for the peroneal compartment and the deep peroneal for the anterior or extensor compartment.

Sympathetic innervation

As with the brachial plexus, a grey ramus communicans connects each nerve root of the lumbar and sacral plexuses with the appropriate ganglion of the sympathetic trunk so that postganglionic fibres can be distributed to each nerve. The preganglionic fibres for the lower limb have come from cell bodies in the lateral horn of spinal cord segments T11–L2, for the supply of blood vessels, sweat glands and arrectores pilorum muscles.

Lumbar and sacral plexuses

Summaries of these plexuses, including all the lower limb branches, begin on page 366, following descriptions of the abdomen and pelvis.

PART THIRTEEN

Summary of lower limb nerve injuries

Peripheral nerve injuries are much less common in the lower limb than in the upper and damage to the lumbar and sacral plexuses is most unusual. The most common injury is to the common peroneal nerve, and the main features of this and other nerve lesions are summarized below, together with notes on the more common exposures if exploration and repair are required.

Femoral nerve

Since the nerve breaks up into a sheaf of branches as soon as it enters the thigh, it is more subject to damage by penetrating injuries of the lower abdomen than of the limb. Pelvic masses such as a haematoma or neoplasm may affect it, and it has been known to be damaged by catheterization of the femoral artery and during laparoscopic repair of inguinal hernia. In a complete lesion extension of the knee by the quadriceps will be lost, with some weakness of hip flexion. There is sensory loss over the front of the thigh; with lesions that cause pain in the nerve the pain may extend as far as the medial side of the foot (saphenous branch). Test for the action of rectus femoris (see p. 124).

Lateral femoral cutaneous nerve

The nerve may be compressed in the iliac fossa or as it passes from abdomen to thigh deep to or through the inguinal ligament and medial to the anterior superior iliac spine (see p. 116), producing meralgia paraesthetica which is recognized by paraesthesia in the lateral part of the thigh. If necessary the nerve may have to be freed from the iliac fascia and inguinal ligament.

Obturator nerve

On account of its deep position, trauma to this nerve is extremely rare, but it may be damaged by obstetric procedures or involved in pelvic disease; e.g. an ovarian tumour may cause pain in the skin on the medial side of the thigh. In obturator paralysis the loss of adduction at the hip is not noticed during walking but when sitting the affected limb cannot be crossed over the other.

Sciatic nerve

The most common cause of damage is (regrettably) by misplaced gluteal injections. Other causes include pelvic disease and severe trauma to the hip (in 7% of dislocations and 16% of fracture dislocations). There is paralysis of the hamstrings and all the muscles of the leg and foot (supplied by the tibial and common peroneal nerves). Paralysis of the hamstrings may be difficult to test because of pain but foot drop will be obvious, and there will be sensory loss below the knee but not on the medial side of the leg or on the upper part of the calf due to the supply from the saphenous branch of the femoral nerve and the posterior femoral cutaneous nerve respectively. Test for plantarflexion and dorsiflexion.

Surgical approach. The sciatic nerve is explored by exposure at the lower border of gluteus maximus, retracting semitendinosus and the long head of biceps medially; from there it can be followed upwards or downwards (retracting biceps laterally).

Common peroneal (fibular) nerve

Direct trauma or pressure by plaster casts at the neck of the fibula make this the most commonly damaged nerve in the lower limb. Foot drop is the most obvious sign, due to paralysis of the extensor muscles supplied by the deep peroneal branch. This results in a high-stepping gait to ensure that the toes do not scrape along the ground. Peroneus longus and brevis in the lateral compartment will also be affected, being supplied by the superficial peroneal branch. Sensory loss in a common peroneal nerve lesion extends over the lower lateral part of the leg and the dorsum of the foot. Test for dorsiflexion.

Surgical approach. The nerve can be exposed by following it down from the lateral side of the popliteal fossa, where it lies medial to the biceps tendon.

Tibial nerve

Damage to this nerve is uncommon. The main effect is paralysis of the calf muscles; sensory loss is on the lower part of the calf and on the sole. Test for standing on tiptoe.

Surgical approach. The nerve is exposed in the middle of the popliteal fossa; it can be followed lower down by splitting gastrocnemius and soleus vertically in the midline.

Saphenous nerve

The lower part of this nerve, in front of the medial malleolus, is at risk of damage during varicose vein surgery and when the great saphenous vein is harvested for arterial bypass procedures.

PART FOURTEEN

Osteology of the lower limb

Innominate (hip bone)

The innominate or hip bone is formed of three bones, which fuse in a Y-shaped epiphysis involving the acetabulum. The **pubis** and **ischium** together form an incomplete bony wall for the pelvic cavity; their outer surfaces give attachment to thigh muscles. The **ilium** forms the pelvic brim between the hip joint and the joint

with the sacrum; above the pelvic brim it is prolonged, broad and wing-like, for the attachment of ligaments and large muscles. The anterior two-thirds of the projecting ilium, thin bone, forms the iliac fossa, part of the posterior abdominal wall. The posterior one-third, thick bone, carries the auricular surface for the sacrum and, behind this, is prolonged for strong sacroiliac ligaments which bear the body weight. The outer surface of the ilium gives attachment to buttock muscles. The ischium and pubis together lie in approximately the same plane; the plane of the ilium is at nearly a right angle with this.

In the anatomical position of the bone the pubic tubercle and anterior superior iliac spine lie in the same vertical plane, and the upper border of the symphysis pubis and the ischial spine lie in the same horizontal plane.

Lateral surface of the hip bone

The hip joint socket, the **acetabulum**, is a concave hemisphere whose axis is not strictly horizontal but is directed also downwards and slightly backwards along the axis of the femoral neck. There is a deficiency at its inferior margin, the *acetabular notch*. The hyaline cartilage lining the inside of the acetabulum is widest over the iliac part of the fossa, opposite the notch; this is the weight-bearing area. The articular cartilage does not cover the whole concavity and the non-articular bone is thin and translucent. Pubis and ischium meet here and their line of union continues down to the notch. Pubis and ilium meet at the iliopubic eminence on the anterior margin of the acetabulum. Ilium and ischium meet at a corresponding low elevation just beyond the posterior margin of the acetabulum.

The convex upper margin of the ilium, the **iliac crest**, extends from the **anterior superior iliac spine** to the **posterior superior iliac spine**. The **tubercle** of the iliac crest lies 5 cm behind the anterior superior spine and forms the most lateral part of the bony pelvis, but not the highest part, which is 7.5 cm behind the tubercle. The line between the highest points of the two iliac crests, the supracristal plane, passes through the spine of L4 vertebra. The tubercle lies at the level of L5 vertebra.

The gluteal surface of the ilium shows three curved gluteal lines. Gluteus maximus, medius and minimus arise from this surface, their sites of attachment being separated by the gluteal lines (Fig. 3.45). Tensor fasciae latae arises from the gluteal surface just below the iliac crest, between anterior superior spine and tubercle. The reflected head of rectus femoris arises from the upper margin of the acetabulum.

The anterior border of the ilium shows a gentle S bend. The inguinal ligament and sartorius are attached

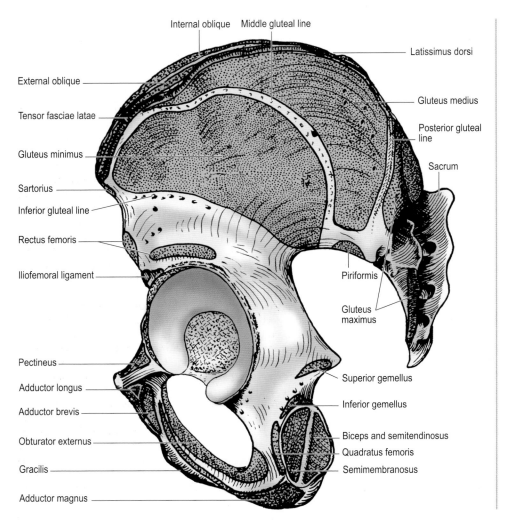

Internal oblique   Middle gluteal line

Latissimus dorsi

External oblique

Tensor fasciae latae

Gluteus minimus

Sartorius

Inferior gluteal line

Rectus femoris

Iliofemoral ligament

Gluteus medius

Posterior gluteal line

Sacrum

Piriformis

Gluteus maximus

Pectineus

Adductor longus

Adductor brevis

Obturator externus

Gracilis

Adductor magnus

Superior gemellus

Inferior gemellus

Biceps and semitendinosus

Quadratus femoris

Semimembranosus

Fig. 3.45 Left hip bone, from the lateral side and behind.

to the anterior superior spine. The straight head of rectus femoris and the iliofemoral ligament are attached to the **anterior inferior iliac spine**.

The posterior border of the ilium is a rounded bar of bone between the posterior superior and posterior inferior spines (see Fig. 6.98, p. 455). It gives attachment to the sacrotuberous ligament. The posterior superior iliac spine makes a characteristic dimple in the skin of the buttock at the level of the second piece of the sacrum.

The posterior part of the **iliac crest** is thicker than the rest. The posterior lamella of the lumbar fascia and the erector spinae muscle are attached here. The aponeurotic origin of latissimus dorsi is fused with the posterior lamella, and muscle fibres are attached further

forward along the iliac crest. Internal to latissimus dorsi, quadratus lumborum and the iliolumbar ligament are attached to the iliac crest. Continuing forwards from here are the attachments of the internal oblique and transversus abdominis muscles side by side, the internal oblique to the centre and the transversus to the inner lip of the crest, both extending to the anterior superior spine. External oblique is attached to the outer lip of the iliac crest in its anterior half. The fascia lata of the thigh is attached along the whole length of the external lip of the iliac crest, splitting to enclose the narrow origin of tensor fasciae latae.

The **body of the pubis**, quadrilateral in shape, is projected laterally as a **superior ramus** which joins the ilium and ischium at the acetabulum and an **inferior ramus** which fuses with the ischium below the obturator foramen. The symphyseal surface of the body is oval in shape; it is coated with a layer of hyaline cartilage for the secondary cartilaginous joint that constitutes the pubic symphysis (see p. 336). The upper border of the body, gently convex, is the **pubic crest**. It is marked laterally by a forward-projecting prominence, the **pubic tubercle**. From the pubic tubercle two ridges diverge laterally onto the superior ramus. The upper ridge, sharp, is the **pectineal line**; it forms part of the pelvic brim, and joins the arcuate line of the ilium. The lower ridge, more rounded, is the **obturator crest**. This passes downwards into the anterior margin of the acetabular notch, where it becomes more prominent. It gives attachment to the pubofemoral ligament. Between these ridges the surface of the superior ramus can be traced to its junction with the ilium, marked by a rounded prominence, the **iliopubic eminence**. Pectineus arises from the pectineal line and the adjacent surface of the superior ramus. Below the obturator crest on the pubic ramus is the obliquely placed **obturator groove**, which lodges the obturator nerve in contact with the bone. The obturator vessels lie below the nerve as the neurovascular bundle passes over the obturator membrane. The inferior ramus of the pubis is marked by an everted crest. The line of junction with the ischial ramus is halfway between the ischial tuberosity and the pubic crest.

The pubic crest gives origin to rectus abdominis and, in front of it, pyramidalis. Lateral to this the conjoint tendon is attached to the pubic crest and along the pectineal line (see Fig. 5.8, p. 235). Anterior to the conjoint tendon, the lacunar ligament is attached to the pectineal line and lateral to this the attachment of the pectineal ligament (of Cooper) (see Fig. 5.5, p. 232) continues along the pectineal line. The pubic tubercle receives the attachment of the inguinal ligament, forming the lateral crus of the superficial ring; the medial crus, in front of the conjoint tendon, is inserted into the front of the pubic crest alongside the symphysis (see Fig. 5.3, p. 231).

The rounded tendon of adductor longus arises from the front of the body of the pubis, in the angle between the pubic crest and symphysis; bone spurs may be found at this attachment (rider's bone). Below it the linear origin of gracilis extends down along the margin of the everted crest of the inferior ramus to reach the ischial ramus. Deep to adductor longus and gracilis the adductor brevis arises from the body of the pubis. Extending up along the inferior ramus the pubic fibres of adductor magnus arise deep to gracilis, and deeper still is the obturator externus (Fig. 3.45). The fascia lata is attached by its deep lamina to the pectineal line over the surface of pectineus (see p. 119), and below the pubic tubercle

along the front of the body of the pubis to the everted crest. It encloses adductor longus and gracilis, and separates them from the external genitalia in the superficial perineal pouch.

The **ischium** is an L-shaped bone. An upper thick portion, the body, joins with pubis and ilium at the acetabulum and extends down to the ischial tuberosity; it supports the sitting weight. A lower, thinner bar, the **inferior ramus**, joins the inferior ramus of the pubis to enclose the obturator foramen.

Behind the acetabulum a low elevation marks the line of fusion of ischium and ilium. The ischiofemoral ligament is attached to the ischium at the margin of the acetabulum. More medially the upper part of the body of the ischium completes the lower part of the greater sciatic notch. The sciatic nerve, with the nerve to quadratus femoris deep to it, lies here on the ischium. This site of emergence of the nerve into the buttock lies one-third of the way up from the ischial tuberosity to the posterior superior iliac spine.

The **spine** of the ischium projects medially to divide the greater from the lesser sciatic notch (Fig. 3.16). The sacrospinous ligament is attached to it, contributing to conversion of the **greater sciatic notch** into the greater sciatic foramen (see Fig. 5.53, p. 300). The pudendal nerve lies on the ligament just medial to the spine (see Fig. 5.69, p. 327). The internal pudendal vessels cross the tip, while the nerve to obturator internus lies on the base of the spine. The superior gemellus takes origin from the spine. The **lesser sciatic notch** lies between the spine and the ischial tuberosity. It is bridged by the sacrotuberous ligament, which with the sacrospinous ligament converts the notch into the lesser sciatic foramen (see Fig. 5.72, p. 334). Obturator internus emerges through this foramen into the buttock, and the internal pudendal vessels and nerve pass forward into the perineum. The lesser sciatic notch is grooved by tendinous fibres on the deep surface of the muscle (Fig. 3.46), which are separated from bone by hyaline cartilage and a bursa. The inferior gemellus arises from the upper margin of the ischial tuberosity, above the hamstrings (Fig. 3.45).

The **ischial tuberosity** is a rugged prominence whose convex posterior surface is divided transversely by a low ridge. An oval smooth area above this is divided by a vertical ridge into two areas, a lateral and a medial (Fig. 3.16). Semimembranosus tendon is attached to the lateral area, semitendinosus and the long head of biceps to the medial area.

Between the semimembranosus area and obturator foramen the lateral surface gives origin to quadratus femoris. Below the transverse ridge the ischial tuberosity shows a longitudinal crest; this supports the sitting body.

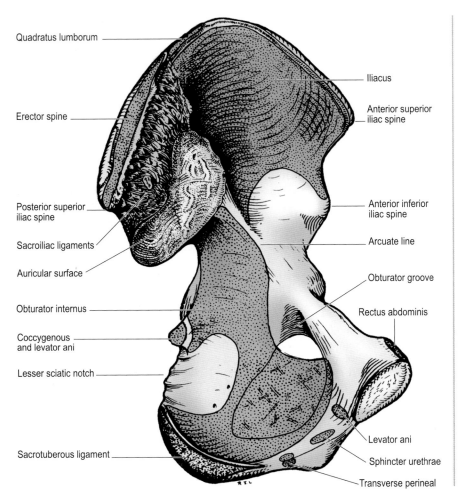

Fig. 3.46 Left hip bone, from the medial side.

Quadratus lumborum

Erector spine

Posterior superior iliac spine

Sacroiliac ligaments

Auricular surface

Obturator internus

Coccygenous and levator ani

Lesser sciatic notch

Sacrotuberous ligament

Iliacus

Anterior superior iliac spine

Anterior inferior iliac spine

Arcuate line

Obturator groove

Rectus abdominis

Levator ani

Sphincter urethrae

Transverse perineal

The fascia lata of the thigh is attached to this ridge. The lateral bevelled surface here gives origin to the fibres of the hamstring part of adductor magnus. The medial bevelled surface receives the sacrotuberous ligament. The ischial tuberosity curves forward from the rugged weight-bearing part into the slender inferior ramus. Adductor magnus has a continuous origin along this ramus for the pubic part of the muscle.

The **obturator foramen** is ringed by the sharp margins of the pubis and ischium, those of the pubis overlapping each other to form the obturator groove. The obturator membrane is attached to the margin of the foramen, but not to the obturator groove. Obturator externus arises from the outer surface of the membrane and the anterior bony margin of the foramen.

Medial surface of hip bone

The pelvic brim is formed by the top of the pubic crest, the pectineal line, the rounded border of the ilium (called the arcuate line) and the top of the auricular surface (Fig. 3.46). This curved pelvic brim slopes up at 60° to the horizontal plane. Below the brim lies the pelvic cavity; above it is the iliac fossa in the abdominal cavity.

The **auricular area** extends from the pelvic brim to the posterior inferior iliac spine. Its surface undulates and is roughened by numerous tubercles and depressions. It articulates with the ala of the sacrum. The anterior sacroiliac ligament is attached to its sharp anterior border.

The **iliac fossa** is a gentle concavity in the ala of the ilium in front of the sacroiliac joint. Its deepest part, high in the fossa, is composed of paper-thin translucent bone. Iliacus arises from the upper two-thirds of this area down to the level of the anterior inferior iliac spine. The lower one-third of the fossa is separated by a large bursa from the overlying iliacus. The fibres of iliacus converge to pass over a broad groove between the iliopubic eminence and the anterior inferior spine. The iliacus fascia is attached around the margins of the muscle: to the iliac crest, the arcuate line and iliopubic eminence. Psoas major passes freely along the pelvic brim and crosses the eminence. The 'psoas' bursa deep to it is the iliacus bursa already mentioned. The psoas fascia is attached to the arcuate line and the iliopubic eminence. Levator ani is attached to the junction of body and inferior ramus on the inner surface of the pubis (see Fig. 5.54, p. 300). More medially the puboprostatic (pubovesical in the female) ligaments are attached at this level. The inferior ramus lies in the perineum. Immediately below the symphyseal surface the arcuate pubic ligament is attached; the deep dorsal vein of the penis (clitoris) lies in the midline below it. Extending down from the symphyseal surface is a ridge of bone to which the perineal membrane is attached. External to this the margin is everted and the crus of the corpus cavernosum and the ischiocavernosus muscle are attached here. Between the perineal membrane and the obturator foramen the inferior ramus forms the wall of the anterior recess of the ischioanal fossa. Sphincter urethrae is attached here, above the perineal membrane.

The inner surface of the **body of the ischium** is smooth. Obturator internus arises from the body of the ischium and the area above it up to the arcuate line on the ilium (pelvic brim) and as far back as the margin of the greater sciatic notch, as well as from the obturator membrane and the ischiopubic ramus (see Fig. 5.64, p. 319). The fascia over obturator internus is attached to bone at the margins of the muscle. The pudendal canal on the obturator internus fascia lies just above the falciform ridge on the ischial tuberosity. This ridge curves forwards from the tuberosity on to the ischial ramus; the falciform process of the sacrotuberous ligament is attached to it (see Fig. 5.69, p. 327). The transverse muscles of the perineum are attached at the anterior edge of the ramus. Levator ani and coccygeus are attached to the inner surface of the ischial spine.

Sex differences

The ala of the ilium has been drawn out to widen the female pelvis; the greater sciatic notch is near a right angle in the female, much less in the male, and the female bone may show a preauricular sulcus below the arcuate line. The female ischial spine lies in the plane of the body of the ischium; the male spine is inverted towards the pelvic cavity. The female obturator foramen is triangular; the male foramen is oval in outline. The distance from the pubic symphysis to the anterior margin of the acetabulum is greater than the diameter of the acetabulum in the female, equal or less in the male bone.

Ossification

The bone develops in cartilage. Three primary centres appear, one for each bone, near the acetabulum. The centre for the weight-bearing ilium appears first, at the second month, followed by the ischium at the third and pubis at the fourth month of fetal life. At birth the acetabulum is wholly cartilage, and while the ilium is a broad blade of bone the ischium and pubis are no more than tiny bars of bone buried in the cartilage. Growth of these three bones causes them later to approximate each other through a Y-shaped cartilage in the acetabulum. The ischial and pubic rami fuse with each other at about 7 years. Secondary centres of ossification begin to appear in the acetabular cartilage at 8 years and by 18 years ossification across the acetabulum is complete. Other centres of ossification occur in the cartilage around the periphery of the bone and these fuse with the main bone by 25 years.

Femur

The femur consists in the main of a long shaft from the proximal end of which a neck proceeds upwards and medially to a rounded head; a greater and a lesser trochanter project from the junction of the shaft and the neck, and the shaft ends distally in a pair of large condyles (Fig. 3.47). In the standing position, the shaft passes downwards and medially and this inclination is evident when the femur is held vertically with both its condyles in contact with a horizontal surface. Femoral obliquity is more in females because of the relatively greater pelvic breadth and the shorter femoral length.

The **head** of the femur, capped with hyaline cartilage, is more than half a sphere. Its medial convexity has a pit, the fovea, for the ligament of the head. Anteriorly the articular cartilage extends slightly onto the neck.

The **neck** of the femur, as it inclines upwards and medially, makes an angle of about 125° with the shaft in the adult male. This angle of inclination is widest at birth and diminishes until adolescence; it is less in females. The neck is also tilted forwards slightly as it passes proximally to the head. This angle of anteversion

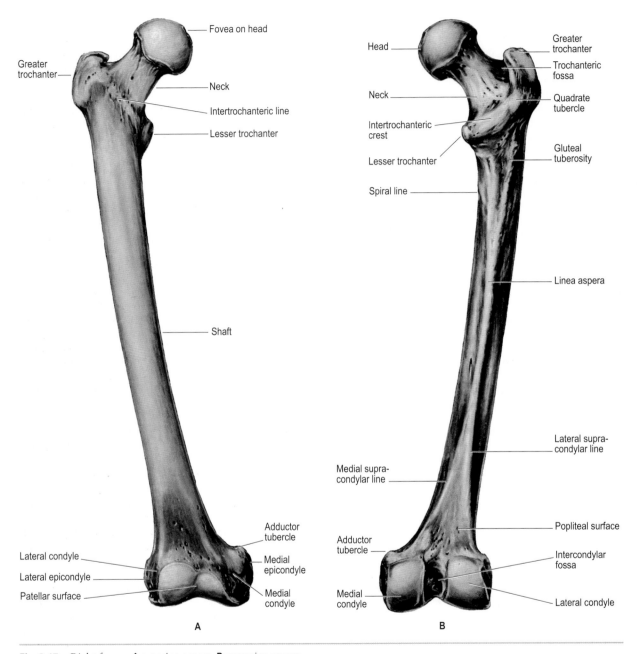

Fig. 3.47   Right femur: **A** anterior aspect; **B** posterior aspect.

is about 10–15°. Ridges on the surface of the neck, particularly on the anterior aspect, indicate the attachment of retinacular fibres of the hip joint capsule which are reflected proximally from the distal attachment of the capsule. Anteriorly the capsule is attached to the **intertrochanteric line,** which extends from the greater to the lesser trochanter where the neck joins the shaft. Posteriorly the capsule is attached halfway along the neck between the articular margin of the head and the prominent **intertrochanteric crest** situated at the junction of the posterior surface of the neck and the shaft. The tendon of obturator externus plays on the relatively smooth bone of the neck distal to the posterior capsular attachment. Many vascular foraminae, directed towards the head, perforate the anterior and posterosuperior surfaces of the neck. In the adult the head receives its blood supply mainly via these foraminae from blood vessels (mostly from the trochanteric anastomosis and particularly from the medial circumflex artery) that run up the neck with the retinacular fibres of the capsule. These vessels and intramedullary vessels running up the neck from the shaft are liable to be ruptured by a transcervical intracapsular fracture and avascular necrosis of the head is a potential hazard. Blood supply to the head from vessels that accompany the ligament to the head is meagre in the adult.

The **greater trochanter** projects up and back from the convexity of the junction of neck and shaft. Its upper border is projected into an inturned apex. Piriformis is attached here on the medial side. More anteriorly on the medial surface of the trochanter the common tendon of obturator internus and the gemelli is inserted. At the bottom of this surface is the trochanteric fossa for the attachment of the obturator externus tendon. The anterior surface of the greater trochanter shows a J-shaped ridge for the gluteus minimus tendon. The lateral surface shows an oblique strip, sloping downwards and forwards for the tendon of gluteus medius. The trochanter's proximal border is level with the centre of the femoral head, and the prominent convexity of the trochanter forms the widest part of the hips. It is covered by the beginning of the iliotibial tract, where gluteus maximus is received. This plays freely over a bursa on the bone. Posteriorly the apex of the trochanter is continued down as the prominent intertrochanteric crest to the lesser trochanter. Nearly halfway down the crest is an oval eminence, the **quadrate tubercle**; quadratus femoris is attached here.

The **lesser trochanter** lies back on the lowest part of the neck. Its rounded surface, facing medially, is smooth for the reception of the psoas major tendon. Iliacus is inserted into the front of the tendon and into the bone below the lesser trochanter.

The **shaft** of the femur has a convex anterior surface and is buttressed by a strong ridge, the **linea aspera**, at the middle third of the concave posterior surface. This narrow ridge has medial and lateral lips. The inter-trochanteric line slopes across the front of the neck and shaft at their junction, and continues down below the lesser trochanter as a *spiral line* that runs into the medial lip of the linea aspera. The medial lip continues on as the *medial supracondylar line* to the adductor tubercle on the medial condyle. On the back of the shaft below the

greater trochanter is a vertical ridge, the **gluteal tuberosity**, for the deep lower quarter of gluteus maximus. It runs down into the lateral lip of the linea aspera, and this lip is continued on as the *lateral supracondylar line* to the lateral epicondyle.

The intertrochanteric line in its lower half gives origin to vastus medialis, which arises in continuity below this along the spiral line, medial lip of the linea aspera and upper one-third of the medial supracondylar line (the lowest part of this muscle comes from the adductor magnus tendon, not from bone). The medial surface of the femoral shaft is bare bone, over which vastus medialis plays. Vastus lateralis arises from the upper half of the trochanteric line, the lower part of the greater trochanter, the lateral edge of the gluteal tuberosity and the lateral lip of the linea aspera. Vastus intermedius arises from the upper two-thirds of the front and lateral surfaces of the shaft, and articularis genu arises below vastus intermedius.

Pectineus is attached to the upper part of the posterior surface of the femur, behind iliacus. Adductor brevis is attached behind pectineus and down to the proximal part of the linea aspera. Adductor magnus is inserted medial to the gluteal tuberosity, below quadratus femoris, and then along the linea aspera to the medial supracondylar line and down to the adductor tubercle. There is a gap in the supracondylar attachment, a hand's breadth above the knee, through which the femoral vessels pass into the popliteal fossa. Between adductor magnus and vastus lateralis, the short head of biceps femoris arises below the gluteal tuberosity from the whole length of the linea aspera. Between adductor magnus and vastus medialis, adductor longus is inserted into the middle third of the linea aspera.

The popliteal surface of the femur between the supracondylar lines is bare. The anterior surface of the lower shaft is likewise bare, with the suprapatellar pouch in contact with periosteum deep to quadriceps tendon for a hand's breadth above the knee joint.

The **lower end** of the femur carries the two *condyles*, separated behind by an *intercondylar fossa* but joined in front by a trochlear surface for the patella. The lateral condyle projects further forward than the medial, thus helping to stabilize the patella (Fig. 3.9). Both are almost flat anteroposteriorly, but boldly curved on the posterior convexities. In the fossa the cruciate ligaments are attached to smooth areas: the anterior cruciate ligament far back on the lateral condyle alongside the articular margin, the posterior far forward on the medial condyle. The **medial condyle** shows on its convex non-articular medial surface a shallow pit for the tibial collateral ligament; this is the *medial epicondyle*. Above it lies the **adductor tubercle** at the lower end of the medial supracondylar line. The medial head of gastrocnemius arises from the back of the medial condyle and the adjacent popliteal surface of the shaft. The **lateral condyle** shows a vertical arrangement of three smooth-floored pits towards the back of its non-articular lateral surface (Fig. 3.23). The upper pit is for the lateral head of gastro-cnemius. Above this, plantaris arises from the lateral supracondylar line (Fig. 3.19). The central pit is at the prominence of the convexity of this surface and is the *lateral epicondyle*, to which the fibular collateral ligament is attached. The lowermost pit receives the popliteus tendon; a groove behind the pit lodges the popliteus tendon when the knee is flexed.

Surgical approach. The shaft can be exposed from the front between rectus femoris and vastus lateralis by incising vastus intermedius vertically down to the bone. The posterolateral approach is in front of biceps, detaching vastus lateralis from the front of the lateral intermuscular septum and following it down to the shaft.

Ossification. Excepting the clavicle, the femur is the first long bone to ossify. It does so in cartilage. A centre in the shaft appears at the seventh week of fetal life. A centre for the lower end appears at the end of the ninth fetal month (at birth) and its presence is acceptable medicolegal evidence of maturity. This is the growing end of the bone and the epiphysis, which bisects the adductor tubercle, unites with the shaft after 20 years. A centre appears in the head during the first year after birth, greater trochanter during the fourth year and lesser trochanter at 12–14 years. These upper epiphyses fuse with the shaft at about 18 years of age.

Patella

This sesamoid bone in the quadriceps tendon plays on the articular surface of the femur. Its edges form a rounded triangle. The anterior surface is gently convex. The lower border is projected down as an apex to the triangle. The posterior surface has a proximal articular area, covered with hyaline cartilage. The articular surface has a vertical ridge dividing it into narrow medial and broader lateral areas (Fig. 3.25). The bone laid down on a table lies on the broad lateral surface of the facet, so the right patella can easily be distinguished from the left. The narrow medial surface is further divided into two vertical strips. The most medial facet is in contact with the medial femoral condyle only in flexion; the larger lateral facet contacts the lateral condyle throughout all phases of knee joint movement (Fig. 3.20). The upper border of the bone receives the quadriceps tendon, the medial border receives the lowest fibres of vastus medialis. The quadriceps tendon covers the front of the bone,

and from each side extensions (patellar retinacula) pass backwards to the collateral ligaments and downwards to the tibial condyles. The patella is attached distally to the tuberosity of the tibia by the patellar ligament. This is attached to the lower border of the patella and to the distal non-articular part of the posterior surface of the bone.

When standing, the lower border of the patella is just proximal to the level of the knee joint (tibial plateau). Stellate fractures may show no displacement of fragments if the overlying quadriceps expansion and retinacula remain intact. The bone can be removed with surprisingly little disability.

Ossification. The bone ossifies in cartilage from several centres that appear at 3–6 years and coalesce quickly. Occasionally one centre may not fuse with the main bone, resulting in a bipartite patella, which must not be mistaken for a fractured patella in a radiograph.

Tibia

The tibia has a large upper end, extended by massive medial and lateral condyles, and a smaller lower end having a prominent medial malleolus projecting distally (Fig. 3.48). The shaft is vertical in the standing position; the femur inclines up from the head of the tibia outwards to the acetabulum. Much of the bone is subcutaneous and easily palpable.

The **superior articular surface** or plateau shows a pair of gently concave condylar articular areas, for articulation with the menisci and the condyles of the femur (Fig. 3.49). The surface on the medial condyle is oval (long axis anteroposterior) in conformity with the medial femoral condyle and meniscus. The lateral surface is a little smaller and more nearly circular, in conformity with the lateral femoral condyle and meniscus. Between the condylar surfaces the plateau is elevated into the **intercondylar eminence**, which is grooved anteroposteriorly to form medial and lateral *intercondylar tubercles*. The non-articular areas in front of and behind the tubercles show well-marked facets for attachment of the horns of the menisci and the cruciate ligaments. The anterior horn of the lateral meniscus is attached just in front of the lateral intercondylar tubercle. Anterior and medial to this is a large smooth area for attachment of the anterior cruciate ligament. Further forward, at the margin of the tibial plateau, is a round smooth facet for the anterior horn of the medial meniscus. The posterior horn of the lateral meniscus is attached just behind the lateral intercondylar tubercle. The posterior horn of the medial meniscus is attached more posteriorly behind the medial intercondylar tubercle. Further back is a shallow groove which extends over the posterior edge

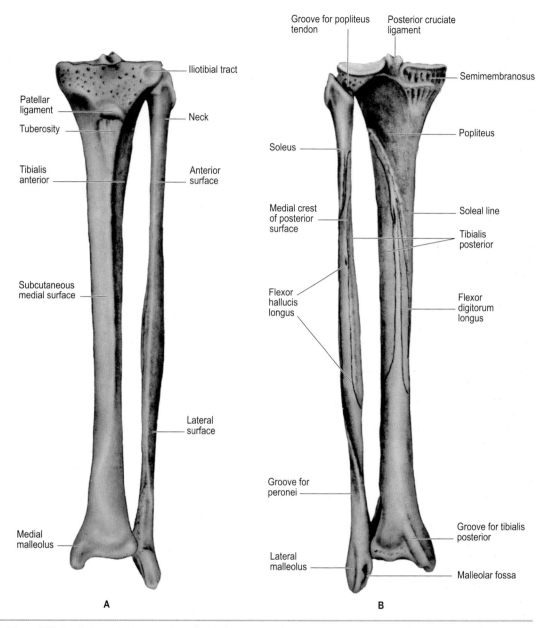

Fig. 3.48   Left tibia and fibula: **A** from the front; **B** from behind.

of the intercondylar area; the posterior cruciate ligament is attached here.

The back of the **medial condyle** is deeply grooved for the semimembranosus insertion; this groove extends around the medial contour of the bone, to receive the expansion of the tendon. The lateral condyle carries the facet for the head of the fibula, facing downwards and posteriorly. Just above this facet the lateral condyle may show a groove for the popliteus tendon, which plays across the bone here, lubricated by the popliteus bursa. The anterior surface of the lateral condyle shows a small smooth facet for the iliotibial tract. Below it a ridge

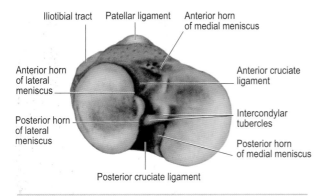

Iliotibial tract   Patellar ligament   Anterior horn of medial meniscus

Anterior horn of lateral meniscus

Posterior horn of lateral meniscus

Anterior cruciate ligament

Intercondylar tubercles

Posterior horn of medial meniscus

Posterior cruciate ligament

Fig. 3.49 Superior surface of the left tibia, with ligamentous attachments indicated.

slopes down to the tuberosity and a similar ridge extends down from the medial condyle; the capsule and patellar retinacula are attached to these ridges. The **tuberosity** shows a smooth oval prominence for the quadriceps insertion via the patellar ligament. The rough triangular area on the lower part of the tuberosity is subcutaneous and covered by the subcutaneous infrapatellar bursa.

The **shaft** of the tibia is triangular in section. Its *anterior* and *posterior borders*, with the medial surface between them, are subcutaneous. The subcutaneous surface receives the tendons of sartorius, gracilis and semitendinosus at its upper part; behind and above these the tibial collateral ligament is attached. The surface is continued at its lower end into the medial malleolus. The anterior border is sharp above, where it shows a medial convexity behind which tibialis anterior is attached to the upper two-thirds of the extensor (lateral) surface. This border becomes blunt below, where it continues into the anterior border of the medial malleolus. The blunt posterior border runs down into the posterior border of the medial malleolus.

On its fibular side the tibia shows a sharp *interosseous border* which near the lower end splits into two. The interosseous border gives attachment to the interosseous membrane, whose oblique fibres slope down to the fibula. The flexor surface of the shaft lies behind the interosseous border. At its upper part the **soleal line** runs down obliquely across this surface from just below the tibiofibular joint to the posterior border one-third of the way down. Popliteus arises from the triangular surface of the tibia above the soleal line. Soleus arises in continuity from the soleal line and the middle third of the posterior border. Below the soleal line the flexor surface shows a vertical ridge on the middle third of the tibia. Tibialis posterior arises between this ridge and the

interosseous border (it crosses the interosseous membrane to arise also from the fibula). Medial to the ridge, between it and the posterior border, flexor digitorum longus arises. The upper part of this surface is perforated by a large nutrient foramen directed downwards.

The **lower end** of the tibia is rectangular in section. Medially the surface is subcutaneous, with the great saphenous vein and nerve crossing in front of the **medial malleolus** (Fig. 3.28). Anteriorly the bare bone is crossed by the tendons of tibialis anterior and extensor hallucis longus and the anterior tibial neurovascular bundle and extensor digitorum longus (Fig. 3.29). Laterally the surface is triangular between the ridges that diverge from the lower end of the interosseous border; this triangular area gives attachment to the strong interosseous tibiofibular ligament. The lower part of this surface may articulate with the fibula as a synovial upward continuation of the ankle joint. Posteriorly there is a groove behind the medial malleolus for the tendon of tibialis posterior, in its synovial sheath (Fig. 3.32). Alongside it is the tendon of flexor digitorum longus, while further to the fibular side the fleshy belly of flexor hallucis longus is in contact with the tibia. The distal surface shows a saddle-shaped facet for the talus, the articular surface extending to the lateral surface of the medial malleolus. The distal surface of the medial malleolus shows a smooth area for the deep lamina of the deltoid ligament, and the superficial part of the ligament is attached more superficially (the deltoid ligament is as thick as the bone of the malleolus).

The fascia lata of the thigh is attached to the ridges running down to the tuberosity, along with the patellar retinacula. The deep fascia of the leg is attached to the anterior and posterior borders of the shaft, down to the medial malleolus, and is fused with the periosteum over the subcutaneous medial surface of the shaft and malleolus. It is thickened at the lower end of the extensor compartment as the superior extensor retinaculum, and from the back of the medial malleolus the flexor retinaculum passes to the calcaneus. The upper limb of the inferior extensor retinaculum is attached to the front of the malleolus.

Surgical approach. The front of the shaft is exposed by incision over tibialis anterior and detachment of the muscle from the bone. The incision is not made over the bone itself as healing over the muscle is better. The posteromedial approach is along the posterior border of the bone, detaching soleus and flexor digitorum longus. A posterolateral approach begins by opening up the interval between peroneus longus and soleus, using the common peroneal nerve as the guide to the interval. Then flexor hallucis longus is stripped off the back of the fibula, and tibialis posterior from the fibula, interosseous

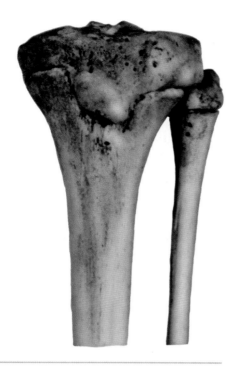

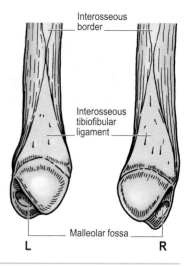

Fig. 3.51 Lower ends of the left and right fibulas, distinguished by the position of the malleolar fossa behind the triangular articular area.

Fig. 3.50 Epiphyseal lines at the upper end of the left tibia and fibula (aged 18 years) from the front. The epiphysis includes the attachment of the patellar ligament and, towards the back, the facet for the superior tibiofibular joint.

membrane and the tibia. By keeping close to the bone when stripping the fibula, the peroneal vessels are displaced with the muscles.

Ossification. The shaft ossifies in cartilage from a primary centre that appears in the eighth week of fetal life. The upper epiphysis (the growing end) shows a centre immediately after birth. At about 10 years, an anterior process from it descends to form the smooth part of the tibial tuberosity to which the patellar ligament is attached (Fig. 3.50). Before the epiphysis has fused with the shaft, at about 20 years, traction on this process by the attached ligament may cause pain and tenderness at this site in young adolescents. The lower epiphysis ossifies in the first year and joins the shaft at about 18 years. The medial malleolus is an extension from the lower epiphysis.

Fibula

The slender shaft of the fibula, the lateral bone of the leg, expands above into a quadrilateral head and below into a flattened malleolus (Fig. 3.48). The triangular articular surface on the medial aspect of the lower end has a pit, the malleolar fossa, behind it. Looking at these features enables the left and right fibulae to be distinguished: the fossa is to the left in the left fibula, to the right in the right fibula (Fig. 3.51).

The **head** of the fibula carries an oval or round facet facing proximally and medially; this articulates with a reciprocal facet on the upper epiphysis of the tibia. The palpable *styloid process* projects upwards from the posterolateral part of the head. The arcuate ligament of the knee joint is attached to it. The fibular collateral ligament and the biceps tendon are attached in front of the styloid process (Fig. 3.21).

The **shaft** has three surfaces, anterior, lateral and posterior, corresponding to the extensor, peroneal and flexor compartments of the leg. The lateral surface between the *anterior* and *posterior borders* is smooth and distally it spirals backwards to become continuous with the groove behind the lateral malleolus. Peroneus brevis arises from the lower two-thirds of this surface and its tendon passes down to groove the back of the malleolus. Peroneus longus arises from the upper two-thirds (behind brevis where they overlap) and its tendon passes down behind that of peroneus brevis. The common peroneal nerve enters peroneus longus at the **neck** of the bone, the part of the shaft adjoining the head; the nerve can be rolled against the bone here, where it may be damaged by a plaster cast or tight bandaging. It also divides here into its superficial and deep branches. The superficial peroneal nerve descends within peroneus longus and brevis, while the deep peroneal nerve pierces the anterior intermuscular septum to reach the extensor compart-ment of the leg. In the lateral compartment, these nerves, though very close to the bone, are not in actual contact with it, being cushioned by a few deep fibres of peroneus longus. The ridges that border the peroneal surface give attachment to the anterior and posterior septa that enclose the peroneal muscles.

Above the malleolar articular facet is a somewhat rough triangular surface for the interosseous tibiofibular ligament. From the apex of this triangular area a short ridge passes upwards and forks into two; the posterior one is the *interosseous border* and the other the anterior border. The anterior surface is between these borders and is extremely narrow, especially at its upper end, where in some bones the anterior and interosseous borders fuse. From the upper three-quarters of this narrow strip extensor digitorum longus takes origin, and here the deep peroneal nerve touches the bone beneath the muscle. In continuity with this muscle peroneus tertius arises from the lower third of the anterior surface. Deep to this (i.e. towards the interosseous border) extensor hallucis longus arises from the middle half of the fibula and the adjacent interosseous membrane.

The posterior surface, between the interosseous and posterior borders, is much wider. The middle third of this surface shows a vertical ridge, the *medial crest*, which runs down towards the interosseous border. It divides this part of the posterior surface into medial and lateral parts. To the medial part, between the medial crest and the interosseous border, tibialis posterior is attached. The lateral part of the posterior surface, between the medial crest and the posterior border, is for flexor hallucis longus. Below the medial crest (i.e. below the origin of tibialis posterior) flexor hallucis longus continues to arise from the whole posterior surface and from the interosseous membrane as far as the inferior tibiofibular joint. Here a spiral twist of the posterior surface matches the spiral twist of the peroneal surface. The upper part of the flexor surface, varying from a quarter to one-third, gives origin to soleus; a roughened 'soleal line' shows on many bones.

The **lateral malleolus** projects further distally than the medial (tibial) malleolus. Its medial surface has a triangular articular surface for the talus. The **malleolar fossa** behind this surface is perforated by foramina. It gives attachment to two ligaments that diverge to the tibia and the talus: the posterior tibiofibular liga-ment, which articulates with the talus and the posterior talofibular ligament. The lateral, triangular subcutaneous area has a rounded lower margin with a smooth area in front for the anterior talofibular ligament and a similar area just in front of the apex for the calcaneofibular ligament (Fig. 3.38). Between the subcutaneous area and the malleolar fossa is a smooth groove on the back of the malleolus for the tendon of peroneus brevis. The superior peroneal retinaculum passes from the tip of the malleolus to the calcaneus.

Surgical approach. The fibula can be exposed from the lateral side, along the interval between peroneus longus and soleus, using the common peroneal nerve at the upper end as the guide to the interval.

Ossification. The fibula ossifies in cartilage by a centre in the shaft which appears in the eighth week. There is an epiphysis at each extremity. The head, the growing end, is exceptional in ossifying later (fourth year) than the lower end (second year). The upper epiphysis fuses with the shaft by 20 years, the lower before this (about 18 years).

Foot

The skeleton of the foot is made up of tarsus, metatarsus and phalanges. The tarsus consists of seven bones arranged in proximal and distal rows. The proximal row comprises the talus and calcaneus. In the distal row are the medial, intermediate and lateral cuneiforms and the cuboid most laterally. Medially the navicular lies between the talus and the medial cuneiform. Only one of the tarsal bones, the calcaneus, rests on the ground. The metatarsus articulates with the tarsus, and the meta-tarsal heads, especially the first and fifth, rest on the ground. The toes lie free to move in front of the meta-tarsal heads, which are weight-bearing, the first taking more weight than the others.

Calcaneus

The calcaneus, the heel bone, is the largest of the tarsal bones. It articulates with the talus above and the cuboid in front. It is a rectangular block of bone, characterized by the sustentaculum tali, a shelf that projects from the upper border of its medial surface (Fig. 3.52).

The **upper surface** carries articular facets on its ante-rior half. The sustentaculum tali and the anterior part of the body show a common articular facet, elongated and concave; this may be separated into two halves, but even so they occupy the one joint cavity with the head of the talus. Behind the sustentacular facet an oblique groove (the floor of the tarsal sinus) widens as it passes laterally and forwards. The groove gives attachment to the talocalcanean interosseous ligaments and the cervical ligament. At the front of the sinus the bifurcate ligament is attached to the anterior margin of the calcaneus. Behind this is the origin of extensor digitorum brevis

Fig. 3.52 Left talus and calcaneus, as seen when the talus is lifted off the calcaneus and turned over to show its undersurface.

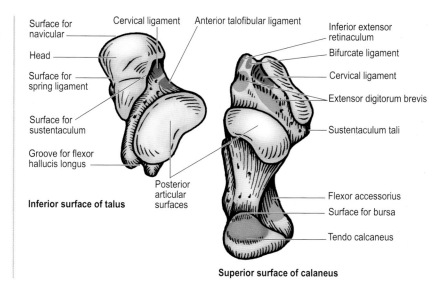

Inferior surface of talus

Surface for navicular
Cervical ligament
Anterior talofibular ligament
Head
Surface for spring ligament
Surface for sustentaculum
Groove for flexor hallucis longus
Posterior articular surfaces

Inferior extensor retinaculum
Bifurcate ligament
Cervical ligament
Extensor digitorum brevis
Sustentaculum tali
Flexor accessorius
Surface for bursa
Tendo calcaneus

Superior surface of calaneus

and, at the lateral margin of the sinus, the inferior extensor retinaculum is attached. Behind the groove is a convex oval articular surface where the talus articulates by a separate joint (talocalcanean). These two joint surfaces on the anterior half of the calcaneus together constitute the inferior surface of the 'subtalar' joint, where inversion and eversion take place. The non-articular posterior half of the upper surface is related to fibrofatty tissue between the tendo calcaneus and the ankle joint.

The **posterior surface** has a smooth upper part for the tendo calcaneus. Its lower part, convex, is grooved longitudinally for attachment of the fibres of the plantar aponeurosis, which sweep back from the undersurface. The uppermost part is bare for a bursa that lies here deep to the tendo calcaneus.

The **inferior surface** has the *calcanean tuberosity* at its posterior end which has medial and lateral processes extending anteriorly (Fig. 3.54). This is the weight-bearing part of the bone. Small muscles of the sole of the foot, and superficial to these the plantar aponeurosis, are attached to these processes. In front of the processes the inferior surface is grooved by the attachment of the long plantar ligament. This surface tapers to the smooth anterior tubercle of the calcaneus with a fossa in front of it. The fossa is filled by the short plantar ligament, which is attached to the anterior tubercle.

The **anterior surface** carries the articular surface for the cuboid.

The **lateral surface** is almost flat but has a small ridge, the *peroneal trochlea*, from which the inferior peroneal retinaculum bridges the sheathed tendons of peroneus brevis in the groove above and peroneus longus in the groove below the trochlea. The calcaneofibular ligament of the ankle joint is attached further back.

The **medial surface** is concave. The fleshy medial head of flexor accessorius occupies this area. Above the concavity the **sustentaculum tali** projects; its undersurface is deeply grooved by the tendon of flexor hallucis longus in its sheath. The rounded medial border of the sustentaculum gives attachment to the spring ligament in front and the superficial part of the deltoid ligament behind (Fig. 3.40). The tendon of flexor digitorum longus lies superficial to the sustentaculum.

The peroneal trochlea is palpable, and the weight-bearing medial and lateral processes can be felt through the thickness of the heelpad.

Talus

The talus carries the whole body weight. It lies on the weight-bearing calcaneus, below the tibia, and communicates thrust from the one to the other. The bone possesses a body which is prolonged forward into a neck and a rounded head.

The upper surface of the **body** carries an articular area, the **trochlea**, which is convex from front to back but with a shallow central groove (i.e. concave from side to side) (Fig. 3.39). The trochlea is broad in front and narrow behind. The trochlear surface is continued down over each side of the body for articulation with the stabilizing malleoli. On the medial surface the articular

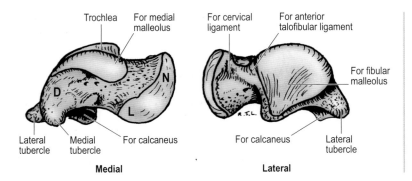

Trochlea   For medial malleolus

For cervical ligament   For anterior talofibular ligament

N

D

L

For fibular malleolus

Lateral tubercle   Medial tubercle   For calcaneus

For calcaneus   Lateral tubercle

Medial   **Lateral**

Fig. 3.53   Left talus from the medial and lateral sides. D, area of attachment of deep part of deltoid ligament; L, surface for articulation with spring ligament; N, area for navicular.

area is comma-shaped, with the broad end anterior (Fig. 3.53); this area articulates with the malleolus of the tibia. In the concavity of the comma curve there are many vascular foramina and behind these the deep lamina of the deltoid ligament is attached. On the lateral surface the articular area is bigger and triangular in outline; this surface articulates with the fibular malleolus.

Behind the trochlea the talus is projected into a **posterior process** which is deeply grooved by the tendon of flexor hallucis longus (Fig. 3.52). The posterior process projects as a pair of tubercles, one on either side of the groove. The *lateral tubercle* is the most posterior part of the talus and gives attachment to the posterior talofibular ligament. The *medial tubercle* gives attachment to the posterior fibres of the deltoid ligament.

The capsule of the ankle joint is attached to the articular margin except in front, where its attachment is further forward on the neck of the talus. The synovial membrane is attached to the articular margin.

The **inferior surface** of the body of the talus has a concave, oval facet for articulation with the calcaneus (Fig. 3.52). In front of this the **neck** is grooved for the tarsal sinus and gives attachment to the interosseous talocalcanean ligament. Laterally the neck gives attachment to the cervical ligament and the anterior talofibular ligament (Fig. 3.38). The neck of the talus is short, and is directed forwards and medially.

The rounded **head** of the talus is capped by a large articular surface facing forwards and downwards. Anteriorly the surface is convex for articulation with the navicular. Inferiorly it is flattened for articulation with the sustentaculum tali and the body of the calcaneus; a low ridge commonly separates this calcanean area into two flat facets. Medial to the calcanean facets the head is covered by hyaline cartilage for articulation with the spring ligament. The head of the talus is the ball of the ball and socket talocalcaneonavicular joint.

No muscles are attached to the talus. Nevertheless the talus has a good anastomotic blood supply within the bone from branches of the dorsalis pedis, posterior tibial and peroneal (fibular) arteries. The intraosseous vessels run mainly from anterior to posterior. In fractures of the talar neck these vessels are disrupted, and avascular necrosis of the body of the talus is a possible complication of a displaced fracture.

Cuboid bone

This bone is narrowest at the lateral margin and broadest medially. Its anterior surface has two facets for articulation with the fourth and fifth metatarsal bones (Fig. 3.54). Medially it articulates with the lateral cuneiform, and usually with the navicular. Its posterior surface has a triangular facet for the calcaneus. The medial surface has an oval facet for the lateral cuneiform and a small facet (sometimes absent) posterior to this for the navicular. The dorsal surface of the bone is bare. The lateral border has a notch which marks the lateral end of the groove on the inferior surface for the tendon of peroneus longus. The posterior margin of the notch has a tuberosity with a facet on it for the sesamoid cartilage or bone in the tendon. The oblique groove crosses the anterior part of the inferior surface. A prominent ridge forms the posterior margin of the groove. The deep fibres of the long plantar ligament are attached to this ridge, while the superficial fibres cross the groove to make a fibro-osseous tunnel that lodges the peroneus longus tendon and its synovial sheath. Behind the ridge is a hollow to which is attached the short plantar ligament and part of the origin of flexor hallucis brevis.

Navicular bone

This bone may be said to be boat-shaped, with a prominent medial tuberosity representing the prow of the boat (Fig. 3.39). The posterior concave articular surface fits the convexity of the head of the talus. The inferior margin of this surface gives attachment to the spring

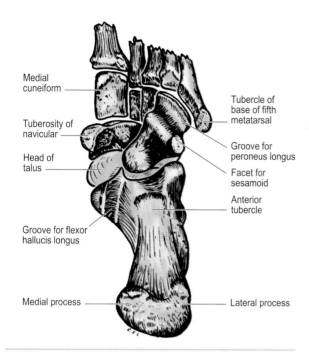

Medial
cuneiform

Tuberosity of
navicular

Head of
talus

Groove for flexor
hallucis longus

Medial process

Tubercle of
base of fifth
metatarsal

Groove for
peroneus longus

Facet for
sesamoid

Anterior
tubercle

Lateral process

Fig. 3.54 Left tarsal bones, from below.

ligament medially, and to the bifurcate ligament laterally. The distal convex articular surface is divided into three facets for the three cuneiform bones. The lateral surface usually has a facet for articulation with the cuboid.

The **tuberosity** is palpable about 2.5 cm below and anterior to the medial malleolus. It gives insertion to tibialis posterior.

Cuneiform bones

The three cuneiform bones, true to their name, are all wedge-shaped. The medial is the largest and lies edge upwards. The intermediate is the smallest and, with the lateral, lies edge downwards. All three articulate posteriorly with the navicular, and anteriorly each articulates with its metatarsal bone, thus completing the medial longitudinal arch (Fig. 3.39).

The medial cuneiform has a facet at the anterior inferior angle of its medial surface; tibialis anterior is inserted into the facet. A small area at the upper limit of the lateral surface articulates with the intermediate cuneiform and the base of the second metatarsal. At the anterior inferior angle of the lateral surface is a low tubercle; peroneus longus is inserted into the tubercle.

The lateral cuneiform articulates laterally with the cuboid, to which it is bound by strong ligaments. It

projects further distally than the intermediate cuneiform, thus also articulating with the base of the second metatarsal.

Metatarsal bones

The **first metatarsal** is a thick bone which transmits thrust in propulsion of the body. Proximally the base articulates with the medial cuneiform and the lateral side of the base articulates with the second metatarsal base. Medially and laterally the base receives part of the insertion of tibialis anterior and peroneus longus respectively.

The second to fifth metatarsals have slender shafts. The metatarsal shafts give attachment to the interosseous muscles. The metatarsal heads are united by a series of deep transverse ligaments that bind them together. The plantar aspects of the bases of the second, third and fourth metatarsals afford origins for the oblique head of adductor hallucis.

The base of the fifth metatarsal is prominent, lateral to the joint with the cuboid, as a proximally directed *tuberosity* which receives the tendon of peroneus brevis (Fig. 3.54). The dorsal surface of the base receives peroneus tertius, whose tendon extends along the top of the shaft for a variable distance (Fig. 3.29).

Phalanges

As in the hand, there are two phalanges for the preaxial digit (big toe) and three each for the others. Each metatarsophalangeal joint is strengthened by a thick pad of fibrocartilage (plantar ligament) on its plantar surface. Four short fibrous bands uniting the plantar ligaments of adjoining metatarsophalangeal joints constitute the deep transverse metatarsal ligament. Collateral ligaments, as in the hand, reinforce the sides of the joints. A similar arrangement exists in the interphalangeal joints.

Ossification of foot bones

All the foot bones ossify in cartilage. Three bones of the tarsus are ossified at birth. The calcaneus begins to ossify in the third month, the talus in the sixth month and the cuboid in the ninth month of fetal life. The navicular and the cuneiforms ossify during the first four years. Metatarsals and phalanges ossify by shaft centres in utero, and their epiphyses are as in the hand (the epiphysis of the first metatarsal is at the base, that of each of the other four is in the head).

There are secondary centres for the posterior surface of the calcaneus and sometimes for the lateral tubercle of the talus, the tubercle at the base of the fifth metatarsal and the tuberosity of the navicular.

Thorax

4

PART ONE

Body wall

The wall of the thorax and the wall of the abdomen are one, topographically and developmentally, the essential difference being the presence of ribs in the part primarily concerned with respiration.

The **skin** varies in texture, tending to be thin in front and thick behind. Distribution of hair varies with sex, age and race. The tension lines run almost horizontally around the body wall (see Fig. 1.2, p. 3).

In the **subcutaneous tissue** over the dilatable part of the body wall, namely the anterior abdominal wall and lower part of the thoracic wall in front of the midaxillary lines, the fibrous septa of the subcutaneous tissue are condensed beneath the fat into a thin but strong membranous layer of superficial fascia, the fascia of Scarpa. This fascia allows the fatty layer of superficial fascia, the fascia of Camper, to slide freely over the underlying thoracic wall, rectus sheath and external oblique aponeurosis. It fades out over the upper thoracic wall and along the midaxillary lines. The fascia of Scarpa is continued over the penis and scrotum as the superficial perineal fascia (of Colles; see p. 328). Below, over the thighs, it is attached to the fascia lata along the flexure skin crease of the hip, extending laterally from the pubic tubercle just below the inguinal ligament (Fig. 4.1).

Blood supply

The intercostal, subcostal and lumbar arteries pass forward in the neurovascular plane (see p. 13) to supply

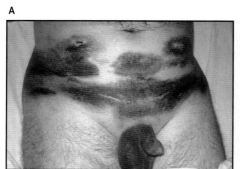
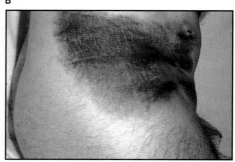

Fig. 4.1 Bilateral damage to the inferior epigastric artery—during the introduction of instruments through both iliac fossae for minimal access surgery—has resulted in blood leaking through the port sites and tracking down in a plane deep to Scarpa's fascia: **A** to the penis and scrotum and **B** to the upper thigh as far as the level of the flexure skin crease of the hip.

the flanks; the internal thoracic and the superior and inferior epigastric arteries supply the ventral midline tissues. From all these arteries cutaneous branches pass to the superficial fat and skin. The venous return from the subcutaneous tissue does not follow the arteries. The blood is collected by an anastomosing network of veins that radiate away from the umbilicus. Below this level they pass to the great saphenous vein in the groin; above the umbilicus they run up to the lateral thoracic vein and so to the axillary vein. From the umbilicus a few paraumbilical veins accompany the ligamentum teres and drain to the left branch of the portal vein; they may distend in portal obstruction, giving rise, if the distension spreads to the subcutaneous veins, to the caput Medusae. A longitudinal channel, the thoracoepigastric vein uniting the lateral thoracic vein with the superficial epigastric vein above the inguinal ligament, provides a communication between superior and inferior venae cavae and often becomes prominent in cases of obstruction of the inferior vena cava.

Lymph drainage

Lymphatic channels from the subcutaneous tissue and skin follow the veins to axillary and superficial inguinal nodes. From above the level of the umbilicus, lymph from the front of the body goes to the anterior (pectoral) group and from the back of the body to the posterior (scapular) group of axillary nodes. From the umbilicus downwards lymph from the anterior aspect of the abdominal wall and perineum goes to the medial group and from the lateral and posterior aspects of the abdominal wall to the lateral group of superficial inguinal nodes.

Nerve supply

Above the second rib and the manubriosternal joint the skin is supplied by supraclavicular branches of the cervical plexus (C4; see Fig. 1.8, p. 13). Below this level a midline and paramedian strip of skin is supplied by the anterior cutaneous branches of the spinal nerves from T2 to L1; the skin in the upper epigastric region is supplied by T7, in the umbilical region by T10 and suprapubic skin by L1. A broad lateral strip is supplied by the lateral cutaneous branches of the spinal nerves from T2 or 3 to L1; these branches emerge in the mid-axillary line. The lateral cutaneous branches of T12 and the iliohypogastric nerve descend over the iliac crest to also supply the skin of the buttock. The ilioinguinal nerve has no lateral cutaneous branch; it is the collateral branch of the iliohypogastric, both coming from L1 nerve. A posterior strip of skin is innervated by the posterior rami of spinal nerves, by their medial branches in the upper thoracic and their lateral branches in the lower thoracic and lumbosacral parts (see Fig. 1.7, p. 12).

PART TWO

Thoracic wall and diaphragm

The skeleton of the thoracic wall consists of the 12 thoracic vertebrae, the 12 pairs of ribs and costal cartilages and the sternum. The thoracic cavity is roofed in above the lung apices by the suprapleural membrane and is floored by the diaphragm. The floor is highly convex (domes of the diaphragm), so that the volume of the thoracic cavity is much less than inspection of the bony cage would suggest. The liver and spleen and the upper parts of the stomach and both kidneys lie in the abdominal cavity wholly or partly covered by ribs.

At the back the ribs articulate with the vertebral column in two places: by their heads (joints of costal heads) and by their tubercles (costotransverse joints). Collectively these form the **costovertebral joints**. At the front the ribs join their costal cartilages (costochondral joints). The upper seven costal cartilages articulate with the sternum at the sternocostal joints, the next three articulate with each other (interchondral joints) and the eighth articulates with the seventh costal cartilage to complete the costal margin; the last two costal cartilages are free. The manubriosternal joint is a symphysis between the manubrium and body of the sternum, and the xiphisternal joint is a symphysis between the body and the xiphoid process.

Joints of costal heads

The head of a typical rib possesses two articular facets that slope away from each other, separated by a ridge. Each facet makes a small synovial joint with a demifacet of a vertebral body; the lower rib facet with the upper costal facet of its own vertebra, and the upper facet with the lower costal facet of the vertebra above (Fig. 4.2). The ridge between the two is attached to the intervertebral disc by the *intra-articular ligament*. The front of the joint capsule is reinforced by the *radiate ligament* which consists of three bands. The upper band passes to the body of the vertebra above, the lower band to the vertebra below, while the central band runs horizontally, deep to the anterior longitudinal ligament, and blends with the intervertebral disc. The first rib articulates with T1 vertebra only, never coming into contact with C7, and the last two ribs also articulate only with their own vertebrae.

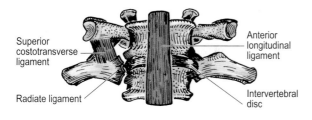

Superior costotransverse ligament

Anterior longitudinal ligament

Radiate ligament

Intervertebral disc

Fig. 4.2 Joints of the heads of the ribs from the front. The upper vertebra shows the articular facet on the transverse process for the costotransverse joint with the tubercle of a rib.

Costotransverse joints

The tubercle of a typical rib (p. 226) has two facets. The medial facet, covered with hyaline cartilage, articulates with a facet near the tip of the transverse process of its own vertebra at a small synovial joint. The lateral facet (non-articular) gives attachment to the *lateral costotransverse ligament* which runs to the tip of the transverse process and is one of three ligaments helping to stabilize the joint. The other two are the *costotransverse ligament*, which occupies the space between the back of the neck of the rib and the front of the transverse process, and the *superior costotransverse ligament*, which passes as two laminae from the crest of the neck of the rib to the undersurface of the transverse process of the vertebra above (Fig. 4.2). The anterior lamina is continuous with the posterior intercostal membrane; the posterior is in the same plane as the external intercostal muscle. The fibres of these two laminae are at right angles to each other, in a similar manner to the fibres of the intercostal muscles. The lower two ribs do not possess tubercles and make no synovial joints with transverse processes.

Costochondral joints

Every rib makes with its costal cartilage a primary cartilaginous joint. The costal cartilage represents no more than the unossified anterior part of a rib.

Interchondral joints

Adjacent surfaces of costal cartilages 6 and 7, 7 and 8, and 8 and 9 are joined to each other by small synovial joints; 9 and 10 are connected by ligamentous fibres.

Sternocostal joints

The first costal cartilage articulates with the manubrium by a primary cartilaginous joint. Thus the manubrium

and the first ribs are fixed to each other and move together as one.

The next six costal cartilages each articulate with the sternum by a synovial joint—a single cavity except in the case of the second, which articulates with the manubrium and body (Fig. 4.3).

Manubriosternal joint

At this symphysis between the manubrium and body of the sternum, the surfaces are covered by hyaline cartilage and there is an intervening disc of fibrocartilage which may become ossified in the elderly. Sometimes (30%) cavitation appears in the disc so that the joint may appear to be synovial, but this is simply a degenerative change that does not alter the fact that the joint is a symphysis.

Xiphisternal joint

This is another symphysis, between the body of the sternum and the xiphoid process. Ossification from middle age onwards is common.

Thoracic muscles

The muscles of the thoracic wall lie in the same three morphological layers as those of the abdominal wall (see p. 229), but in the thoracic region they have become divided up by the presence of ribs. They are innervated segmentally by anterior rami. In the outer thoracic layer the external intercostal muscles correspond to the external oblique in the abdomen and in the middle layer the internal intercostals correspond to the internal oblique. The inner layer is broken up into three muscles, the subcostals, innermost intercostals and the transversus thoracis. This incomplete layer corresponds to the transversus abdominis. Between it and the middle layer is the neurovascular plane, continuous with that of the abdominal wall; in it run intercostal vessels and nerves, with their collateral branches (see Fig. 1.6, p. 12).

Outer layer

Two small muscles of the external layer have migrated posteriorly, and lie on the surface of the erector spinae mass. They are the posterior serratus muscles and are supplied by anterior rami. Each arises from four spinous processes, two in the thorax and two beyond it, and each is inserted into four ribs.

Serratus posterior superior arises from the spinous processes of the lowest two cervical and the upper two thoracic vertebrae and is inserted just lateral to the

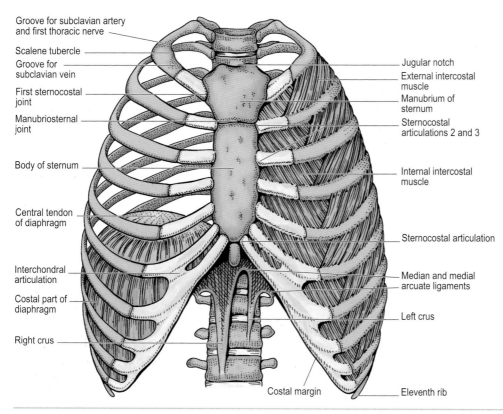

Groove for subclavian artery
and first thoracic nerve

Scalene tubercle

Groove for
subclavian vein

First sternocostal
joint

Manubriosternal
joint

Body of sternum

Central tendon
of diaphragm

Interchondral
articulation

Costal part of
diaphragm

Right crus

Jugular notch

External intercostal
muscle

Manubrium of
sternum

Sternocostal
articulations 2 and 3

Internal intercostal
muscle

Sternocostal articulation

Median and medial
arcuate ligaments

Left crus

Eleventh rib

Costal margin

Fig. 4.3 Chest wall, including diaphragm: anterior aspect.

angles of ribs 2–5. Many tendinous fibres in the sheet of muscle give it a characteristic glistening appearance which provides a useful landmark in exposures of this region. The dorsal scapular nerve and vessels run down on the posterior surface of the muscle, between it and the rhomboids (see Fig. 2.5, p. 44).

Serratus posterior inferior arises from the lower two thoracic and the upper two lumbar spinous processes and is inserted just lateral to the angles of the lowest four ribs.

The serratus posterior muscles are weak muscles of respiration. The superior muscle elevates the upper ribs (inspiration) while the inferior muscle depresses the lower ribs (expiration).

Although morphologically associated with the muscles of the back (see p. 445), the **levator costae** muscles are functionally classified as thoracic muscles. Each one of each of the 12 pairs is fan-shaped, spreading down from the tip of a transverse process (from C7 to T11 vertebra) to be inserted into the upper border of the rib below,

lateral to its tubercle (see Fig. 6.82, p. 446), and presumably helps to elevate it. They are supplied by the posterior rami of spinal nerves (from C8 to T11).

The chief muscles of the outer layer are the **external intercostals**. The fibres of the external intercostal muscles pass obliquely downwards and forwards from the sharp lower border of the rib above to the smooth upper border of the rib below. Each muscle extends from the superior costotransverse ligament at the back of the intercostal space as far forwards as the costochondral junction; here it is replaced by the *anterior intercostal membrane* (see Fig. 1.6, p. 12). This extends to the side of the sternum. Between the bony ribs is muscle; between the costal cartilages is membrane.

Middle layer

This consists of the **internal intercostal muscles**. The fibres run downwards and backwards, from the costal groove to the upper border of the rib below (Fig. 4.4).

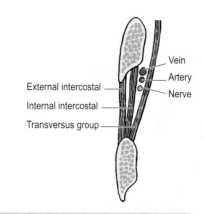

External intercostal

Internal intercostal

Transversus group

Vein

Artery

Nerve

Fig. 4.4 Vertical section through an intercostal space. The neurovascular structures (vein, artery, nerve from above downwards) lie between the internal intercostals and the transversus group. The small collateral branches (not shown) are in the same plane just above the lower rib.

Each muscle, unlike an external intercostal, extends as far forwards as the side of the sternum; it is replaced posteriorly by the *posterior intercostal membrane*, which extends from the angle of the rib to the superior costotransverse ligament at the posterior limit of the space (see Fig. 1.6, p. 12).

Inner layer

Of the three groups of muscles in this layer the innermost intercostals line the rib cage at the side, while the subcostals are at the back, and the transversus thoracis at the front. They all cross more than one intercostal space.

Lying in the paravertebral gutter are the **subcostal muscles** attached to the inner surfaces of ribs. They are separated from the posterior border of the innermost intercostals by a space across which the intercostal nerves and vessels are in contact with the parietal pleura.

The **innermost intercostal muscles** (intercostales intimi) are attached to the inner surfaces of ribs on the lateral part of the thoracic wall.

Transversus thoracis arises from the posterior surface of the lower part of the sternum, whence digitations diverge on each side to the second to the sixth costal cartilages. This muscle was formerly called sternocostalis, which was a more exact name. The *transversus thoracis group* is the best inclusive name for all three muscles of the inner layer because it conforms with the transversus abdominis muscle.

Intercostal spaces

The intercostal spaces (between the ribs) are filled in by the muscles of the three layers described above. Running in the plane between the intermediate and inner layers are the intercostal nerves and vessels (Fig. 4.4). The vein, artery and nerve lie in that order from above downwards, under cover of the downward projection of the lower border of the rib. Thus a needle or trocar for pleural drainage (see p. 220) is inserted just above the rib that forms the lower boundary of the space, in order to avoid the main nerve and vessels that are at its upper boundary. The collateral branches of nerve and vessels that run along the upper border of a rib are small and can be ignored.

Intercostal nerves

The mixed **spinal nerve**, having emerged from the intervertebral foramen and given off its posterior ramus, passes around in the neurovascular plane, between the internal intercostal and the transversus thoracis group of muscles (see Fig. 1.6, p. 12). This intercostal nerve gives off a collateral and a lateral cutaneous branch before it reaches the costal angle. The **collateral branch** runs along the inferior border of its space and supplies the muscles of the space, the parietal pleura and the periosteum of the ribs. The **lateral cutaneous branch** pierces the intercostal muscles and the overlying muscles of the body wall along the midaxillary line, and divides into an anterior and posterior branch to supply the skin over the space. The intercostal nerve ends as an **anterior cutaneous nerve**, which in the upper six spaces passes anterior to the internal thoracic artery and pierces the intercostal muscles to reach the skin. In its course around the space the intercostal nerve lies below the vein and artery, but in its course around the body wall the main nerve lies in a wider circle that embraces the narrower circle of the intercostal vessels. Hence, at the back of the intercostal space where the nerve crosses the intercostal artery, the nerve lies behind the artery; at the front of the space the nerve crosses in front of the internal thoracic artery.

The lower five intercostal nerves and their collateral branches slope downwards behind the costal margin into the neurovascular plane of the abdominal wall, which they supply (see p. 233).

The anterior ramus of T1 ascends across the neck of the first rib to enter the brachial plexus. Before it does so it gives off the small **first intercostal nerve**, which courses around beneath the flat inferior surface of the first rib (see Fig. 6.9B, p. 360) and supplies the intercostal muscles of the first space, the adjacent pleura and rib periosteum.

The lateral cutaneous branch of the second intercostal nerve crosses the axilla to the medial side of the arm as the intercostobrachial nerve (see p. 63).

The **subcostal nerve** (twelfth thoracic), although arising in the thorax, quickly leaves by passing behind the lateral arcuate ligament of the diaphragm into the abdomen, below the subcostal artery and vein.

Intercostal arteries

Arteries enter intercostal spaces at the back and front. At the back the upper two spaces are supplied by the **superior intercostal artery**. This is the descending branch of the costocervical trunk, which comes off from the second part of the subclavian artery behind scalenus anterior. It enters the thorax by passing across the front of the neck of the first rib; here it has the sympathetic trunk on its medial side, while the first thoracic nerve passes laterally across the first rib to join the brachial plexus (Fig. 6.9B). The small first posterior intercostal vein lies between the artery and the sympathetic trunk. At this point the first thoracic sympathetic ganglion is frequently fused with the inferior cervical ganglion to form the cervicothoracic (stellate) ganglion.

The remaining nine intercostal spaces are supplied each with a separate branch of the descending thoracic aorta. All 11 arteries constitute the **posterior intercostal arteries**. Each gives off a small collateral branch, which passes around in the neurovascular plane at a lower level than the main trunk.

At the front of the intercostal space the internal thoracic artery in the upper six spaces and the musculo-phrenic artery in the seventh, eighth and ninth spaces give off two **anterior intercostal arteries** that pass backwards and anastomose with the posterior vessels. There are no anterior intercostal arteries in the last two spaces.

Intercostal veins

In each space there are one **posterior** and two **anterior intercostal veins**, accompanying the arteries of the same names. The anterior veins drain into the musculophrenic and internal thoracic veins. The posterior veins are not regular. In the lower eight spaces they drain into the azygos system: the azygos vein on the right and the hemiazygos and accessory hemiazygos on the left. The first posterior intercostal vein opens either into the verte-bral vein or the brachiocephalic vein of its own side. The second and third posterior intercostal veins, and sometimes the fourth, form a single trunk on each side, the **superior intercostal vein**. That on the right drains simply into the azygos vein (Fig. 4.12). That on the left runs forward over the arch of the aorta, superficial to the

vagus nerve and deep to the phrenic nerve, to empty into the left brachiocephalic vein (Fig. 4.13).

Lymph drainage

The lymph vessels of the intercostal spaces follow the arteries. From the front of the space vessels pass to the anterior intercostal (parasternal) nodes that lie along the internal thoracic artery; from the back of the space they drain to posterior intercostal nodes.

Internal thoracic artery

From the first part of the subclavian artery, the internal thoracic artery (formerly the internal mammary) passes vertically downwards about 1 cm lateral to the border of the sternum (Fig. 4.5). It gives off two *anterior inter-costal arteries* in each intercostal space. At the costal margin it divides into the *superior epigastric* and *musculophrenic arteries*. The former passes between the xiphisternal and highest costal fibres of the diaphragm to enter the rectus sheath behind the muscle. The latter passes along the costodiaphragmatic gutter and gives off two anterior intercostal arteries in each space till it ends by piercing the diaphragm in the ninth space to ramify on its abdominal surface. The internal thoracic artery is accompanied by two venae comitantes that empty into the brachiocephalic vein.

The artery gives off a *pericardiacophrenic branch* that runs with the phrenic nerve and supplies branches to the nerve itself, pleura and fibrous and parietal pericardium.

Perforating branches emerge towards the surface from each intercostal space. They are especially large in the second, third and fourth spaces of the female for supply of the breast. Thus the internal thoracic artery supplies the anterior body wall from the clavicle to the umbilicus.

Suprapleural membrane

This is a rather dense fascial layer (Sibson's fascia) attached to the inner border of the first rib and costal cartilage and the transverse process of C7 vertebra (Fig. 4.5). It is not attached to the neck of the first rib. It has the cervical dome of the pleura attached to its undersurface, and when traced medially it is found to thin out and disappear into the mediastinal pleura. It lies in the oblique plane of the thoracic inlet, and the subclavian vessels arch upwards and laterally over it. The membrane gives rigidity to the thoracic inlet and prevents the neck structures being 'puffed' up and down during respiration. Damage to the suprapleural mem-brane during surgical procedures at the root of the neck

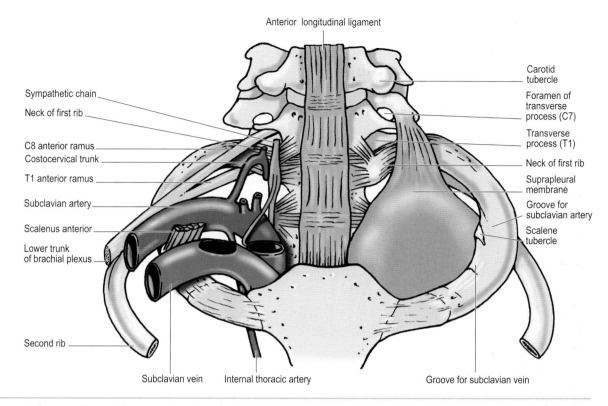

Anterior longitudinal ligament

Sympathetic chain

Neck of first rib

C8 anterior ramus

Costocervical trunk

T1 anterior ramus

Subclavian artery

Scalenus anterior

Lower trunk
of brachial plexus

Second rib

Subclavian vein   Internal thoracic artery

Carotid tubercle

Foramen of transverse process (C7)

Transverse process (T1)

Neck of first rib

Suprapleural membrane

Groove for subclavian artery

Scalene tubercle

Groove for subclavian vein

Fig. 4.5   Thoracic inlet and the suprapleural membrane.
(The membrane on the right and the subclavian vessels on the left are not shown.)

will usually result in the development of a pneumothorax on the same side.

Diaphragm

The diaphragm is a domed fibromuscular sheet that separates the thoracic and abdominal cavities. Its purpose is essentially for inspiration.

Morphologically the diaphragm is a derivative of the inner (transversus) layer of the muscles of the body wall, and its fibres arise in continuity with those of transversus abdominis from within the costal margin. It is completed behind the costal origin by fibres that arise from the arcuate ligaments and the crura. From the circumference of this oval origin the fibres arch upwards into a pair of domes and then descend to a central tendon which lies at the level of the xiphisternal joint. Viewed from in front the diaphragm curves up into right and left domes. The right dome of the diaphragm is higher than the left, ascending in full expiration as high as the nipple (fourth space), while the left dome reaches the fifth rib.

Viewed from the side the profile of the diaphragm resembles an inverted J, the long limb extending up from the crura (upper lumbar vertebrae) and the short limb attached to the xiphisternum (level of T8 vertebra). Viewed from above the outline is kidney shaped, in conformity with the oval outline of the body wall which is indented posteriorly by the vertebral column (see Fig. 1.6, p. 12).

The **crura** are strong tendons attached to the antero-lateral surfaces of the bodies of the upper lumbar vertebrae. The **right crus** is fixed to the upper three lumbar vertebrae and the intervening discs; the **left crus** likewise to the upper two lumbar vertebrae. Muscle fibres radiate from each crus, overlap, and pass vertically upwards before curving forwards into the central tendon. Some of the fibres of the *right* crus pass up on the abdominal surface of fibres from the left crus and surround the oesophageal orifice in a sling-like loop (Fig. 4.6; see also Fig. 5.26, p. 260). Tendinous fibres from the medial edge of each crus unite with one another in front of the aorta at the level of T12 vertebra to form the *median arcuate*

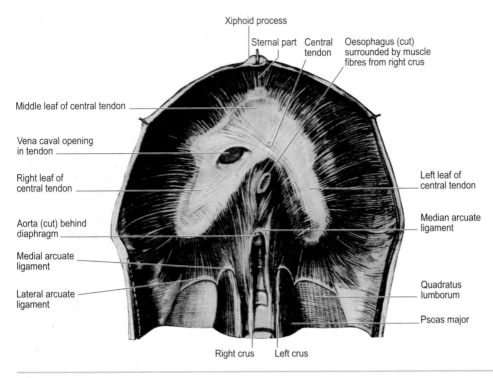

Xiphoid process

Sternal part Central tendon Oesophagus (cut) surrounded by muscle fibres from right crus

Middle leaf of central tendon

Vena caval opening in tendon

Right leaf of central tendon

Aorta (cut) behind diaphragm

Medial arcuate ligament

Lateral arcuate ligament

Left leaf of central tendon

Median arcuate ligament

Quadratus lumborum

Psoas major

Right crus   Left crus

Fig. 4.6   Diaphragm: abdominal aspect.

ligament. The *medial arcuate ligament* is a thickening in the psoas fascia. It extends from the side of the body of L1 or L2 vertebra to a ridge on the anterior surface of the transverse process of L1 vertebra, at the lateral margin of psoas. From here the *lateral arcuate ligament* extends across to the middle of the lower margin of the twelfth rib; it is a thickening in the anterior layer of the lumbar fascia on the front of quadratus lumborum. Further laterally a digitation arises from the internal surfaces of each of the lower six costal cartilages and ribs, interdigitating with the slips of origin of transversus abdominis. In front, the diaphragm arises from the back of the xiphisternum.

The **central tendon** has a trefoil shape, having an anteriorly situated middle leaf fused on each side to lateral leaves that extend back towards the paravertebral gutters. The tendon is inseparable from the fibrous pericardium, both having the same embryological origin.

Openings in the diaphragm

For the passage of structures between thorax and abdomen there are three large openings in the diaphragm and several smaller ones.

The **aortic opening** is opposite T12 vertebra, in the midline, behind the median arcuate ligament. It transmits the aorta with the azygos vein to the right and the thoracic duct leading up from the cisterna chyli between them.

The **oesophageal opening** is opposite T10 vertebra, usually 2.5 cm to the left of the midline behind the seventh left costal cartilage. It lies in the fibres of the left crus, but a sling of fibres from the right crus loop around it. The transversalis fascia on the undersurface of the diaphragm extends up through the opening, blends with the endothoracic fascia above the diaphragm, and is attached to the oesophagus about 2–3 cm above the oesophagogastric junction. This fascial cone is the phreno-oesophageal ligament. It becomes stretched in the 'sliding' type of hiatus hernia (see p. 194). The vagal trunks and the oesophageal branches of the left gastric artery, veins and lymphatics accompany the oesophagus as it passes through the diaphragm. The venous drainage from this site passes caudally to the portal venous system and cranially to the azygos venous system, constituting a major site of portal–systemic anastomosis.

The **vena caval foramen** is opposite T8 vertebra just to the right of the midline, behind the sixth right costal cartilage. It lies between the middle and right leaves of the central tendon, the fibres of which fuse firmly with the adventitial wall of the inferior vena cava (Fig. 4.12). The right phrenic nerve passes through the central tendon alongside the inferior vena cava at this opening.

Other structures make their own smaller openings. The *hemiazygos vein* passes through the left crus. The *greater*, *lesser*, and *least splanchnic nerves* pierce each crus. The *sympathetic trunk* passes behind the medial arcuate ligament. The *subcostal nerve and vessels* pass behind the lateral arcuate ligament. The *left phrenic nerve* pierces the muscle of the left dome. The *neurovascular bundles* of the seventh to the eleventh intercostal spaces pass between the digitations of the diaphragm and transversus abdominis into the neurovascular plane of the abdominal wall. The *superior epigastric vessels* pass between the xiphisternal and costal (seventh) fibres of the diaphragm. Extraperitoneal *lymph vessels* on the abdominal surface pass through the diaphragm to lymph nodes lying on its thoracic surface, mainly in the posterior mediastinum.

At the posterior part of the diaphragm there may be a gap between the lowest costal fibres and those arising from the lateral arcuate ligament. The posterior surface of the kidney and its perirenal fascial covering is then separated from the pleura only by areolar tissue.

Blood supply

The costal margin of the diaphragm is supplied by the lower five intercostal and the subcostal arteries. The main mass of fibres rising up from the crura are supplied on their abdominal surface by right and left inferior phrenic arteries from the abdominal aorta (see Fig. 5.43, p. 285). The pericardiacophrenic and musculophrenic branches of the internal thoracic artery and the superior phrenic branches of the thoracic aorta make small contributions to the blood supply of the diaphragm.

Nerve supply

The motor nerve supply is solely from the phrenics (C3, 4, 5 but predominantly C4). Each half of the diaphragm is supplied by its own phrenic nerve and the fibres of the right crus that loop to the left around the oesophageal opening are supplied by the left phrenic. The lower intercostal nerves give proprioceptive fibres to the periphery of the diaphragm, proprioceptive supply to the central part coming from the phrenics. On reaching the abdominal surface of the diaphragm, both nerves divide into anterior, lateral and posterior branches which run radially, giving off branches that enter the muscle from below.

Associated with a lifetime of constant activity, about 55% of diaphragmatic muscle fibres (and 65% of intercostal muscle fibres) are of the slow twitch fatigue-resistant variety.

Actions

The major role of the diaphragm is inspiratory, but it is used also in abdominal straining.

Inspiration. When the fibres contract in tranquil inspiration only the domes descend; this sucks down the lung bases and does not disturb the mediastinum. In a deeper breath further descent of the domes, below the level of the central tendon, can depress the central tendon from T8 to T9 level. This stretches the mediastinum (traction on pericardium and great vessels) and no further descent of the tendon is possible. Further contraction of the muscle (maximum inspiration) now everts the ribs of the costal margin in a 'bucket handle'-like movement with widening of the subcostal angle.

As the diaphragm contracts intra-abdominal pressure tends to rise, and the vena caval foramen (in the central tendon) is pulled widely open to assist venous return via the inferior vena cava. The oesophageal opening is held closed by the pinch-like action resulting from contraction of the muscle sling of the right crus, to discourage regurgitation of stomach contents. The aortic opening is unaffected.

Hiccup is a (repeated) spasmodic contraction of the diaphragm, its contraction being followed immediately by closure of the glottis and subsequent release of the trapped air to produce the characteristic sound.

Expiration. Whether expiration is tranquil or forced (coughing, sneezing, blowing, etc.) the diaphragm is wholly passive, its relaxed fibres being elongated by pressure from below.

Abdominal straining. For evacuation of a pelvic effluent (defecation, micturition, parturition) diaphragmatic contraction aids that of the abdominal wall in raising intra-abdominal pressure. It is much weaker than the powerful obliques, transversus and recti, so for maximum pressure a deep breath is taken, the glottis is closed and the diaphragm is prevented from undue elevation by being held down by a cushion of compressed air. Forcible escape of some of this air causes the characteristic grunt.

During heavy lifting in the stooping position abdominal straining is beneficial. With the breath held and intracoelomic pressure raised as above, the vertebral column cannot easily flex; it is as though an inflated football filled the body from pelvic brim to thoracic inlet. The weight of the stooping trunk is supported on the football, freeing erector spinae to use all its power to lift the weight. Such acts are similarly accompanied on occasion by the characteristic grunt.

Development

The diaphragm develops from four sources. The *septum transversum* (p. 26) gives rise to most of the central tendon. Prior to its descent the transverse septum becomes invaded by muscle cells derived from the third, fourth and fifth *cervical myotomes*. The muscle cells carry their own nerve supply with them, hence the motor supply from the phrenic nerves. Mesodermal folds, the *pleuroperitoneal membranes*, which close the connection between the thoracic and abdominal parts of the coelom, and the *oesophageal mesentery* also contribute to the development of the diaphragm. Failure of pleuroperitoneal membrane development is the most common cause of congenital diaphragmatic hernia. The defect (Bochdalek's foramen) is posteriorly placed and clinically manifests more often on the left side, probably due to the presence of the liver on the right side. Another possible but smaller hernial site is at the junction of the costal and xiphoid origins—Morgagni's foramen.

Diaphragmatic hernia

The congenital types of diaphragmatic hernia have just been mentioned. Of the acquired varieties, the most common is the *sliding* type of hiatus hernia, through the oesophageal opening. Here the oesophagogastric junction rises up into the thorax. In the much rarer *paraoesophageal* (*rolling*) type, the oesophagogastric junction remains in the abdomen, but a pouch of peritoneum containing a part of the stomach projects upwards alongside the oesophagus.

Thoracic movements and respiration

The diaphragm is the main muscle of inspiration. The external intercostals are most active in inspiration and the internal intercostals in expiration, but the intercostals are more important for stiffening of the chest wall and preventing paradoxical movement of the interspaces. In expiration, elastic recoil of the lungs assisted by contraction of the muscles of the abdominal wall makes the relaxed diaphragm regain its domed form.

During maximal inspiratory efforts, other muscles too are active. The scalene muscles and sternocleidomastoid elevate the first rib and manubrium. The twelfth rib is fixed by quadratus lumborum and may even descend.

The erector spinae extend the spine, and muscles connecting the trunk to the upper limbs, such as pectoralis major, contribute to chest expansion when the arms are fixed. In forced expiratory efforts, latissimus dorsi contracts, compressing the lower ribs.

All three diameters of the thorax—anteroposterior, transverse and vertical—are increased during inspiration. The anteroposterior diameter increases because the sternum moves forwards as the ribs are raised since their anterior ends are at a lower level than their heads (see Fig. 4.33, p. 226). This sternal movement is facilitated by the hinge movement (up to about 7°) at the manubriosternal joint. If this joint becomes ankylosed, thoracic expansion due to sternocostal movement is virtually lost (as in emphysema) and only diaphragmatic respiration is possible. As each rib forms the arc of a circle, which is larger than that formed by the rib above, elevation of the ribs during inspiration increases the transverse diameter of the thorax. Change in the vertical extent of the thoracic cavity is due to diaphragmatic movement (Figs 4.7 and 4.8).

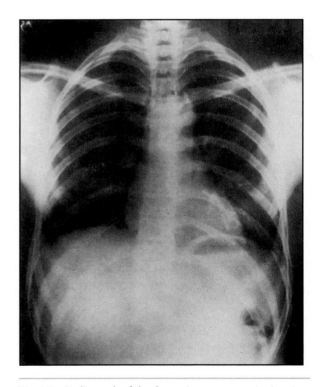

Fig. 4.7   Radiograph of the thorax in extreme expiration, in a healthy male aged 21 years.

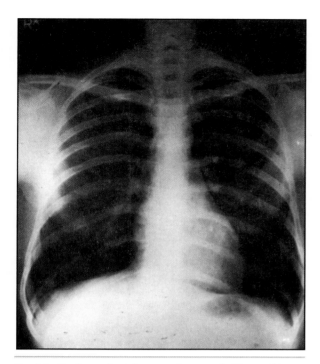

Fig. 4.8   Radiograph of the same thorax as in Figure 4.7 taken in full inspiration. The anterior ends of the ribs are elevated and the lower ribs everted. The descent of the domes of the diaphragm is greater than that of the central tendon.

Movements of the abdominal wall

Since the volume of the abdominal cavity remains constant, the abdominal wall moves in accordance with changes in the thoracic cavity. Diaphragmatic inspiration and rib inspiration occur simultaneously, but each in itself produces opposite movements in the abdominal wall. In purely diaphragmatic breathing, with the ribs motionless, descent of the diaphragm is accompanied by passive protrusion of the relaxed abdominal wall. Ascent of the diaphragm is accompanied by retraction of the abdominal wall; indeed, it is the active contraction of the abdominal wall muscles that forces the relaxed diaphragm up. This to-and-fro movement of the abdominal wall is usually called 'abdominal respiration'.

In 'thoracic respiration' the movements of the abdominal wall are purely passive. When the ribs are elevated in inspiration the diaphragm is elevated with the up-going costal margin and the abdominal wall is sucked in. With descent of the costal margin in expiration the abdominal wall moves forwards again.

The ordinary simultaneous rib and diaphragm movements can be so balanced that the abdominal wall does not move at all. Thus respiration may function quite well in tight corsets, plaster casts, etc. In children and many women thoracic movement is greater than diaphragmatic movement. In men diaphragmatic movement is greater, especially as the years go by.

Thoracotomy

Surgical access to thoracic structures involves some kind of thoracotomy. In the *anterolateral* or *posterolateral* type, skin and underlying muscles are incised along the line of the chosen rib (often fifth or sixth) and the periosteum stripped off the rib (keeping away from the intercostal nerve and vessels which run immediately below a rib). With or without resection of the rib, the periosteal bed of the rib is then incised to enter the pleural cavity. The nerve to serratus anterior may have to be sacrificed when incising that muscle in order to obtain the necessary exposure.

In anterior thoracotomy, or *median sternotomy*, the whole length of the sternum is split vertically in the midline, the sternal origin of the diaphragm detached, and the tissues behind the sternum freed by blunt dissection. Damage to the pleural sacs is avoided, remembering that the right pleura may extend a little to the left of the midline (see p. 220).

In the combined *thoracoabdominal incision*, the line of approach is through the eighth or ninth rib bed or intercostal space, dividing the cartilage at the costal margin and incising the anterior abdominal wall. The diaphragm is incised circumferentially near its periphery or radially towards the point of entry of the phrenic nerve, thus minimizing damage to the branches of the nerve (see p. 193).

PART THREE

Thoracic cavity

The cavity of the thorax is completely filled laterally by the lungs, each lying in its pleural cavity. The space between the pleural cavities occupying the centre of the thoracic cavity is the **mediastinum**. It contains the heart and great blood vessels, oesophagus, trachea and its bifurcation, thymus, thoracic duct, lymph nodes, phrenic and vagus nerves. The loose connective tissue between these structures connects freely with that of the neck. Mediastinitis may complicate infections in the neck.

Divisions of the mediastinum

There is a plane of division to which the whole topography of the mediastinum can be related, namely a plane passing horizontally through the sternal angle (of Louis), i.e. the manubriosternal joint (Fig. 4.9). From the second costal cartilages, this plane passes backwards to the lower border of T4 vertebra. Above, between it and the thoracic inlet, lies the *superior mediastinum*. Below the plane, the *inferior mediastinum* is divided into three compartments by the fibrous pericardium: a part in front, the *anterior mediastinum*; a part behind, the *posterior mediastinum*; and the *middle mediastinum* in between containing the pericardium and heart together with the adjoining parts of the great vessels and the lung roots. The anterior and posterior mediastina are in direct continuity with the superior mediastinum; their separation from it is purely descriptive, not anatomical. The plane passes through the bifurcation of the trachea, the concavity of the arch of the aorta, and just above the bifurcation of the pulmonary trunk. On the plane the azygos vein enters the superior vena cava, and the thoracic duct reaches the left side of the oesophagus in its passage upwards from the abdomen. Also lying in the plane are the ligamentum arteriosum, with the left recurrent laryngeal nerve recurring below it, and the superficial and deep parts of the cardiac plexus.

The prevertebral and pretracheal fasciae extend from the neck into the superior mediastinum. The former fuses with the anterior longitudinal ligament over T4 vertebra; the latter blends with the pericardium over the front upper part of the heart. Thus, neck infection in front of the pretracheal fascia is directed into the anterior mediastinum, while infection behind the prevertebral fascia is imprisoned in the superior mediastinum in front of the vertebral bodies (Fig. 4.9). From elsewhere in the neck infection may extend through the superior into the posterior mediastinum.

PART **FOUR**

Superior mediastinum

General topography

The superior mediastinum is wedge shaped (Fig. 4.9). The anterior boundary is the manubrium. The posterior boundary is much longer, due to the obliquity of the thoracic inlet. It consists of the bodies of the first four thoracic vertebrae; this wall is concave towards the mediastinum.

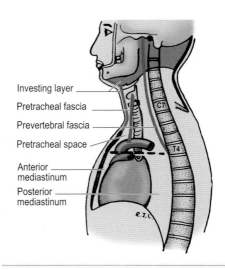

Fig. 4.9 Divisions of the mediastinum, showing the continuity with the tissue spaces of the neck. The superior mediastinum is above the interrupted line passing from the sternal angle to the lower border of T4 vertebra. The anterior mediastinum is continuous through the superior mediastinum with the pretracheal space of the neck, up to the hyoid bone. The posterior mediastinum is continuous with the retropharyngeal and paratracheal space of the neck, up to the base of the skull.

At the *thoracic inlet* (Fig. 4.10; and Fig. 6.9A, p. 360), often called clinically the thoracic *outlet*, the oesophagus lies against the body of T1 vertebra. The trachea lies on the oesophagus and may touch the jugular notch of the manubrium. The midline of the inlet is thus wholly occupied by these two tubes. At the inlet the apices of the lungs lie laterally, separated by the trachea and oesophagus and by vessels and nerves passing between the neck and the superior mediastinum. Below the inlet, the trachea slopes back and the manubrium slopes forward; the brachiocephalic trunk, the left brachiocephalic vein and the thymus occupy the space thus provided. The concavity of the arch of the aorta lies in the plane of the sternal angle, and the arch of the aorta lies wholly in the superior mediastinum, behind the manubrium. It arches over the beginning of the left bronchus and the bifurcation of the pulmonary trunk. The brachiocephalic trunk begins as a midline branch from the arch and diverges to the right as it ascends in front of the trachea (Fig. 4.10). The two other branches of the arch, the left common carotid and left subclavian arteries, pass upwards on the left side of the trachea (Fig. 4.11). These great arteries keep the left vagus nerve and apex of the left lung away from contact with the

Fig. 4.10 Superior mediastinum and thoracic inlet, after removal of the sternum, costal cartilages and clavicles. The left brachiocephalic vein crosses in front of the three great arteries to join its fellow to form the superior vena cava.

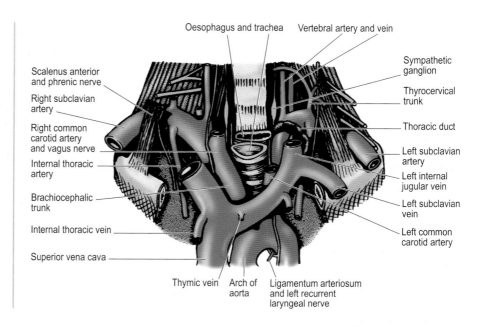

Oesophagus and trachea

Vertebral artery and vein

Sympathetic ganglion

Thyrocervical trunk

Thoracic duct

Left subclavian artery

Left internal jugular vein

Left subclavian vein

Left common carotid artery

Scalenus anterior and phrenic nerve

Right subclavian artery

Right common carotid artery and vagus nerve

Internal thoracic artery

Brachiocephalic trunk

Internal thoracic vein

Superior vena cava

Thymic vein

Arch of aorta

Ligamentum arteriosum and left recurrent laryngeal nerve

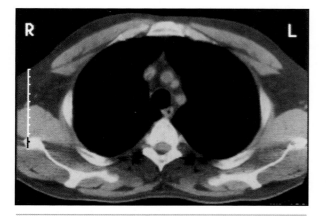

Fig. 4.11 CT scan above the level of the aortic arch. Viewed from below, the oesophagus with a rather small round lumen is seen in front of the vertebral column, and the round translucency in front of the oesophagus is the trachea. The four opacities adjacent to the trachea are, from the right side of the body to the left, the superior vena cava, brachiocephalic trunk, left common carotid artery and left subclavian artery.

trachea (Fig. 4.13). On the right side there is no structure to separate the trachea from the right vagus (Fig. 4.12) and apex of the right lung.

The veins entering the superior mediastinum are the right and left brachiocephalic veins, each formed by the confluence of the internal jugular with the subclavian vein. They lie in front of the arteries and are asymmetrical. The right brachiocephalic vein passes vertically downwards; the left vein runs across the superior mediastinum, above the arch of the aorta, to join the right (Fig. 4.10). The confluence of the brachiocephalic veins produces the superior vena cava, which passes vertically downwards behind the right edge of the sternum, anterior to the right pulmonary hilum (Fig. 4.12). The right phrenic nerve descends in contact with the lateral aspect of the right brachiocephalic vein and superior vena cava.

Great vessels

Arch of the aorta

Emerging from the pericardium the ascending aorta approaches the manubrium and then at the level of the manubriosternal joint becomes the arch, which passes backwards over the left bronchus to reach the body of T4 vertebra just to the left of the midline. From its upper convexity, which reaches as high as the midpoint of the manubrium, arise the three great arteries for the head and upper limbs: the brachiocephalic trunk, and the left common carotid and left subclavian arteries (Figs 4.10 and 4.13). The arch is crossed on its left side by the phrenic and vagus nerves as they pass downwards in front of and behind the lung root respectively. Between them lie the sympathetic and vagus branches to the superficial part of the cardiac plexus. The left superior intercostal vein passes forwards across the arch

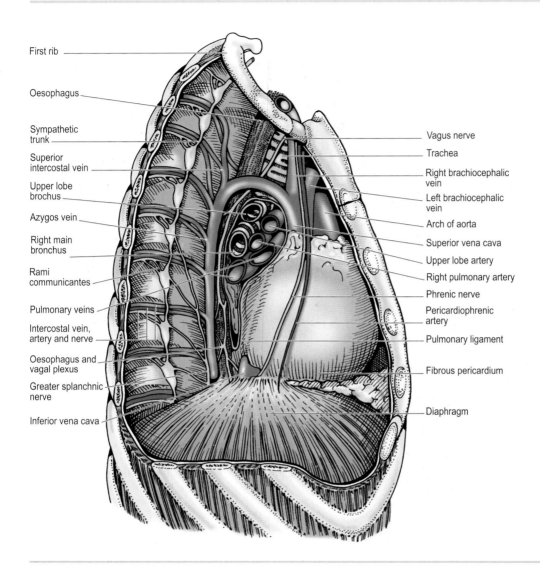

First rib

Oesophagus

Sympathetic
trunk

Superior
intercostal vein

Upper lobe
brochus

Azygos vein

Right main
bronchus

Rami
communicantes

Pulmonary veins

Intercostal vein,
artery and nerve

Oesophagus and
vagal plexus

Greater splanchnic
nerve

Inferior vena cava

Vagus nerve

Trachea

Right brachiocephalic
vein

Left brachiocephalic
vein

Arch of aorta

Superior vena cava

Upper lobe artery

Right pulmonary artery

Phrenic nerve

Pericardiophrenic
artery

Pulmonary ligament

Fibrous pericardium

Diaphragm

Fig. 4.12   Mediastinum: right aspect.

superficial to the vagus, deep to the phrenic, to empty into the left brachiocephalic vein. The left recurrent laryngeal nerve hooks around the ligamentum arteriosum to pass upwards on the right side of the arch of the aorta, in the groove between the trachea and oesophagus. The pulmonary trunk bifurcates into right and left pulmonary arteries in the concavity of the arch. On the right side of the arch lie the trachea and oesophagus.

The adventitial layer of the arch contains baroreceptors (like the carotid sinus in the wall of the internal carotid artery, see p. 355) innervated by vagal nerve fibres,

which are concerned with the reflex control of the heart rate. Under the arch in the region of the ligamentum arteriosum there are some very small masses of tissue, the aortic bodies (also supplied by vagal fibres), which like the carotid bodies (see p. 355) are chemoreceptors concerned with respiratory reflexes.

The **brachiocephalic trunk** (innominate artery) arises in or a little to the left of the midline of the body. It slopes upwards across the trachea to the back of the right sternoclavicular joint, where it divides into the right common carotid and right subclavian arteries.

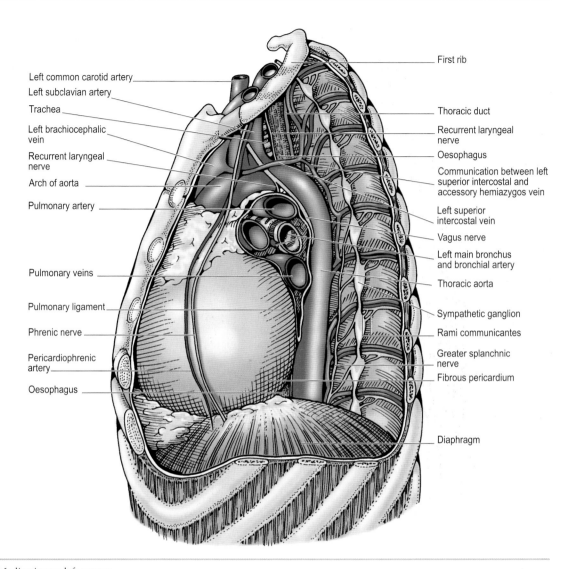

Fig. 4.13 Mediastinum: left aspect.

It has no branches apart from the rare thyroidea ima artery, which may arise from it or directly from the arch of the aorta. The termination of the left brachiocephalic vein lies in front of the artery (Fig. 4.10).

The **left common carotid artery** arises just behind the brachiocephalic trunk from the upper convexity of the aortic arch. It passes straight up alongside the trachea into the neck (Fig. 4.13). It has no branches in the mediastinum.

The **left subclavian artery** arises just behind the left common carotid; the two run upwards together. The subclavian artery arches to the left over the pleura and

the apex of the lung, which it deeply grooves. It moves away from the left common carotid at a point directly behind the left sternoclavicular joint. It has no branches in the mediastinum.

Ligamentum arteriosum

This is the fibrous remnant of the ductus arteriosus of the fetus, a channel that short-circuited the lungs. It passes from the commencement of the left pulmonary artery to the concavity of the aortic arch (Fig. 4.10), beyond the point where the left subclavian artery branches off. It lies almost horizontally. The left recurrent laryngeal nerve hooks around it. The superficial part of the cardiac plexus lies anterior to it, and the deep part is on its right, between the aortic arch and tracheal bifurcation.

Surgical approach. When the ductus persists after birth (patent ductus arteriosus) and requires surgical interruption the pleura over the aortic arch is incised behind the vagus nerve and upwards towards the origin of the left subclavian artery. The pleural flap is reflected forwards with the vagus and its left recurrent laryngeal branch to give sufficient access to the ductus.

Brachiocephalic veins

The brachiocephalic (innominate) veins are formed behind the sternoclavicular joints by confluence of the internal jugular and subclavian veins. In the neck the internal jugular vein lies lateral to the common carotid artery, in front of the upper part of scalenus anterior. The subclavian vein lies lateral to and then in front of the lower part of the muscle. Medial to scalenus anterior, these veins have joined to form the brachiocephalic vein, which lies in front of the first part of the subclavian artery. This part of each brachiocephalic vein thus receives tributaries corresponding to the branches of the first part of the subclavian artery (vertebral, inferior thyroid, internal thoracic and, on the left side only, superior intercostal).

The **right brachiocephalic vein** commences behind the right sternoclavicular joint and runs downwards. At its commencement it receives the right jugular, subclavian and bronchomediastinal lymph trunks separately or their confluent channel, the right lymphatic duct.

The **left brachiocephalic vein** passes to the right with a downward inclination, across the superior mediastinum, above the arch of the aorta, behind the thymus and the upper half of the manubrium. In the infant the left brachiocephalic vein projects slightly above the jugular notch, and may do so in the adult if the vein is distended, especially if the head and neck are thrown back. The vein is then vulnerable to suprasternal incisions (e.g. tracheotomy). The commencement of the vein receives the thoracic duct, which often divides into two or three branches that join the vein separately. In addition to the vertebral and internal thoracic veins the left brachiocephalic vein receives most of the inferior thyroid veins, the left superior intercostal vein, and a large thymic vein (Figs 4.10 and 4.13).

The pretracheal fascia (see p. 343) passes down behind the vein and directs a retrosternal goitre into the space between the vein and the brachiocephalic trunk and trachea.

Superior vena cava

This vessel commences at the lower border of the first right costal cartilage by confluence of the two brachiocephalic veins (Figs 4.10 and 4.12). It passes vertically downwards behind the right border of the sternum and, piercing the pericardium at the level of the second costal cartilage, enters the upper border of the right atrium at the lower border of the third right costal cartilage. Behind the sternal angle it receives the azygos vein, which has arched forwards over the root of the right lung. There are no valves in the superior vena cava, the brachiocephalic veins or the azygos system of veins.

Cardiac plexus

The cardiac plexus consists of sympathetic, parasympathetic and afferent fibres and small ganglia. It is divided into superficial and deep parts, but functionally they are one. Their branches enter the pericardium to accompany the coronary arteries (vasomotor) and to reach the myocardium, in particular the SA and AV nodes (cardio-inhibitor and cardioaccelerator).

The **superficial part** of the cardiac plexus lies in front of the ligamentum arteriosum. The **deep part** of the cardiac plexus is larger and lies to the right of the ligamentum arteriosum, in front of the bifurcation of the trachea and behind the aortic arch.

The cardiac plexus receives sympathetic fibres from the three cervical and the upper four or five thoracic sympathetic ganglia of both sides, and parasympathetic fibres from both vagi in their cervical course and both recurrent laryngeal nerves. The sympathetic fibres accelerate the heart and dilate the coronary arteries; the parasympathetic fibres slow the heart and constrict the coronary arteries.

The vagi carry afferent fibres concerned with cardiovascular reflexes. Pain fibres run with sympathetic nerves, reaching any of the cervical and upper thoracic sympathetic ganglia. The pain fibres pursue the usual pathway to the central nervous system, passing through the sympathetic ganglia to the spinal nerves via white rami communicantes (see Fig. 1.14C, p. 20). The connection with cervical and thoracic spinal nerves presumably explains the referral of cardiac pain to the arm, chest or neck.

Trachea

The trachea is the continuation of the larynx and commences in the neck below the cricoid cartilage at the level of C6 vertebra, 5 cm above the jugular notch. Entering the thoracic inlet in the midline it passes downwards and backwards behind the manubrium to bifurcate into the two principal or main bronchi a little to the right of the midline, level with the upper border of T5 vertebra (Fig. 4.14). The trachea is about 10 cm long and 2 cm in diameter. In the first year of life the tracheal diameter is only 3 mm and in childhood it is about equal in millimetres to the age in years. In full inspiration the trachea may stretch to 15 cm and the bifurcation descend to the level of T6 vertebra.

The **cervical part** of the trachea is described on page 353.

The **thoracic part** runs through the superior mediastinum in front of the oesophagus. In front of this part are the manubrium with sternohyoid and sternothyroid muscles attached, remnants of the thymus, the inferior thyroid and left brachiocephalic veins, and the brachiocephalic and left common carotid arteries as they diverge to either side (Figs 4.10 and 4.15). The right vagus is in contact with the right side of the trachea, which is separated from the right lung by the pleura and the arch of the azygos vein as it hooks forwards over the right bronchus (Fig. 4.12). The right brachiocephalic vein and superior vena cava are anterolateral to the trachea. On the left, the left common carotid and subclavian arteries (Fig. 4.13) prevent the pleura and the left vagus nerve from coming into contact with the trachea; the arch of

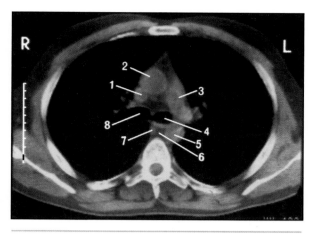

Fig. 4.14 CT scan at the T5 vertebra level, just below the tracheal bifurcation, viewed from below: 1, superior vena cava; 2, ascending aorta; 3, left pulmonary artery; 4, left main bronchus; 5, thoracic aorta; 6, oesophagus; 7, azygos vein; 8, right main bronchus.

Fig. 4.15 Thoracic contents, seen after removal of the anterior thoracic wall. The thymus lies in front of the upper pericardium and great vessels.

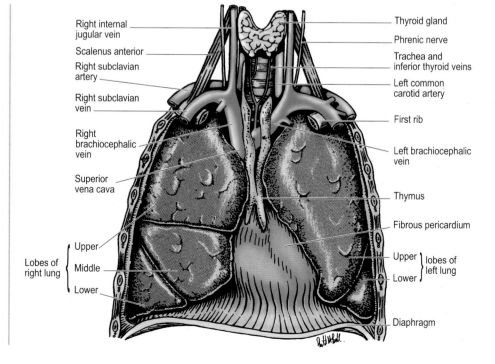

Right internal jugular vein

Scalenus anterior

Right subclavian artery

Right subclavian vein

Right brachiocephalic vein

Superior vena cava

Lobes of right lung { Upper / Middle / Lower

Thyroid gland

Phrenic nerve

Trachea and inferior thyroid veins

Left common carotid artery

First rib

Left brachiocephalic vein

Thymus

Fibrous pericardium

Upper } lobes of / Lower } left lung

Diaphragm

the aorta curves backwards over the left bronchus, and the left recurrent laryngeal nerve passes upwards in the groove between trachea and oesophagus.

The pulmonary trunk branches into the right and left pulmonary arteries to the left of the tracheal bifurcation, in front of the left bronchus, and the right pulmonary artery crosses the midline (in front of the oesophagus) just below the tracheal bifurcation (Fig. 4.29).

Blood supply

Branches from the inferior thyroid and bronchial arteries form anastomotic networks in the tracheal wall. Veins drain to the inferior thyroid vein.

Lymph drainage

Lymphatic channels pass to pre- and paratracheal nodes and to inferior deep cervical nodes.

Nerve supply

The mucous membrane is supplied by afferent (including pain) fibres from the vagi and recurrent laryngeal nerves. Sympathetic fibres from upper ganglia of the sympathetic trunks supply the smooth muscle and blood vessels.

Structure

The patency of the trachea as an airway, its essential function, is maintained by 15–20 horseshoe-shaped hyaline cartilages. The gaps in the rings are at the back, where there is smooth muscle, mostly transversely placed (the *trachealis* muscle). There is a high content of elastic fibres to facilitate the necessary elastic recoil during respiration. The mucous membrane is of typical respiratory type, with pseudostratified columnar ciliated epithelium and goblet cells, mucous glands and scattered lymphoid nodules.

Function

The cartilaginous rings keep the airway open, mucus traps particles, cilia beat upwards to clear debris, and glandular secretion helps to humidify the passing air. During swallowing the trachea is stretched as the larynx moves upwards (the bifurcation does not move) and elasticity restores the normal position. The trachealis muscle controls the diameter of the tube. During coughing there is a 30% increase in transverse diameter produced by compressed air in the trachea while the vocal cords are shut, but the trachea narrows to 10% less than the resting diameter at the instant the cords open. Like the choke barrel of a shotgun this greatly increases the explosive force of the blast of compressed air.

Phrenic and vagus nerves

Phrenic nerve

Arising principally from C4 in the neck, the nerve passes down over the anterior scalene muscle across the dome of the pleura behind the subclavian vein. It crosses anterior to the vagus and runs through the mediastinum in front of the lung root. Each nerve is in contact laterally with the mediastinal pleura throughout the whole of its course.

The **right phrenic nerve** is related medially with venous structures throughout its thoracic course (Fig. 4.12). The right brachiocephalic vein, the superior vena cava, the pericardium over the right atrium, and the inferior vena cava, lie to its medial side. It reaches the undersurface of the diaphragm by passing through the central tendon alongside the inferior vena cava, piercing the tendon fibres that fuse with the caval wall.

The **left phrenic nerve** is related medially to arterial structures throughout its thoracic course (Fig. 4.13). It has the left common carotid and left subclavian arteries that arise from the arch of the aorta to its medial side. It crosses the arch lateral to the superior intercostal vein and in front of the vagus nerve, and then runs laterally down the pericardium over the left ventricle towards the apex of the heart. It reaches the undersurface of the diaphragm by piercing the muscular part just to the left of the pericardium.

About two-thirds of the phrenic nerve fibres are motor to the diaphragm. The rest are sensory to the diaphragm (except for the most peripheral parts which receive intercostal afferent fibres), and to the mediastinal pleura, the fibrous pericardium, the parietal layer of serous pericardium, and the central parts of the diaphragmatic pleura and peritoneum. Pain referred from the diaphragmatic peritoneum is classically felt in the shoulder tip (C4), but pain from thoracic surfaces supplied by the phrenic nerve (pleura, pericardium) is usually only vaguely located there.

Vagus nerve

In their descent through the thorax, the **right vagus** (Fig. 4.12) is in contact with the trachea, while the **left vagus** (Fig. 4.13) is held away from that structure by great arteries that spring from the arch of the aorta. The left nerve crosses the arch medial to the left superior intercostal vein, and the right nerve lies on the trachea medial to the arch of the azygos vein. Each vagus passes down behind the lung root, dividing into branches which contribute to the pulmonary plexuses and pass onwards to form a plexus around the oesophagus. On the arch of the aorta the left vagus nerve flattens out and gives off its **recurrent laryngeal branch** (Fig. 4.13). This nerve hooks around the ligamentum arteriosum, and, passing up on the right side of the aortic arch, ascends in the groove between trachea and oesophagus. The right recurrent laryngeal nerve is given off at the root of the neck and hooks around the right subclavian artery (Fig. 4.10). Both recurrent laryngeal nerves give branches to the deep part of the cardiac plexus. Both recurrent laryngeal nerves supply the whole trachea and the adjacent oesophagus (i.e. above the lung roots), and proceed to supply the larynx (see p. 411).

The *oesophagus* lies against the vertebrae at the back of the superior mediastinum. The *thoracic duct* lies to its left. Both structures pass through the posterior mediastinum; they are described on pages 215 and 217.

PART FIVE

Anterior mediastinum

This space, little more than a potential one, lies between the pericardium and sternum. It is overlapped by the anterior edges of both lungs. It contains the thymus (or its remnants), sternopericardial ligaments, a few lymph nodes and branches of the internal thoracic vessels.

Thymus

The thymus may appear to be a single organ, but in fact it consists of right and left lobes closely applied to each other for much of their extent (Fig. 4.15). It is usually most prominent in children, where it may extend from the level of the fourth costal cartilages to the lower poles of the thyroid gland. In front of it lie the sternohyoid and sternothyroid muscles, the manubrium and upper part of the body of the sternum and their adjacent costal cartilages. Behind it are the pericardium, the arch of the aorta with its three large branches, the left brachiocephalic vein and the trachea.

Blood supply

Small branches enter the thymus from the inferior thyroid and internal thoracic arteries, and there are corresponding veins. Frequently a large short thymic vein enters the left brachiocephalic vein (Fig. 4.10) and needs to be secured before the thymus is retracted after median sternotomy.

Lymph drainage

Efferent channels drain into parasternal, tracheo-bronchial and brachiocephalic nodes. The thymus does not receive any afferent lymphatics.

Development

The epithelium of the thymus develops mainly from the endoderm of the third branchial pouch. Some of the epithelial cells become the thymic (Hassall's) corpuscles; others form a network of epithelial reticular cells believed to be the source of thymic hormones concerned with the differentiation of T lymphocytes. Connective tissue elements are derived from surrounding mesoderm, but the original colonizing lymphocytes have migrated from the bone marrow. The developing thymus descends from the neck into the mediastinum in front of all the major contents. It doubles its weight rapidly after birth and then maintains that level although the lymphoid content decreases with age, being replaced by fat and fibrous tissue. However, the secretion of thymic hormones and its influence on lymphocytes that migrate to it continue throughout life.

Surgical approach

Median sternotomy provides surgical access to the thymus.

PART SIX

Middle mediastinum and heart

The middle mediastinum (a term not frequently used) contains the pericardium and heart, the adjoining parts of the great vessels, the lung roots, the phrenic nerves, and the deep part of the cardiac plexus.

Pericardium

Fibrous pericardium

Unlike the pleura and peritoneum, the pericardium has an outer single-layered fibrous sac that encloses the heart and the roots of the great vessels, fusing with the adventitia of these vessels. Its broad base overlies the central tendon of the diaphragm, with which it is in-separably blended, both being derived from the septum transversum. The phrenic nerves lie on the surface of the fibrous pericardium and the mediastinal pleura is adherent to it, wherever the two membranes are in contact with each other. The fibrous pericardium is connected to the back of the sternum by weak *sterno-pericardial ligaments*. It is supplied with blood by the internal thoracic arteries.

Serous pericardium

A serous layer lines the inside of the fibrous pericardium, whence it is reflected around the roots of the great vessels to cover the entire surface of the heart, where it forms the epicardium. Between these parietal and visceral layers there are two sinuses: the transverse sinus and the oblique sinus of the pericardium. The **transverse sinus** is a passage above the heart, between the ascending aorta and pulmonary trunk in front and the superior vena cava, left atrium and pulmonary veins behind. The **oblique sinus** is a space behind the heart, between the left atrium in front and the fibrous pericardium behind, posterior to which lies the oesophagus. A hand passed from below easily enters the oblique sinus, but the fingertips can only pass up as far as a double fold of serous pericardium that separates the oblique and transverse sinuses from each other (Fig. 4.16). It is through the transverse sinus that a temporary ligature is passed to occlude pulmonary trunk and aorta during pulmonary embolectomy and cardiac operations.

Nerve supply

The fibrous pericardium is supplied by the phrenic nerve. The parietal layer of serous pericardium that lines it is similarly innervated, but the visceral layer on the heart surface is insensitive. Pain from the heart (angina) originates in the muscle or the vessels and is transmitted by sympathetic nerves (see p. 200). The pain of pericarditis originates in the parietal layer only, and is transmitted by the phrenic nerve.

Blood supply

Pericardial blood supply is derived from the internal thoracic artery, its pericardiophrenic and musculophrenic branches, bronchial arteries and the thoracic aorta. The veins drain into the azygos system.

Pericardial drainage

A needle inserted in the angle between the xiphoid process and the left seventh costal cartilage and directed upwards at an angle of 45°, towards the left shoulder, passes through the central tendon of the diaphragm into the pericardial cavity. The creation of a small pericardial window surgically through the same route, or through

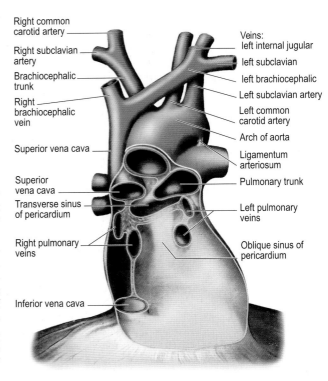

Fig 4.16   Posterior wall of serous pericardial sac: viewed from in front after removal of the heart.

the anterior end of the fourth intercostal space, provides more effective drainage.

Heart

The heart is the muscular pump responsible for blood circulation. It is an organ with four chambers: right and left atria, and right and left ventricles. The two atria receive blood, the left from the lungs and the right from the rest of the body. The right ventricle propels blood to the lungs and the left ventricle propels blood around the rest of the body (the systemic circulation).

Position

As the heart lies obliquely in the thorax, with its long axis passing downwards and to the left to the apex, and as the heart has undergone a degree of rotation during development, these chambers are not located strictly in the positions that their names suggest. The right-sided chambers are mainly anterior to their left-sided counterparts and the atria are mainly to the right of their

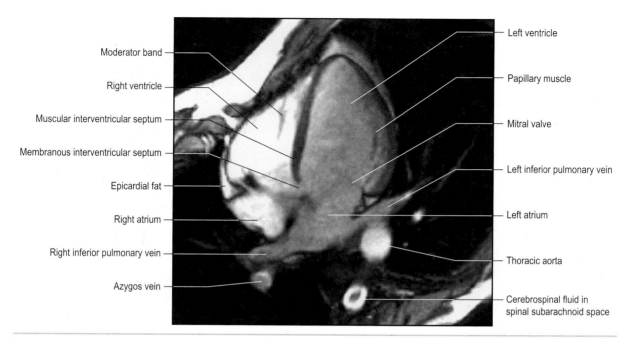

Left ventricle

Papillary muscle

Mitral valve

Left inferior pulmonary vein

Left atrium

Thoracic aorta

Cerebrospinal fluid in
spinal subarachnoid space

Moderator band

Right ventricle

Muscular interventricular septum

Membranous interventricular septum

Epicardial fat

Right atrium

Right inferior pulmonary vein

Azygos vein

Fig. 4.17 Oblique axial magnetic resonance image (MRI) showing a four-chamber view of the heart, viewed from below. (Courtesy of Dr R.A. Coulden, Papworth Hospital.)

respective ventricles (Fig. 4.17). The atrial and ventricular septa thus lie at about 45° to the sagittal plane, while the plane of the atrioventricular valve orifices lies almost vertically at about 90° to the septal plane. As seen from the front, the heart is described as having right, inferior (acute) and left (obtuse) borders, an anterior or sternocostal surface, an inferior or diaphragmatic surface, a base or posterior surface, and an apex at its left inferior corner.

The **right border** consists entirely of the right atrium (Fig. 4.18). The **inferior border** is made up mostly of right ventricle with a small portion of left ventricle, which forms the **apex**, at the junction of the inferior and left borders. The **left border** is mostly left ventricle, with the auricle of the left atrium forming the uppermost part of this border. The anterior or **sternocostal surface** consists mainly of the right ventricle, with the right atrium on its right side and a narrow strip of the left ventricle on the left border. The tip of the left auricular appendage peeps over the top of this border. The inferior or **diaphragmatic surface** is made up of one-third right ventricle and two-thirds left ventricle, separated by the posterior interventricular branch of the right coronary artery. The **posterior surface** (or base) of the heart

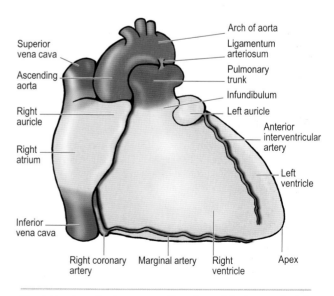

Superior
vena cava

Ascending
aorta

Right
auricle

Right
atrium

Inferior
vena cava

Arch of aorta

Ligamentum
arteriosum

Pulmonary
trunk

Infundibulum

Left auricle

Anterior
interventricular
artery

Left
ventricle

Right coronary
artery

Marginal artery

Right
ventricle

Apex

Fig. 4.18 Anterior (sternocostal) surface of the heart. The left auricle is shown somewhat enlarged.

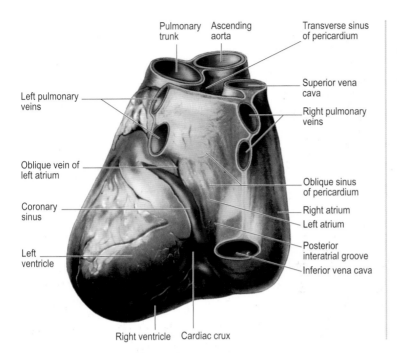

Pulmonary trunk

Ascending aorta

Transverse sinus of pericardium

Superior vena cava

Right pulmonary veins

Left pulmonary veins

Oblique vein of left atrium

Coronary sinus

Left ventricle

Oblique sinus of pericardium

Right atrium

Left atrium

Posterior interatrial groove

Inferior vena cava

Right ventricle   Cardiac crux

Fig. 4.19 Posterior and inferior (diaphragmatic) surfaces of the heart. The cardiac crux is the junction of the posterior interatrial, atrioventricular and interventricular grooves.

(Fig. 4.19) consists almost entirely of the left atrium, receiving the four pulmonary veins. From it the left ventricle converges to the left towards the apex. A narrow strip of right atrium forms the horizon on the right.

Surface markings

About one-third of the heart lies to the right of the midline. The right border of the heart extends from the lower border of the right third costal cartilage to the lower border of the right sixth costal cartilage, just beyond the right margin of the sternum and describing a slight convex curve between these points. The inferior border passes from the right sixth costal cartilage to the apex, which is normally in the left fifth intercostal space in the midclavicular line. From the apex the left border extends upwards to the lower border of the left second costal cartilage about 2 cm from the sternal margin. These are the borders as seen in a typical radiograph of the normal heart, although the area of cardiac dullness as determined by percussion will be smaller.

Fibrous skeleton

The two atria and the two ventricles are attached to a pair of conjoined fibrous rings which, in the form of a figure 8, bound the atrioventricular orifices. To this

fibrous skeleton the muscle of the heart is attached; the muscle fibres encircle the chambers of the heart in a series of whorls and spirals. The atria lie to the right and the ventricles to the left of the fibrous skeleton and there is no muscular continuity between the two. The atrioventricular conducting bundle is the only physiological connection between atria and ventricles across the fibrous ring. The membranous part of the interventricular septum is attached to the fibrous skeleton, and so are the bases of the cusps of the tricuspid, mitral and aortic valves; the region where they meet is termed the central fibrous body.

Right atrium

This elongated chamber lies between the superior and inferior venae cavae, and forms the right border of the heart (Fig. 4.18). Its lower end is almost completely occupied by the orifice for the inferior vena cava but its upper end is prolonged to the left of the superior vena cava as the **right auricle**. This large, triangular appendage overlies the commencement of the aorta and the upper part of the right atrioventricular groove and, with the left auricle, it clasps the infundibulum of the right ventricle. The left atrium lies behind the right atrium. From the angle between the superior vena cava and the right auricle a shallow groove sometimes

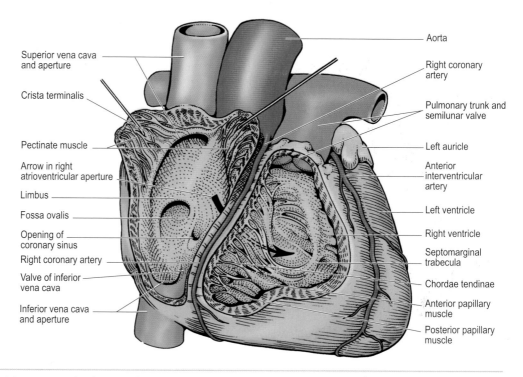

Superior vena cava and aperture

Crista terminalis

Pectinate muscle

Arrow in right atrioventricular aperture

Limbus

Fossa ovalis

Opening of coronary sinus

Right coronary artery

Valve of inferior vena cava

Inferior vena cava and aperture

Aorta

Right coronary artery

Pulmonary trunk and semilunar valve

Left auricle

Anterior interventricular artery

Left ventricle

Right ventricle

Septomarginal trabecula

Chordae tendinae

Anterior papillary muscle

Posterior papillary muscle

Fig. 4.20   Interior of right atrium and right ventricle.

descends; this is the *sulcus terminalis*. It is produced, when present, by the projection into the cavity of the right atrium of a vertical ridge of heart muscle, the *crista terminalis*. The interior of the right atrium is smooth to the right of the crista terminalis, but between the crista and the blind extremity of the auricle the myocardium is projected into a series of horizontal ridges like the teeth of a comb: the *pectinate muscles* (Fig. 4.20). This rough area represents the true auricular chamber of the embryonic heart. The smooth-walled remainder of the atrial cavity is produced by incorporation of the right horn of the sinus venosus (see p. 32).

The opening of the inferior vena cava is partly bounded by a small, crescentic ridge, the remains of the valve of the inferior vena cava, that is continued upwards towards the *opening of the coronary sinus*. This opening lies above the septal cusp of the tricuspid valve, and to the left of the inferior vena caval orifice.

The **interatrial septum** forms the posterior wall of the right atrium above the opening of the coronary sinus. Towards its lower part is a shallow saucer-shaped depression, the *fossa ovalis*. This is the primary septum of the fetal heart. The crescentic upper margin of the fossa ovalis is called the *limbus*, and indicates the lower edge

of the secondary septum. Failure of fusion of the two septa gives rise to a persistent foramen ovale (see p. 213).

Right ventricle

This chamber projects to the left of the right atrium (Figs 4.18 and 4.20). The *atrioventricular groove* between the two is almost vertical over the front of the heart and anteroposterior on the diaphragmatic surface. It lodges the right coronary artery and is usually filled with fat. The right ventricle narrows as it passes upwards towards the commencement of the pulmonary trunk.

The walls are thrown into a series of muscular ridges, the *trabeculae carneae*, which project into the cavity of the ventricle. One of these ridges has broken free and lies in the cavity attached by its two ends to the interventricular septum and the anterior papillary muscle. This is the *septomarginal trabecula* (also called the moderator band); it contains part of the right branch of the conducting bundle. Other projections into the lumen from the ventricular walls form the *papillary muscles* which are connected to the cusps of the tricuspid valve.

The **tricuspid valve** guards the right atrioventricular orifice. It has three cusps and admits the tips of three

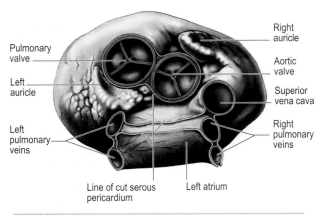

Pulmonary valve

Left auricle

Left pulmonary veins

Right auricle

Aortic valve

Superior vena cava

Right pulmonary veins

Line of cut serous pericardium   Left atrium

Fig. 4.21   Superior aspect of the heart; the aorta and pulmonary trunk have been removed, exposing their valves.

fingers. The three *cusps*, called *anterior*, *posterior* and *septal*, are attached by their bases to the fibrous atrio-ventricular ring and lie against the sternocostal, diaphragmatic and septal walls of the ventricle. The cusps of both the tricuspid and mitral valves often appear to be subdivided but without forming complete additional leaflets. The edges and ventricular surfaces of the cusps receive the attachments of the *chordae tendineae*, collagenous cords which diverge from the papillary muscles and prevent the cusps from being everted when the ventricle contracts. The main papillary muscles are anterior, inferior (posterior) and septal in location and each is connected to more than one cusp.

The cavity of the ventricle continues upwards into a narrowing funnel-shaped approach to the pulmonary orifice. The walls of this part, the *infundibulum* or *conus*, are thin and smooth.

The three semilunar cusps of the **pulmonary valve** are attached at the junction of the infundibulum and the commencement of the pulmonary trunk. In the adult heart there are two anterior (right and left) and one posterior cusp (Fig. 4.21). The official anatomical nomenclature (*Terminologia Anatomica*, 1998) refers to them as anterior, posterior and septal cusps in accordance with their position in the fetus. The pulmonary orifice lies almost in the horizontal plane and is at a higher level than the aortic orifice.

Left atrium

The left atrium forms the posterior surface (base) of the heart, and lies behind the right atrium (Fig. 4.19). The inferior margin of the left atrium lies a little above that of the right atrium, whose posterior wall here receives

the coronary sinus. From the left atrium the left ventricle slopes away to the apex. A small, bent *left auricle* projects from its upper border and curves round to the front on the left side of the infundibulum (Fig. 4.18). The four pulmonary veins enter the left atrium symmetrically, one above the other on each side.

The cavity of the left atrium is smooth-walled except in the auricle; here muscular ridges indicate that the appendage was the original auricular chamber of the embryonic heart. All the smooth-walled portion is derived by incorporation of the embryonic pulmonary veins into the atrial cavity.

The bicuspid **mitral valve** admits the tips of two fingers. The *cusps* are named *anterior* and *posterior*. The base of the anterior cusp is attached to one-third, and that of the posterior cusp to two-thirds of the margin of the fibrous atrioventricular ring; but sometimes they fail to meet and a small accessory cusp fills the gap between them. The anterior cusp of the mitral valve is thicker and more rigid than the posterior cusp. The anterior cusp lies between the mitral and aortic orifices and thus lies between the inflow and outflow tracts of the left ventricle (Fig. 4.22).

Left ventricle

The walls of this cavity are three times as thick as those of the right ventricle. The *trabeculae carneae* are well developed. There are two *papillary muscles*, *anterior* and *posterior*, the anterior being the larger. Both are connected by *chordae tendineae* to each valve cusp (Fig. 4.22). The posterior cusp receives the chordae on both its margin and its ventricular surface, but since blood is squirted across both surfaces of the anterior cusp the chordae are attached to it only along its margins.

The **interventricular septum** bulges forwards into the cavity of the right ventricle, so that in cross-section the lumen of the left ventricle is circular and that of the right crescentic. The upper and right end of the septal wall is smooth, thinner and more fibrous; this is the *membranous* part of the septum. As the left ventricle is larger than the right ventricle and the right atrium is larger than the left atrium, the membranous part of the septum lies between the left ventricle and the right atrium. Between the membranous part and the anterior cusp of the mitral valve is the aortic vestibule, which leads up to the aortic orifice.

The aortic orifice is guarded by the **aortic valve**, at the entrance to the ascending aorta. It lies at a lower level than the pulmonary orifice, to its right side (Fig. 4.21), and is more obliquely placed. It has three semilunar *cusps*. In the adult heart these cusps are in anterior, left posterior and right posterior positions. In the

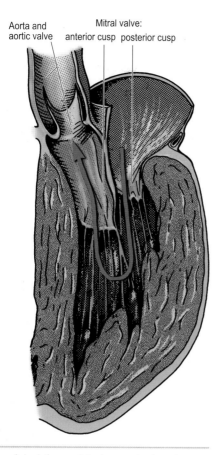

Aorta and aortic valve

Mitral valve: anterior cusp posterior cusp

Fig. 4.22 Interior of the left ventricle, in a sagittal section viewed from the left, to show the cusps of the mitral valve. The arrow indicates the path of blood, entering from the left atrium behind the anterior cusp and leaving the ventricle in front of the anterior cusp to pass through the aortic valve.

Terminologia Anatomica (1998) the corresponding cusps are named right, left and posterior in keeping with their fetal positions. Cardiac surgeons refer to the same cusps as right coronary, left coronary and non-coronary in accordance with the origins of the coronary arteries. Fibrous continuity between the left coronary and non-coronary aortic cusps and the anterior mitral cusp is termed the subaortic curtain.

Structure of heart valves

The cusps of the tricuspid and mitral valves are flat and their free edges are serrated. On closure of the valves during ventricular systole the cusps do not meet edge to edge, but come into mutual contact on their auricular surfaces near the serrated margins. This contact and the pull of the marginal chordae prevent eversion of the free edges into the cavity of the atrium, while the centrally attached chordae limit the amount of ballooning of the cusps towards the atrium. The tricuspid and mitral valves are kept competent by active contraction of the papillary muscles, which pull on the chordae during ventricular systole.

The cusps of the pulmonary and aortic valves are cup shaped. The free edge of each cusp contains a central fibrous nodule from each side of which straight edges slope at 120° from each other to the attached base of the cusp. Three cusps lying edge to edge thus close the circular orifice (Fig. 4.21). During ventricular systole the bulge of the aortic sinuses (see below) above the cusps prevents the cusps from becoming flattened against the walls of the sinuses; the residual blood in the sinuses forms vortices which help the elastic recoil of the cusps at the end of systole. During ventricular diastole pressure of blood above the valves distends the cusps, so that their free edges are forced together. Competence of the pulmonary and aortic valves is thus a passive phenomenon, the result of mutual pressure between the distended cusps, and is dependent on the integrity of their straight edges.

Microscopically the valves of the heart are composed of a core of collagenous fibrous tissue covered on each surface by vascular endothelium (endocardium).

Surface markings of valves

All the valves of the heart lie behind the sternum, making a line with each other that is nearly vertical (Fig. 4.23). The bases of tricuspid and mitral valves, attached to the atrioventricular ring, are indicated by vertical lines over the lower part of the sternum. The tricuspid valve lies behind the midline of the lower sternum, the mitral valve, overlapping it, lies higher and somewhat to the left opposite the fourth left costal cartilage. The aortic and pulmonary orifices lie behind the left border of the sternum at the level of the third intercostal space and the third costal cartilage, respectively.

The normal heart sounds are produced by closure of heart valves, and the opening snap of the mitral valve may also be audible. They are heard best (Fig. 4.23) where the corresponding chambers or channels lie nearest to the chest wall. For the tricuspid valve this is over its surface, but for the mitral valve it is at the apex beat. For the aortic valve it is where the ascending aorta lies nearest the surface, at the right sternal margin in the second intercostal space, and for the pulmonary valve at the left sternal margin at the same level, over the pulmonary trunk.

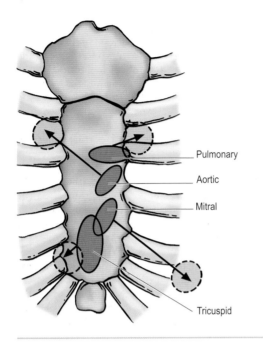

Pulmonary

Aortic

Mitral

Tricuspid

Fig. 4.23   Surface markings of the heart valves. The arrows indicate the directions in which the sounds of the closing valves are propagated, and the circles indicate the generally preferred sites for auscultation. Mitral valve sounds are best heard over the apex of the heart at the fifth left intercostal space in the midclavicular line.

Great vessels

In their course through the pericardial cavity the great vessels are invested with a reflexion of serous pericardium. The ascending aorta and pulmonary trunk share a common sleeve of serous pericardium in which they lie in front of the transverse sinus (Fig. 4.19). The whole of the ascending aorta and the entire pulmonary trunk, each about 5 cm in length, are inside the fibrous pericardium.

The six veins share another common sleeve of serous pericardium (Fig. 4.19). The four pulmonary veins and the inferior vena cava are all 1 cm or less in length within the pericardium, but the superior vena cava courses for about three times that distance through the pericardial cavity before entering the right atrium.

Ascending aorta

Immediately above the aortic orifice the wall of the ascending aorta bulges to form the *aortic sinuses* (of Valsalva), one above each cusp and similarly named.

From the sinus that lies anteriorly in the adult heart the right coronary artery emerges, and from the left posterior sinus, the left coronary artery. Above the sinuses the aorta runs to the right behind the infundibulum of the right ventricle (Fig. 4.18) and as it passes upwards it slants a little forward towards the manubrium, before curving backwards at the commencement of the arch. Here the fibrous pericardium is blended with its wall.

Pulmonary trunk

Commencing at the summit of the infundibulum at a slightly higher level than the aortic orifice (Fig. 4.23), the wide pulmonary trunk arches backwards initially in front of and then to the left of the ascending aorta. The two vessels make a gentle spiral enclosed in the common sleeve of serous pericardium in front of the transverse sinus. The fibrous pericardium blends with the wall of the pulmonary trunk as it divides—to the left of the midline (Fig. 4.29), under the concavity of the aortic arch and in front of the left main bronchus—into the *right* and *left pulmonary arteries*.

Catheterization. Various aspects of cardiorespiratory function can be monitored by pulmonary artery catheterization. The catheters are introduced into the right atrium, usually via the internal jugular or subclavian veins (see pp 356 and 360) and carried on through the tricuspid valve into the right ventricle and pulmonary trunk, and then into the right pulmonary artery.

Conducting (conduction) system

The conducting system of the heart consists of the sinuatrial node (SA node), the atrioventricular node (AV node), the atrioventricular bundle (of His), the right and left limbs or branches of the bundle, and the subendocardial Purkinje fibres. From the SA node, which, like the AV node and its extensions, is composed of a specialized type of cardiac muscle fibres (not nervous tissue), impulses are conducted to the AV node by atrial cardiac muscle fibres. The AV node, bundle, branches and subendocardial fibres form one continuous mass of conduction tissue.

The **sinuatrial node**, or pacemaker of the heart, is a small mass of histologically distinctive myocardial cells. It is subepicardially situated in the wall of the right atrium, just below the superior vena cava, at the top of the sulcus terminalis. It has no macroscopic or palpable features that indicate its location. The **atrioventricular node** is also a small mass of specialized myocardial cells. It is situated in the right atrium on the interatrial septum, above the attachment of the septal cusp of the

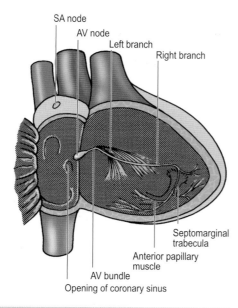

SA node
AV node
Left branch
Right branch
Septomarginal trabecula
Anterior papillary muscle
AV bundle
Opening of coronary sinus

Fig. 4.24 Conducting system of the heart, from the front after removal of parts of the right atrium and the ventricles. This diagrammatic representation illustrates that the left and right branches of the AV bundle, which pass down their respective sides of the interventricular septum, are very different. The left branch rapidly breaks up into a sheaf of subendocardial fibres, but the right continues towards the septomarginal trabecula; part of the branch enters it to reach the anterior papillary muscle. Only the more proximal parts of the subendocardial fibres are shown.

tricuspid valve, to the left of the opening of the coronary sinus (Fig. 4.24).

From the AV node, the **AV bundle** runs along the inferior border of the membranous part of the interventricular septum, where it divides into right and left branches. Since the fibrous framework of the heart separates the muscles of the atria from those of the ventricles, the bundle is the only means of conducting the contractile impulse from atria to ventricles. The *right branch* runs at first within the muscle of the septum and then becomes subendocardial on the right side of the septum. Much of it continues into the septomarginal trabecula (moderator band) to reach the anterior papillary muscle and the anterior wall of the ventricle, and its Purkinje fibres then spread out beneath the endocardium. The *left branch* reaches the septal endocardium of the left ventricle and rapidly breaks up into a sheaf of branches which spread out subendocardially over the septum and the rest of the ventricular wall.

Blood supply of the heart

The heart is supplied by the two **coronary arteries** and their branches (Fig. 4.25). Variations occur occasionally in their origins and patterns of distribution; the account that follows describes the usual arrangement. The right and left coronary arteries arise from aortic sinuses at the beginning of the ascending aorta. Each coronary artery is the main source of supply to its same side atrium and ventricle, but also supplies the opposite side chambers to some extent. The veins that drain the myocardium do not have names that correspond to the arteries; in this respect the heart resembles the brain.

Right coronary artery. Arising from the anterior aortic sinus the artery passes between the right auricle and the infundibulum of the right ventricle (Fig. 4.20). Running downwards in the atrioventricular groove the artery turns backwards at the inferior border of the heart and runs posteriorly. It gives off branches to both atrium and ventricle. One of the highest branches is the *conus artery* which passes upwards and medially on the front of the conus (infundibulum) of the right ventricle. It frequently anastomoses with a similar branch from the left coronary artery to form an anastomosis around the origin of the pulmonary trunk. Another high atrial branch is usually the *SA nodal artery* which passes back between right auricle and the aorta and forms a vascualr ring around the termination of the superior vena cava. It supplies the SA node in about 60% of hearts. At the inferior border the *right marginal artery* passes to the left along the right ventricle, although it often has a much higher origin and passes obliquely down over the front of the ventricle. On the diaphragmatic surface of the heart the *posterior interventricular* branch—also called the posterior descending artery—is given off. This large vessel passes along the interventricular groove towards the apex of the heart. The right coronary artery has a characteristic loop where the posterior interventricular artery is given off and the *AV nodal artery* arises here. Having given off one or more left ventricular (*right posterolateral*) branches, the remaining and much smaller right coronary artery anastomoses with the termination of the circumflex branch of the left coronary artery to a varying extent.

Left coronary artery. Arising from the left posterior aortic sinus behind the pulmonary trunk the vessel emerges between the left auricle and the infundibulum of the right ventricle. After this short course it divides into its two terminal (circumflex and anterior interventricular) branches (Fig. 4.25). The *circumflex branch* continues round the left margin to the back of the heart in the atrioventricular groove, giving off various ventricular and atrial branches and anastomosing variably

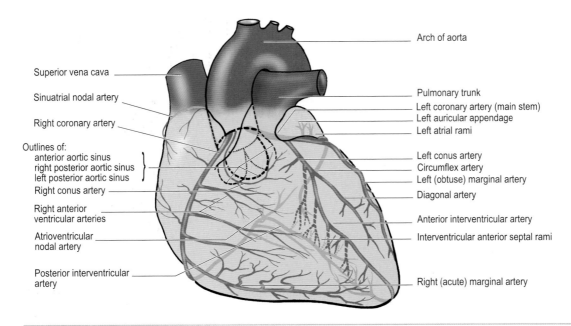

Fig. 4.25   Coronary arteries and their main branches. The ascending aorta and pulmonary trunk are depicted in the same pink colour as the heart to enable the visualization of the origins and early branches of the coronary arteries. The right conus artery is seen arising directly from the anterior aortic sinus as it may do in one third of individuals.

with the end of the right coronary. One large *left marginal artery* frequently runs down the rounded left border of the heart. In about 40% of hearts the circumflex artery gives off the *SA nodal artery* which passes to the right behind the ascending aorta. The *anterior interventricular artery*, also called the left anterior descending artery, is the cardiac vessel most often affected by disease. It runs down in the interventricular groove to anastomose under the apex with the posterior interventricular branch of the right coronary. Near its origin it gives a *conus branch* and further towards the left several ventricular branches. One is often large; this *diagonal artery* may arise separately from the left coronary trunk, which then ends by trifurcation.

In about 10% of hearts the right coronary is shorter than usual and the posterior interventricular artery is replaced by a continuation of the circumflex artery, which also supplies the AV node; in this case the heart is said to show 'left dominance'. In the more common 'right dominance' the posterior interventricular comes from the right coronary; the artery giving off the posterior interventricular branch is defined as the dominant artery. In a 'balanced' circulation, branches of both arteries run in or near the interventricular groove.

Anastomoses of the coronary arteries. Anastomoses exist at the arteriolar level between the terminations of

the right and left coronary arteries in the atrioventricular groove and between their interventricular and conus branches. The time factor in occlusion is all important; in slow occlusion there is time for healthy arterioles to open up, in abrupt occlusion there is not. Potential anastomoses exist between the coronary arteries and pericardial arteries around the roots of the great vessels.

Veins of the heart. The veins of the heart (Fig. 4.26) are the coronary sinus with its five normal tributaries: the great, middle and small cardiac veins, the posterior vein of the left ventricle and the oblique vein of the left atrium, the anterior cardiac veins and the venae cordis minimae. The coronary sinus receives most of the heart's blood.

The **coronary sinus** is a wide vessel that lies in the posterior part of the atrioventricular groove (Fig. 4.19), covered by a thin layer of myocardium, and opens at its right end into the posterior wall of the right atrium to the left of the inferior vena caval opening (Fig. 4.20). The *great cardiac vein* accompanies the anterior interventricular and circumflex arteries to enter the left end of the sinus, receiving in its course a number of left ventricular tributaries. The *middle cardiac vein* accompanies the posterior interventricular artery and opens near the termination of the coronary sinus. The *small cardiac vein* opens into the lower end of the coronary

Fig. 4.26 Cardiac veins, seen from the front. The vessels not on the anterior surface are shown in interrupted line. The middle cardiac vein usually opens into the coronary sinus nearer its termination.

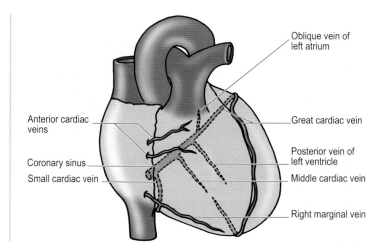

Oblique vein of left atrium

Anterior cardiac veins

Great cardiac vein

Posterior vein of left ventricle

Coronary sinus

Small cardiac vein

Middle cardiac vein

Right marginal vein

sinus near its atrial end. The *posterior vein of the left ventricle* joins the sinus to the left of the middle cardiac vein, and the small *oblique vein of the left atrium* runs downwards into the sinus near its left end.

The *anterior cardiac veins* are a series of parallel veins that run across the surface of the right ventricle to open into the right atrium. The right marginal vein passes to the right along the inferior cardiac margin and joins the small cardiac vein, or drains directly into the right atrium in the manner of an anterior cardiac vein.

The *venae cordis minimae* are very small veins in the walls of all four chambers of the heart that open directly into the respective chambers. They are most frequent in the right atrium.

Lymph drainage

The lymphatics of the heart drain back along the coronary arteries, emerge from the fibrous pericardium along with the aorta and pulmonary trunk, and empty into the tracheobronchial and brachiocephalic lymph nodes.

Nerve supply

The heart is innervated by the cardiac plexus, which has been described on page 200 together with the pathways for cardiac pain.

Development

The earliest stages of cardiac development have been mentioned on page 31.

The original single atrium becomes partitioned by the formation of two septa. The *primary septum* (septum primum) grows down towards the endocardial cushions (see below) at the atrioventricular orifice but does not immediately fuse with them; the gap remaining above the cushions is the *primary foramen* (ostium primum). Before this foramen becomes obliterated by further downgrowth of the septum, a new foramen (*secondary foramen*, ostium secundum) appears as a result of breakdown of the upper part of the primary septum. The right and left parts of the atrium thus still remain in communication. Now a further septum appears (*secondary septum*, septum secundum), on the right of the primary septum, overlapping the secondary foramen. It does not grow down as far as the cushions but ends at a curved posteroinferior border. The gap under the secondary septum which leads through to the secondary foramen in the primary septum is the **foramen ovale**, allowing fetal blood to flow from the right to the left side. At birth when the lungs begin to function, the pressure in the left atrium increases, forcing the primary septum against the left side of the secondary septum so that they fuse, making a complete *interatrial septum*. The lower edge of the secondary septum remains as the *limbus* of the *fossa ovalis*; the floor of the fossa is the part of the primary septum not overlapped by the secondary septum. Sometimes, although the septa overlap, fusion is incomplete and a small cleft remains; this has no functional significance, but a catheter introduced into the right atrium may be manipulated between the septa into the left atrium-a condition known as *probe-patent foramen ovale*. The right horn of the sinus venosus becomes incorporated into the wall of the right atrium, forming its smooth part and accounting for the drainage of the superior and inferior venae cavae into this chamber; the auricle with the pectinate muscles represents the original atrium. The rest of the sinus venosus persists as the *coronary sinus*, with the left horn being represented by the *oblique vein of the left atrium* (vein of Marshall).

The left atrium incorporates the ends of the pulmonary veins to such an extent that only the auricle represents the original atrium.

The channel between the original atrium and ventricle (atrioventricular canal) becomes constricted by internal dorsal and ventral swellings, the *endocardial cushions*, and these meet to convert what was a single passage into the two atrioventricular orifices. Subendocardial tissue at these sites produces the mitral and tricuspid valves.

In the floor of the original ventricle, a partition grows upwards to become the *muscular part* of the *interventricular septum*. It does not grow as far as the endocardial cushions, but leaves a gap which becomes filled in by the *membranous part* of the septum. The muscular part of the septum arises from the junction of the ventricle and the bulb (see p. 32), so that the original ventricle becomes the left ventricle and the adjacent part of the bulb becomes the rough (trabecular) part of the right ventricle. The lower part of the bulb forms the smooth (outflow) part of the right ventricle, which continues upwards into the part of the bulb called the *truncus arteriosus*. This becomes divided into two by internal swellings, the right and left *bulbar ridges*, which meet to form the *aorticopulmonary septum*, so that from the single tube both the ascending aorta and pulmonary trunk are formed. The bulbar ridges are not vertical but assume a spiral form, hence the way the aorta and pulmonary trunk curl round one another. It is the fusion of the lower ends of the bulbar ridges with the posterior endocardial cushion which creates the fibrous part of the interventricular septum.

The junction of the truncus arterious and the definitive ventricles is the site where the *aortic* and *pulmonary valves* develop from the bulbar ridges and the aortic and pulmonary trunk walls.

The SA node develops from sinus venosus tissue but the AV node and bundle are derived from the original atrium.

Congenital defects. Among the more common congenital defects of cardiac development are malformations of the interatrial and interventricular septa, and Fallot's tetralogy. Most *atrial septal defects* are due to maldevelopment of the primary or secondary septa. Most *ventricular septal defects* are in the fibrous part. *Fallot's tetralogy* is due to the unequal division of the truncus arteriosus, giving a small pulmonary trunk and a large ascending aorta, and hence the tetrad of (1) pulmonary stenosis, (2) right ventricular hypertrophy,

(3) a defect of the fibrous part of the interventricular septum, and (4) an over-riding aorta (sitting astride both ventricles because of the septal defect).

Other anomalies, such as patent ductus arteriosus and coarctation of the aorta, although commonly classified as 'cardiac' defects, are strictly speaking anomalies of the great vessels, and are considered on page 29.

Surgical approach

Many operations on the heart are carried out through a median sternotomy, although some require a left thoracotomy. In the former, after splitting the sternum and dividing the thymus into its two lobes, the pericardium is incised in the lines of an inverted T, with the vertical incision extending as high as the pericardial reflexion from the aorta and the transverse incisions along the reflexions from the diaphragm. For *cardiopulmonary bypass* (to keep the circulation going during open heart surgery), the superior and inferior venae cavae are cannulated through the wall of the right atrium, in order to deliver blood to the oxygenating machine. The oxygenated blood is delivered to the aorta through a cannula in the aortic arch proximal to the brachiocephalic trunk. Some of this blood will pass downwards into the ascending aorta and so perfuse the coronary vessels whose openings are just above the aortic valves (kept closed by the pressure of the incoming blood).

In earlier *coronary artery bypass* operations, a suitable length of great saphenous vein was anastomosed at one end to the ascending aorta and at the other to the appropriate coronary vessel distal to the site of blockage. The vein, of course, must be turned upside down so that any valves in the chosen segment do not obstruct the arterial flow. Current opinion now often favours the use of the internal thoracic artery, particularly for the left anterior descending artery; the proximal end remains intact at its subclavian origin and the cut lower end is anastomosed to the coronary vessel. Three or four coronary arteries may be bypassed in the same patient utilizing both internal thoracic arteries and vein grafts or free arterial segments (such as from the radial artery).

In percutaneous transluminal *coronary angioplasty*, following vascular access through the femoral artery in the groin, a catheter is passed retrograde to the site of coronary arterial obstruction and a balloon at the tip of the catheter inflated; patency may be maintained by the placement of a stent.

For the repair of atrial septal defects, the right atrium is incised along its right border, avoiding the region of the SA node. For ventricular septal defects the front of the right ventricle can be incised vertically or transversely avoiding any obvious arteries or veins. For operations on the mitral valve, the left atrium is entered from the right through an incision behind the interatrial groove and in front of the two pulmonary veins.

Transplantation. The patient's heart is removed by incisions through the aorta, pulmonary trunk and both atria. The incision line through the right atrium leaves the two venae cavae, the posterior wall of the atrium and the region of the SA node in situ. The posterior part of the left atrium with the four pulmonary vein orifices is also left intact. The donor heart is trimmed through the atria to match up with the remains of the patient's atria, although the lower end of the donor superior vena cava remains attached to the right atrium so that the donor heart retains its own SA node. For combined heart–lung transplantation, the donor block is removed through the trachea, right atrium and aorta, and sutured to the recipient in that order.

PART SEVEN

Posterior mediastinum

The posterior mediastinum is the space posterior to the pericardium and to the domed upper surface of the diaphragm. It is continuous directly, via the posterior part of the superior mediastinum, with the tissue spaces behind the pretracheal fascia and in front of the prevertebral fascia in the neck. It is bounded posteriorly by thoracic vertebrae 5 to 12 and anteriorly by the pericardium and the sloping fibres of the diaphragm (Fig. 4.9). It contains the oesophagus, thoracic aorta, azygos, hemiazygos and accessory hemiazygos veins, thoracic duct and lymph nodes.

Thoracic (descending) aorta

This large arterial trunk commences at the lower border of T4 vertebra, where the arch of the aorta ends (Fig. 4.13). At first to the left of the midline, the vessel slants gradually to the midline and leaves the posterior mediastinum at the level of T12 vertebra by passing behind the diaphragm between the crura (i.e. behind the median arcuate ligament). It gives off nine pairs of posterior intercostal arteries (see p. 190), a pair of subcostal arteries (see p. 286), bronchial arteries (see p. 224), oesophageal vessels (see below) and a few small pericardial and phrenic branches.

Oesophagus

This muscular tube begins at the lower border of the cricoid cartilage (at the level of C6 vertebra), passes through the diaphragm at the level of T10 vertebra and ends in the abdomen at the cardiac orifice of the stomach at the level of T11 vertebra. It is 25 cm long.

The cervical portion of the oesophagus (see p. 354) commences in the midline in front of the prevertebral fascia, then inclines slightly to the left of the midline, enters the thoracic inlet and passes downwards through the superior mediastinum. At the level of T5 vertebra the oesophagus returns to the midline, but at T7 it deviates again to the left and curves forward to pass in front of the descending thoracic aorta and pierce the diaphragm 2.5 cm to the left of the midline (a thumb's breadth from the side of the sternum), at the level of the seventh left costal cartilage. Here fibres from the right crus of the diaphragm sweep around the oesophageal opening in a sling-like loop (see p. 191). The intra-abdominal part of the oesophagus (see p. 257) varies in length according to the tone of its muscle and the degree of distension of the stomach; it averages 1 to 2 cm.

In the superior mediastinum the oesophagus is crossed by the arch of the aorta on its left side, and the vena azygos on its right (Figs 4.12 and 4.13). Throughout its length the trachea is a direct anterior relation of the oesophagus. Just below the bifurcation of the trachea, in the posterior mediastinum, it is crossed anteriorly by the left main bronchus and the right pulmonary artery (Fig. 4.29). Below that the pericardium (separating it from the left atrium) and the posterior sloping fibres of the diaphragm are in front of the oesophagus. The thoracic duct is posterior to the oesophagus, at first to its right, then ascending directly behind it and lying to its left in the superior mediastinum. On a more posterior plane, the hemiazygos, accessory hemiazygos and right posterior (aortic) intercostal arteries cross the midline behind the oesophagus. The mediastinal pleura touches the oesophagus on both sides, and there is a pocket of right pleura behind the oesophagus and in front of the azygos vein and vertebral column.

Constrictions. The narrowest part of the oesophagus is its commencement at the cricopharyngeal sphincter (see p. 400), 15 cm from the incisor teeth. Other sites where slight constrictions may be expected are where it is crossed by the aortic arch, 22 cm, by the left principal bronchus, 27 cm, and where it passes through the opening in the diphragm, 38 cm from the incisor teeth. Although the left atrium is in front of the lower part below the left bronchus, it is only when enlarged that the atrium causes an indentation in the oesophagus.

Blood supply

The upper oesophagus is supplied by the inferior thyroid arteries, the middle portion by oesophageal branches from the aorta and by the bronchial arteries, and the lower part by the oesophageal branches of the left gastric artery. Venous return from the upper part is to the brachiocephalic veins, from the middle part to the azygos system of veins, and from the lower reaches by oesophageal tributaries of the left gastric vein, which empties into the portal vein. Thus there exists, in the lower part of the oesophagus, an anastomosis between portal and systemic venous systems. This anastomosis lies level with the central tendon (T8 vertebra) well above the oesophageal hiatus in the diaphragm. In cases of portal obstruction varicosities of these veins occur and their rupture may give rise to serious or fatal haemorrhage.

Lymph drainage

Lymph channels from the cervical oesophagus drain to deep cervical nodes, from the thoracic oesophagus to the tracheobronchial and posterior mediastinal nodes, and from the abdominal part to left gastric and coeliac nodes. However, within the oesophageal walls there are lymphatic channels which enable lymph to pass for long distances within the viscus so that drainage from any given area does not strictly follow the above pattern.

Nerve supply

The upper part of the oesophagus is supplied by the recurrent laryngeal nerves and by sympathetic fibres from cell bodies in the middle cervical ganglia running in on the inferior thyroid arteries. The middle and lower parts receive fibres from the thoracic sympathetic trunks and greater splanchnic nerves, while the parasympathetic supply is from the vagus nerves which form a plexus on the surface of the oesophagus. Over the last few centimetres of the thoracic oesophagus the anterior and posterior vagal trunks (see p. 259) form from this plexus. The anterior trunk contains predominantly left vagal fibres and the posterior mainly right fibres, but both trunks have fibres from both vagi.

The motor supply is from the vagus, from cell bodies in the nucleus ambiguous for the upper striated muscle part, and from the dorsal motor nucleus with relay in plexuses in the wall for the lower visceral muscle part. The glands receive secretomotor fibres from the vagus. Pain fibres appear to run with both the vagal and the vasomotor sympathetic supply. As with cardiac pain, oesophageal pain can be referred to the neck, arm and thoracic wall.

Structure

The muscular wall of the oesophagus consists of an inner circular and an outer longitudinal layer, which are of skeletal muscle in the upper part and smooth muscle in the lower part. There is no sharp line of demarcation between these two areas and there is considerable overlap of the two types of muscle in the middle part. The skeletal muscle provides rapid contraction so that the bolus is quickly passed well into the oesophaus, and the larynx may safely open to resume breathing. The thicker longitudinal layer forms a continuous outer coat except at the top, where two tendinous bands ascend within the lower border of the inferior constrictor of the pharynx (see Fig. 6.41, p. 405) and get attached to the midline ridge on the back of the lamina of the cricoid cartilage (see Fig. 6.47, p. 409). The circular muscle of the oesophagus reaches higher than the longitudinal muscle to be continuous with the cricopharyngeus muscle (see p. 400). Except for the short intra-abdominal segment, there is no serous covering of the tube. The mucous membrane is thick and in the collapsed state thrown into longitudinal folds. There is a thick muscularis mucosae. The surface epithelium of the mucous membrane is non-keratinized stratified squamous. This is replaced by columnar epithelium at the gastro-oesophageal junction, but the change may not take place strictly at the cardiac orifice and columnar epithelium may line the lowermost oesophagus. But an oesophagus that has the squamocolumnar junction 3 cm or more above the gastro-oesophageal junction is abnormal (Barrett's oesophagus), metaplastic change having occurred in response to reflux from the stomach. In the submucosa are mucous glands that are rather sparse and found for the most part at the upper and lower ends of the tube. Although there is no anatomical thickening of muscle at the lower end of the oesophagus, there is a zone of high pressure (lower oesophageal sphincter) approximately 3 cm in length, which helps to prevent reflux of stomach contents but relaxes during swallowing.

Surgical approach

The cervical part of the oesophagus is approached usually from the left side of the neck by opening up the interval between the trachea and the carotid sheath. In the thorax, a long length of oesophagus is readily accessible on the right side in front of the vertebral column, after transecting the azygos arch (Fig. 4.12). The posterior intercostal vessels and thoracic duct are at risk when mobilizing the oesophagus posteriorly. The lower part is more easily approached from the left side, above the diaphragm (Fig. 4.13) in the interval between the pericardium in front and the aorta behind. The gastro-oesophageal junction may be approached through the abdomen (see p. 258) and maximal access to the lower oesophagus and stomach is obtained via a thoracoabdominal incision with division of the diaphragm (see p. 195).

Lymphatic drainage of the thorax

The superficial lymphatics of the thoracic wall drain mainly to axillary nodes. Lymph vessels close to the sternum pass between the costal cartilages to parasternal nodes and a few lymphatics from the pectoral region ascend across the clavicle to inferior deep cervical nodes. Lymphatic drainage from the deeper tissues of the thoracic wall goes to intrathoracic lymph nodes.

Parasternal (internal thoracic) nodes are situated at the anterior ends of the upper five intercostal spaces, along the internal thoracic artery. Their efferents drain to the bronchomediastinal lymph trunks. They may become involved in cancer of the breast.

Intercostal nodes lie at the posterior ends of the intercostal spaces. Efferents from upper intercostal nodes pass to the thoracic duct or right lymphatic duct. Lower nodes of both sides drain downwards to the cisterna chyli in the abdomen.

Diaphragmatic nodes are on the thoracic side of the diaphragm in anterior, lateral and posterior groups. In addition to draining the diaphragm, the lateral nodes on the right receive lymph from the liver. Efferents from diaphragmatic nodes pass to parasternal and posterior mediastinal nodes.

Posterior mediastinal nodes are situated behind the pericardium on the oesophagus and descending aorta. They receive afferents from the oesophagus, pericardium and diaphragm. Their efferents pass mainly to the thoracic duct.

Tracheobronchial nodes drain the lungs and the heart. Superior tracheobronchial nodes lie on both sides in the angles between the trachea and the main bronchi, while inferior tracheobronchial (subcarinal or carinal) nodes are in the angle between the bronchi.

Paratracheal nodes lie on the front and sides of the trachea. They receive afferent lymphatics from the tracheobronchial nodes and their efferents pass to the bronchomediastinal lymph trunks.

Brachiocephalic nodes are in the superior mediastinum anterior to the brachiocephalic veins. They drain the thyroid, thymus, pericardium and heart. Their efferents join with those of the paratracheal and parasternal nodes to form the *bronchomediastinal lymph trunks*. The right trunk drains to the right lymphatic duct and the left to the thoracic duct, or they may each open directly into the junction of the internal jugular and subclavian veins on their respective sides.

Thoracic duct

The thoracic duct commences at the upper end of the cisterna chyli (Fig. 4.27 and see p. 288), on a level with the body of T12 vertebra between the aorta and the azygos vein. It passes upwards, with these structures, between the crura of the diaphragm and comes to lie against the right side of the oesophagus. At the level of T5 vertebra it inclines to the left and passes behind the oesophagus. In the superior mediastinum it lies to the left of the oesophagus on a posterior plane. As the duct ascends in the thorax it lies anterior to the right aortic intercostal arteries and the terminal parts of the hemiazygos and accessory hemiazygos veins. Passing vertically upwards in the superior mediastinum it lies posterior to the arch of the aorta and the left subclavian artery. At the root of the neck it arches forwards and to the left, behind the carotid sheath and its contents, crossing over the dome of the pleura and the left subclavian artery to enter the point of confluence of the left internal jugular and subclavian veins (Fig. 4.10). It may divide into two or three separate branches, all of which open at the angle between these two veins. The thoracic duct has several valves.

Carrying all the lymph from the lower half of the body, the duct receives in its course through the thorax lymph from the posterior mediastinal and left intercostal nodes, and from the left bronchomediastinal trunk. In the neck it receives the left *jugular* and *subclavian lymph trunks* and thus finally comes to drain all the lymph of the body except that from the right upper limb and the right halves of the thorax and the head and neck.

The *right lymphatic duct* drains the right intercostal nodes and the right bronchomediastinal trunk. It may receive the right jugular and subclavian lymph trunks before it opens into the commencement of the right brachiocephalic vein, or they may remain separate and open independently into the jugulosubclavian junction.

Azygos system of veins

The thoracic wall and upper lumbar region are drained by the posterior intercostal and lumbar veins into the azygos system of veins.

Azygos vein

The azygos vein is usually formed by the union of the ascending lumbar vein with the subcostal vein of the right side. The vessel goes through the aortic opening

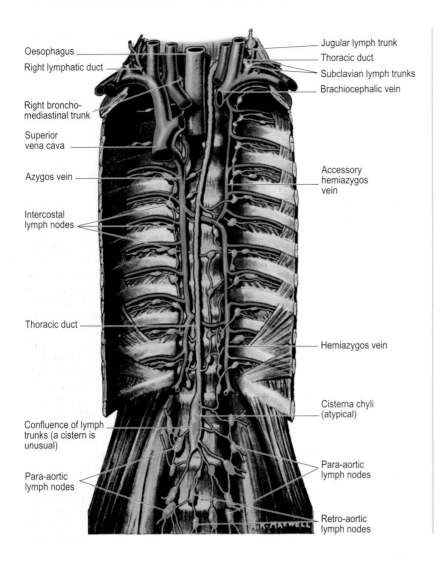

Oesophagus
Right lymphatic duct
Right broncho-mediastinal trunk
Superior vena cava
Azygos vein
Intercostal lymph nodes
Thoracic duct
Confluence of lymph trunks (a cistern is unusual)
Para-aortic lymph nodes

Jugular lymph trunk
Thoracic duct
Subclavian lymph trunks
Brachiocephalic vein
Accessory hemiazygos vein
Hemiazygos vein
Cisterna chyli (atypical)
Para-aortic lymph nodes
Retro-aortic lymph nodes

Fig. 4.27   Azygos system of veins and thoracic duct on the posterior wall of the thorax. The hemiazygos vein is shown draining into the azygos vein at a lower level than usual.

of the diaphragm under shelter of the right crus, lateral to the thoracic duct, and passes upwards lying on the sides of the vertebral bodies, on a plane posterior to that of the oesophagus. At the level of T4 vertebra the azygos vein arches forwards over the hilum of the right lung and ends in the superior vena cava (Fig. 4.12). It receives the lower eight posterior intercostal veins and at its convexity the superior intercostal vein of the right side. It receives the bronchial veins from the right lung, pericardial veins and some veins from the middle third of the oesophagus. The two hemiazygos veins usually join it at the levels of T7 and 8 vertebrae.

Hemiazygos veins

These two veins lie longitudinally on the left side of the bodies of the thoracic vertebrae. They may communicate with each other, but characteristically drain separately from their adjoining ends behind the oesophagus into the azygos vein (Fig. 4.27). They receive the left lower eight posterior intercostal veins, four each. The inferior vein, the **hemiazygos vein,** is formed in the abdomen by the union of the left ascending lumbar and subcostal vein (and often communicates with the left renal vein). It passes up through the left crus of the diaphragm and receives veins from the lower oesophagus. The superior vein is the **accessory hemiazygos vein**; it receives the bronchial veins from the left lung.

Thoracic sympathetic trunk

The thoracic part of the sympathetic trunk (Figs 4.12 and 4.13) lies posterior to the costovertebral pleura and is hence not a content of the posterior mediastinum. It contains about 12 ganglia, most of which lie anterior to the heads of ribs. The first thoracic ganglion is frequently fused with the inferior cervical ganglion, forming the cervicothoracic (stellate) ganglion, and lies anterior to the neck of the first rib. The lowest three ganglia lie lateral to the corresponding vertebral bodies. Each ganglion receives a preganglionic white ramus from the anterior ramus of its corresponding spinal nerve. After relay in the ganglion a postganglionic grey ramus returns to each thoracic nerve, usually medial to the white ramus. Postganglionic sympathetic fibres also pass to the cardiac and pulmonary plexuses, trachea, oesophagus, thoracic aorta and its branches.

The splanchnic nerves, three in number, come from the lower eight ganglia and consist mainly of pre-ganglionic fibres. The lowest, or *least splanchnic nerve* leaves the twelfth ganglion; the *lesser splanchnic nerve* comes from the tenth and eleventh ganglia. The *greater splanchnic nerve* is formed by branches from the fifth to the ninth ganglia. Each pierces the crus of its own side. Their abdominal course and distribution are described on page 291).

The thoracic trunk continues downwards into the abdomen by passing behind the medial arcuate ligament of the diaphragm.

Upper thoracic ganglionectomy

Interruption of the sympathetic outflow to the upper limb from the upper thoracic ganglia (see Fig. 1.15, p. 21) is used in the treatment of Raynaud's syndrome and palmar hyperhidrosis. This can be effected through a cervical approach at the root of the neck, or by an axillary transthoracic route through the third intercostal space, or by a minimal access procedure through a thoracoscope. The cervical approach requires division of the suprapleural membrane and separation of the pleura from the heads and necks of the ribs. In transthoracic approaches the pleural cavity is entered and the costo-vertebral pleura is then divided to expose the sympa-thetic chain that lies behind it. The sympathetic chain is interrupted below the third ganglion and the rami com-municantes of the second and third ganglia are divided, or these ganglia are removed with the intervening chain.

The first thoracic ganglion is preserved intact to avoid the occurrence of Horner's syndrome.

PART EIGHT

Pleura

The pleura is a thin membrane of fibrous tissue surfaced by a single layer of flat cells (mesothelium). It clothes each lung and lines the thoracic cavity.

The *parietal layer* of the pleura lines the thoracic wall (rib cage, vertebrae and diaphragm), from which it is separated by loose areolar tissue, the endothoracic fascia. But the parietal pleura is attached to the inferior surface of the suprapleural membrane, at the thoracic inlet, and to the mediastinal surface of the fibrous pericardium. The pleura is one continuous sheet. From its mediastinal layer a cuff of membrane is projected around the lung root and passes on to invest the surface of the lung. This is the *visceral layer* of the pleura; it extends into the depths of the interlobar clefts and is adherent to the lung surface. The pleural cavity is a completely closed space. The visceral pleura on the lung surface is in contact with parietal pleura, the surfaces being lubricated by a thin film of tissue fluid. The parietal pleura, however, extends further than the inferior lung edge, to allow space for lung expansion. In these situa-tions the costal parietal pleura is in contact with mediastinal and diaphragmatic parietal pleura.

The cuff of pleura projected around the lung root is too big for it, as a coat cuff is too big for the wrist. It hangs down below as an empty fold, the *pulmonary ligament*. It provides 'dead space' into which the lung root descends with descent of the diaphragm, and allows for expansion of vessels in the lung root, especially the inferior pulmonary vein.

Vessels and nerves

The vessels and nerves of the parietal pleura are derived from somatic sources. The arterial supply is from the intercostal, internal thoracic and musculophrenic arteries. The venous drainage is to the azygos system of veins. The lymphatics pass to the intercostal, parasternal, diaphrag-matic and posterior mediastinal nodes. Intercostal nerves supply the costovertebral pleura. The diaphragmatic pleura is supplied by the phrenic nerve over the domes, and by intercostal nerves around its periphery. The mediastinal pleura is supplied by the phrenic nerve.

The arterial supply and venous drainage of the visceral pleura are provided by the bronchial vessels.

The lymphatics join those of the lung (see p. 224). The visceral pleura has an autonomic nerve supply and is insensitive to ordinary stimuli.

Surface markings

The parietal pleura lines the costal walls of the thorax; seen from in front its lateral surface marking is the horizon of the thoracic cage (Fig. 4.28). It projects up to 2.5 cm above the junction of the middle and medial thirds of the clavicle. Due to the obliquity of the thoracic inlet, the pleura does not extend above the neck of the first rib, which lies well above the clavicle.

Tracing the pleura now (Fig. 4.28) from behind the sternoclavicular joint, downwards behind the sternum and around the costodiaphragmatic gutter, there is a point to be noted at each of the even-numbered ribs (2, 4, 6, 8, 10, 12) as follows. The line of pleural reflexion slopes downwards from the sternoclavicular joint to meet its fellow at the *second* rib level, that is, at the sternal angle. Lying together, or even overlapping, they pass vertically behind the sternum down to the *fourth* costal cartilage. Here the right pleura continues vertically, but the left arches out and descends lateral to the border of the sternum, half-way to the apex of the heart. Each turns laterally at the *sixth* costal cartilage, and passing around the chest wall crosses the mid-clavicular line at the *eighth* rib, and the midaxillary at the *tenth* rib. This lower border crosses the *twelfth* rib at the lateral border of erector spinae and passes in horizontally to the lower border of the *twelfth* thoracic vertebra. There is thus a triangle of pleura in the costo-vertebral angle below the medial part of the twelfth rib, behind the upper pole of the kidney, a fact to be noted in incisions and wounds in this region (see Fig. 5.48, p. 293).

The lungs do not extend as far down as the pleural reflection, and below the level of the lungs the costal and diaphragmatic pleura are separated by a narrow space, the costodiaphragmatic recess.

Pleural aspiration and drainage

The anatomy of an intercostal space determines the route for removing fluid (or air) from the pleural cavity. Aspiration needles or drainage tubes are passed through the chest wall close to the upper border of a rib (lower part of an intercostal space) to avoid the vessels and

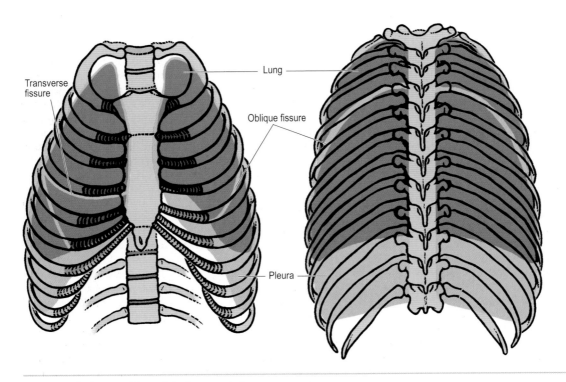

Fig. 4.28 Surface markings of the lungs and pleurae.

nerve which course along the lower border of a rib (upper part of a space) (Fig. 4.4). The choice of space may be determined by the localization of fluid, e.g. a walled-off abscess, but for general purposes the fourth space in or just in front of the midaxillary line is often chosen. A needle, trocar and cannula or drainage tube inserted here is not near any major structure and is high enough to avoid the dome of the diaphragm.

PART NINE

Lungs

Each lung, consisting of two lobes on the left and three on the right, lies within its own side of the thoracic cavity and is surrounded by the visceral layer of the pleura. Each has a principal or main bronchus, one pulmonary artery and two pulmonary veins, all of which undergo subdivisions within the lung substance, together with bronchial vessels, nerves and lymphatics. The region of the mediastinum where the lung is connected to the trachea and heart is the root of the lung, and the region of the lung where the bronchi and pulmonary vessels enter or leave is the hilum.

The lung surface is mottled, and in colour is pink or grey according to the atmosphere in which it has lived. It is crepitant to the touch.

The lung conforms to the shape of the cavity which contains it. It has a convex costal surface and a concave diaphragmatic surface, separated from each other by a sharp inferior border. The posterior border of each lung is generously rounded to fit the paravertebral gutter, and is continued up to the convex apex. The anterior border is thin and sharp; on the left side the lower part of this border is deeply concave—the cardiac notch. The mediastinal surfaces differ somewhat. On the left side the cardiac notch is seen to be the anterior margin of a deep concavity produced by the pericardium in front of the hilum; the arch and ascending aorta make a deep groove on the lung surface around the hilum. Above the aortic arch are vertical impressions made by the subclavian artery and (behind the artery) the oesophagus. On the right the cardiac impression is much shallower; a groove for the azygos vein curves over the hilum to meet the impression made by the superior vena cava. Above the azygos arch and behind the vena cava is a shallow groove for the trachea and right vagus. The apices are grooved by the subclavian arteries (Fig. 4.10). Inferiorly, in front of the lower end of the pulmonary ligament, both lungs may have shallow impressions, on the left lung for the oesophagus and on the right lung for the inferior vena cava.

Lung roots

The left and right lung roots are similar but not identical.

In the **left lung root** (Fig. 4.13) the upper part is occupied by the left pulmonary artery lying within the concavity of the arch of the aorta. Below it is the left bronchus. There are two pulmonary veins, one in front of and the other below the bronchus. These structures are enclosed in a sleeve of pleura continuous below with the pulmonary ligament.

In the **right lung root** (Fig. 4.12) the general arrangement of structures is similar to that on the left, but the bronchus to the upper lobe and the branch of the pulmonary artery to the upper lobe originate outside the lung. Thus the upper lobe bronchus and its accompanying artery are found above the level of the main bronchus and pulmonary artery, the arteries lying in front of their respective bronchi. The two pulmonary veins are disposed as on the left side, in front of and below the main bronchus. The root of the right lung lies within a sleeve of pleura with a dependent pulmonary ligament, as on the left.

In addition to the above large structures, each root contains bronchial vessels, autonomic nerves and lymph nodes and channels.

Pulmonary arteries

The *left pulmonary artery* attached to the undersurface of the aortic arch by the ligamentum arteriosum, quickly spirals over the top of the left bronchus. The *right pulmonary artery*, longer than the left, passes below the carina anterior to the oesophagus, and at the lung root is anterior to the right main bronchus (Fig. 4.29). It gives off its branch to the upper lobe and then enters the hilum.

Fissures

The *oblique fissure* (Figs 4.30 and 4.31) extends from the surface of the lung to the hilum and divides the organ into separate upper and lower lobes which are connected only by the lobar bronchi and vessels. In some lungs the fissure may not be complete. On the right lung a *horizontal fissure* (Fig. 4.30) passes from the anterior margin into the oblique fissure to separate a wedge-shaped middle lobe from the upper lobe. The visceral pleura, clothing the surface of the lung, extends inwards to line the depths of the fissures. The middle lobe of the right lung may not be completely separate from the upper lobe, the fissure separating it from the upper lobe being incomplete or even absent. In the left lung the lowest and most medial part of the upper lobe that

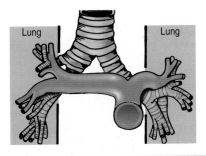

Fig. 4.29   Bifurcation of the pulmonary trunk and the pulmonary arteries. The trunk divides in front of the left main bronchus. The left pulmonary artery spirals over the main bronchus to descend behind the lobar bronchi. The right pulmonary artery crosses below the tracheal bifurcation (in front of the oesophagus), and its descent behind the lower lobe bronchus is delayed because the artery is held anterior at the lung root by the upper lobe bronchus.

overlaps the front of the pericardium is the lingula and forms the boundary of the cardiac notch.

Surface markings

The hilum of each lung lies approximately behind the third and fourth costal cartilages at the sternal margin, and level with T5–7 vertebrae.

On upper costal walls and the supraclavicular region, the surface markings of the lungs coincide with those

of the pleura (Fig. 4.28). The anterior border of the right lung falls very little short of the pleura, lying within the lateral margin of the sternum; that of the left lung in contrast curves laterally to uncover the area of superficial cardiac dullness from the fourth costal cartilage out to the fifth intercostal space just medial to the midclavicular line. The lower border of the lung lies nearly horizontally around the chest wall, but two ribs higher than the pleural reflexion, i.e. in the midclavicular line at the sixth rib, midaxillary line at the eighth rib, and at the lateral border of erector spinae at the tenth rib.

The oblique fissures of each lung are indicated by a line joining the spine of the T3 vertebra, which is opposite the posterior end of the fifth rib, to the sixth rib in the midclavicular line. More simply, this is approximately the line of the fifth rib, or level with the vertebral border of the scapula when the arm is fully abducted above the head. On the right the fourth costal cartilage overlies the horizontal fissure between the upper and middle lobes; continued horizontally this line meets the oblique fissure in the midaxillary line.

Lobar and segmental bronchi

Because the left lung grows into a smaller cavity than the right, the way bronchi divide to supply segments of lung is not identical on the two sides, although there are close similarities.

From the bifurcation of the trachea each **main bronchus** (Fig. 4.32) passes downwards and laterally to

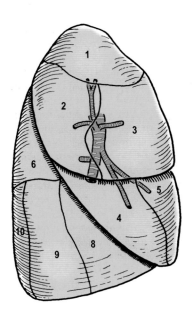
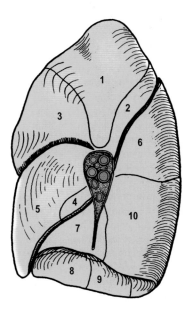

Fig. 4.30   Bronchopulmonary segments of the right lung, lateral and medial surfaces. Note the distribution of the upper and middle lobe bronchi and the posterior origin of the superior bronchus of the lower lobe (6).

Fig. 4.31 Bronchopulmonary segments of the left lung, lateral and medial surfaces. Note the distribution of the lingular bronchi of the upper lobe and the posterior origin of the superior bronchus of the lower lobe (6), as in the right lung.

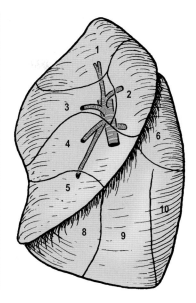
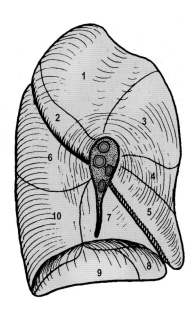

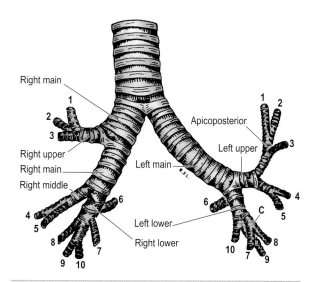

Fig. 4.32 Main, lobar and segmental bronchi. The main and lobar bronchi are named, the segmental bronchi are given their numbers as listed in the text, and the common stem for the left 7 and 8 bronchi is labelled C.

enter the hilum of the lung. The right main bronchus is 2.5 cm long and shorter, wider and more vertical than the left, which is 5 cm long. At the bifurcation the lowest tracheal cartilage has a hook-shaped process, the carina, which curves backwards between the bronchi and raises

an anteroposterior internal ridge that lies to the left of the midline. Foreign bodies that fall down the trachea are more likely to enter the right bronchus.

Each main bronchus gives rise to **lobar bronchi** (Fig. 4.32) that supply the lobes of the lung. The right main bronchus gives off the upper lobe bronchus outside the hilum and ends within the hilum by dividing into middle and lower lobe bronchi. The left main bronchus divides within the hilum into upper and lower lobar bronchi. The tissues of the bronchi are supplied by the bronchial arteries. The veins of the right main bronchus drain to the azygos vein and those of the left to the accessory hemiazygos vein.

Each lobar bronchus gives rise to further branches, the **segmental bronchi** (Fig. 4.32), for each segment of the lung. There are typically 10 **bronchopulmonary segments** in each lung and therefore 10 segmental bronchi; some left segmental bronchi may share a common stem. Each lung segment is roughly pyramidal in shape, with its apex towards the hilum and base towards the surface of the lung. The bronchopulmonary segments are given the same names and numbers as the segmental bronchi, which are listed as follows:

Right lung	Left lung
Upper lobe	*Upper lobe*
1. Apical	1. Apical
2. Posterior	2. Posterior
3. Anterior	3. Anterior

Middle lobe
4. Lateral
5. Medial

4. Superior lingular
5. Inferior lingular

Lower lobe
6. Apical (superior)
7. Medial basal (cardiac)
8. Anterior basal
9. Lateral basal
10. Posterior basal

Lower lobe
6. Apical (superior)
7. Medial basal (cardiac)
8. Anterior basal
9. Lateral basal
10. Posterior basal.

From the above it can be seen that the bronchi and segments of the two lungs are very similar. The upper lobe of the right lung bronchus arises from the lateral aspect of the main bronchus and divides into three segmental bronchi. The middle lobe bronchus arises from the front of the main bronchus and divides into lateral and medial segmental bronchi. The upper lobe of the left lung has five segments, the uppermost two being supplied by bronchi that have a common apicoposterior stem. The lingular part of the left upper lobe has segments called superior and inferior; otherwise the names on the two sides are identical. Both lower lobes have five segmental bronchi and segments. On the left the medial and anterior basal segments and the lateral and posterior basal segments arise from common stem bronchi which subsequently subdivide.

On both sides the apical segment of the lower lobe is supplied by a bronchus (6) which is the highest to arise from the posterior surface of the bronchial tree. Material aspirated by a supine, comatose or anaesthetized patient would tend to gravitate into the apical segment of the right lower lobe, which is consequently a common site for aspiration pneumonia and abscess formation.

Blood supply

The bronchial tree receives its own arterial supply by the *bronchial arteries*. There are usually three: two on the left which are direct branches from the aorta, and one on the right coming from the third right posterior intercostal artery. They supply the bronchi from the carina to the respiratory bronchioles and the visceral pleura. The *bronchial veins* fall into a superficial system draining from the hilar region and visceral pleura into the azygos vein on the right and the accessory hemiazygos on the left, and a deep system from the deeper lung substance draining to a main pulmonary vein or directly into the left atrium (thus mixing venous with arterial blood). The alveoli contain within their walls a rich capillary plexus which is fed with deoxygenated blood by the *pulmonary artery*. The pulmonary artery divides with the bronchi; every bronchus is accompanied by a branch of the artery. The artery supplies no bronchus but it does supply the alveoli, giving them all they need except oxygen, of which they have more than enough. There is some anastomosis between the bronchial and pulmonary arteries at precapillary level. The *pulmonary veins* are formed from tributaries which do not closely follow the bronchi but tend to run in the intersegmental septa. Two pulmonary veins leave each hilum, one from above and one from below the oblique fissure.

Lymph drainage

Lymphatic vessels in the lung originate in a superficial subpleural plexus and a deep submucosal plexus. They drain along the lung surface and with the pulmonary vessels to *bronchopulmonary*, or *hilar*, *nodes* in the hilum of each lung. Efferents from bronchopulmonary nodes run to tracheobronchial nodes. Lymphatics from the upper and middle lobes tend to drain to superior, and those from the lower lobes to inferior, tracheobronchial nodes, but these connections are not exclusive.

Nerve supply

Autonomic nerve fibres from the cardiac plexuses, and directly from the thoracic vagus and sympathetic chain, pass to the pulmonary plexuses, which are situated anterior and posterior to other hilar structures, the anterior plexus being much smaller than the posterior. From here nerve fibres pass into the lung with the bronchi and vessels. The parasympathetic (vagal) fibres are afferent (cell bodies in the inferior ganglion) and efferent (cell bodies in dorsal nucleus, with relay in the bronchial mucosa). They provide the afferent fibres for the cough reflex (see p. 411), important for clearing excess secretions and inhaled substances from the tracheobronchial tree; the receptors are unmyelinated endings in the epithelium. Included among the afferent fibres are those subserving pain. The vagal efferents are bronchoconstrictor, vasodilator and secretomotor to mucous glands. The sympathetic fibres relay in the upper thoracic ganglia; their connector cells lie in the lateral horn of the T2–4 segments of the cord. The sympathetic efferents are bronchodilator and vasoconstrictor.

Structure

Bronchi have smooth muscle and hyaline cartilage in their walls and are lined by the typical respiratory type of epithelium, pseudostratified columnar ciliated, with mucous glands. By successive divisions they become smaller and smaller; when cartilage disappears (at a diameter of about 1 mm) bronchi become *bronchioles*.

After repeated branching, a *lobular bronchiole* enters each lung lobule and divides into *terminal bronchioles* which are the most distal air passages lined by typical respiratory epithelium. They subdivide into *respiratory bronchioles*, so called because some *alveoli* (air sacs) open directly off their walls. Beyond the respiratory bronchioles are *alveolar ducts* which have a lining of cubical epithelium (but no cilia) and also many alveoli. Finally there are the *alveolar sacs* which have walls studded with alveoli.

The walls of the alveoli are lined by two types of epithelial cells covering a layer of connective tissue which contains capillaries. Over 90% of the lining consists of squamous *type I alveolar cells* through which gaseous exchange can occur. The rest of the alveolar wall is lined by smaller, rounded *type II alveolar cells*, containing lamellar bodies with a high phospholipid content; when discharged from the cell they produce the surfactant effect (reducing surface tension). Migratory macrophages are also present on the epithelial surface and within the alveolar lumen.

Development

Each lung develops from a bud at the lower end of the laryngotracheal tube that grows down from the floor of the primitive pharynx (see Fig. 1.20, p. 26). These endodermal buds form the epithelial part of the lung; the connective tissue, cartilage and muscle of the bronchial tree are derived from the surrounding mesoderm. By the fifth month the lung has a glandular appearance, with clumps of epithelial cells and hardly any recognizable lumina. The cell groups proliferate, become canalized and lie adjacent to capillaries so that by the seventh month there are sufficient alveoli to sustain a viable infant following premature birth at this time. Surfactant begins to be secreted about the sixth month.

In the fetus the lungs are not just a mass of collapsed air spaces but are full of fluid, largely secreted by the lungs but with a contribution from swallowed amniotic fluid. At the time of birth some is squeezed out by thoracic pressure and the rest escapes into blood capillaries and lymphatics, assisted by surfactant action. After birth there is no new development of any kind of bronchioles, but more than 80% of the adult number of alveoli are budded off during about the first 8 years of life.

Surgical approach

For *pneumonectomy* the approach on each side is usually a posterolateral thoracotomy through the bed of the sixth rib. It is necessary to divide the main pulmonary artery, both pulmonary veins and the main bronchus, but the sequence in which these principal structures are divided varies in accordance with their ease of isolation and the pathological indication for pneumonectomy. On the left the vagus is divided distal to the recurrent laryngeal branch, and the pulmonary artery is divided distal to the ligamentum arteriosum. The nearness of the aortic arch may make closure of the bronchus difficult. On the right the arch of the azygos vein is preserved if possible, as it affords collateral circulation if the superior vena cava is obstructed. The latter may have to be displaced forwards to allow satisfactory ligation of the pulmonary artery.

PART TEN

Osteology of the thorax

Sternum

The sternum consists of an uppermost manubrium, an intermediate body and a small lowermost xiphoid process (Fig. 4.3). The manubrium and body are connected by a secondary cartilaginous joint (see p. 187). Like the ribs, most of the sternum is made of cancellous bone which throughout life is filled with haemopoietic marrow.

The **manubrium** is a flat four-sided bone broader above than below (Fig. 4.5). Its upper margin is concave, the *jugular notch*, on which lies the adherent interclavicular ligament. The two layers of the investing layer of deep cervical fascia are attached to the anterior and posterior borders of the notch (see p. 342). Each upper angle of the manubrium is scooped out into a concavity for the sternoclavicular joint, an atypical synovial joint (see p. 45). Below this the lateral border is excavated for the first costal cartilage, which articulates here by a primary cartilaginous joint (see p. 187). At the inferior angle is a small facet for articulation (synovial) with the upper part of the second costal cartilage. Between the first and second costal cartilages the internal intercostal muscle is attached to the lateral border. The anterior surface is mainly covered by the attachment of pectoralis major but also gives attachment to the tendon of sternocleidomastoid. Sternohyoid and sternothyroid are attached to the upper part of the posterior surface. The manubrium forms the anterior wall of the superior mediastinum.

The **body of the sternum** has articular facets along its lateral border for the lower part of the second costal cartilage and for the third to seventh costal cartilages, all these articulations being synovial joints (Fig. 4.3).

Between the costal facets the lateral border gives attachment to the anterior intercostal membrane and the internal intercostal muscle. Pectoralis major arises widely from the anterior surface almost to the midline, and transversus thoracis arises from the posterior surface low down. From the posterior surface weak sterno-pericardial ligaments pass to the fibrous pericardium.

From the posterior margin of the lower end of the sternal body the xiphoid process (xiphisternum) projects downwards for attachment of the linea alba. It articulates with the body by a symphysis which usually ossifies in middle age.

Surface markings

The sternal angle is palpable and the second costal cartilage can be felt at either side of the angle; the ribs can be counted down from here. On account of the downward inclination of the ribs, the jugular notch lies at the level of the upper border of the third, the sternal angle at the lower border of the fourth, and the lower end of the sternum at the lower border of the eighth thoracic vertebral bodies.

Ribs

A typical rib

A typical rib from the middle of the series has a head, a neck and a shaft; a tubercle projects posteriorly from the lateral end of the neck (Fig. 4.33).

The **head** is bevelled by two articular facets that slope away from a dividing ridge. The lower facet is vertical; it articulates with its own vertebra and the upper facet articulates with the vertebra above. Each makes a synovial joint, and the cavities are separated by a ligament attached to the ridge on the head and to the intervertebral disc.

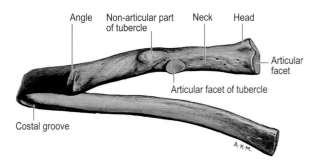

Costal groove · Angle · Non-articular part of tubercle · Neck · Head · Articular facet · Articular facet of tubercle · A.K.M.

Fig. 4.33 Typical left rib: posterior aspect.

The **neck** is flattened, with a sharp crest forming the upper border. The two laminae of the superior costo-transverse ligament are attached to the crest (Fig. 4.2). The neck of the rib inclines backwards when traced from head to tubercle.

The **tubercle** shows two facets. The smooth medial facet makes a synovial joint with the transverse process of its own vertebra. The rough lateral facet gives attachment to the lateral costotransverse ligament.

The **shaft** slopes down and back to the angle and there twists forward in its characteristic curvature. Anterior to the angles the shafts of ribs are curved to form arcs of circles whose diameters increase from above downwards. On account of torsion at their angles, the heads of ribs lie at a higher level than their anterior ends; the degree of torsion is most marked in the seventh to ninth ribs. The upper border of a rib is blunt. It gives attachment in its whole length to the external and from the angle forwards to the internal intercostal muscles. The lower border of the shaft is sharp and hangs down to produce a well-marked *costal groove* on the inner surface. The external intercostal muscle arises from the sharp lower border and the internal intercostal is attached to the costal groove. The transverse thoracic group of muscles are attached to the inner surface of the shaft. The neurovascular bundle lies between this layer and the internal intercostal muscle, deep to the costal groove (Fig. 4.4). The anterior end of the rib is excavated into a concave fossa which is plugged by the costal cartilage in an immovable primary cartilaginous joint.

Atypical ribs

First rib

The first rib (Fig. 4.34) is the strongest, broadest, flattest and most curved rib. Its superior surface is part of the root of the neck; its inferior (pleural) surface is part of the roof of the thoracic cavity. The neck slopes upwards, backwards and laterally from the head to the tubercle. Hence if the rib is laid on the table, the head and anterior extremity both touch the surface, but laid upside down the head lies above the table; this enables right and left sides to be identified. The plane of the shaft is at 45° to the horizontal, with the tubercle the most posterior and highest part of the rib.

The **head** is small and carries a single facet for the synovial joint it makes with the upper part of the body of T1 vertebra. The sympathetic trunk (or cervicothoracic ganglion) lies in contact with the anterior border of the neck alongside the head. Lateral to it the first posterior

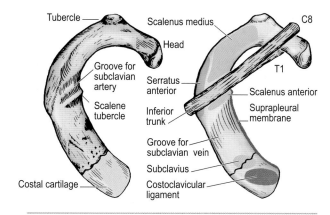

Fig. 4.34 Right first rib, from above, and attachments.

intercostal vein and then the superior intercostal artery lie in contact, and more lateral still the first thoracic nerve lies in front of the neck and inner border of the shaft. The cervical dome of the pleura and the apex of the lung hold these vessels and nerves against the front of the neck of the rib.

The rib broadens at the junction of neck and shaft, where a prominent **tubercle** projects back to form the most posterior convexity of the rib. It is a fusion of tubercle and angle. Medially it has a cylindrical facet for a corresponding concavity on the first transverse process. The lateral prominent part of the tubercle receives the lateral costotransverse ligament.

The undersurface of the **shaft**, crossed obliquely by the small first intercostal nerve and vessels, is covered by adherent parietal pleura. The external and internal intercostal muscles are attached together to the outer rim of this surface. The outer border is blunt between the tubercle and subclavian groove and the first digitation of serratus anterior is attached to the anterior part of this blunt area. The concave internal border of the shaft gives attachment to the suprapleural membrane in front of the subclavian groove (Fig. 4.5).

The upper surface of the **shaft** is grooved obliquely at its greatest lateral convexity. Called the groove for the subclavian artery, it lodges the lower trunk of the brachial plexus as well, behind the artery. The fibres in contact with the rib are all T1, the C8 fibres lying above them. Between the groove and the tubercle the large quadrangular area of the upper surface gives attachment to scalenus medius. At the front of the groove the inner border is projected into a small spur, the **scalene tubercle**. The tendon of scalenus anterior is attached to the tubercle and extends along a triangular impression on the upper surface which may be more discernable than the tubercle itself. Anterior to the attachment of scalenus anterior is another groove on the upper surface of the shaft in which the subclavian vein lies. The anterior end of the shaft expands into a concavity for the first costal cartilage. From the upper surface of this junction subclavius arises from both bone and cartilage.

Eleventh rib

The eleventh rib has a head, with a single facet for T11 vertebra, a short neck, no tubercle, a slight angle and a shallow costal groove.

Twelfth rib

The twelfth rib varies in length. The head has a single facet for T12 vertebra. A short constriction forms a neck which passes imperceptibly into the shaft. There is no tubercle, no angle and no costal groove. The inner surface of the shaft faces slightly upwards.

Ossification of the sternum

In two longitudinal cartilaginous plates that fuse in the midline, a variable number of primary centres appear at about the fifth fetal month and later. There are one or two in the manubrium, and one or two in each of the four pieces (*sternebrae*) that will form the body of the sternum. The double centres coalesce, and fusion between sternebrae occurs between puberty and 25 years. Sternal foramina ('bullet holes') in the adult sternum are the result of incomplete fusion of double centres. The cartilaginous xiphoid process may ossify any time after the third year but often not until later life.

Ossification of ribs

Primary ossification centres appear at the eighth week of fetal life at the angle, and ossification proceeds anteriorly and posteriorly from here. At birth the unossified anterior end remains as the costal cartilage. Secondary centres for the head and tubercle appear at puberty and fuse with the shaft after 20 years.

Costal cartilages

These form primary cartilaginous joints at the extremities of all twelve ribs. The *first* is short and thick, and forms also a primary cartilaginous joint with the manubrium. It articulates also with the clavicle and gives attachment to the sternoclavicular disc and the costoclavicular ligament.

Below this the cartilages increase in length down to the seventh, which is the longest. From the fifth to the tenth they are bent from a downward slope in line with the rib to an upward slope towards the sternum (Fig. 4.3). Their medial ends form synovial joints with the sternum or the cartilage above (see p. 187). The cartilages of the eleventh and twelfth ribs have free pointed anterior ends. All cartilages, especially the first, tend to calcify and even ossify in patches after middle age.

Abdomen

5

PART ONE

Anterior abdominal wall

The skin and subcutaneous tissues of the anterior abdominal wall have been dealt with as part of the body wall (see p. 185).

For clinical purposes, such as the description of sites of pain, swellings, and incisions, the abdomen is divided into regions that are defined by lines on the surface of the anterior abdominal wall. Usually nine regions are delineated by two vertical and two horizontal lines (Fig. 5.1). The vertical line on each side corresponds to the **midclavicular line**; when extended downwards it reaches the **midinguinal point**, which is midway between the pubic symphysis and the anterior superior iliac spine. The lower transverse line is drawn between the tubercles of the iliac crests (**intertubercular plane**) and the upper transverse line is in the **transpyloric plane** (see p. 242), midway between the jugular notch and the top of the pubic symphysis. (Some clinicians use the *subcostal plane* which is a little lower—level with the lowest part of the costal margin). Using these four lines, three central regions are defined from above downwards: *epigastric*, *umbilical* and *hypogastric* (or suprapubic). Similarly there are three lateral regions on each side: *hypochondrial*, *lumbar* and *iliac*.

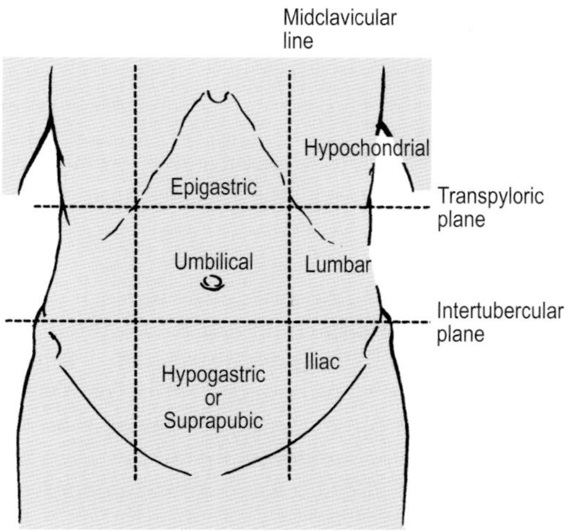

Anterolateral abdominal muscles

The three muscle layers of the body wall (see p. 187) are separate in the flanks, where they are known as the external oblique, internal oblique and transversus abdominis muscles. The layers have fused ventrally to form the rectus abdominis muscle.

External oblique

The muscle arises by eight digitations, one from each of the lower eight ribs just lateral to their anterior extremities. The lower four slips interdigitate with the costal fibres of latissimus dorsi and the upper four with digitations of serratus anterior. From its fleshy origin the muscle fans out to a very wide insertion, much of which is aponeurotic. The muscle has a free posterior border which extends from the twelfth rib to its insertion as fleshy fibres into the anterior half of the outer lip of the iliac crest. Muscular fibres are replaced by an aponeurosis

Fig. 5.1 Regions of the abdomen.

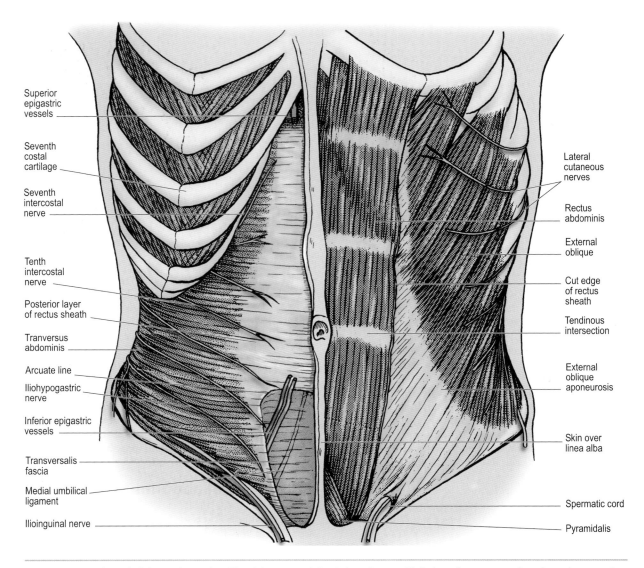

Superior epigastric vessels

Seventh costal cartilage

Seventh intercostal nerve

Tenth intercostal nerve

Posterior layer of rectus sheath

Tranversus abdominis

Arcuate line

Iliohypogastric nerve

Inferior epigastric vessels

Transversalis fascia

Medial umbilical ligament

Ilioinguinal nerve

Lateral cutaneous nerves

Rectus abdominis

External oblique

Cut edge of rectus sheath

Tendinous intersection

External oblique aponeurosis

Skin over linea alba

Spermatic cord

Pyramidalis

Fig. 5.2   Anterolateral abdominal muscles. The right rectus abdominis and pyramidalis have been removed to show the posterior wall of the rectus sheath, the arcuate line and the ends of the intercostal nerves.

below a line joining the anterior superior iliac spine to the umbilicus, and medial to a vertical line drawn from the tip of the ninth costal cartilage (Fig. 5.2). The limit of the fleshy fibres is visible in an athlete as a graceful curve. The aponeurotic fibres, directed obliquely downwards and forwards, interdigitate with each other across the front of the rectus abdominis along the whole length of the linea alba. (This description is adequate for all practical purposes although detailed studies of cadaveric material have revealed that the aponeurotic fibres are in superficial and deep layers, the fibres in the superficial layer running obliquely upwards and those in the deep layer at right angles downwards. The fibres continue across the midline after decussation, the fibres from the deep layer passing to the superficial layer on the contralateral side of the abdominal wall and vice versa.) The free horizontal upper border of this aponeurosis extends from the fifth rib to the xiphisternum. It is the only structure in the anterior sheath of the rectus muscle above the costal margin.

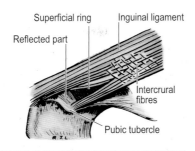

Fig. 5.3 Left superficial inguinal ring, after removal of the external spermatic fascia which is continuous with the margins of the ring.

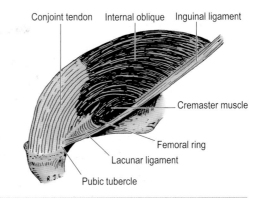

Fig. 5.4 Left conjoint tendon and lacunar ligament. The lowest fibres of the internal oblique arise from the inguinal ligament and arch medially to reach the conjoint tendon, forming as they do so the roof of the inguinal canal. They cover up the similar fibres of transversus abdominis, shown in Figure 5.5. Note that the nearly vertical conjoint tendon lies at right angles to the nearly horizontal lacunar ligament.

The posterior border of the muscle is free, and forms the anterior boundary of the **lumbar triangle** (of Petit) that is floored in by the internal oblique and bounded behind by the anterior border of latissimus dorsi and below by the iliac crest. The triangle may be the site of a rare lumbar hernia (see Fig. 2.4, p. 43).

The lower border, lying between the anterior superior iliac spine and the pubic tubercle, forms the **inguinal ligament** (of Poupart). Its edge is rolled inwards to form a gutter; the lateral part of this gutter gives origin to part of the internal oblique and transversus abdominis muscles. The fascia lata of the thigh is attached to the inguinal ligament and when the thigh is extended the fascia lata pulls the inguinal ligament downwards into a gentle convexity.

Just above and lateral to the pubic tubercle is an oblique, triangular gap, the *superficial inguinal ring*, in the aponeurosis (Fig. 5.3). The base of the gap is the pubic crest, and the margins are the crura of the ring.

From the medial end of the inguinal ligament the triangular **lacunar ligament** (of Gimbernat) extends horizontally backwards to the pectineal line on the pubis (see Fig. 3.1, p. 116). A fibrous band, the pectineal ligament (of Astley Cooper) extends further along the pectineal line. The crescentic free lateral edge of the lacunar ligament is the medial margin of the femoral ring (see p. 122).

From the pubic tubercle, fibres may be traced upwards and medially, behind the spermatic cord, to interdigitate in the linea alba with those of the opposite side. This is the *reflected part* of the ligament (Fig. 5.3). Near the apex of the superficial inguinal ring are fibres running at right angles to those of the aponeurosis, the *intercrural fibres*, that prevent the crura from separating.

Internal oblique

Fleshy fibres of the muscle arise from the whole length of the lumbar fascia, from the intermediate area of the anterior two-thirds of the iliac crest and from the lateral two-thirds of the inguinal ligament. From the lumbar fascia the muscle fibres run upwards along the costal margin, to which they are attached, becoming aponeurotic at the tip of the ninth costal cartilage. Below the costal margin, the aponeurosis splits around the rectus muscle, the two layers rejoining at the linea alba. Halfway between the umbilicus and the pubic symphysis the posterior layer ends in a curved free margin, the arcuate line. Below this point, the aponeurosis passes wholly in front of the rectus muscle, to the linea alba (Fig. 5.6) (but see p. 232).

The muscle fibres that arise from the inguinal ligament are continued into an aponeurosis that is attached to the crest of the pubic bone and, more laterally, to the pectineal line (Fig. 5.4). This aponeurosis is fused with a similar arrangement of the transversus aponeurosis to form the conjoint tendon. The internal oblique therefore has a free lower border, which arches over the spermatic cord: laterally the margin consists of muscle fibres in front of the cord; medially the margin consists of tendinous fibres behind the cord.

Transversus abdominis

The muscle arises in continuity from the lateral third of the inguinal ligament, the anterior two-thirds of the inner lip of the iliac crest, the lumbar fascia, the twelfth rib, and from the inner aspects of the lower six costal cartilages where it interdigitates with the diaphragm.

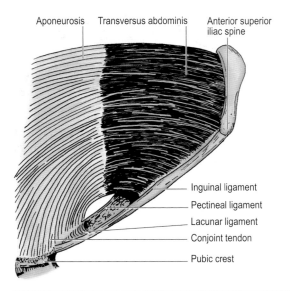

Aponeurosis   Transversus abdominis   Anterior superior iliac spine

Inguinal ligament

Pectineal ligament

Lacunar ligament

Conjoint tendon

Pubic crest

Fig. 5.5 Left transversus abdominis, showing the lowest fibres arching medially to join the conjoint tendon.

The muscle fibres become aponeurotic and pass behind the rectus to fuse with the internal oblique aponeurosis in the linea alba. Below the arcuate line the aponeurosis passes wholly in front of the rectus muscle. (As in the case of external oblique, detailed cadaveric studies have shown that the aponeurotic fibres of transverse abdominis that contribute to the rectus sheath are in two layers at right angles to each other.) In the upper part of the abdomen the outer margin of the aponeurosis is more medial, and muscular fibres lie behind the lateral part of rectus abdominis. The lower fibres of the aponeurosis curve downwards and medially with those of the internal oblique as the **conjoint tendon**, to insert on the pubic crest and the pectineal line (Fig. 5.5).

Rectus abdominis and pyramidalis

Rectus abdominis arises by two heads: a medial from in front of the pubic symphysis and a lateral from the upper border of the pubic crest. The two muscles lie edge to edge in the lower part, but broaden out above, and are there separated from each other by the linea alba (Fig. 5.2). They are inserted on to the front of the fifth to seventh costal cartilages. Typically three *tendinous intersections* are found in the muscle, one at the umbilicus, one at the xiphisternum, and one between these two; one or two incomplete intersections are sometimes found below the umbilicus. The tendinous intersections blend inseparably with the anterior layer of the rectus sheath.

They occupy only the superficial part of the rectus and do not penetrate to the posterior surface of the muscle, which is thus not connected to the posterior layer of the sheath. The contracting rectus abdominis can be seen as bulgings between the tendinous intersections in an individual who is not too fat.

The small triangular **pyramidalis** muscle arises from the pubis and the symphysis between rectus abdominis and its sheath. It converges with its fellow into the linea alba 4 cm or so above its origin.

Between the two recti all the aponeuroses that form the rectus sheath fuse to form the **linea alba**, a strong midline fibrous structure which is firmly attached to the xiphoid process above and the pubic symphysis below (Fig. 5.2). Above the symphysis it is very narrow, for here the two recti are in contact with one another behind it. From just below the umbilicus to the xiphisternum it broadens out between the recti. Here the fibres form a tough felted membrane.

Rectus sheath

The aponeurosis of the internal oblique splits into anterior and posterior layers to enclose the rectus muscle (Fig. 5.6B). The external oblique aponeurosis fuses with the anterior layer to form the anterior layer of the sheath, and the transversus aponeurosis fuses with the posterior layer to form the posterior layer of the sheath. From halfway between the umbilicus and the pubic symphysis all three aponeuroses pass in front of the muscle (Fig. 5.6C). The posterior layer thus has a free lower margin concave downwards, the *arcuate line* or *semicircular line* (of Douglas). The aponeuroses of internal oblique and transversus fuse completely but that of the external oblique fuses only to the most medial part of the sheath. The posterior layer of the sheath is attached to the costal margin (seventh, eighth and ninth costal cartilages). Above the costal margin the anterior layer of the sheath consists only of the external oblique aponeurosis (Fig. 5.6A).

The splitting of the internal oblique aponeurosis along the lateral border of the rectus muscle forms a relatively shallow groove, the *semilunar line*. It curves up from the pubic tubercle to the costal margin at the tip of the ninth costal cartilage in the transpyloric plane.

Detailed studies indicate that the aponeuroses of external oblique, internal oblique and transversus abdominis are each bilaminar, giving six layers in all; three form the anterior and three the posterior layers of the rectus sheath. These layers decussate across the midline. There may not be a well-defined arcuate line but a gradual diminution of aponeurotic fibres with increasing thickness of the transversalis fascia. The

Fig. 5.6 Formation of the rectus sheath as seen in horizontal sections: **A** above the costal margin—only the external oblique and its aponeurosis exist here; **B** between the umbilicus and the costal margin—the aponeurosis of the internal oblique splits around the rectus, taking the external oblique aponeurosis to join the anterior layer and that of transversus to join the posterior layer; **C** below the arcuate line—all three aponeuroses pass in front of the rectus muscle. See text for other possibilities.

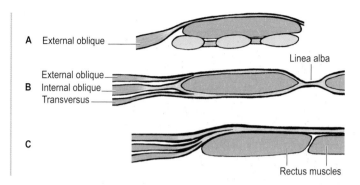

lower thickened part of the transversalis fascia, between the iliac crest and pubis just above the inguinal ligament, is called the *iliopubic tract*.

Contents. Apart from the rectus and pyramidalis muscles, the sheath contains the ends of the lower six thoracic nerves and their accompanying posterior intercostal vessels, and the superior and inferior epigastric arteries.

The **intercostal nerves** (T7–11; see p. 189) pass from their intercostal spaces into the abdominal wall between the internal oblique and transversus muscles, and run round in this neurovascular plane to enter the sheath by piercing the posterior layer of the internal oblique aponeurosis. They then proceed behind the rectus muscle to about its midline (Fig. 5.2), where they pierce the muscle, supply it, and pass through the anterior layer of the sheath to become the anterior cutaneous nerves. In the sheath T7 runs upwards just below the costal margin, T8 transversely and the others obliquely downwards. Before they reach the sheath the nerves give off their lateral cutaneous branches, which pierce the internal and external oblique to reach the skin.

The lowest thoracic nerve, T12 or subcostal, is described on page 289.

The **superior epigastric artery**, a terminal branch of the internal thoracic (see p. 190), enters the sheath by passing between the sternal and highest costal fibres of the diaphragm. It supplies the rectus muscle and anastomoses within it with the **inferior epigastric artery**. This vessel leaves the external iliac at the inguinal ligament (Fig. 5.8), passes upwards behind the conjoint tendon, slips over the arcuate line and so enters the sheath. Veins accompany these arteries, draining to internal thoracic and external iliac veins respectively.

A pedicled flap of the upper part of the rectus muscle based on the superior epigastric artery—or a free flap of the lower part with anastomosis of the divided inferior epigastric artery to the internal thoracic artery—is used in *reconstructive breast surgery*.

Blood supplies

Apart from the intercostal and epigastric vessels mentioned above, the anterolateral abdominal muscles also receive a blood supply from the lumbar and deep circumflex iliac arteries. The lumbar arteries are described on page 286; they end among the flat anterolateral muscles and do not reach the rectus sheath.

The **deep circumflex iliac artery** arises from the external iliac (see p. 286) behind the inguinal ligament (Fig. 5.8), and runs laterally towards the anterior superior iliac spine in a sheath formed by the transversalis and iliac fasciae where they meet. It continues along the inner lip of the iliac crest, pierces the transversus muscle to reach the neurovascular plane and anastomose with branches of the iliolumbar and superior gluteal arteries. At the anterior superior iliac spine it gives off an ascending branch which may be at risk in a gridiron incision (see p. 241).

Lymph drainage

The superficial tissues of the anterolateral abdominal wall drain in quadrants: to the pectoral group of axillary nodes above the umbilicus on each side, and to superficial inguinal nodes below that level. The deeper parts of the wall drain into vessels in the extraperitoneal tissues. Above the umbilicus these pierce the diaphragm to reach mediastinal nodes, and below it they run to the external iliac and para-aortic nodes.

Nerve supplies

The rectus muscle and external oblique are both supplied by the lower intercostal and subcostal nerves (T7–T12), and the internal oblique and transversus by those same nerves but with the addition of the iliohypogastric and ilioinguinal nerves (L1). The lowest fibres of the internal oblique and transversus that continue medially as the conjoint tendon receive the L1 innervation, which thus helps to maintain the integrity of the inguinal canal (see below). Pyramidalis is supplied by the subcostal nerve (T12).

Actions of abdominal muscles

The muscles of the anterior abdominal wall have four main roles: (1) to move the trunk, (2) to depress the ribs (expiration), (3) to compress the abdomen (evacuation, expiration, heavy lifting), and (4) to support the viscera (intestines only). The abdominal wall, moving to and fro with breathing, conforms to the volume of the abdominal contents. Its *shape* is determined by the tonus of its own muscles. The subumbilical pull of healthy flank muscles keeps its lower part flat by holding back the lower recti.

Moving the trunk. As the muscles are attached to the thoracic cage and the bony pelvis their action is to approximate the two. They are flexors of the vertebral column in its lumbar and lower thoracic parts. Rectus abdominis is the most powerful flexor. The oblique muscles are also lateral flexors and rotators of the trunk.

Depressing the ribs. The recti and obliques approximate the ribs to the pelvic girdle. If erector spinae prevents thoracolumbar flexion this provides a powerful expiratory force (e.g. coughing, blowing the trumpet). Added to this is the abdominal compression (aided by transversus) that elevates the diaphragm to increase the expiratory effort.

Compressing the abdomen. While flexion of the vertebral column is prevented by the erector spinae muscles, the oblique muscles compress the abdominal cavity; in this they are aided strongly by transversus abdominis, which has no flexing action on the spine. The recti play little part in compression. If the diaphragm is relaxed, it is forced up, as in expiration. At the same time levator ani helps to hold the pelvic effluents closed. The reverse occurs in evacuation of the pelvic effluents. Here the diaphragm contracts to resist upward displacement, but it is a far weaker muscle than the abdominal wall, and in forceful compression it is prevented from rising by holding the breath, i.e. by closure of the glottis, and perhaps of the mouth and nostrils (see p. 411).

Supporting and protecting viscera. If the anterior abdominal wall is incised or removed, only the intestines spill out. The upper abdominal viscera, such as the liver, spleen and kidneys, do not require the support of the wall. Reflex contraction in response to a blow helps to protect all viscera.

Tests. Rectus abdominis can be tested by lying flat on the back and raising the head (without using the arms). There are no specific tests for the other flat muscles. The abdominal reflex and Beevor's sign have been referred to on page 18.

Inguinal canal

The inguinal canal is an oblique intermuscular slit about 4 cm long lying above the medial half of the inguinal ligament. It commences at the deep inguinal ring, ends at the superficial inguinal ring, and transmits the spermatic cord and ilioinguinal nerve in the male and the round ligament of the uterus and ilioinguinal nerve in the female. Its anterior wall is formed by the external oblique aponeurosis (Fig. 5.2), assisted laterally by the internal oblique muscle (Fig. 5.7). Its floor is the inrolled lower edge of the inguinal ligament, reinforced medially by the lacunar ligament (Fig. 5.4). Its roof is formed by the lower edges of the internal oblique and transversus muscles, which arch over from in front of the cord laterally to behind the cord medially, where their conjoined aponeuroses, constituting the conjoint tendon, are inserted into the pubic crest and the pectineal line of the pubic bone. The posterior wall of the canal is formed by the strong conjoint tendon medially and the weak transversalis fascia throughout.

The integrity of the inguinal canal depends upon the strength of the anterior wall in the lateral part and of the posterior wall in the medial part, provided the abdominal muscles are of good tone and their aponeuroses unyielding. The deep and superficial inguinal rings lie at opposite ends of the inguinal canal and the intervening part of the canal is pressed flat when the aponeuroses are under tension and the intra-abdominal pressure raised. The conjoint tendon lies posterior to the superficial inguinal ring and helps to reinforce this area. Laterally the transversalis fascia in the posterior wall is strengthened by the presence in front of it of tendinous, and sometimes muscular, fibres derived from the transversus abdominis muscle. These fibres constitute the *interfoveolar ligament* (Fig. 5.8). They arch down from the lower border of transversus around the vas to the inguinal ligament, and constitute the functional medial edge of the deep ring.

The **deep inguinal ring** lies about 1.25 cm above the midpoint of the inguinal ligament and is an opening in the transversalis fascia. From the margins of this opening the transversalis fascia is projected along the canal, like a sleeve, the internal spermatic fascia, around the structures that pass through the ring. These are the vas (ductus) deferens and its artery, the testicular artery and the accompanying veins (usually double at this level, Fig. 5.10), the obliterated remains of the processus vaginalis, the genital branch of the genitofemoral nerve, autonomic nerves and lymphatics. These structures

Fig. 5.7 Right inguinal canal after division of the external oblique aponeurosis and fasciae. The ilioinguinal nerve has been displaced downwards with the lower flap of the aponeurosis.

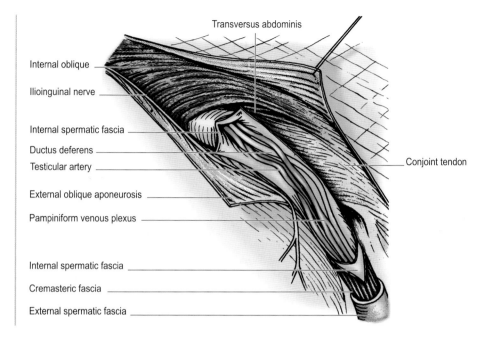

Transversus abdominis

Internal oblique

Ilioinguinal nerve

Internal spermatic fascia

Ductus deferens

Testicular artery

External oblique aponeurosis

Pampiniform venous plexus

Internal spermatic fascia

Cremasteric fascia

External spermatic fascia

Conjoint tendon

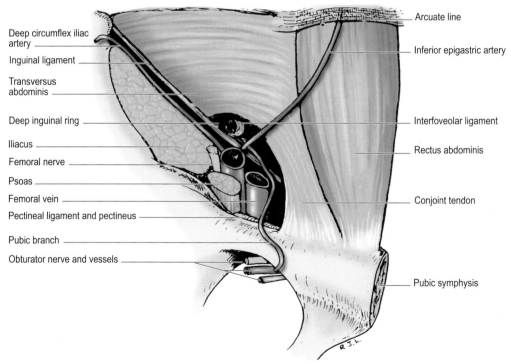

Deep circumflex iliac artery

Inguinal ligament

Transversus abdominis

Deep inguinal ring

Iliacus

Femoral nerve

Psoas

Femoral vein

Pectineal ligament and pectineus

Pubic branch

Obturator nerve and vessels

Arcuate line

Inferior epigastric artery

Interfoveolar ligament

Rectus abdominis

Conjoint tendon

Pubic symphysis

Fig. 5.8 Left inguinal region viewed from within the abdomen. The deep inguinal ring lies lateral to the inferior epigastric artery. The femoral ring lies medial to the external iliac (femoral) vein; the lacunar ligament which is at the medial border of the ring is here obscured by the conjoint tendon.

constitute the spermatic cord; in the female they are re-placed by the obliterated processus vaginalis, the round ligament and lymphatics from the uterus. The ilio-inguinal nerve, although a content of the inguinal canal, does not enter the canal through the deep ring, but by piercing the internal oblique muscle, i.e. it slips into the canal from the side, not from the back. The nerve lies in front of the cord and leaves the canal through the superficial ring to supply skin of the inguinal region, upper part of the thigh, anterior third of the scrotum (or labium majus) and root of the penis.

Structures deep to the posterior wall

Crossing the posterior wall at the medial edge of the deep inguinal ring is the inferior epigastric artery. Lateral to the artery the ductus deferens in the male and the round ligament of the uterus in the female enter the canal by hooking around the interfoveolar ligament. At the deep ring the inferior epigastric artery gives off the cremasteric branch to supply that muscle and the coverings of the cord. The area bounded laterally by the inferior epigastric artery, medially by the lateral border of the rectus muscle, and below by the inguinal ligament is the *inguinal triangle* (of Hesselbach). By definition a hernial sac passing lateral to the artery (i.e. through the deep ring) is an *indirect hernia*, one passing medial to the artery (through the inguinal triangle) is a *direct hernia*; the latter stretches out the conjoint tendon over itself and is therefore seldom large. As an inguinal hernia emerges through the superficial inguinal ring it lies above and medial to the pubic tubercle, while the neck of a femoral hernia (see p. 122) is below and lateral to the pubic tubercle.

Spermatic cord

The spermatic cord has three coverings and six (groups of) constituents.

Of the three coverings of the spermatic cord (Fig. 5.9), the *internal spermatic fascia* is derived from the transversalis fascia at the deep inguinal ring. As the cord passes through the ring into the inguinal canal, it picks up a second covering, the *cremaster muscle* and *cremasteric fascia*. This loosely arranged layer consists of striated muscle bundles united by areolar tissue. The muscle arises laterally from the inguinal ligament, the internal oblique and transversus abdominis muscles. The fibres spiral down the cord (the longest reaching as far as the tunica vaginalis of the testis) and loop back to become attached to the pubic tubercle. The third covering, the *external spermatic fascia*, is acquired from the external oblique aponeurosis as the cord passes between the crura of the superficial ring.

The cremaster muscle can elevate the testis towards or even into the inguinal canal; although the fibres are skeletal the action is reflex rather than voluntary. This cremasteric reflex is particularly active in the infant and child and must be borne in mind when examining the scrotum in the young, to avoid an erroneous diagnosis of undescended testis.

The constituents of the cord consist of:

- The *ductus deferens*, which usually lies in the lower and posterior part of the cord.
- Arteries, the largest of which is the *testicular artery* (see below), with the *artery to the ductus* (from the superior or inferior vesical), and the *cremasteric artery* (from the inferior epigastric, Fig. 5.8) to the coverings.
- Veins—the *pampiniform plexus* (see below).

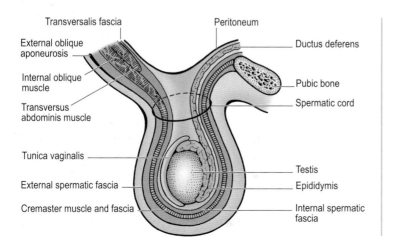

Tunica vaginalis

External spermatic fascia

Cremaster muscle and fascia

Transversalis fascia

External oblique aponeurosis

Internal oblique muscle

Transversus abdominis muscle

Peritoneum

Ductus deferens

Pubic bone

Spermatic cord

Testis

Epididymis

Internal spermatic fascia

Fig. 5.9 Formation of the sheaths of the spermatic cord, testis and epididymis.

- *Lymphatics*, essentially those from the testis draining to para-aortic nodes, but including some from the coverings which drain to external iliac nodes.
- Nerves, in particular the *genital branch* of the *genitofemoral nerve* which supplies the cremaster muscle. Other nerves are *sympathetic* twigs which accompany the arteries.
- The *processus vaginalis*, the obliterated remains of the peritoneal connection with the tunica vaginalis of the testis. When patent it forms the sac of an indirect inguinal hernia.

Testis

The testis (Fig. 5.12) is an oval organ possessing a thick covering of fibrous tissue, the *tunica albuginea*. The *epididymis* is attached to its posterolateral surface; this is an important point to remember when trying to distinguish between swellings of these two structures. The vas (ductus deferens) arises from the lower pole of the epididymis (see p. 239) and runs up medial to it behind the testis. The front and sides of the testis lie free in a serous space formed by the overlying *tunica vaginalis*, a remnant of the fetal processus vaginalis. This serous membrane covers also the anterolateral part of the epididymis and lines a slit-like space, the *sinus of the epididymis*, which lies between testis and epididymis. Testis, epididymis and tunica vaginalis lie in the scrotum surrounded by thin membranes, adherent to each other,

that are downward prolongations of the coverings of the spermatic cord (Fig. 5.9). Right and left sides are separated by the median scrotal septum (see p. 331). Average testicular dimensions are 5 cm (length), 2.5 cm (breadth), 3 cm (anteroposterior diameter). The *appendix testis* is a minute sessile cyst attached to the upper pole of the testis within the tunica vaginalis. It is a remnant of the paramesonephric duct (see p. 315).

Blood supply

The **testicular artery**, from the aorta, runs in the spermatic cord, gives off a branch to the epididymis, and reaches the back of the testis, where it divides into medial and lateral branches. These do not penetrate the mediastinum testis (see below), but sweep around horizontally within the tunica albuginea. Branches from these vessels penetrate the substance of the organ. In the region of the epididymis there is an anastomosis between the testicular, cremasteric and ductal arteries; but if the main artery is divided, the smaller vessels may not completely sustain the testis and atrophy may occur, though ischaemic necrosis is unlikely. Venules reach the mediastinum, from which several veins pass upwards in the spermatic cord as a mass of intercommunicating veins, the **pampiniform plexus** (Fig. 5.10), which surround the testicular artery. In the inguinal canal the plexus separates out into about four veins which join to form two that leave the deep inguinal ring, becoming single

Fig. 5.10 Right testicular venogram.

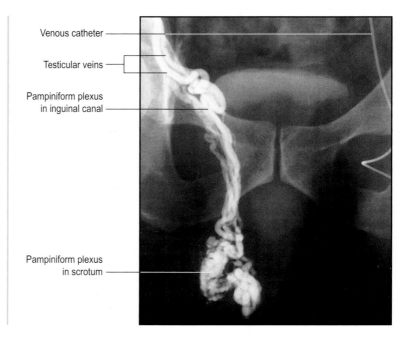

Venous catheter

Testicular veins

Pampiniform plexus in inguinal canal

Pampiniform plexus in scrotum

on psoas major on the posterior abdominal wall. The left vein invariably joins the left renal vein at a right angle and the right drains directly into the inferior vena cava at an acute angle. The testicular veins usually have valves. *Varicocele* (varicosities of the pampiniform and cremasteric veins) occurs much more frequently on the left side than the right.

Lymph drainage

Lymphatics from the testis run back with the testicular artery to para-aortic nodes lying alongside the aorta at the level of origin of the testicular arteries (L2 vertebra), i.e. just above the umbilicus. The testicular lymph therefore does not drain to inguinal nodes, although the overlying scrotal skin does.

Nerve supply

The testis is supplied by sympathetic nerves. Most of the connector cells lie in T10 segment of the cord. Passing in the greater or lesser splanchnic nerve to the coeliac ganglia the efferent fibres synapse there. Postganglionic grey fibres reach the testis along the testicular artery. Sensory fibres share the same sympathetic pathway. They run up along the testicular artery and through the coeliac plexus and lesser splanchnic nerve and its white ramus to cell bodies in the posterior root ganglion of T10 spinal nerve.

Structure

The upper pole of the epididymis is attached high up on the posterolateral surface of the testis. Here there is a fibrous mass, the *mediastinum testis*, from which septa radiate to reach the tunica albuginea. The septa divide the testis into some 200–300 *lobules*, each of which contains 1–4 highly convoluted *seminiferous tubules*. The cut surface of the organ bulges with protruding tubules. The seminiferous tubules open into the *rete testis*, which is a network of intercommunicating channels lying in the mediastinum testis. From the rete 12–20 *vasa efferentia* enter the commencement of the canal of the epididymis, thus attaching the head of the epididymis to the testis.

The seminiferous tubules have several layers of cells. The outermost layer consists of *spermatogonia*, which divide to produce the *primary spermatocytes*. These divide to form *secondary spermatocytes*. They have a very short life and divide almost immediately to form *spermatids*. These do not divide but undergo a metamorphosis into *spermatozoa*. The whole process of producing spermatozoa from spermatogonia is termed *spermatogenesis*.

Among the developing germ cells are the supporting or *sustentacular cells* (of Sertoli). The Sertoli cells secrete an androgen binding protein (ABP) which keeps a high concentration of testosterone in the germ cell environment.

Scattered among the cells of the connective tissue between the tubules (outside them) are the *interstitial cells* (of Leydig). Larger than fibroblasts, they constitute the endocrine portion of the testis and secrete testosterone.

Apart from spermatozoa, the testis makes only a small contribution to semen (seminal fluid); most of it (60%) comes from the seminal vesicles (see p. 311) and prostate (30%; see p. 309).

Development and descent of the testis

The testis develops from the gonadal ridge, formed by proliferation of the coelomic epithelium and a condensation of underlying mesoderm, on the medial side of the mesonephros (see p. 25). Primordial germ cells from the yolk sac migrate to the gonadal ridge and become incorporated in the developing gonad. At first the testis and mesonephros are situated on the posterior abdominal wall, attached by the urogenital mesentery. As the testis enlarges its cranial end degenerates and the remaining organ lies at a more caudal location. Most of the mesonephros atrophies. Derivatives of the remaining mesonephric tubules include the vasa efferentia of the testis and the *paradidymis* (a small collection of tubules above the epididymis at the lower end of the spermatic cord). In the male, the mesonephric duct forms the canal of the epididymis, ductus deferens, ejaculatory duct and the *appendix of the epididymis* (a small appendage on the head of the epididymis).

A condensation of mesodermal cells, the *gubernaculum*, connects the lower pole of the testis to the region of the anterior abdominal wall that later forms the scrotum (Fig. 5.11). It traverses the site of the future inguinal canal, which is formed around it by the developing muscles of the abdominal wall. A sac of peritoneum, the *processus vaginalis*, protrudes down the inguinal canal anterosuperior to the gubernaculum. By the seventh month of fetal life the testis is in the deep inguinal ring and thereafter it progresses rapidly through the inguinal canal into the scrotum before birth. As the testis descends it is accompanied by the processus vaginalis. The testis projects into the distal part of the processus, which forms the tunica vaginalis. The rest of this peritoneal sac usually gets obliterated. Persistence of the whole, or proximal part, of the sac maintaining its connection with the peritoneal cavity constitutes a hernial sac, a clinical hernia occurring when intra-abdominal contents enter the sac. Persistence of an intervening segment of

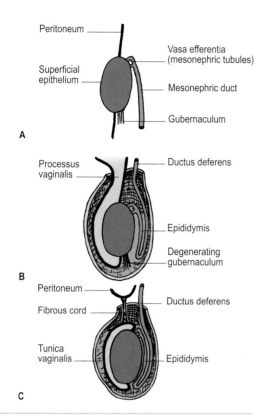

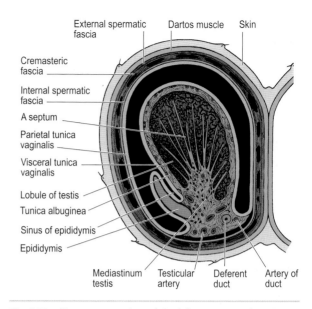

Fig. 5.12 Transverse section of the left scrotum and testis.

Fig. 5.11 Stages of testicular descent: **A** in the fetus, the testis projects through the peritoneum into the coelomic cavity—the ductus deferens (mesonephric duct) runs downwards; **B** in the neonate, the testis has reached the scrotum together with the tube-like prolongation of the peritoneal cavity, the processus vaginalis; **C** the end result, with the testis partly surrounded by the tunica vaginalis derived from the processus, and the rest of the processus reduced to a fibrous cord.

the processus may lead to the development of a hydrocele of the cord. Accumulation of serous fluid between the layers of the tunica vaginalis forms the much more common hydrocele of the testis.

Sometimes the testis is not fully descended at birth, but enters the scrotum during the first few months thereafter. Failure to descend may result in *cryptorchid testis*, where it remains in the abdomen, or descent may be arrested anywhere from the deep inguinal ring downwards. Undescended testes are peculiarly liable to malignant disease; spermatogenesis is defective or absent but androgenic activity is not. They must be distinguished from *retracted testes*, where the cremaster muscle draws them back into the canal, especially in the young under the influence of cold examining hands!

Epididymis and ductus deferens

The **epididymis** is a firm structure, attached behind the testis, with the ductus deferens to its medial side. It consists of a single highly coiled tube packed together by fibrous tissue. It has a large head at its upper end, connected by a body to a pointed tail at its lower end. The head is connected to the upper pole of the testis by the vasa efferentia and the tail to the lower pole by loose connective tissue. The body is partly separated from the testis by a recess which is open laterally, the sinus of the epididymis (Fig. 5.12). The lateral surface of the epididymis is covered by the tunica vaginalis, which also lines the sinus.

From the tail the **ductus (vas) deferens**, a direct continuation of the canal of the epididymis, provided with a thick wall of smooth muscle, passes up medially. It enters the spermatic cord, passes through the inguinal canal, across the side wall of the pelvis just under the peritoneum, and crosses the pelvic cavity. It pierces the prostate and opens by the ejaculatory duct into the prostatic urethra. Its pelvic course is described on page 311.

Blood supply

The epididymis is supplied by a branch of the testicular artery. This enters the upper pole and runs down to the lower pole. It anastomoses with the tiny artery to the ductus.

Venous and lymphatic drainage are as for the testis.

Nerve supply

The epididymis is supplied, like the testis, by sympathetic fibres from the coeliac ganglion via the testicular artery.

Structure

The epithelial lining of the coiled tube that forms the epididymis is columnar in type, with long microvilli called stereocilia. The thin wall has a single layer of circular smooth muscle.

Development

The whole length of the single tube constituting the epididymis and ductus is a persistent and much elongated part of the **mesonephric** (Wolffian) **duct** of the embryo. This duct receives the efferent tubules of the mesonephros (see p. 296). When the mesonephros is replaced by the metanephros and disappears, some of its tubules persist and attach to the developing testis, forming the vasa efferentia and draining the products of the testis into the commencement of the mesonephric duct. Some mesonephric tubules persist without serving any function of drainage. Thus, above and below the epididymis blind tubules, the *vasa aberrantia*, open into its canal. Their bulbous blind ends may form small swellings; an upper one is relatively constant, the *appendix of the epididymis*. Above the epididymis, at the lower extremity of the spermatic cord, a mass of tubules, blind at each end, persists as the *paradidymis* (organ of Giraldès). A cyst formed from an aberrant tubule will contain spermatozoa and thus be opalescent. A cyst formed from a tubule of the paradidymis cannot contain spermatozoa, and its fluid is thus crystal clear.

The **paramesonephric** (Müllerian) **duct**, developing into the uterine tube and uterus (see p. 315), disappears in the male except at its two ends. The upper end persists as the *appendix testis*, the conjoined lower ends of the two ducts persist as the *prostatic utricle* (*utriculus masculinus*) (see p. 309).

Vasectomy

The 'vas' is now renamed the 'ductus deferens' but sterilization of the male by division and ligation of the tube is still popularly known as 'vasectomy'. The spermatic cord containing the firm tubular ductus is palpated between the thumb and fingers at the top of the scrotum

and a transverse incision made so that the ductus can be dissected out and a small length of it removed. Each remaining cut end is turned back on itself and ligated, and the same procedure is then carried out on the opposite side.

Abdominal incisions

The simplest abdominal incision is the **midline incision**, above or below the umbilicus, and passing through skin and subcutaneous tissues, the linea alba, transversalis fascia, extraperitoneal fat and peritoneum. No major vessels or nerves are involved, but a few small vessels may cross the midline of the peritoneum. In the lower abdomen the linea alba is very narrow and the two rectus muscles may lie very close together; here poor suture technique predisposes to incisional hernias. In the suprapubic region the bladder must not be damaged. For laparoscopic surgery, the incision for insertion of the needle to induce pneumoperitoneum is usually made in the midline, just above or below the umbilicus, and the instrument is first directed down towards the pelvic cavity to avoid damaging the aorta. Separate incisions are made for other instruments, often lateral to the rectus sheath but not too low, to avoid the inferior epigastric vessels; transillumination from within the peritoneal cavity helps to avoid them. Other openings can be made above the umbilicus to the left of the midline (to avoid the falciform ligament which lies increasingly towards the right), or in the midclavicular or midaxillary lines below the costal margin. Sites below the umbilicus or at the lateral border of the rectus sheath are also used for the insertion of a trocar and cannula for the drainage of peritoneal fluid (paracentesis) or a peritoneal dialysis catheter.

In a **paramedian incision**, the anterior wall of the rectus sheath is incised vertically 2 cm from the midline and the rectus muscle retracted laterally so that the posterior wall of the sheath can be incised. The tendinous intersections in the rectus muscle at and above the umbilicus have to be dissected off the anterior wall of the sheath; they may contain vessels. Above the umbilicus on the right the falciform ligament may have to be divided. In a rectus split incision, through a vertical incision 3 cm from the midline the rectus is split instead of being retracted. The small part of the muscle medial to the split will be denervated and devascularized but this usually does not cause problems. The lack of a posterior wall of the sheath below a point midway between the umbilicus and pubic symphysis implies that sound healing depends on proper closure of the sheath's anterior wall.

The **right subcostal (Kocher's) incision** is made 3 cm parallel to and below the right costal margin, from the midline to beyond the lateral border of the rectus sheath. The incision is often made more horizontal than parallel to the subcostal margin. The anterior layer of the sheath (with the external oblique) and the rectus muscle are divided in the line of the skin incision, with ligation of the superior epigastric vessels and/or their branches. The posterior layer of the sheath is then incised, continuing laterally into the internal oblique and transversus and through to the peritoneum. The seventh intercostal nerve follows the costal margin upwards and is usually above the incision line, although the eighth or ninth nerve may have to be cut, with little effect on the rectus muscle. Cutting more than two nerves (paralysing more of the rectus) should be avoided.

The double Kocher or curved **rooftop incision**, combining subcostal incisions on both sides, gives a very wide exposure of the upper abdomen.

The **gridiron (McBurney's) incision** is a right lower oblique muscle-splitting incision, long used for appendicectomy. The skin incision runs downwards and medially through the junction of the outer and middle thirds of a line drawn from the anterior superior iliac spine to the umbilicus. The external oblique muscle and its aponeurosis are divided in the line of their fibres and then the internal oblique and transversus are split transversely (in the line of their own fibres). The two muscles are close and may appear as one; the transversus becomes aponeurotic at this level and adheres to the transversalis fascia. The peritoneum can then be incised. The iliohypogastric and ilioinguinal nerves may be seen between the internal oblique and transversus and must not be damaged, to avoid weakening the protective effect that the muscles exert upon the inguinal canal. Extending the incision laterally may cut the deep circumflex iliac artery's ascending branch, which runs upwards above the anterior superior iliac spine between the internal oblique and transversus.

For cosmetic reasons the gridiron incision is often replaced by a more **transverse muscle-splitting incision** in a skin crease starting above and medial to the anterior superior iliac spine and extending nearly to the lateral border of the rectus sheath.

The **oblique muscle-cutting incision** (Rutherford Morison's) is similar to the gridiron but after incising the external oblique in the line of its fibres the internal oblique and transversus are cut in the same line (not in the line of their own fibres).

Transverse muscle-cutting incisions can be made at or about the level of the umbilicus, cutting the rectus sheaths and the obliques and transversus muscles. The rectus muscle is retracted medially and rarely requires division. Intercostal nerves run obliquely through the lower abdominal wall, but more than one is not likely to be cut by this incision.

The lower abdominal **transverse incision** (Pfannenstiel's) is commonly used for approach to the pelvic organs. A skin crease incision is made above the pubic symphysis, just below the hairline, as far as the lateral borders of the rectus sheaths. The anterior layers of the rectus sheaths are divided in the line of the skin incision and flaps dissected off the muscles both upwards and downwards, including midline tissue and with the pyramidalis muscles included in the lower flap. The rectus muscles which at this level lie close together are separated to expose transversalis fascia which is incised with the peritoneum, care being taken to avoid the bladder. Transverse division of the rectus muscles gives wider exposure, and the incisions can be extended laterally into the flat muscles.

A **lumbar incision** is used for extraperitoneal approach to the kidney and upper ureter. The incision extends below the twelfth rib from the lateral border of erector spinae towards the anterior superior iliac spine. Latissimus dorsi and external oblique are incised and their cut edges retracted so that the internal oblique and transversus merging with the lumbar fascia can also be incised. The subcostal nerve deep to internal oblique should be preserved but the vessels can be ligated. The transversalis fascia and extraperitoneal fat in the posterior part of the incision are separated to expose the renal fascia. The peritoneal cavity is not entered. Proper identification of the twelfth rib is essential to avoid entering the pleural cavity, which extends below its medial part (see p. 220).

PART TWO

Abdominal cavity

The abdominal cavity is much more extensive than the impression gained from examination of the anterior abdominal wall. Much of it lies under cover of the lower ribs, for the domes of the diaphragm arch high above the costal margin. Hidden by the lower ribs are the liver and spleen, much of the stomach, and the upper poles of the kidneys and both suprarenals. The volume of the thoracic cavity is, correspondingly, much less than examination of the bony thorax would suggest. Furthermore, an appreciable amount of the abdominal cavity projects backwards into the pelvis, just in front of the buttocks. A perforating wound of the buttock can easily involve the pelvic cavity. The pelvic cavity accommodates not only its own pelvic organs (rectum, uterus, bladder, etc.), but also a goodly volume of intestine (sigmoid colon and ileum).

General topography of the abdomen

The alimentary canal and its two chief derivatives the liver and pancreas (and also the spleen) are developed in fetal mesenteries which later alter their disposition as a result of fusion of adjacent leaves of peritoneum. The liver and spleen remain invested in peritoneum, but the pancreas becomes retroperitoneal.

The alimentary canal is invested unevenly. Parts of it are suspended in the abdominal cavity by peritoneal folds ('mesenteries'); other parts become plastered down to the posterior abdominal wall. The stomach is fixed at its two ends, but is elsewhere suspended by 'mesenteries'. The duodenum is plastered down to the posterior abdominal wall, while the whole length of small intestine swings free on its own mesentery. The ascending and descending colon are both adherent to the posterior abdominal wall, but between the colic flexures the transverse colon is mobile on its own mesentery, the transverse mesocolon. The sigmoid (pelvic) colon swings free on a mesentery, while the rectum is plastered by peritoneum to the hollow of the sacrum.

The suprarenals, kidneys and ureters lie behind the peritoneum. The aorta and inferior vena cava also lie behind the peritoneum, and intestinal vessels run through the mesenteries to reach the gut.

The **transpyloric plane** bisects the body between the jugular notch and the pubic symphysis. This level is approximately midway between the xiphisternum and the umbilicus, or about a hand's breadth below the xiphisternal joint (Fig. 5.1). It cuts each costal margin at the tip of the ninth costal cartilage, which is at the lateral border of the rectus abdominis (semilunar line); deep to this point on the right side lies the fundus of the gallbladder. The plane passes through the lower border of the first lumbar vertebra, where the spinal cord ends at the conus medullaris.

As its name implies, the plane usually passes through the pylorus, but the pylorus is free on a mesentery, and therefore mobile. The plane passes along the head, neck and body of the pancreas, just above the attachment of the transverse mesocolon. The supracolic compartment (liver, spleen, fundus of stomach) lies above the plane, the infracolic compartment (small intestine, colon) below it. The superior mesenteric artery leaves the aorta, and the splenic vein joins the superior mesenteric vein to form the portal vein at this level. The hilum of each kidney lies at the plane, the right just below and the left just above it.

PART THREE

Peritoneum

The peritoneum is a serous membrane which lines the abdominal cavity; it covers the anterior and posterior walls, the undersurface of the diaphragm and the walls and floor of the pelvic cavity. All this is the **parietal peritoneum**. In places it leaves the posterior abdominal wall or diaphragm or pelvic floor to form a partial or complete investment for viscera; this is the **visceral peritoneum**, which forms the serous covering for many viscera.

Peritoneum consists of a single layer of flattened cells, with phagocytic properties, overlying areolar tissue which varies in both thickness and density in different places. Over expansile parts this areolar tissue is loose and cellular (e.g. transversalis fascia on the lower anterior abdominal wall) while over non-expansile parts it is often thick (e.g. iliac fascia, psoas fascia, parietal pelvic fascia); but loose or dense, thin or thick, these variously named fasciae are part of the one continuous extra-peritoneal connective tissue lying between the parietal peritoneum and the walls of the abdominal and pelvic cavities.

Various folds or reflexions of peritoneum connect viscera to the abdominal walls or to one another. Some of these are properly called *folds*, but others are called mesentery, omentum or ligament. The double fold supporting the small intestine is *the mesentery*; the mesenteries supporting the transverse colon, sigmoid colon and appendix are the *transverse mesocolon, sigmoid mesocolon* and *mesoappendix*. The *lesser omentum* connects the stomach to the liver, and the *greater omentum* hangs down from the lower border of the stomach. The various *ligaments* associated with the liver, stomach and spleen are simply peritoneal folds attached to them, and the broad ligament stretches out on either side of the uterus.

Peritoneal folds of the anterior abdominal wall

On the posterior surface of the anterior abdominal wall the peritoneum is raised into six folds, one above and five below the umbilicus. The **falciform ligament** consists of two adherent layers of peritoneum connecting the liver to the supraumbilical part of the anterior abdominal wall and the inferior surface of the diaphragm. Its concave, inferior margin, which contains the ligamentum teres (the obliterated remains of the left umbilical vein, see p. 33), deviates to the right and is attached to the notch for this ligament on the inferior border of the liver.

Below the umbilicus there is a central fold with a pair on either side. Centrally is the *median umbilical fold*, containing the *median umbilical ligament* (the obliterated remains of the urachus; see p. 308). On each side, and also running as far as the umbilicus, is the *medial umbilical fold*, containing the *medial umbilical ligament* (the obliterated remains of the umbilical artery; p. 33). Farther laterally is the *lateral umbilical fold*, containing the *inferior epigastric vessels*, which enter the rectus sheath by passing across the arcuate line; although called umbilical folds, this lateral pair do not reach as far as the umbilicus.

Peritoneal cavity: greater and lesser sacs

The serous-coated organs fill the abdominal cavity so that visceral surfaces are in contact with one another or with the parietal peritoneum. The space between them is only potential, not actual, and it contains only a few millilitres of tissue fluid which lubricates adjacent surfaces so they can glide over one another. This is the general peritoneal cavity or **greater sac**.

The *omental bursa*, or **lesser sac**, is a subsection or diverticulum of the peritoneal cavity behind the stomach. It opens into the greater sac through a slit-like aperture in front of the inferior vena cava, the epiploic foramen (see p. 245). The anterior wall of the lesser sac is formed by the posterior layer of the lesser omentum, the peritoneum over the posterior aspect of the stomach and the posterior of the anterior two layers of the greater omentum (Fig. 5.13). The posterior wall is formed by the anterior of the two posterior layers of the greater omentum which adheres to, but is surgically separable from, the anterior surface of the transverse colon and the transverse mesocolon. Above the attachment of the transverse mesocolon to the anterior border of the pancreas, the posterior wall is formed by the peritoneum that covers the front of the neck and body of pancreas, upper part of left kidney, left suprarenal gland, commencement of abdominal aorta, coeliac artery (plexus and nodes) and part of the diaphragm (Fig. 5.14). Theoretically the cavity of the lesser sac should extend down between the anterior two layers and the posterior two layers of the greater omentum, but because of fusion of these layers the cavity does not extend much below the transverse colon. The narrow upper border of the lesser

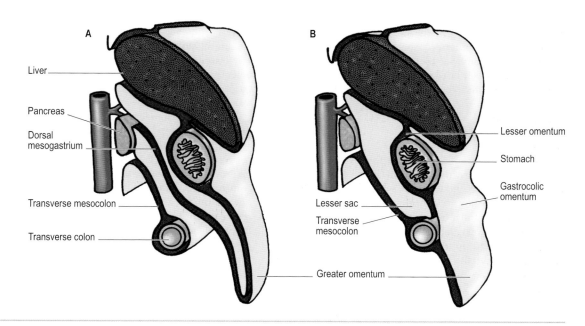

Fig. 5.13 Peritoneum of the lesser sac and greater omentum, as seen in diagrammatic sagittal sections looking towards the left: **A** the theoretical developmental condition, with the two layers of the dorsal mesogastrium overlying the two layers of the transverse mesocolon (containing the transverse colon) and forming a fold (the greater omentum) doubling back to the greater curvature of the stomach; **B** the end result, with fusion of adjacent double peritoneal layers.

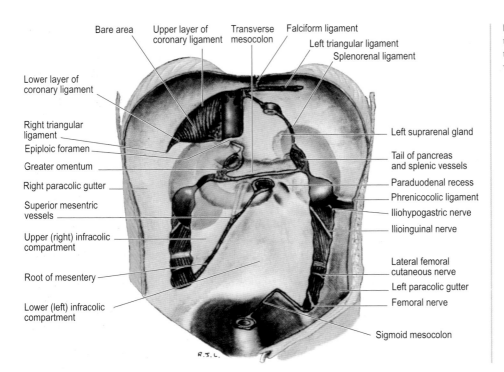

Bare area   Upper layer of coronary ligament   Transverse mesocolon   Falciform ligament   Left triangular ligament   Splenorenal ligament

Lower layer of coronary ligament

Right triangular ligament

Epiploic foramen

Greater omentum

Right paracolic gutter

Superior mesentric vessels

Upper (right) infracolic compartment

Root of mesentery

Lower (left) infracolic compartment

Left suprarenal gland

Tail of pancreas and splenic vessels

Paraduodenal recess

Phrenicocolic ligament

Iliohypogastric nerve

Ilioinguinal nerve

Lateral femoral cutaneous nerve

Left paracolic gutter

Femoral nerve

Sigmoid mesocolon

R.J.L.

Fig. 5.14 Attachments of the parietal peritoneum to the posterior abdominal wall.

sac is at the right side of the abdominal oesophagus, where the peritoneum of the posterior wall is reflected anteriorly on the inferior aspect of the diaphragm to form the posterior layer of the lesser omentum. Above the pancreas the left border of the lesser sac is formed by the splenorenal and gastrosplenic ligaments (see below and Fig. 5.49).

Greater omentum

The greater omentum is a double sheet of peritoneum, folded on itself to form four layers (Fig. 5.13). The anterior two layers descend from the greater curvature of the stomach (where they are continuous with the peritoneum on the anterior and posterior surfaces of the stomach) like an apron, overlying coils of intestine, and then turn round and ascend up to the transverse colon where they loosely blend with the peritoneum on the anterior surfaces of the transverse colon and the transverse mesocolon above it. The four layers of the greater omentum below the transverse colon fuse with each other to form an integral structure. This contains adipose tissue of variable amount, depending on the nutritional status of the patient and numerous macrophages.

The part of the greater omentum between the stomach and the transverse colon is often referred to as the

gastrocolic omentum. The right and left gastroepiploic vessels run between the layers of the gastrocolic omentum, close to the greater curvature of the stomach. The lesser sac may be accessed through the gastrocolic omentum. Other routes of surgical access to the lesser sac are through the lesser omentum and through the transverse mesocolon.

Below the stomach the left border of the greater omentum envelops the spleen, except for a small bare area at the hilum. The spleen therefore lies in the general peritoneal cavity. Two double-layered folds of peritoneum, the *gastrosplenic* and *splenorenal ligaments*, connect the hilum of the spleen to the greater curvature of the stomach and the anterior surface of the left kidney respectively. The splenic vessels and pancreatic tail lie in the splenorenal ligament and the short gastric and left gastroepiploic vessels run in the gastrosplenic ligament (Fig. 5.49).

Lesser omentum

The two layers of peritoneum that extend between the liver and the upper border (lesser curvature) of the stomach constitute the lesser omentum or *gastrohepatic omentum*). It can usually only be seen when the liver is lifted up, away from the stomach. Its attachment to the stomach extends from the *right* side of the abdominal oesophagus and along the *lesser* curvature to the first 2 cm of the duodenum (Fig. 5.35). The liver attachment is L-shaped (Fig. 5.32B), to the *fissure for the ligamentum venosum* and the *porta hepatis*. Between the duodenum and the liver it has a right free margin, where the anterior and posterior layers of peritoneum become continuous. This fold forms the anterior boundary of the epiploic foramen.

The **epiploic foramen** (of Winslow, or the *aditus to the lesser sac*, Fig. 5.35) is a vertical slit about 2.5 cm at the right border of the lesser sac. Its upper boundary is the caudate process of the liver (Fig. 5.32B). The lower boundary is the first part of the duodenum. The posterior boundary is the inferior vena cava, covered by the parietal peritoneum of the posterior abdominal wall which, continuing to the left through the foramen, becomes the peritoneum of the posterior wall of the lesser sac. Anteriorly the foramen is bounded by the right free margin of the lesser omentum containing between its two peritoneal layers the portal vein, and anterior to it the hepatic artery and bile duct, with the duct to the right of the artery, as well as autonomic nerves, lymphatics and nodes.

Traced downwards over the stomach, the two layers of the lesser omentum become the greater omentum (Fig. 5.13). Traced upwards, the two layers enclose the liver and then spread on to the diaphragm and anterior abdominal wall as the coronary, triangular and falciform ligaments (Fig. 5.14).

Peritoneal compartments

The peritoneal cavity is descriptively divided into compartments called supracolic, infracolic and pelvic.

The dividing line between the supracolic and infracolic compartments is the attachment of the **transverse mesocolon** to the posterior abdominal wall, or rather to the organs that lie on the abdominal wall at this level (Figs 5.13 and 5.14). The transverse mesocolon is a double fold of peritoneum passing from the transverse colon to the front of the second part of the duodenum, and to the anterior aspect of the head and the anterior border of the body of the pancreas. The transverse colon and transverse mesocolon are adherent to the posterior surface of the greater omentum. When the greater omentum is lifted up over the costal margin, the stomach, transverse colon and mesocolon are lifted upwards with it, and the posterior surface of the mesocolon brought into view (Fig. 5.15).

The attachments of the liver to the diaphragm and abdominal wall define the subdivisions of the supracolic compartment (Figs 5.16 and 5.32). To the right and

left of the falciform ligament are the **right** and **left subphrenic (subdiaphragmatic) spaces**. These two spaces are closed above by the superior layer of the coronary ligament and the anterior layer of the left triangular ligament respectively. Behind the right lobe of the liver and in front of the right kidney is the **right subhepatic space** or **hepatorenal pouch** (of Morison). This space is closed above by the inferior layer of the coronary ligament and the small right triangular ligament. To the right it is bounded by the abdominal surface of the diaphragm. On the left side the space communicates through the epiploic foramen with the lesser sac or **left subhepatic space**. Below it is continuous with the right paracolic gutter (see below).

When lying supine, the hepatorenal pouch is the lowest part of the peritoneal cavity (with the sole exception of the pelvis), and hence is an area where intraperitoneal fluid is likely to accumulate.

The infracolic compartment, below the level of the transverse mesocolon, is divided into two by the attachment of the **root of the mesentery** of the small intestine (Fig. 5.14), which passes down from left to right at an angle of about 45°. It begins on the left at the duodeno-jejunal junction, crosses the third part of the duodenum where the superior mesenteric vessels enter between its two layers, and then continues downwards across the aorta, inferior vena cava, right psoas muscle and ureter to the right iliac fossa. This attachment is 15 cm long. The intestinal border of the mesentery is plicated like the hem of a very full skirt and measures about 6 m long. The depth of the mesentery (from root to gut) is greatest at the central part, about 20 cm.

In the retroperitoneal tissue in the region of the root of the mesentery there are numerous Pacinian corpuscles. It is well established that tension and traction on peritoneal folds in the upper abdomen produce a fall of blood pressure by undue stimulation of these encapsulated mechanoreceptors.

To the right of the root of the mesentery is the triangular **right infracolic space** (Fig. 5.14). Its apex lies below, at the ileocaecal junction. Its right side is the ascending colon, and its base is the attachment of the transverse mesocolon.

Lateral to the ascending colon is the **right paracolic gutter**. It can be traced upwards into the hepatorenal pouch and downwards into the pelvis—pathways for the gravitation of fluid.

The **left infracolic space** is larger than the right infracolic compartment and is quadrilateral in shape. It widens below where it is continuous across the pelvic brim with the cavity of the pelvis (Fig. 5.14). Its upper border is the attachment of the transverse mesocolon, and its left side is the descending colon.

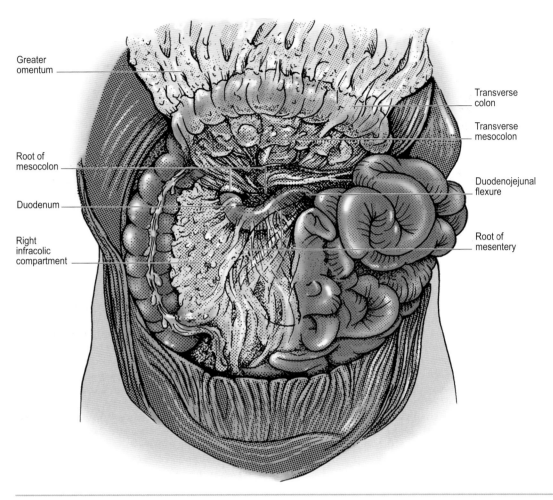

Fig. 5.15   Infracolic compartment of peritoneum. The greater omentum, transverse mesocolon and transverse colon have been lifted up and the small intestine pulled towards the left side of the peritoneal cavity, to show the root of the transverse mesocolon, root of the mesentery and the upper (right) infracolic compartment.

Lateral to the descending colon is the **left paracolic gutter** (Fig. 5.14). It is limited above by a small transverse fold of peritoneum between the left (splenic) flexure of the colon and the diaphragm, the *phrenicocolic ligament*. Traced downwards the gutter leads to the left of the attachment of the lateral limb of the sigmoid mesocolon at the pelvic brim.

At the lower end of the left infracolic compartment is the attachment of the **sigmoid mesocolon** (Fig. 5.14). It is Λ-shaped and the two limbs diverge from each other at the bifurcation of the common iliac vessels, on the

pelvic brim over the left sacroiliac joint. The lateral limb passes forwards along the pelvic brim (over the external iliac vessels) halfway to the inguinal ligament (i.e. about 5 cm), while the medial limb slopes down into the hollow of the sacrum, where it reaches the midline in front of S3 vertebra, at the commencement of the rectum. At the apex of the attachment of the pelvic mesocolon, just beneath the peritoneum and lying over the bifurcation of the common iliac artery, is the left ureter, with the inferior mesenteric vessels medial to it, the vein lying between the ureter and the artery.

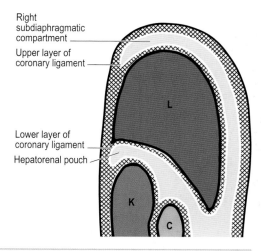

Right subdiaphragmatic compartment

Upper layer of coronary ligament

L

Lower layer of coronary ligament

Hepatorenal pouch

K

C

Fig. 5.16 Sagittal section through the right lobe of the liver (L), kidney (K) and transverse colon (C), showing peritoneal reflections and the formation of the hepatorenal pouch.

Nerve supply

The parietal peritoneum is supplied segmentally by the spinal nerves that innervate the overlying muscles. Thus the diaphragmatic peritoneum is supplied centrally by the phrenic nerve (C4)—hence referred pain and hyperaesthesia from this area to the tip of the shoulder—and peripherally by intercostal nerves. The remainder of the parietal peritoneum is supplied segmentally by intercostal and lumbar nerves. In the pelvis the obturator nerve is the chief source of supply. The visceral peritoneum is innervated by afferent nerves which travel with the autonomic supply to the viscera. Pain from diseased viscera is due to ischaemia, muscle spasm and stretching of the visceral peritoneum, including mesenteric folds or involvement of the parietal peritoneum.

Retroperitoneal space

Several major structures lie on the posterior abdominal wall behind the peritoneum. These include the aorta and inferior vena cava with a number of their branches and tributaries; the cisterna chyli, lymph nodes and vessels; nerves (mostly branches of the lumbar plexus) including the sympathetic trunks; the kidneys, ureters, pancreas, ascending and descending colon and most of the duodenum and suprarenal glands. All these can be said to lie in the **retroperitoneal space**, though the term is often used to apply only to the area of the posterior abdominal wall behind the peritoneum that

is not occupied by the major viscera and great vessels, e.g. over parts of psoas and other muscles. Haemorrhage and infection may develop in it and blood and pus may be confined to the retroperitoneal space.

PART FOUR

Development of the gut

The disposition of the gut and its mesenteries in the early embryo is simple. The more complex arrangement in the adult is due to elongation and consequent coiling of the alimentary canal and to fusion of certain adjacent peritoneal surfaces.

Gut arteries

Just before the sixth week of embryonic life the alimentary canal is a simple tube passing through to the hind end, its whole length supported by a dorsal mesentery attached in the midline in front of the aorta (Fig. 5.17). Three gut arteries leave the aorta and pass ventrally to supply the tube. The most cranial passes in the *dorsal mesogastrium* to supply the foregut, the next passes through the dorsal mesentery to supply the midgut and the last passes through the dorsal mesocolon to supply the hindgut. They are the coeliac, the superior mesenteric and the inferior mesenteric arteries respectively, and they continue to supply the derivatives of these parts of the alimentary canal in the adult.

The *foregut* possesses, in addition, a *ventral mesogastrium* (derived from the septum transversum, see p. 26) attached in the midline to the undersurface of the diaphragm and the anterior abdominal wall down to the umbilicus (Fig. 5.17). Its caudal free edge is crescentic and carries the left umbilical vein.

The derivatives of the foregut (liver and pancreas) and also the spleen are supplied with blood by the artery of the foregut, the coeliac artery. The liver develops as an outgrowth from the foregut at its junction with the midgut. A tube grows ventrally into the ventral mesogastrium, bifurcates, and cells proliferate from the blind end of the two divisions to form the two lobes of the liver, which are thus enclosed between the two layers of the ventral mesogastrium. The pancreas develops as two outgrowths, one into the ventral and one into the dorsal mesogastrium. These two parts subsequently fuse and exchange ducts by anastomosis, but the double origin of the pancreas is imprinted on the adult by the persistence of two pancreatic ducts, the main and the accessory. The spleen develops by proliferation of cells in the left leaf of the dorsal mesogastrium. It is not

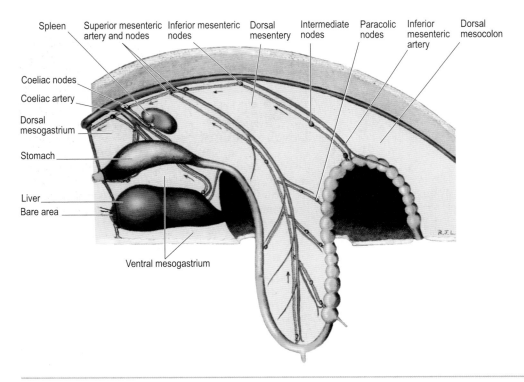

Fig. 5.17   Representation of the developing alimentary canal, viewed from the left, at the stage of herniation of the midgut. Lymphatics run back along the gut arteries to preaortic nodes.

a derivative of the foregut itself. The coeliac artery supplies the stomach and these three organs in the adult, where it is properly called the coeliac trunk.

Lymph drainage

Lymph from the alimentary canal drains by lymph vessels that run with the arteries and end ultimately in lymph nodes that lie in front of the aorta at the roots of the three gut arteries. Lymph from the mucous membrane of the alimentary canal passes through several filters. In the mucous membrane itself, from tonsils to anal margin, are lymphoid follicles. In the mesentery, at its gut margin, are lymph nodes (the 'para-' group, e.g. paracolic). In the mesentery between its gut margin and root are further intermediate nodes. The preaortic nodes, inferior mesenteric, superior mesenteric, and coeliac, are interconnected by lymph vessels. All the lymph thus ultimately reaches the coeliac nodes, whence it passes to the cisterna chyli. This simple lymphatic arrangement persists in the adult.

Herniation of the gut

By the end of the sixth week the liver has enlarged greatly and the gut has elongated, both to such an extent that the more leisurely growing abdominal walls cannot accommodate them. A loop of gut extrudes into the umbilical cord as the *physiological hernia* (Fig. 5.17). The loop remains in the umbilical cord for a full month. At the end of the tenth week the abdominal walls have grown enough to accommodate the abdominal contents and the hernia is reduced.

The herniated loop of gut is that supplied by the superior mesenteric artery and it is defined as the *midgut*. It is destined to produce all the small intestine from the distal part of the duodenum (i.e. distal to the entry of the bile duct) and the proximal part of the colon, almost as far as the left colic flexure. The apex of the loop is at the attachment of the vitellointestinal duct (see p. 26), the site of the ileal (Meckel's) diverticulum. The main trunk of the superior mesenteric artery is directed to the apex of the loop. Many branches run from it to the proximal limb of the loop, extending from the ventral pancreatic bud to Meckel's diverticulum. They persist as the jejunal and ileal branches. Only three branches run to the distal limb of the loop; all three persist in the adult as the ileocolic, right colic and middle colic arteries. Their directions are altered considerably after the reduction of the physiological hernia and the rotation of the gut.

Rotation of the midgut

As the loop of midgut in the physiological hernia returns to the abdominal cavity it rotates so that the distal limb goes up on the left and the proximal limb goes down on the right, i.e. to the observer looking at the front of the abdomen, in an anticlockwise direction (Fig. 5.18). The distal loop, developing into colon, thus comes to lie anterior to the commencement of the proximal loop. The commencement of the proximal loop becomes, after some rotation, plastered to the posterior abdominal wall as the duodenum, and the mesentery of the transverse colon thus comes to lie across it (Fig. 5.19). The last part of the midgut to be reincluded within the abdominal cavity is the caecum, which lies first near the midline, high up. It grows then to the right, turns downwards at the right colic flexure and stops elongating at the right iliac fossa. It leaves a trail of large intestine to indicate its migration and drags the attached lower end of the ileum with it.

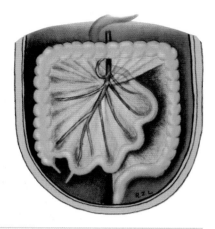

Fig. 5.19 Return of the physiological hernia and completion of rotation of the midgut, viewed from the front. The midgut loop rotates altogether through 270°: 90° during herniation and 180° during return into the abdominal cavity.

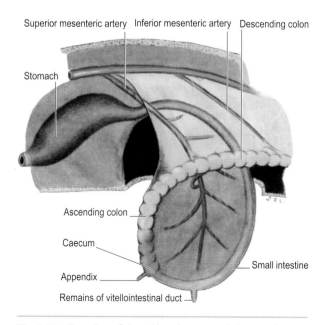

Fig. 5.18 Rotation of the midgut loop round the superior mesenteric artery, viewed from the left.

Rotation of the midgut loop occurs around the axis of the superior mesenteric artery, so in the adult the branches to the proximal loop (jejunal and ileal arteries) come off its left side while the three branches to the distal loop (colic arteries) leave its right side (Figs 5.19 and 5.23).

The simple dorsal mesentery of the midgut containing the superior mesenteric artery is, of course, much twisted and distorted during the return of the rotated loop of midgut and the subsequent migration of the caecum. Its attachment to the proximal loop causes it to pass across the posterior abdominal wall from the commencement of the loop (duodenum) to the ileocaecal junction (Fig. 5.14). The dorsal mesentery of the distal loop of the midgut hinges like a door across from the midline to the right. It comes into contact with the parietal peritoneum in the right paravertebral gutter, with which it fuses, the colic vessels lying immediately deep to it and in front of everything else on the posterior abdominal wall. The dorsal mesentery of the most distal part of the distal loop, pulled across transversely, does not fuse completely with the parietal peritoneum and persists, with the middle colic artery between its layers, as the transverse mesocolon (Fig. 5.19).

Movement of the hindgut

As the midgut loop returns to the abdominal cavity, the *hindgut* swings on its dorsal mesocolon like a door across to the left (Fig. 5.20), and the mesocolon fuses with the parietal peritoneum of the left paravertebral

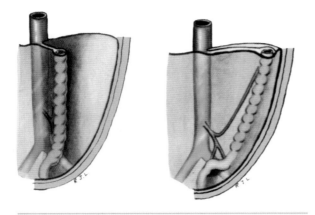

Fig. 5.20 Hindgut before and after return of the midgut hernia, viewed from the front. The mesocolon fuses with the peritoneum of the posterior abdominal wall except at the pelvic brim, where part of the embryonic mesocolon persists as the sigmoid mesocolon.

gutter; a white line (of Toldt) marks the site of fusion along the left side of the descending colon. Hence the left colic vessels lie in front of everything else on the posterior abdominal wall. At the pelvic brim fusion of the layers is not complete and a small part of the intestinal edge of the dorsal mesocolon of the hindgut remains free as the sigmoid mesocolon of the adult.

Growth of the liver

The liver grows apace, and soon outstrips the ventral mesogastrium in which it lies. It grows caudally into the

free edge of the ventral mesogastrium, which it pushes down until the left umbilical vein (*ligamentum teres* in the adult) notches its inferior border and is enclosed in a deep groove on its undersurface. This encroachment of the liver over the crescentic free margin of the ventral mesogastrium divides the latter into two separate parts, namely the *falciform ligament* between liver and anterior abdominal wall and the *lesser omentum* (gastrohepatic omentum) between liver and stomach (Fig. 5.17). The lesser omentum is attached to the liver along a fissure that runs backwards behind the fissure for the ligamentum teres (Fig. 5.33), and lodges the fibrous remnant of the ductus venosus (*ligamentum venosum*).

Rotation of the foregut

Coincident with the growth of the liver, the foregut rotates. The liver originally was ventral to the foregut, in the ventral mesogastrium, and both lie in the midline. As the liver grows it swings to the right, taking the ventral mesogastrium with it. The stomach swings across to the left and in doing so rotates (Fig. 5.21). It has already elongated and broadened, with its dorsal border becoming convex, and its ventral border concave. The distal end of the foregut, destined to become the duodenum (i.e. proximal to the entry of the bile duct), does not dilate in this manner, and its dorsal mesentery shortens. The duodenal part of the gut elongates into a loop which swings to the right and becomes plastered to the posterior abdominal wall (like the ascending and descending parts of the colon). At the same time its walls grow asymmetrically so that the ventral bile duct

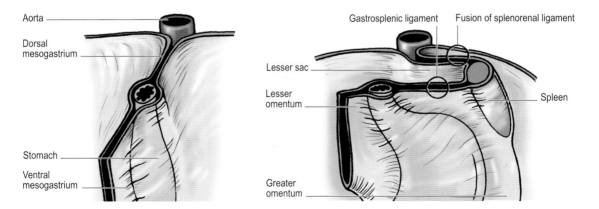

Fig. 5.21 Rotation of the stomach, viewed from the front after removal of the liver (kidney and pancreas not shown). The dorsal mesogastrium balloons down and to the left (and the spleen develops within it), and the stomach rotates through 90° so that its left surface becomes anterior, and its right surface becomes posterior, at the front of the lesser sac, with the spleen at the left margin of the sac.

and pancreatic duct are carried around to open on the medial wall (Fig. 5.40) in line with the duct of the dorsal diverticulum. The duodenum is now fixed in position; so, too, is the oesophagus at the diaphragm. Between these two fixed points as an axis, the dorsal convexity of the stomach rotates to the left. The dorsal convexity becomes the greater curvature, and the original left side of the stomach now faces anteriorly. The concave ventral border becomes the lesser curvature, attached by the lesser omentum (originally the ventral mesogastrium) to the liver, and to the diaphragm between liver and oesophagus. The original right surface of the stomach now lies behind, and faces the peritoneum of the posterior abdominal wall. The space behind the stomach and the lesser omentum is the lesser sac, and the free edge of the lesser omentum lies over the opening from the greater sac into this space. The rotation of the stomach accounts for the left and right vagal nerve trunks becoming anterior and posterior, respectively, in relation to the stomach.

Meanwhile changes have occurred in the disposition of the dorsal mesogastrium. As the dorsal border of the stomach swings to the left the dorsal mesogastrium hinges to the left from this attachment and adheres to the parietal peritoneum as far left as the front of the left kidney. From the front of the left kidney, and from the diaphragm above it, the two layers of the dorsal mesogastrium pass to the oesophagus and the upper part of the greater curvature of the stomach. They form part of the greater omentum, and constitute the left boundary of the lesser sac behind the stomach. The spleen projects from the left leaf into the greater sac, and it divides this part of the greater omentum into *gastrosplenic and splenorenal ligaments* (Fig. 5.21).

The more caudal part of the dorsal mesogastrium is attached to the lower part of the greater curvature of the stomach, the inferior border of the pylorus and the first 2 cm of the duodenum. Its dorsal attachment, in the midline, hinges to the left and becomes plastered to, and fused with, the peritoneum on the posterior abdominal wall over the pancreas. Below this it balloons down like an apron from the greater curvature, over the transverse mesocolon and transverse colon, and returns to the posterior abdominal wall (Fig. 5.13). The deeper part of the double layer fuses with the upper leaf of the transverse mesocolon and with the transverse colon itself, forming the inferior limit of the lesser sac. The superficial part hangs down from the greater curvature to the transverse colon, to which it adheres, forming the gastrocolic omentum, a part of the greater omentum, which is the anterior wall of the lower part of the lesser sac.

From the transverse colon the dependent dorsal mesogastrium hangs down over the front of the coils

of small intestine as a fat-containing apron, the main *greater omentum*.

PART FIVE

Vessels and nerves of the gut

Blood supply of the foregut

Coeliac trunk

This is the artery of the foregut, and its three branches—the left gastric, splenic and common hepatic arteries—supply not only the gut from the lower part of the oesophagus down to the opening of the bile duct into the duodenum, but also the foregut derivatives (the liver and pancreas) and the spleen. It arises from the front of the abdominal aorta between the crura of the diaphragm a little below the median arcuate ligament, at the level of the body of T12 vertebra. It is usually a short wide trunk, flanked by the coeliac group of preaortic lymph nodes. The coeliac ganglia lie one on each side and they send to the artery sympathetic nerves which are carried along all its branches.

At the upper border of the pancreas the trunk divides into its three branches behind the peritoneum of the posterior wall of the lesser sac (Fig. 5.22).

The **left gastric artery** runs upwards across the left crus towards the oesophageal opening in the diaphragm. It gives off oesphageal branches and turns antero-inferiorly, raising a small fold of peritoneum, the left gastropancreatic fold. It then runs to the right in the lesser omentum along the lesser curvature and supplies the stomach.

The **splenic artery** passes to the left. It is usually very tortuous; the crests of its waves appear above the pancreas, and the troughs lie hidden behind its upper border. It runs across the left crus and left psoas to the hilum of the left kidney, where it turns forward in the splenorenal ligament to the hilum of the spleen. Apart from the spleen it is the main supply to the pancreas. Before breaking up into its terminal splenic branches it gives off about 6 **short gastric arteries** which run in the gastrosplenic ligament, and the **left gastroepiploic artery** which runs to the right in the greater omentum, a little distance away from the greater curvature, from where it gives branches to the stomach and the omentum. From the middle part of its course the splenic artery may give off a posterior gastric artery to the stomach.

The **common hepatic artery** passes over the upper border of the pancreas, downwards and to the right behind the peritoneum of the posterior abdominal wall

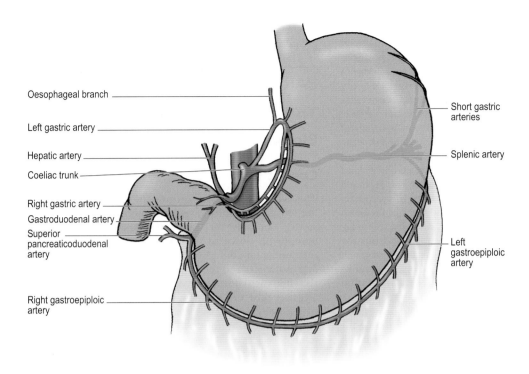

Oesophageal branch

Left gastric artery

Hepatic artery

Coeliac trunk

Right gastric artery

Gastroduodenal artery

Superior pancreaticoduodenal artery

Right gastroepiploic artery

Short gastric arteries

Splenic artery

Left gastroepiploic artery

Fig. 5.22   Arterial supply of the stomach, from the three branches of the coeliac trunk.

as far as the first part of the duodenum. It then turns forward, raising a small fold of peritoneum, the right gastropancreatic fold, and curves upwards between the two layers of the lesser omentum as the **hepatic artery**. Here it meets the bile duct and lies on its left side, both in front of the portal vein surrounded by the peritoneum at the free edge of the lesser omentum. On reaching the porta hepatis, the hepatic artery divides into right and left branches to supply the right and left halves of the liver. These branches and the associated aberrant or accessory hepatic arteries are described on page 271.

The common hepatic usually gives off the right gastric and gastroduodenal arteries.

The **right gastric artery** leaves the common hepatic as it turns forwards into the lesser omentum. It runs to the left along the lesser curvature and anastomoses with the left gastric artery.

The **gastroduodenal artery** passes down behind the first part of the duodenum, where it may be eroded by a duodenal ulcer. At the lower border of the duodenum it divides into two. The **right gastroepiploic artery** passes forward between the first part of the duodenum and the pancreas, and turns to the left between the two leaves

of the greater omentum. It runs close to the greater curvature of the stomach and anastomoses with the left gastroepiploic artery.

The other branch of the gastroduodenal artery is the **superior pancreaticoduodenal artery**. It divides into a smaller anterior and a larger posterior branch, which may arise directly from the gastroduodenal artery; they anastomose with similar branches of the inferior pancreaticoduodenal branch of the superior mesenteric artery. The pancreaticoduodenal arteries supply the duodenum, head of the pancreas and bile duct. The entrance of the bile duct marks the junction of foregut and midgut, and is the meeting place of the arterial distributions of their respective arteries, coeliac and superior mesenteric.

One or two small *supraduodenal arteries* may arise from the common hepatic artery or its branches.

Venous drainage of the foregut

Right and left gastric, right and left gastroepiploic and the short gastric veins run with the corresponding arteries. All this blood reaches the liver via the portal vein (see p. 276) and, with the arterial blood of the hepatic artery, passes through the liver to be carried via the hepatic veins to the inferior vena cava.

The lower third of the oesophagus in the posterior mediastinum drains downwards by **oesophageal veins**, through the oesophageal opening in the diaphragm, to the left gastric vein. The oesophagus above this level drains into the azygos system of veins.

The **left gastric vein** runs to the left along the lesser curvature up to the oesophagus, then passes medially behind the peritoneum of the posterior wall of the lesser sac to join the portal vein at the upper border of the first part of the duodenum. The **right gastric vein** runs along the lesser curvature to the pylorus and empties into the portal vein. It receives the *prepyloric vein* which ascends in front of the pylorus.

The **short gastric** and **left gastroepiploic veins** run with the arteries through the gastrosplenic ligament and greater omentum to the hilum of the spleen, where they empty into the splenic vein.

The **splenic vein** begins in the hilum of the spleen by confluence of half a dozen tributaries from that organ. Having received the short gastric and left gastroepiploic veins, it passes with the tail of the pancreas, below the splenic artery, in the splenorenal ligament to lie over the hilum of the left kidney. It is a large straight vein which passes to the right, posterior to the body of the pancreas (Fig. 5.26), which it grooves. In its course it lies on the hilum of the left kidney, the left psoas muscle and left sympathetic trunk, the left crus of the diaphragm, the aorta and superior mesenteric artery and the inferior vena cava. It lies in front of the left renal vein along the upper border of that vessel. In front of the inferior vena cava it joins the superior mesenteric vein at a right angle to form the portal vein. It receives many tributaries from the tail, body, neck and head of the pancreas. As it lies in front of the left crus of the diaphragm it receives the inferior mesenteric vein from the hindgut.

The **right gastroepiploic vein** runs to the right in the greater omentum and descends over the front of the pancreas to join the superior mesenteric vein at the lower border of the neck of the pancreas.

The **superior pancreaticoduodenal vein** ascends behind the head of the pancreas to join the portal vein at the upper border of the pancreas.

Blood supply of the midgut

Superior mesenteric artery

This is the artery of the midgut and supplies the gut from the entrance of the bile duct to a level just short of the splenic flexure of the colon. The artery arises from the front of the aorta a centimetre below the coeliac trunk,

at the level of the lower border of L1 vertebra. It is directed steeply downwards behind the splenic vein and the body of the pancreas, with the superior mesenteric vein on its right side. It lies anterior to the left renal vein, the uncinate process of the pancreas and the third part of the duodenum, in that order from above downwards (Fig. 5.26). With its vein it enters the upper end of the mesentery of the small intestine and passes down to the right along the root of the mesentery (Fig. 5.23). Pressure of the superior mesenteric artery on the left renal vein may produce left-sided varicocele, and pressure on the duodenum may give symptoms of chronic duodenal ileus.

The **inferior pancreaticoduodenal artery** is its first branch, arising from the posterior surface; it may come off the first jejunal branch. It divides into anterior and posterior branches which run in the curve between the duodenum and the head of the pancreas, supply both, and anastomose with the terminal branches of the superior pancreaticoduodenal artery.

The **jejunal and ileal branches** arise from the left of the main trunk and pass down between the two layers of the mesentery. The pattern of anastomosing arcades from which vessels enter the gut wall is described with the jejunum and ileum (see p. 263).

The **ileocolic artery** (Fig. 5.23) arises from the right side of the superior mesenteric trunk low down in the base of the mesentery. It descends to the right iliac fossa and divides into superior and inferior branches. The superior branch runs up along the left side of the ascending colon to anastomose with the right colic artery. The inferior branch runs to the ileocolic junction, and gives off anterior and posterior caecal arteries, an appendicular artery, and an ileal branch which ascends to the left on the ileum to anastomose with the terminal branch of the superior mesenteric artery.

The **right colic artery** (Fig. 5.23) arises from the right side of the superior mesenteric artery, or in common with the ileocolic artery. It runs to the right across the right psoas muscle, gonadal vessels, ureter and genitofemoral nerve, and quadratus lumborum, just behind the peritoneal floor of the right infracolic compartment. It divides near the left side of the ascending colon into two branches. The descending branch runs down to anastomose with the superior branch of the ileocolic artery. The ascending branch runs up across the inferior pole of the right kidney to the hepatic flexure where it anastomoses with a branch of the middle colic artery.

The **middle colic artery** (Fig. 5.23) arises from the right side of the superior mesenteric artery, as the artery emerges at the lower border of the neck of the pancreas, and descends between the two leaves of the transverse mesocolon. It lies to the right of the midline and at the

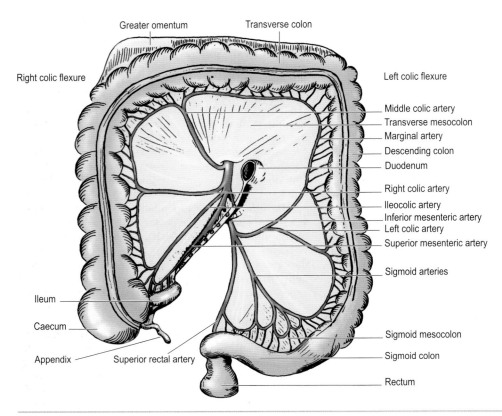

Fig. 5.23 Distribution of the superior and inferior mesenteric arteries to the large intestine. The transverse colon has been displaced upwards to expose the inferior layer of the transverse mesocolon; the middle colic artery thus appears to be running upwards, but in the normal position it passes downwards.

intestinal border of the transverse mesocolon it divides into right and left branches which run along the margin of the transverse colon. The right branch anastomoses with the ascending branch of the right colic artery. The left branch supplies the transverse colon almost to the splenic flexure (the distal part of the midgut) where it anastomoses with a branch of the left colic artery. As the middle colic lies to the right of the midline it leaves a large avascular window to its left in the transverse mesocolon. This window is the site of election for surgical access to the lesser sac and the posterior wall of the stomach (Fig. 5.23).

Venous drainage of the midgut

Each branch of the superior mesenteric artery is accompanied by a vein. All these veins flow into the **superior mesenteric vein**, a large trunk which lies to the right of the artery. It crosses the third part of the duodenum and the uncinate process of the pancreas. Behind the neck of

the pancreas it is joined by the splenic vein to form the portal vein. This continues upwards behind the first part of the duodenum. The superior mesenteric and portal veins represent a single continuing venous trunk, named portal vein above, and superior mesenteric vein below, the level of entry of the splenic vein (Fig. 5.26).

Blood supply of the hindgut

Inferior mesenteric artery

This is the artery of the hindgut; its area of supply extends as far as the upper third of the anal canal, i.e. to the level of the pectinate (dentate) line (see p. 325). The inferior mesenteric artery arises from the front of the aorta behind the inferior border of the third part of the duodenum, opposite L3 vertebra, at the level of the umbilicus, 3 or 4 cm above the aortic bifurcation. It is smaller than the superior mesenteric artery. It runs obliquely down to the pelvic brim, immediately beneath the peritoneal floor of the left infracolic compartment. It gives off the left colic and sigmoid arteries. It crosses the pelvic brim at the bifurcation of the left common iliac vessels over the sacroiliac joint, at which point it converges towards the ureter, with the inferior mesenteric vein lying between them, at the apex of the Λ-shaped attachment of the sigmoid mesocolon. Its branches cross to the left in front of the ureter and the other structures in the posterior abdominal wall of the left infracolic compartment. Beyond the pelvic brim it continues along the pelvic wall in the root of the sigmoid mesocolon as the **superior rectal artery** (see p. 304).

The **left colic artery** leaves the trunk and passes upwards and to the left behind the peritoneum. After a short course it divides into an ascending and a descending branch. The ascending branch continues laterally and upwards, crossing the left psoas muscle, gonadal vessels, ureter and genitofemoral nerve, and quadratus lumborum. It is crossed anteriorly by the inferior mesenteric vein. The descending branch passes laterally and downwards. The branches of these two arteries anastomose with each other as well as (above) with the left branch of the middle colic artery and (below) with the highest sigmoid artery, thus contributing to an anastomotic channel along the inner margin of the colon (Fig. 5.24 and p. 267).

The **sigmoid arteries** are two to four branches which pass between the layers of the sigmoid mesocolon, in which they form anastomosing loops. The last sigmoid branch anastomoses with the first branch of the superior rectal artery.

Venous drainage of the hindgut

The superior rectal vein runs up in the root of the sigmoid mesocolon, on the left of the superior rectal artery, to the pelvic brim, above which it is named the **inferior mesenteric vein**. This receives tributaries identical with the branches of the inferior mesenteric artery. The vein itself runs vertically upwards well to the left of the artery, beneath the peritoneal floor of the left infracolic compartment. It lies on the left psoas muscle, in front of the gonadal vessels, ureter and genitofemoral nerve. At the upper limit of the left infracolic compartment, just below the attachment of the transverse mesocolon, it lies to the left of the duodenojejunal flexure. Here it curves towards the right and often raises up a ridge of peritoneum. This ridge may be excavated by a small recess of peritoneum, thus making a shallow cave, the paraduodenal recess (see p. 263).

The inferior mesenteric vein now passes behind the lower border of the body of the pancreas, in front of the left renal vein, and joins the splenic vein. Occasionally it curves to the right more sharply, and passes behind the pancreas, below and parallel with the splenic vein, in front of the superior mesenteric artery, to open directly into the superior mesenteric vein.

Fig. 5.24 Inferior mesenteric arteriogram. Excretion of the contrast medium through the urinary system has commenced.

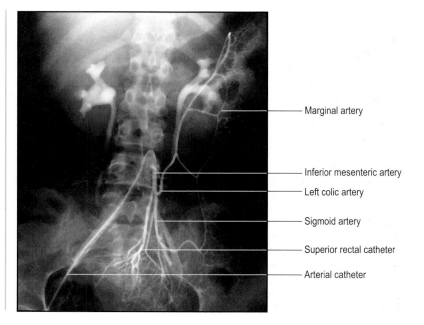

— Marginal artery

— Inferior mesenteric artery

— Left colic artery

— Sigmoid artery

— Superior rectal catheter

— Arterial catheter

Lymph drainage of the gastrointestinal tract

From the whole length of the gastrointestinal tract the lymph vessels pass back along the arteries to lymph nodes that lie in front of the aorta at the origins of the gut arteries (Fig. 5.17). These comprise the coeliac, superior mesenteric and inferior mesenteric groups of lymph nodes. They drain into each other from below upwards, the coeliac group itself draining by two or three lymph channels into the cisterna chyli.

These preaortic lymph nodes are the last in a series of lymph node filters that lie between the mucous membrane of the gut and the cisterna chyli. The first filtering mechanism consists of isolated *lymphoid follicles* which lie in the mucous membrane of the alimentary canal from mouth to anus. They are not very numerous in the oesophagus, are more numerous in the stomach, and become increasingly so along the small intestine (the MALT, see p. 10). In the lower reaches of the ileum they become aggregated together into *Peyer's patches* visible through the muscular wall. These lie on the anti-mesenteric border of the ileum and are oval in shape, with their long axes lying longitudinally along the ileum. In the large intestine the lymphoid follicles in the mucous membrane are numerous, but isolated from each other. In the appendix they are aggregated as in a tonsil.

Lymph vessels pass from the follicles in the mucous membrane through the muscle wall of the gut to nearby nodes. The various groups of nodes are considered with the individual organs and have particular significance for the stomach and large intestine in view of the prevalence of carcinoma at these sites. However, it is convenient to note here that the small and large intestines have a common pattern of three groups of nodes. The first group lies in the peritoneum adjacent to the margin of the gut, the *mural nodes* in the mesentery of the small intestine, and the *paracolic nodes* of the large intestine. The second group of *intermediate nodes* lies along the main blood vessels of supply, and the third are the *preaortic nodes* at the origins of the coeliac and the superior and inferior mesenteric arteries. The large intestine has some additional nodes which lie on the external surface of the gut wall (and occasionally within appendices epiploicae); these are the *epicolic nodes*.

Nerve supply of the gastrointestinal tract

All parts of the gut and its derivatives are innervated by parasympathetic and sympathetic nerves, which travel together along the gut arteries to reach their destination. Most come from the coeliac plexus and connected plexuses on the abdominal aorta (see p. 291), but the inferior hypogastric (pelvic) plexus (see p. 322) contributes parasympathetic fibres to the hindgut.

From the middle third of the oesophagus to the rectum, nerve cells and fibres that supply muscle, blood vessels and glands are concentrated in two plexuses. The **myenteric plexus** (of Auerbach) is situated between the two muscle layers of the gut and the **submucous plexus** (of Meissner) is in the submucosa. Collectively the plexuses form the **enteric nervous system**. The system receives postganglionic sympathetic (inhibitory) and preganglionic parasympathetic (excitatory) fibres, but is unique in being able to function without these extrinsic efferent supplies, which do not pass directly to the gut muscle; the enteric system always intervenes. Afferent fibres connect with the spinal cord (by the sympathetic trunks) and with the brainstem (by the vagus). Pain impulses are transmitted by sympathetic and parasympathetic fibres, while impulses mediating sensations of distension pass in parasympathetic fibres.

PART SIX

Gastrointestinal tract

General structural features

The alimentary canal has its embryological origin in the yolk sac. It is lined by epithelium derived from the endoderm, and outgrowths from this epithelium (liver and pancreas) are thus endodermal in origin.

Macroscopically the alimentary canal is a tube of muscle lined with mucous membrane and covered, for the most part, with peritoneum.

The **muscular wall** of the alimentary canal, from the upper end of the oesophagus to the lower end of the rectum, is in two separate layers, an inner circular and an outer longitudinal. This arrangement is characteristic of all tubes that empty by orderly peristalsis and not by a mass contraction. In reality the muscle is in two spiral layers. The inner layer forms a closewound spiral and is known as the *circular layer*, while the outer layer spirals in such gradual fashion that its fibres are virtually longitudinal, the *longitudinal layer*. The latter is mostly separated into three discrete bundles, the taeniae coli, in the colon. An innermost third layer reinforces the body of the stomach.

The two layers of the upper third of the oesophagus (cervical and superior mediastinal parts) consist of striated muscle. In the lower two-thirds of the oesophagus this is gradually replaced by visceral muscle, which constitutes the two layers of the remainder of the alimentary canal.

The **mucous membrane** of the alimentary tube consists of three components: *epithelium*, an underlying connective tissue layer or *lamina propria*, and a thin layer of visceral muscle, the *muscularis mucosae*.

A variety of neuroendocrine cells are scattered in the mucosa of the alimentary tract from oesophagus to anal canal. The number of these cells progressively decreases in an anal direction. They all produce peptides and/or amines, which are active as hormones or neuro-transmitters. They are a part of the *amine precursor uptake and decarboxylation (APUD) cell series*, and they modulate autonomic activity as well as each other. The substances produced by these cells include gastrin, vasoactive intestinal polypeptide (VIP), cholecystokinin (CCK), motilin, secretin, somatostatin, substance P (SP), serotonin and endorphins.

Oesophagus

The epithelium is stratified squamous non-keratinizing, like that of most of the pharynx and mouth. The muscularis mucosae, which is absent from the uppermost part, is characteristically thicker in the oesophagus than in any other part of the alimentary tract. Small groups of mucus-secreting glands may be present at the upper and lower ends, in both the mucosa and submucosa.

Stomach

At the gastro-oesophageal junction (cardia), or a few centimetres above it, there is an abrupt change from stratified to single-layered columnar epithelium which continues all the way to the anal canal, but with differing cell types and configuration in the different organs. Throughout, the epithelium is not a flat layer but dips down into the connective tissue lamina propria to form myriads of glands. In the main part of the stomach, the body, the mucus-secreting surface cells dip down to form the gastric pits which in turn continue downwards as the straight test-tube-like glands whose cells include the peptic and parietal cells secreting pepsin and hydrochloric acid respectively. The parietal cells also secrete intrinsic factor, which is necessary for the intestinal absorption of vitamin B_{12}. For about a 1 cm ring at the cardia, the glands are shorter and the cells all mucus-secreting. In the pyloric region the glands are like coiled test-tubes and again the cells are all mucus-secreting. This part of the stomach contains most of the gastrin-producing endocrine G cells, as well as D cells which secrete somatostatin. Chromaffin endocrine cells in both body and pyloric regions produce serotonin and endorphin.

Small intestine

In the whole length of the small intestine, the columnar epithelium not only dips down to form glands (otherwise known as the crypts of Lieberkühn) but is also thrown up between the gland openings into villi, which consist of finger-like or leaf-like connective tissue cores covered by epithelium. Some of the villous cells are mucus-secreting goblet cells; others are the absorbing cells or enterocytes. Both types are derived from progenitors in the crypts and are constantly being shed and renewed, every few days. (So are other alimentary epithelial cells but at slower rates.) At the bases of the crypts are the granular Paneth cells which secrete lysozyme. Scattered among the other crypt cells are various neuroendocrine cells responsible for the production of intestinal hormones, including secretin, somatostatin and CCK, as well as chromaffin cells.

The duodenum is distinguished from the rest of the small intestine in having mucus-secreting glands (of Brunner) in the submucosa. In the terminal ileum there are groups of lymphoid follicles in the mucosa forming Peyer's patches, in contrast to single follicles which can be found throughout the alimentary canal from mouth to anus.

Large intestine

In the large intestine there are no villi, only glands (crypts) containing a high proportion of goblet cells. In the appendix the glands are rather shallower and less closely packed than in the rest of the large intestine, and there are numerous lymphoid follicles in the mucosa and submucosa.

In the upper part of the anal canal, the columnar epithelium gives place to the stratified squamous type, but here the junction is not as clear cut as the change at the cardia (see p. 258).

Oesophagus

The abdominal oesophagus, about 1 to 2 cm in length, turns forwards and to the left immediately below the diaphragmatic opening and grooves the posterior surface of the left lobe of the liver. The anterior and posterior vagal trunks are related to the respective oesophageal surfaces here (see p. 259). It is covered on its front and left side by peritoneum which passes from it on the right to the diaphragm as the uppermost part of the lesser omentum, and on the left forms the uppermost part of the greater omentum. The posterior wall of the oesophagus is rather shorter than the anterior, for the orifice in the diaphragm lies very nearly vertical. The left inferior phrenic artery lies behind the oesophagus.

The oesophagus enters the stomach at the cardiac orifice. The right margin is continuous with the lesser curvature, while the left margin makes an acute angle with the gastric fundus, the cardiac notch. The fibres of the right crus that pass to the left of the diaphragmatic opening form a sling around the abdominal oesophagus. Various factors contribute towards guarding against the reflux of gastric contents; these include the contraction of these right crus fibres, the angle of entry of the oesophagus into the stomach, the longitudinal folds of the oesophageal mucosa, a high pressure zone in the lower 3 cm of oesophagus and the effect of positive intra-abdominal pressure on the abdominal segment of the oesophagus.

Stomach

The stomach is the most dilated part of the alimentary tract, interposed between the oesophagus and duodenum in the upper part of the abdominal cavity. Lying mainly in the left hypochondrial, epigastric and umbilical regions, much of it is under cover of the lower ribs. It is a muscular bag, relatively fixed at both ends but otherwise subject to great variations in size depending on the volume of its contents. The gastro-oesophageal junction is the *cardia*, the most fixed part of the organ, and lies 2.5 cm to the left of the midline at the level of T10 vertebra. It is 40 cm from the incisor teeth. The gastroduodenal junction is the *pylorus*. In the recumbent position with the stomach empty this is usually a little to the right of the midline at the level of L1 vertebra but may be considerably lower.

The main parts of the stomach are the fundus, body and pyloric part, with the *greater* and *lesser curvatures* forming the left and right borders respectively. The stomach is completely invested by peritoneum, which passes in a double layer from the lesser curvature to the liver as the lesser omentum, and hangs down from the fundus and greater curvature as the greater omentum.

The *fundus* is the part which projects upwards above the level of the cardia, and is in contact with the left dome of the diaphragm. It is usually full of swallowed air.

The largest part of the stomach is the *body*, extending from the fundus to the notch, the *angular incisure*, on the lower part of the lesser curvature. Variable amounts of the body will be above and below the costal margin, in contact with the diaphragm and anterior abdominal wall. Likewise the lowest part of the greater curvature may be above or below umbilical level.

The pyloric part extends from the angular notch to the gastroduodenal junction, and consists of the proximal *pyloric antrum* which narrows distally as the *pyloric canal* (Fig. 5.25). The circular muscle of the distal end of the canal is palpably thickened to form the *pyloric sphincter*, whose position is indicated on the anterior surface by the prepyloric vein (of Mayo). The pyloric canal lies on the head and neck of the pancreas.

Behind the stomach are a group of structures comprising the *stomach bed* (Fig. 5.26). The posterior wall of the stomach is covered by peritoneum of the anterior wall of the lesser sac, and the bed is covered by the lesser sac's posterior wall. Apart from the left crus and dome of the diaphragm the bed consists of the splenic artery, body of pancreas, transverse mesocolon, upper part of left kidney, left suprarenal gland, spleen and left colic flexure. To the right of the lesser curvature in the midline lies the aorta with the coeliac trunk, the coeliac plexus and ganglia, and coeliac lymph nodes.

Blood supply

The stomach is supplied by branches from the coeliac trunk. Along the lesser curvature between the two layers of the lesser omentum the left gastric artery anastomoses with the right gastric; these arteries may be double. The fundus and upper left part of the greater curvature receive about six short gastric arteries from the splenic artery in the gastroplenic ligament. The rest of the curvature is supplied by the left and right gastroepiploic vessels, which run between the two layers of the greater omentum and anastomose with each other. The right gastroepiploic artery is closer to the greater curvature than the left gastroepiploic artery. During partial gastrectomy the greater omentum is divided below the right and above the left gastroepiploic arteries; the blood supply to the omentum usually remains intact as the larger omental branches of the left gastroepiploic artery are preserved.

Veins of the same name accompany the arteries and drain into the portal vein itself or its splenic and superior mesenteric tributaries. The prepyloric vein (unaccompanied by an artery) drains into the right gastric vein.

Lymph drainage

All lymph from the stomach eventually reaches coeliac nodes after passing through various outlying groups (Fig. 5.27A). Lymph vessels anastomose freely in the stomach wall, but there are valves in the vessels that direct lymph in such a way that a line drawn parallel to

Fig. 5.25 Radiograph of the stomach and duodenum after a barium meal.

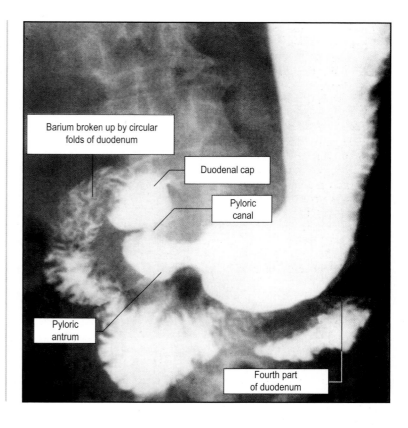

the greater curvature and two-thirds of the way down the anterior surface indicates a 'watershed' (Fig. 5.27B). From the largest zone above and to the right of this line, lymph passes to left and right gastric nodes along the left and right gastric arteries. From the upper left quadrant lymph flows via left gastroepiploic nodes and directly to pancreaticosplenic nodes at the splenic hilum, and at the upper border and posterior surface of the pancreas, accompanying the splenic artery. From the rest of the greater curvature region of the stomach lymph reaches nodes along the right gastroepiploic vessels, which drain to subpyloric nodes near the gastroduodenal artery. The pyloric part of the stomach drains to hepatic nodes in the porta hepatis and to subpyloric and right gastric nodes. In cases of gastric carcinoma, the left supra-clavicular nodes may rarely become palpably involved (*Troisier's sign*), presumably by spread along the thoracic duct.

Nerve supply

Sympathetic fibres (vasomotor) accompanied by afferent (pain) fibres run with the various arterial branches to the stomach, but of greater importance is the para-sympathetic supply from the vagi which control motility and secretion (although 90% of vagal fibres below the diaphragm are afferent for reflex activities, not pain). At the oesophageal opening in the diaphragm the **anterior vagal trunk** (comprising mainly left vagal fibres from the oesophageal plexus in the posterior mediastinum) lies in contact with the anterior oesophageal wall (Fig. 5.28), usually nearer its right margin; sometimes this trunk is double or triple. Each anterior trunk gives off one or two hepatic branches, which run in the upper part of the lesser omentum to join the plexus on the hepatic artery and portal vein, and then turn down in the anterior wall of the epiploic foramen to reach the pylorus. The anterior vagus also gives off several gastric branches which supply the fundus and body, and one large branch (greater anterior gastric nerve or anterior nerve of Latarget) which runs down in the lesser omentum near the lesser curvature with the left gastric artery, and subdivides in the manner of a crow's foot to supply the antrum and pyloric sphincter. The **posterior vagal trunk** (comprising mainly right vagal fibres) lies in loose tissue a little behind and to the right, not in contact with the

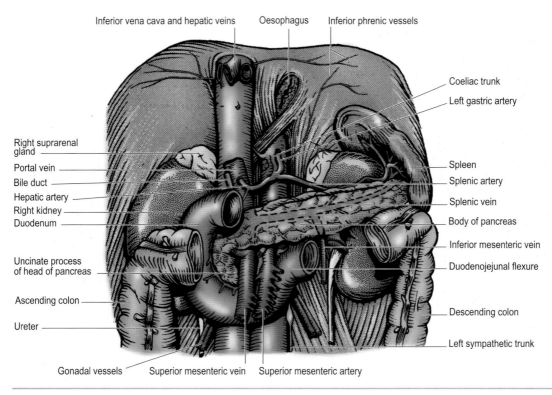

Inferior vena cava and hepatic veins · Oesophagus · Inferior phrenic vessels

Coeliac trunk
Left gastric artery

Right suprarenal gland
Portal vein
Bile duct
Hepatic artery
Right kidney
Duodenum

Uncinate process of head of pancreas

Ascending colon

Ureter

Spleen
Splenic artery
Splenic vein
Body of pancreas
Inferior mesenteric vein
Duodenojejunal flexure

Descending colon

Left sympathetic trunk

Gonadal vessels · Superior mesenteric vein · Superior mesenteric artery

Fig. 5.26 Retroperitoneal viscera on the posterior abdominal wall.

posterior surface of the oesophagus (Fig. 5.28). It gives coeliac branches that run backwards along the left gastric artery to the coeliac plexus. It also gives gastric branches to the fundus and body, and a large branch (greater posterior gastric nerve or posterior nerve of Latarget) which runs in the lesser omentum behind the anterior trunk to reach the antrum but not the pyloric sphincter.

Vagotomy. Truncal vagotomy involves cutting the trunks at the level of the abdominal oesophagus. In *selective vagotomy* the vagal trunks are cut distal to the hepatic branch of the anterior vagus and the coeliac branches of the posterior vagus. Although effective in diminishing gastric secretion, truncal and selective vagotomy are often accompanied by gastric stasis, so that an antral drainage procedure is required. *Highly selective vagotomy* (parietal cell vagotomy) attempts to avoid stasis by cutting only the branches to the fundus and body, leaving the antral and pyloric branches intact. Arterial branches run into the lesser curvature trans-

versely but nerve branches approach it obliquely. Ligating vessels will inevitably sever some nerve branches but not all, as not all nerves accompany vessels closely, and any individual nerves that can be identified must be cut also.

Structure

The main histological features are referred to on page 257. Although the angular notch is usually taken as the dividing line between the body and pyloric parts of the stomach, this does not necessarily indicate exactly where the body-type of mucosa with its parietal (acid-secreting) cells gives way to the pyloric-type with its concentration of G cells (producing gastrin). The *outer longitudinal* and *inner circular* muscle coats completely invest the stomach. They are reinforced by an incomplete *innermost oblique* muscle layer; its fibres loop over the fundus, being thickest at the notch between oesophagus and stomach, helping to maintain the angle here.

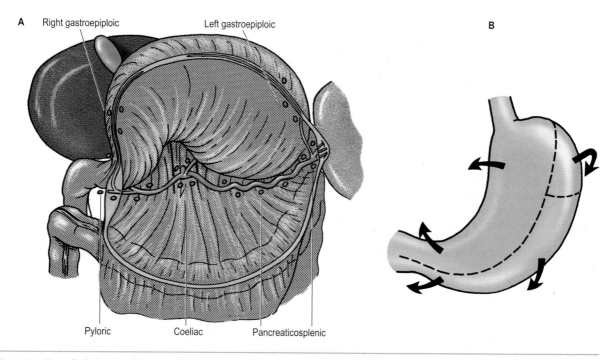

Fig. 5.27 Lymph drainage of the stomach: **A** the lesser sac has been opened up by cutting the gastrocolic omentum above the transverse colon, to show lymph nodes associated with branches of the coeliac trunk; **B** direction of lymph flow from the stomach, as described in the text.

Fig. 5.28 Anterior and posterior vagal trunks and their main branches.

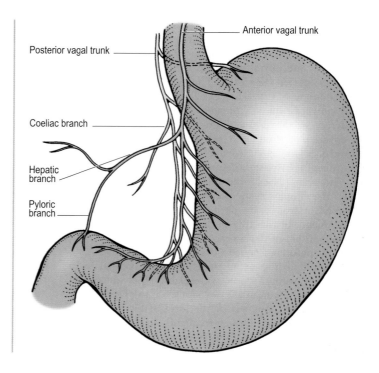

Small intestine

The small intestine consists of the duodenum, jejunum and ileum, although clinically the term small intestine often excludes the duodenum.

Duodenum

The duodenum is a C-shaped tube lying in front of, and to the right of the inferior vena cava and aorta (Fig. 5.26). The first 2.5 cm are contained between the peritoneum of the lesser and greater omenta, but the remainder is retroperitoneal. It is divided into four parts, superior, descending, horizontal and ascending, or more simply first, second, third and fourth. The total length is 25 cm (10 in), the lengths of the parts being easily remembered in inches as 2, 3, 4 and 1 but less conveniently in centimetres (5, 7.5, 10 and 2.5).

The duodenum makes its C-shaped loop round the head of the pancreas, which is opposite the body of L2 vertebra, so the first part may be said to lie at the level of L1 vertebra, the second on the right side of L2, the third crosses in front of L3, and the fourth is on the left of L2.

The *first part* of the duodenum runs to the right, upwards and backwards from the pylorus; a foreshortened view is consequently obtained in anteroposterior radiographs (Fig. 5.25). The first 2.5 cm (i.e. the duodenal cap, see below) lies between the peritoneal folds of the greater and lesser omenta; it forms the lowermost boundary of the opening into the lesser sac (Fig. 5.35A). It lies in front of the gastroduodenal artery, bile duct, and portal vein, and behind these structures lies the inferior vena cava. The gallbladder is anterior to the duodenal cap. The next 2.5 cm passes backwards and upwards on the upper part of the head of the pancreas to the medial border of the right kidney. It is covered in front with peritoneum, and the inferior surface of the right lobe of the liver lies over this peritoneum. Its posterior surface is bare of peritoneum.

The *second part* of the duodenum curves downwards over the hilum of the right kidney (Fig. 5.26). It is covered in front with peritoneum and crossed by the attachment of the transverse mesocolon, so that its upper half lies in the supracolic compartment to the left of the hepatorenal pouch (in contact with the liver) and its lower half lies in the right infracolic compartment medial to the inferior pole of the right kidney (in contact with coils of jejunum). It lies alongside the head of the pancreas, approximately at the level of L2 vertebra in a textbook cadaver, though frequently lower in life.

Its posteromedial wall receives the common opening of the bile duct and main pancreatic duct at the *hepatopancreatic ampulla* (of Vater), which opens on the summit of the *major duodenal papilla*, halfway along the second part, 10 cm from the pylorus. It is overlapped by a semilunar flap of mucous membrane. Two centimetres proximal is the small opening of the accessory pancreatic duct (on the *minor duodenal papilla*).

The *third part* of the duodenum curves forwards from the right paravertebral gutter over the slope of the right psoas muscle (gonadal vessels and ureter intervening) and passes over the forwardly projecting inferior vena cava and aorta to reach the left psoas muscle (Fig. 5.26). As its inferior border crosses the aorta it lies on the commencement of the inferior mesenteric artery. Its upper border hugs the lower border of the pancreas. It is covered by the peritoneum of the posterior abdominal wall just below the transverse mesocolon. It is crossed by the superior mesenteric vessels and by the leaves of the commencement of the mesentery of the small intestine sloping down from the duodenojejunal flexure. It lies, therefore, in both right and left infracolic compartments (Fig. 5.14). Its anterior surface is in contact with coils of jejunum.

The *fourth part* of the duodenum ascends to the left of the aorta, lying on the left psoas muscle and left lumbar sympathetic trunk, to reach the lower border of the body of the pancreas. It is covered in front by the peritoneal floor of the left infracolic compartment and by coils of jejunum. It breaks free from the peritoneum that has plastered it down to the posterior abdominal wall and curves forwards and to the right as the *duodenojejunal flexure*. This pulls up a double sheet of peritoneum from the posterior abdominal wall, the mesentery of the small intestine, which slopes down to the right across the third part of the duodenum and posterior abdominal wall (Fig. 5.29).

The duodenojejunal flexure is fixed to the left psoas fascia by fibrous tissue and may be further supported by the *suspensory muscle of the duodenum* (muscle or ligament of Treitz). This is a thin band of connective tissue which may contain muscle—skeletal muscle fibres that run from the left crus of the diaphragm to connective tissue around the coeliac trunk and smooth muscle fibres that run from there, behind the pancreas and in front of the left venal vein, to the muscle coat of the flexure.

Internally the mucous membrane of most of the duodenum, like the rest of the small intestine, is thrown into numerous circular folds (plicae circulares or valvulae conniventes). But the walls of the first 2.5 cm are smooth, hence the smooth outline of the full shadow of barium in the 'duodenal cap' at radiographic examination (Fig. 5.25). From the duodenal cap onwards the plicae break up the barium and its shadow.

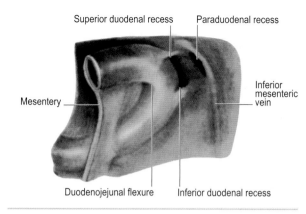

Superior duodenal recess   Paraduodenal recess

Mesentery

Inferior mesenteric vein

Duodenojejunal flexure   Inferior duodenal recess

Fig. 5.29   Peritoneal recesses of the duodenum. They are only occasionally present. The paraduodenal recess has the inferior mesenteric vein at the front of its opening.

Paraduodenal recesses. To the left of the duodeno-jejunal flexure certain peritoneal folds may cover recesses or fossae. The *paraduodenal recess* proper (Fig. 5.29) lies behind a fold raised by the upper end of the inferior mesenteric vein; an incarcerated hernia in this fossa may obstruct and thrombose the vein, and there is danger of dividing the vein if the peritoneum has to be divided at operation to free the hernia. Horizontal folds of peritoneum may cover *superior* and *inferior duodenal* recesses and a *retroduodenal* recess may be found behind the flexure. The mouths of these four recesses or fossae all face towards each other.

Blood supply

The duodenum is supplied by the superior and inferior pancreaticoduodenal arteries, but the first 2 cm, the usual site of ulceration, receives blood from the hepatic, gastroduodenal, supraduodenal, right gastric and right gastroepiploic arteries. Venous drainage is to tributaries of the superior mesenteric and portal veins.

Lymph drainage

Duodenal lymph drains by channels that accompany the superior and inferior pancreaticoduodenal vessels to coeliac and superior mesenteric nodes.

Jejunum and ileum

The jejunum is wider-bored and thicker-walled than the ileum. The thick wall of the jejunum feels double (the mucous membrane can be felt through the muscle wall,

'a shirt sleeve felt through a coat sleeve'); the thin wall of the ileum feels single.

The lower reaches of the ileum are distinguished by the presence on the antimesenteric border of elongated whitish plaques in the mucous membrane, usually but not always visible through the muscle wall. These are the aggregated lymphoid follicles (Peyer's patches). The jejunum lies coiled in the upper part of the infracolic compartment, the ileum in the lower part thereof and in the pelvis.

The jejunum and ileum together lie in the free margin of the mesentery. Total length varies greatly, from about 4 to 6 metres. The jejunum constitutes rather less than half the total length, say two-fifths, allowing three-fifths for the ileum.

An **ileal (Meckel's) diverticulum** is present in 2% of individuals, 60 cm (2 ft) from the caecum, and is 5 cm (2 in) long, according to a popular mnemonic but the length of the diverticulum is variable and its site may be more proximal. Its blind end may contain gastric mucosa or liver or pancreatic tissue; ulceration and perforation of the tip can occur. It represents the intestinal end of the vitellointestinal duct, and its apex may be adherent to the umbilicus or connected thereto by a fibrous cord, a further remnant of the duct.

Blood supply

Numerous jejunal and ileal branches arise from the left side of the superior mesenteric artery and enter the mesentery by passing between the two layers of the root. The jejunal branches join each other in a series of anastomosing loops to form *arterial arcades*: single for the upper jejunum and double lower down. From the arcades, *straight arteries* pass to the mesenteric border of the gut (Fig. 5.30). These vessels are long and close together, forming high narrow 'windows' in the intestinal border of the mesentery, visible because the mesenteric fat does not reach thus far. The straight vessels pass to one or other side of the jejunum and sink into its wall. Occlusion of a straight artery may lead to infarction of the segment supplied because these are end arteries, but occlusion of arcade vessels is usually without effect due to their numerous anastomotic connections.

The ileal arteries are similar but form a larger series of arcades—three to five, the most distal lying near the ileal wall so that the straight vessels branching off the arcades are shorter. There is more fat in this part of the mesentery, so the windows characteristic of the jejunal part are not seen; this is a useful feature in identifying loops of the bowel.

The end of the superior mesenteric artery itself supplies the region of the ileal diverticulum (if present),

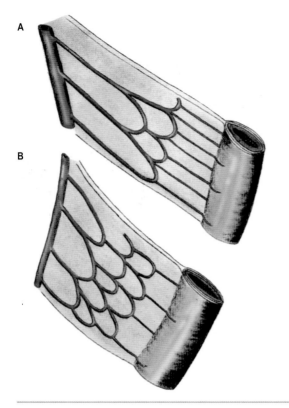

A

B

Fig. 5.30 Arcades of the superior mesenteric artery: **A** in the jejunum; **B** in the ileum. Compare the high narrow windows between the straight arteries running to the wall of the jejunum with the low broad windows between those of the ileum.

and anastomoses with the arcades and with the ileocolic branch to supply the terminal ileum.

The veins all correspond to the arteries and thus drain to the superior mesenteric.

Lymph drainage

Jejunal and ileal lymph drains to superior mesenteric nodes via mural and intermediate nodes in the mesentery.

Nerve supply

Autonomic nerves reach the wall of the small intestine with its blood vessels. The parasympathetic vagal supply augments peristaltic activity and intestinal secretion. There are many afferent fibres whose function is uncertain. The sympathetic supply, which is vasoconstrictor and normally inhibits peristalsis, is from the lateral horn

cells of spinal segments T9 and 10. Pain impulses use sympathetic pathways mainly and small intestinal pain is usually felt in the umbilical region of the abdomen.

Large intestine

The large intestine consists of the caecum with the (vermiform) appendix, the ascending, transverse, descending and sigmoid parts of the colon, the rectum and the anal canal.

Caecum and appendix

Caecum

This blind pouch of the large intestine projects downwards from the commencement of the ascending colon, below the ileocaecal junction (Fig. 5.31A). It is usually completely covered by peritoneum. The serous coat behind it is reflected downwards to the floor of the right iliac fossa and the retrocaecal peritoneal space may be shallow or deep, according to the distance of the retrocaecal fold from the lower end of the caecum. Often there are two peritoneal folds from either side of the posterior wall of the caecum, forming between them the *retrocaecal recess* in which the appendix may lie. As in the rest of the colon, the longitudinal muscle of the caecum is concentrated into three flat bands, the taeniae coli, within which is the circular muscle layer of the sacculated wall. The taeniae lie one anterior, one posteromedial and one posterolateral. All three converge on the base of the appendix, to which they are a useful guide.

Internally the ileocaecal junction is guarded by the *ileocaecal valve* (Fig. 5.31B), whose almost transverse lips may help to prevent some reflux into the ileum, but any possible sphincteric action is poor.

In the infant the caecum is conical and the appendix extends downwards from its apex. The lateral wall outgrows the medial wall and bulges down below the base of the appendix in the adult; the base of the appendix thus comes to lie in the posteromedial wall of the caecum above its lower end and the three taeniae coverage to this point.

The caecum lies on the peritoneal floor of the right iliac fossa, over the iliacus and psoas fasciae and the femoral and lateral femoral cutaneous nerves. Its lower end lies at the pelvic brim. When distended its anterior surface touches the parietal peritoneum of the anterior abdominal wall; when collapsed, coils of ileum lie between the two.

Blood supply. Branches of the anterior and posterior caecal arteries (branches of the ileocolic artery) fan out

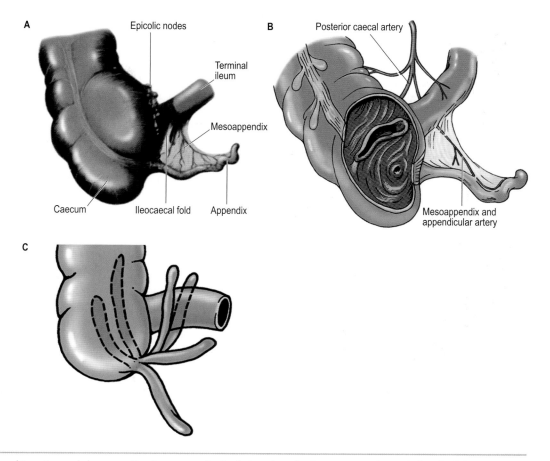

Fig. 5.31 Ileocaecal junction and the appendix: **A** a group of epicolic lymph nodes is present on the medial wall of the caecum, and there is a small ileocaecal fold passing from the terminal ileum to the mesoappendix; **B** the anterior wall of the caecum has been removed, and the opening of the appendix is seen 2 cm below the transverse lips of the ileocaecal valve; **C** various positions of the appendix, including (in interrupted line) retrocaecal, retrocolic and retroileal positions. The appendix may also be paracaecal in position beside the right side of the caecum.

over the respective surfaces of the caecum. The posterior caecal artery is larger and gives a branch to the base of the appendix. There are corresponding veins.

Lymph drainage. Lymph passes to nodes associated with the ileocolic artery.

Appendix

The vermiform (worm-shaped) appendix is a blind-ending tube (Fig. 5.31) varying in length (commonly about 6–9 cm), which opens into the posteromedial wall of the caecum 2 cm below the ileocaecal valve (Fig. 5.31B). On the surface of the abdomen this point (McBurney's) lies one-third of the way up the oblique line that joins the right anterior superior iliac spine to the umbilicus.

While the position of its base is constant in relation to the caecum, the appendix itself may lie in a variety of positions (Fig. 5.31C). The most common, as found at operation, is the retrocaecal position, with the pelvic position next in order of frequency; but recent scanning studies suggest that a retroileal site is the most common in the absence of disease.

The three taeniae of the caecum merge into a complete longitudinal muscle layer for the appendix. The sub-mucosa contains many lymphoid masses and the lumen is thereby irregularly narrowed. This lumen is wider in the young child and may be obliterated in old age.

The appendix has its own short mesentery, the *mesoappendix*, which is a triangular fold of peritoneum from the left (inferior) layer of the mesentery of the terminal ileum (Fig. 5.31A). A small fold of peritoneum extends from the terminal ileum to the front of the mesoappendix. This is the ileocaecal fold (or 'bloodless fold of Treves', although it sometimes contains blood vessels) and the space between it and the mesoappendix is the inferior ileocaecal recess. Another fold lies in front of the terminal ileum, between the base of the mesentery and the anterior wall of the caecum. This fold is raised up by the contained anterior caecal artery and is called the vascular fold of the caecum. The space behind it is the superior ileocaecal recess.

Blood supply. The appendicular artery is normally a branch of the inferior division of the ileocolic artery, which runs behind the terminal ileum to enter the meso-appendix. As it does so it gives off a recurrent branch which anastomoses with a branch of the posterior caecal artery. The appendicular artery runs first in the free margin of the mesoappendix and then close to the appendicular wall, where it may be thrombosed in appendicitis, leading to ischaemic necrosis and perhaps rupture of the appendix; there is no collateral circula-tion, for the appendicular artery is an end artery. There are corresponding veins.

Lymph drainage. As from the caecum, lymph passes to nodes associated with the ileocolic artery.

Appendicectomy. Exposure of the appendix during appendicectomy is through a McBurney or transverse muscle-splitting incision (see p. 241). If it is not imme-diately obvious, tracing any of the taeniae down over the caecal wall will lead to the base of the appendix.

Colon

Of the four parts of the colon, the transverse and sigmoid parts are suspended in mesenteries—the trans-verse mesocolon and sigmoid mesocolon respectively—but the ascending and descending colon are plastered on to the posterior abdominal wall so that they have posterior 'bare areas' devoid of peritoneum.

Ascending colon

This first part of the colon, about 15 cm in length, ex-tends upwards from the ileocaecal junction to the right colic (hepatic) flexure. The latter lies on the inferolateral part of the anterior surface of the right kidney, in contact with the inferior surface of the liver. The ascending colon lies on the iliac fascia and the anterior layer of the lumbar fascia. Its front and both sides possess a serous coat, which runs laterally into the paracolic gutter and medially into the right infracolic compartment. The original embryonic mesentery is retained in about 10% of adults.

The *taeniae coli* lie, in line with those of the caecum, anteriorly, posterolaterally and posteromedially. These consist of longitudinal muscle fibres and the circular muscle coat is exposed between them. The ascending colon is sacculated, due to the three taeniae being 'too short' for the bowel. If the taeniae are divided between the sacculations the latter can be drawn apart and the bowel wall flattened.

Small pouches of peritoneum, distended with fat, the *appendices epiploicae*, project in places from the serous coat. The blood vessels supplying them from the mucosa perforate the muscle wall. Mucous membrane may herniate through these vascular perforations, a condition known as diverticulosis. Diverticulitis is inflammation of these mucosal herniae.

Transverse colon

This part of the colon, normally over 45 cm long, extends from the hepatic to the splenic flexure in a loop which hangs down to a variable degree between these two fixed points, anterior to coils of jejunum and ileum. The convexity of the greater curvature of the stomach lies in its concavity, the two being connected by the gastrocolic omentum. Because of the fusion between the greater omentum and the transverse colon, the rest of the greater omentum appears to hang down from its lower convexity. The transverse colon is completely invested in peritoneum; it hangs free on the transverse mesocolon, which is attached from the inferior pole of the right kidney across the descending (second) part of the duodenum and the pancreas to the inferior pole of the left kidney. The splenic flexure lies, at a higher level than the hepatic flexure, well up under cover of the left costal margin.

The taeniae coli continue from the ascending colon. Due to the looping downwards and forwards of the transverse colon from the flexures, which lie well back in the paravertebral gutters, some rotation of the gut wall occurs at the flexures, and the anterior taenia of ascending and descending colons lies posteriorly, while the other two lie anteriorly, above and below. The appendices epiploicae are larger and more numerous than on the ascending colon.

Descending colon

Less than 30 cm long, this extends from the splenic flexure to the pelvic brim, and in the whole of its course is plastered to the posterior abdominal wall by perito-neum (like the ascending colon), though a mesentery is present in about 20% of adults. The splenic flexure lies on the lateral surface of the left kidney, below and in contact with the tail of the pancreas and the spleen. A fold of peritoneum, the phrenicocolic ligament (see p. 246), attaches the splenic flexure to the diaphragm at the level of the tenth and eleventh ribs. *Surgical mobilization* of the splenic flexure requires division of this ligament. During this manoeuvre the spleen needs to be safeguarded as it lies in contact with the upper surface of the ligament. The descending colon lies on the lumbar fascia and the iliac fascia. It ends at the pelvic brim about 5 cm above the inguinal ligament. Mobilization of the descending colon is conveniently carried out by dividing the peritoneum along the white line of Toldt (see p. 250).

The three taeniae coli, in continuity with those of the transverse colon, lie one anterior and two posterior (medial and lateral). Appendices epiploicae are numerous and diverticulosis is common in this part of the colon.

Sigmoid colon

Formerly known as the pelvic colon, this extends from the descending colon at the pelvic brim to the commencement of the rectum in front of the third piece of the sacrum. It is usually less than 45 cm long, though great variations in length are common. It is completely invested in peritoneum and hangs free on a mesentery, the sigmoid mesocolon. The attachment of the pelvic mesocolon to the pelvic brim and the sacrum has been described on page 250. Congenital peritoneal adhesions are frequently found between the lateral aspect of the pelvic mesocolon and the parietal peritoneum of the floor of the left iliac fossa; they need to be divided during *surgical mobilization* of the sigmoid colon.

Like the rest of the large intestine, the commencement of the sigmoid colon is sacculated by three taeniae coli, but these muscular bands are wider than elsewhere in the large gut, and meet to clothe the terminal part of the sigmoid in a complete longitudinal coat. The sigmoid colon possesses well-developed appendices epiploicae, and diverticulosis is most common in this part of the colon. It lies, usually, in the pelvic cavity, coiled in front of the rectum, lying on the peritoneal surface of the bladder (and uterus).

Blood supply of the colon

The ascending colon and the proximal two-thirds of the transverse colon are supplied by the ileocolic, right colic and middle colic branches of the superior mesenteric artery, and the remainder of the colon by the left colic and sigmoid branches of the inferior mesenteric. The anastomotic branches near the inner margin of the whole colon form the *marginal artery* (of Drummond)

from which short vessels run into the gut wall (Fig. 5.23). The weakest link in this marginal chain of vessels is near the left colic flexure, between the middle and left colic branches, i.e. between midgut and hindgut vessels. An inner arterial arc (of Riolan) between the ascending branch of the left colic artery and the trunk of the middle colic artery may supplement the blood supply to the colon in this region.

The veins correspond to the arteries, and thus reach the portal vein via the superior or inferior mesenteric veins. There is some anastomosis between portal and systemic venous drainage where the ascending and descending colon are in contact with the posterior abdominal wall.

Lymph drainage

As is usual the lymph channels follow the arteries, so that drainage is to superior or inferior mesenteric nodes.

Nerve supply

Being derived from the midgut (up to near the splenic flexure) and the hindgut (from there onwards), the parasympathetic supply to the large intestine is partly from the vagi and partly from the pelvic splanchnic nerves (see p. 292). The sympathetic supply is derived from spinal cord segments T10–L2. The pain fibres that accompany these vasoconstrictor nerves give rise to periumbilical pain if from midgut derivatives (e.g. the appendix) but to hypogastric pain if from the hindgut. As from the rectum, some pain fibres from the descending and sigmoid colon appear to run with the parasympathetic nerves (see p. 305).

Colectomy

The vessel pattern with the accompanying lymphatics determines the extent of partial resections of the colon for carcinoma. For a *right hemicolectomy* the resection extends from the terminal ileum to the proximal part of the transverse colon, with ligation of the ileocolic and right colic vessels adjacent to their superior mesenteric parent. In a *transverse colectomy* the transverse colon and the right and left colic flexures are removed together with the transverse mesocolon and greater omentum with ligation of the middle colic vessels. For a *left hemicolectomy* the resection is from the left end of the transverse colon to part of the sigmoid colon, with ligation of left colic and upper sigmoid vessels. For *sigmoid colectomy* the removal extends from the lower descending colon to the rectum, with ligation of lower left colic and sigmoid vessels. Resections for diverticular disease (as opposed to neoplasia) can be more localized.

The **rectum** is considered with the pelvic organs on page 302, and the **anal canal** with the perineum on page 324.

PART SEVEN

Liver and biliary tract

Liver

The liver, the largest gland in the body, weighs approximately 1500 g and receives about 1500 mL of blood per minute. The wedge-shaped organ (Figs 5.32 and 5.33) occupies most of the right hypochondrium and epigastrium. It has two *surfaces, diaphragmatic* and *visceral*. The diaphragmatic surface is boldly convex, moulded to the undersurface of the diaphragm, and is descriptively subdivided into anterior, superior, posterior and right surfaces which merge into one another without any clear demarcations. A sharp *inferior border* separates the right and anterior surfaces from the visceral surface, which slopes upwards and backwards from here to merge with the posterior surface. Most main vessels and ducts enter or leave at the porta hepatis which is on the visceral surface, but the hepatic veins emerge from the posterior surface.

From the diaphragmatic and visceral surfaces peritoneal folds pass respectively to the diaphragm and to the stomach; these persist from the ventral mesogastrium into which the developing liver grows (Fig. 5.17).

The inferior border is notched by the ligamentum teres which lies in the free lower margin of the falciform ligament (see p. 242). From here the attachment of the falciform ligament ascends on the anterior surface to reach the superior surface where a reduplication of the left leaf forms the *left triangular ligament* (Fig. 5.32A). The right leaf of the falciform ligament passes to the

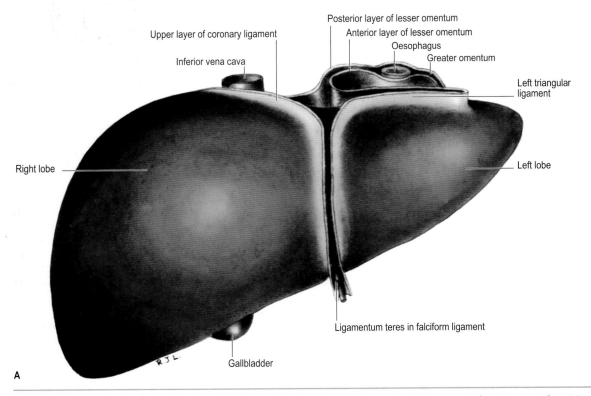

Upper layer of coronary ligament
Posterior layer of lesser omentum
Anterior layer of lesser omentum
Oesophagus
Greater omentum
Inferior vena cava
Left triangular ligament
Right lobe
Left lobe
Ligamentum teres in falciform ligament
Gallbladder
A

Fig. 5.32 Liver and peritoneal reflections. **A** In the anterior view the oesophagus is pulled upwards from its normal position behind the left lobe to show the peritoneal attachments. All peritoneal edges seen here are attached to the diaphragm. **B** Posterior view (posterior and visceral surfaces). The lesser omentum, whose cut edges are seen in the fissure for the ligamentum venosum and which continues round the structures in the porta hepatis, is attached to the lesser curvature of the stomach. All other peritoneal edges seen here are attached to the diaphragm. The caudate process connects the caudate lobe to the right lobe.

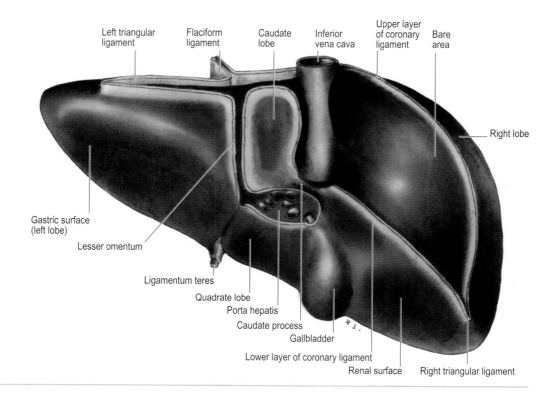

Left triangular ligament Flaciform ligament Caudate lobe Inferior vena cava Upper layer of coronary ligament Bare area

Right lobe

Gastric surface (left lobe)

Lesser omentum

Ligamentum teres

Quadrate lobe

Porta hepatis

Caudate process

Gallbladder

Lower layer of coronary ligament

Renal surface Right triangular ligament

Fig. 5.32 B

right, in front of the inferior vena cava, and becomes the upper layer of the coronary ligament.

When the posterior and visceral surfaces are viewed together (Fig. 5.32B), an H-shaped pattern of structures is seen. Centrally lies the porta hepatis (the hilum of the liver), the cross-piece of the H. The right limb of the H is made by the inferior vena cava (on the posterior surface) and the gallbladder (inferior surface), while the left limb is made by the continuity of the *fissures for the ligamentum venosum and ligamentum teres*. The vena cava lies in a deep groove or sometimes a tunnel, on the convexity of the posterior surface. To the right of the vena cava is the triangular *bare area*, with the vena cava as its base and with sides formed by the superior and inferior layers of the *coronary ligament*. The apex where these two layers meet is the small *right triangular ligament*. From the inferior layer, the line of peritoneal attachment passes in front of the inferior vena cava, and thence up along its left side to the summit of the liver. Here it meets the diverging right leaf of the falciform ligament (Fig. 5.32B). The two peritoneal layers are attached to the bottom of a deep groove that runs to the left from the inferior vena cava and lodges the

ligamentum venosum. This fissure and the contained ligament turn at a right angle and run downwards on the posterior surface to the left end of the porta hepatis, outlining a rectangular area of the liver, the caudate lobe, between the fissures, the porta and the inferior vena cava. The two layers of the lesser omentum are attached to the bottom of the fissure along the left margin of the caudate lobe. Due to the depth of the fissure, which passes obliquely into the substance of the liver, the caudate lobe is partly separated from the rest of the liver and has an anterior surface that forms the posterior wall of the fissure. The caudate lobe thus lies behind the right part of the lesser omentum, as a content of the lesser sac. A narrow caudate process extends to the right between the porta hepatis and the inferior vena cava (Fig. 5.32B).

At the **porta hepatis** the two layers of the lesser omentum deviate to the right to enclose the right and left hepatic ducts and the right and left branches of the hepatic artery and portal vein. They lie in the order vein–artery–duct (VAD) with the ducts in front and thereby more accessible in surgery. Also present in the porta are several lymph nodes and the nerves of the liver.

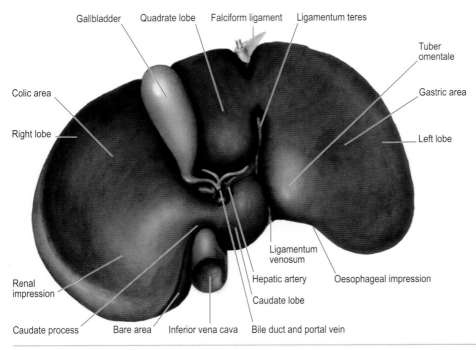

Gallblader   Quadrate lobe   Falciform ligament   Ligamentum teres

Tuber omentale

Colic area

Gastric area

Right lobe

Left lobe

Ligamentum venosum

Renal impression

Hepatic artery   Oesophageal impression

Caudate lobe

Caudate process   Bare area   Inferior vena cava   Bile duct and portal vein

Fig. 5.33   Visceral surface of the liver, as seen when looking into the abdomen with the lower border of the liver lifted up towards the costal margin.

The gallbladder lies in a shallow fossa on the down-sloping visceral surface, with its cystic duct close to the right end of the porta hepatis. Its neck is highest, its fundus lowest, frequently projecting below the inferior border. The quadrate lobe lies between the gallbladder and the fissure for the ligamentum teres.

The bare area is in contact with the diaphragm and the right suprarenal gland. The visceral surface is related, with peritoneum intervening, to the stomach, duodenum, hepatic flexure of the colon and right kidney, and these organs may leave impressions on the liver surface. To the right of the gastric impression a slight bulge, the omental tuberosity, is in contact with the lesser omentum, which separates it from a similar eminence on the body of the pancreas. The oesophagus makes a shallow impression on the posterior surface of the liver.

The liver is suspended by the hepatic veins and the inferior vena cava. The hepatic veins are entirely intra-hepatic and enter the vena cava while it is clasped in the deep groove on the posterior surface. The visceral surface rests on the underlying viscera, particularly the stomach and hepatic flexure of the colon. The left triangular ligament needs to be divided surgically, before the left lobe of the liver can be retracted to the right,

to expose the abdominal oesophagus and upper part of stomach.

Surface marking

The upper margin of the liver is approximately level with the xiphisternal joint, arching slightly upwards on each side. On the left it reaches the fifth intercostal space 7–8 cm from the midline, and on the right to the fifth rib, curving down to the right border which extends from ribs 7 to 11 in the midaxillary line. The inferior border is along a line joining the right lower and upper left extremities; some of it thus lies approximately level with the right costal margin, while centrally it crosses behind the upper abdominal wall between the costal margins about a hand's breadth below the xiphisternal joint.

Lobes

The liver was customarily divided by anatomists into a larger **right** and a smaller **left lobe** utilizing the line of attachment of the falciform ligament anteriorly and the fissures for the ligamentum teres and ligamentum venosum on the visceral surface. The **caudate lobe**, lying between the inferior vena cava and the fissure for the ligamentum venosum, and the **quadrate lobe**, lying between the gallbladder fossa and the fissure for the ligamentum teres, were consequently considered to be part of the right lobe. This subdivision of the liver is not in accordance with the arrangement of the vascular and biliary channels within the liver. The functional division of the liver into right and left halves is along an oblique plane that runs through the centre of the bed of the gallbladder and the groove for the inferior vena cava. The middle hepatic vein lies in this plane and is a useful landmark in radiological and ultrasonographic investigations.

Segments

On the basis of blood supply and biliary drainage, there are four main hepatic sectors (also called sections): left lateral; left medial; right anterior; and right posterior. The *left lateral sector* lies to the left of the attachment of the falciform ligament and the grooves for the ligamentum teres and ligamentum venosum. The *left medial sector* lies between this demarcating line and the planes of the gallbladder and inferior vena cava. The line of division between the *right anterior* and *right posterior sectors* has no external marking; it runs in an oblique direction posteriorly and medially from the middle of the front of the right lobe towards the vena caval groove, and the right hepatic vein lies in this plane. These four sectors are further subdivided into eight segments, which are customarily numbered using Roman numerals (Fig. 5.34); the International Hepato-Pancreatico-Biliary Association has, however, recommended the use of Arabic numerals.

Segment I is the caudate lobe of the liver. Despite lying to the left of the plane between the two functional lobes of the liver, the caudate lobe is an autonomous segment receiving blood from right and left branches of the hepatic artery and portal vein, draining bile into right and left hepatic ducts and having independent venous drainage into the inferior vena cava. The left lateral sector contains segment II posteriorly and segment III anteriorly, with the left hepatic vein being between them. Segment IV is recognized on the visceral surface as the quadrate lobe. Segments V and VI are the inferior segments of the right anterior and right posterior sectors respectively. Segments VII and VIII are the superior segments of the right posterior and right anterior sectors respectively. When the visceral surface of the liver is viewed from below (Fig. 5.33), the hepatic segments appear to be arranged in an approximately anticlockwise direction around the porta hepatis. Further segmental subdivision partitions segment IV into IVa (superior) and IVb (inferior) segments, the latter coinciding more accurately with the quadrate lobe. Similarly the caudate lobe (segment I) is subdivided into right and left parts and the caudate process.

Blood supply

The liver receives blood from two sources. Arterial (oxygenated) blood is furnished by the **hepatic artery**, which divides into right and left branches in the porta hepatis. The right branch of the hepatic artery normally passes behind the common hepatic duct and in the liver divides into anterior and posterior sectoral branches; the left branch divides into medial and lateral sectoral branches. Sometimes the common hepatic artery arises from the superior mesenteric artery or the aorta (instead of the coeliac trunk), in which case it usually runs behind the portal vein. The right hepatic artery may arise from the superior mesenteric artery (15%), and the left hepatic artery from the left gastric artery (20%) as aberrant or accessory arteries; i.e. they may either replace the normal branches or exist in addition to them.

Venous blood is carried to the liver by the **portal vein** (see p. 276) which divides in the porta hepatis into right and left branches which in turn give sectoral branches like the arteries; this portal blood is laden with the products of digestion which have been absorbed from the alimentary canal, and which are metabolized by the liver cells.

There is no communication between right and left halves of the liver; indeed, even within each half the arteries are end arteries (hence infarction of the liver). Although infarction may illustrate this point, in the presence of disease there are often enough anastomoses with phrenic vessels (e.g. across the bare area) to provide a collateral circulation that is sufficient to allow ligation

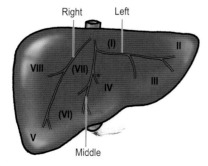

Right   Left

(I)   II

VIII   (VII)

IV   III

(VI)

V

Middle

Fig. 5.34   Main hepatic veins and approximate positions of surgical segments, indicated by Roman numerals (posterior segments are in brackets). See text for explanation.

of the hepatic artery, a procedure that has been used to induce metastases to regress without compromising normal liver tissue (though with less success than was hoped).

The venous return differs in that it shows a mixing of right and left halves of the liver. Three main **hepatic veins** (Fig. 5.34) drain into the inferior vena cava. A large central vein runs in the plane between right and left halves and receives from each. Further laterally lie a right and left vein; the middle vein frequently joins the left very near the vena cava. All the veins have no extrahepatic course and enter the vena cava just below the central tendon of the diaphragm. Several small accessory hepatic veins enter the vena cava below the main veins, including a separate vein from the caudate lobe. There is some anastomosis between portal venous channels in the liver and the azygos system of veins above the diaphragm across the bare area of the liver.

Lymph drainage

The lymphatics of the liver drain into three or four nodes that lie in the porta hepatis (*hepatic nodes*). These nodes also receive the lymphatics of the gallbladder. They drain downwards alongside the hepatic artery to pyloric nodes as well as directly to coeliac nodes. Lymphatics from the bare area of the liver communicate with extraperitoneal lymphatics which perforate the diaphragm and drain to nodes in the posterior mediastinum. Similar communications exist along the left triangular and falciform ligaments from the adjacent liver surfaces.

Nerve supply

The nerve supply of the liver is derived from both the sympathetic and vagus, the former by way of the coeliac ganglia, whence nerves run with the vessels in the free edge of the lesser omentum and enter the porta hepatis. Vagal fibres from the hepatic branch of the anterior vagal trunk reach the porta hepatis via the lesser omentum.

Structure

The classic description of liver morphology is centred on the *hepatic lobule*, a region of liver tissue of something like pinhead size and hexagonal shape, with a central vein and plates or cords of hepatocytes, separated by vascular spaces or sinusoids radiating from the vein to the periphery of the lobule. At the corners of the lobules are the *portal triads* consisting of small branches of the hepatic artery and portal vein and bile ductules. In the human liver, however, such a classical lobule is not usually present. The arrangement is that of a polygonal

territory with a portal triad at the centre and tributaries of the hepatic veins at the boundary. This is termed a *portal lobule* and corresponds to sections of at least three 'classic' lobules.

The *sinusoids* intervening between the cords of hepatocytes are lined by endothelial cells which show frequent intercellular spaces and fenestrations. These allow plasma (but not blood cells) to leave the sinusoids and enter the perisinusoidal spaces between the endothelium and hepatocytes, so that exchange of materials can take place between plasma and liver cells. Many of the endothelial lining cells are capable of phagocytic activity, constituting the *Kupffer cells* of the reticulo-endothelial system. Bile manufactured by hepatocytes first enters the biliary canaliculi which are situated between apposing sides of adjacent hepatocytes. Collectively the canaliculi form a meshwork which drains into the bile ductules of the portal triads, and these in turn unite to form the larger intrahepatic ducts.

The liver is enclosed in a thin capsule of connective tissue from which sheaths pass into the liver at the porta hepatis, surrounding the branches of the hepatic artery, portal vein and bile ducts. Inside the liver smaller branches of these vascular and biliary channels run within connective tissue trabeculae, termed *portal canals*.

Development

The liver develops by proliferation of cells from the blind ends of a Y-shaped diverticulum which grows from the foregut into the septum transversum. The cranial part of the septum transversum becomes the pericardium and diaphragm. The caudal part becomes the ventral mesogastrium (Fig. 5.17), and it is into this that the liver grows (see p. 247).

The original diverticulum from the endoderm of the foregut (Fig. 5.40A–C) becomes the bile duct; its Y-shaped bifurcation produces the right and left hepatic ducts. A blind diverticulum from the bile duct becomes the cystic duct and gallbladder. The hepatic ducts divide and redivide to become the interlobular and intralobular bile ductules. Hepatic circulation in the fetus is referred to on page 33.

Biopsy, lobectomy and transplantation

Needle *biopsy* of the liver is carried out through the right eighth or ninth intercostal space in the midaxillary line; the needle path is below the level of the lung but traverses the costodiaphragmatic recess of the pleura before going through the diaphragm and crossing the peritoneal cavity to enter the liver. The needle must not penetrate more than 6 cm from the skin to avoid entering the inferior vena cava. A misplaced needle could damage the kidney, colon or pancreas, and pneumothorax is another possible complication. When the liver lesion is malignant, needle biopsy can lead to the seeding of cancer cells along the needle track.

A *right hepatic lobectomy* involves dividing liver tissue along a line from the left of the gallbladder to the right edge of the inferior vena cava, ligating vessels and ducts along the way, so that the right lobe and the gallbladder can be removed. The middle and left hepatic veins are preserved. For *left lobectomy*, the left lobe together with most of the caudate and quadrate lobes are removed. The gallbladder may be removed or left intact, and the line of resection at the back is level with the left edge of the vena cava. The right and usually the middle hepatic veins are preserved. In more extensive procedures left lobectomy is combined with removal of segments V and VIII (right anterior sector) or right lobectomy with the removal of segment IV. Alternatively, the more restricted removal of segments is carried out when pathological involvement of the liver is limited.

In liver **transplantation** the patient's liver is removed, usually with the attached segment of the inferior vena cava, utilizing a venovenous bypass between the portal vein and left femoral vein to the left axillary vein. The suprahepatic inferior vena cava of the donor liver is sutured to the patient's, followed by the infrahepatic caval anastomosis and thereafter the portal vein anastomosis. The venous clamps are released in the same sequence and venovenous bypass interrupted. The hepatic artery anastomosis is made and biliary tract continuity established by end-to-end common bile duct anastomosis, or by anastomosing the donor bile duct to the recipient's jejunum. Particularly in children, in whom it may not be possible to use a venovenous shunt, preservation of the patient's inferior vena cava may be necessary. The donor liver is then attached to the recipient's inferior vena cava by a 'piggy-back' technique.

Biliary tract

The extrahepatic biliary tract consists of the three hepatic ducts (right, left and common), the gallbladder and cystic duct, and the bile duct. The **right and left hepatic ducts** exit from the liver and join to form the **common hepatic duct** near the right end of the porta hepatis. In a surgical sense, it is only the confluence of the hepatic ducts which is accessible without dissection into the liver substance. But prior to its emergence from the liver, the left hepatic duct may run along the base of the quadrate lobe only partly surrounded by the liver substance. The *common hepatic duct* so formed passes down between the two peritoneal layers at the free edge of the lesser omentum. The common hepatic duct is soon joined on its right side at an acute angle by the cystic duct from the gallbladder, to form the bile duct (Fig. 5.35A). When the liver is retracted at operation the ducts are seen to descend below the liver, but at rest they lie in loose contact with the porta hepatis.

Gallbladder

The gallbladder stores and concentrates the bile secreted by the liver. It is a globular or pear-shaped viscus (Fig. 5.33) with a capacity of about 50 mL, and consists of three parts: fundus; body; and neck. It lies in the gallbladder fossa on the visceral surface of the right lobe of the liver, adjacent to the quadrate lobe.

Its bulbous blind end, the **fundus**, usually projects a little beyond the sharp lower border of the liver and touches the parietal peritoneum of the anterior abdominal wall at the tip of the ninth costal cartilage, where the transpyloric plane crosses the right costal margin, at the lateral border of the right rectus sheath (Fig. 5.1). This is the *surface marking* for the fundus and the area of abdominal tenderness in gallbladder disease. (The fundus of the normal gallbladder is not palpable but may become so if distended by biliary tract obstruction.) The fundus lies on the commencement of the transverse colon, just to the left of the hepatic flexure. The **body** passes backwards and upwards towards the right end of the porta hepatis and is in contact with the first part of the duodenum. The upper end of the body narrows into the **neck** which, when the liver is in its normal position (not retracted upwards), lies at a higher level than the fundus. The neck continues into the **cystic duct**, which is 2 to 3 cm long and 2 to 3 mm in diameter. It runs backwards, downwards and to the left to join the common hepatic duct, usually in front of the right hepatic artery and its cystic branch (but variations are common). The wall of the neck where it joins the cystic duct may show a small diverticulum (Hartmann's pouch). This is not a feature of the normal gallbladder and is always associated with a pathological condition; it may be the site of impaction of a gallstone.

The fundus and body of the gallbladder are usually firmly bound to the undersurface of the liver by connective tissue; small cystic veins pass from the gallbladder into the liver substance. Small bile ducts may also pass from the liver to the gallbladder, and if undetected they may drain bile into the peritoneal cavity after cholecystectomy. The peritoneum covering the liver passes smoothly over the gallbladder. Occasionally the gallbladder hangs free on a narrow 'mesentery' from the undersurface of the liver. Rarely the gallbladder may be

A

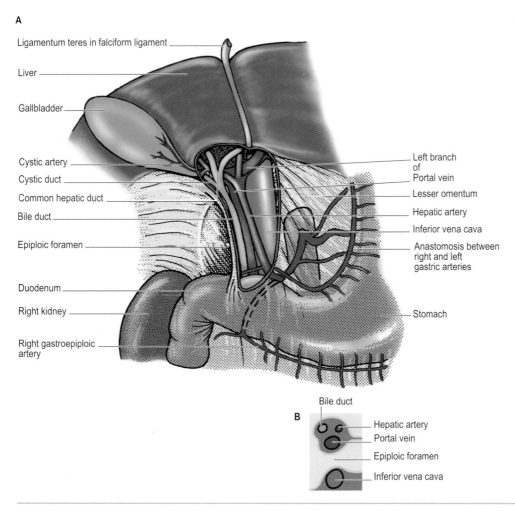

Ligamentum teres in falciform ligament

Liver

Gallbladder

Cystic artery

Cystic duct

Common hepatic duct

Bile duct

Epiploic foramen

Duodenum

Right kidney

Right gastroepiploic artery

Left branch of Portal vein

Lesser omentum

Hepatic artery

Inferior vena cava

Anastomosis between right and left gastric arteries

Stomach

Bile duct

B

Hepatic artery

Portal vein

Epiploic foramen

Inferior vena cava

Fig. 5.35   Lesser omentum and the epiploic foramen. **A** Part of the omentum has been cut away to display the bile duct and hepatic artery in front of the portal vein. Interrupted lines indicate gastroduodenal artery behind first part of duodenum. **B** Transverse section of the right free margin at the level of the epiploic foramen, viewed from below, showing the foramen bounded in front and behind by the two great veins.

embedded within the liver. Very rarely the gallbladder may be absent.

The gallbladder varies in size and shape. In rare cases it is duplicated with single or double cystic ducts. It may be septate with the lumen divided into two chambers. The fundus may be folded in the manner of a Phrygian cap; this is the most common congenital abnormality.

Blood supply

The cystic artery is usually a branch of the right hepatic. It runs across the triangle formed by the liver, common hepatic duct and cystic duct (Calot's triangle), to reach the gallbladder. Variations in the origin of the artery are common. It may arise from the main trunk of the hepatic artery, from the left branch of that vessel or from the gastroduodenal artery, and in either case may pass in front of the cystic and bile ducts.

Venous return is by multiple small veins in the gallbladder bed into the substance of the liver and so into the hepatic veins. One or more cystic veins may be present but these are uncommon; they run from the neck of the gallbladder into the right branch of the portal vein. Cystic veins do not accompany the cystic artery.

Lymph drainage

Lymphatic channels from the gallbladder drain to nodes in the porta hepatis, to the cystic node (in Calot's triangle at the junction of the common hepatic and cystic ducts), and to a node situated at the anterior boundary of the epiploic foramen. From these nodes lymph passes to the coeliac group of preaortic nodes.

Structure

The gallbladder is a fibromuscular sac which, histologically, shows a surprisingly small amount of smooth muscle in its wall. Its mucous membrane is a lax areolar tissue lined with a simple columnar epithelium. It is projected into folds which produce a honeycomb appearance in the body of the gallbladder, but are arranged in a more or less spiral manner in the neck and cystic duct (the '*spiral valve*' of Heister). Mucus is secreted by the columnar epithelium but there are no goblet cells, and mucus-secreting glands are present only in the neck.

Common hepatic duct

The *right* and *left hepatic ducts* emerge from the porta hepatis and unite near its right margin in a Y-shaped manner to form the common hepatic duct. This is joined, usually after about 3 cm, by the cystic duct to form the bile duct. The right branch of the hepatic artery normally passes behind the common hepatic duct but may run in front of it. The site of union of the cystic and common hepatic ducts is usually on the right side of the common hepatic duct about 1 to 2 cm above the duodenum, but sometimes the cystic duct runs parallel to and on the right of the hepatic duct for a variable distance before uniting with it, and it may also spiral round behind the hepatic duct before joining it on its left side. Rarely the cystic duct may be absent and the gallbladder drains directly into the common hepatic duct. Another anomaly is an accessory right hepatic duct which may open into the common hepatic duct, cystic duct or gallbladder. All these possibilities must be borne in mind during cholecystectomy and other operations on the biliary tract.

Bile duct

The bile duct (formerly called the common bile duct) is about 6 to 8 cm long and its normal diameter does not exceed 8 mm. It is best described in three parts or thirds. The upper (supraduodenal) third lies in the free edge of the lesser omentum (Fig. 5.35) in the most accessible position for surgery—in front of the portal vein and to the right of the hepatic artery, where the lesser omentum forms the anterior boundary of the epiploic foramen. The middle (retroduodenal) third runs behind the first part of the duodenum (Fig. 5.26) and slopes down to the right, away from the almost vertical portal vein which now lies to the left of the duct with the gastroduodenal artery. The inferior vena cava is behind the duct. The lower (paraduodenal) third slopes further to the right in a groove between the back of the head of the pancreas and the second part of the duodenum (it may even be embedded in a tunnel of pancreatic tissue) and in front of the right renal vein. Neoplasms of the head of the pancreas may obstruct the duct here. It joins the pancreatic duct (Fig. 5.40D) at an angle of about 60° at the **hepatopancreatic ampulla** (of Vater). The ampulla and the ends of the two ducts are each surrounded by sphincteric muscle, the whole constituting the *ampullary sphincter* (of Oddi). Sometimes the muscle fibres surrounding the ampulla and the pancreatic duct are absent, leaving only the bile duct sphincter. When all three are present the arrangement allows for independent control of flow from bile and pancreatic ducts. The ampulla itself opens into the posteromedial wall of the second part of the duodenum at the major duodenal papilla, which is situated 10 cm from the pylorus.

Blood supply of the biliary tract

The extrahepatic biliary tract receives small branches from the cystic and right hepatic arteries and the posterior branch of the superior pancreaticoduodenal artery; they form anastomotic channels on the duct. Small veins from the biliary tract drain to the portal vein or enter the liver.

Nerve supply of the biliary tract

Parasympathetic fibres, mainly from the hepatic branch of the anterior vagal trunk, stimulate contraction of the gallbladder and relax the ampullary sphincter, and sympathetic fibres from cell bodies in the coeliac ganglia (with preganglionic cells in the lateral horn of spinal cord segments T7–9) inhibit contraction, but the hormonal control of gallbladder activity (by CCK from neuroendocrine cells of the upper small intestine) is much more important than the neural. Afferent fibres including those subserving pain (e.g. from a duct distended by a gallstone) mostly run with right-sided sympathetic fibres and reach spinal cord segments T7–9, but some from the gallbladder may run in the right phrenic nerve (C3–5), through connections between this nerve and the coeliac plexus. Any afferent vagal fibres are probably concerned with reflex activities, not pain. Biliary tract

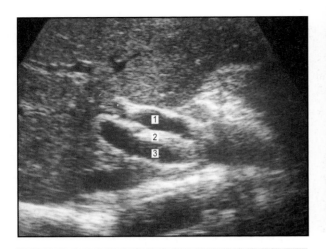

Fig. 5.36 Ultrasound image of normal structures at porta hepatis: 1, common bile duct; 2, hepatic artery; 3, portal vein.
(Provided by D. J. Lomas, Department of Radiology, Cambridge University Hospital.)

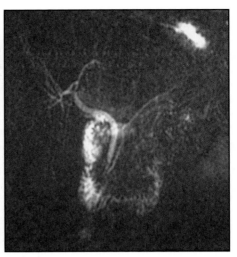

Fig. 5.37 Magnetic resonance cholangiopancreaticogram. Coronal view showing normal intra and extrahepatic bile ducts and main pancreatic duct. Fluid in these channels and in the alimentary tract enables their visualization without the use of contrast medium by this non-invasive technique.
(Provided by D. J. Lomas, Department of Radiology, Cambridge University Hospital.)

pain is usually felt in the right hypochondrium and epigastrium, and may radiate round to the back in the infrascapular region, in the area of distribution of spinal nerves T7–9. The phrenic nerve supply explains the occasional referral of pain to the right shoulder region.

Imaging of the biliary tract

The gallbladder and biliary ducts can be demonstrated by ultrasound (Fig. 5.36), and this technique has largely replaced the visualization of these structures by radiography after the administration of radio-opaque substances which are excreted by the liver into bile. Under direct vision through an endoscope, a catheter can be inserted into the hepatopancreatic ampulla and radio-opaque contrast medium injected, resulting in the radiographic delineation of the bile and pancreatic ducts (endoscopic retrograde cholangiopancreatography). These ducts can now also be demonstrated by the non-invasive technique of magnetic resonance imaging (Fig. 5.37).

Portal vein

The portal vein is the upward continuation of the superior mesenteric vein, which changes its name to portal after it has received the splenic vein behind the neck of the pancreas (Fig. 5.38). It lies in front of the inferior vena cava, as it lies behind the pancreas and the first part of the duodenum but loses contact with the inferior vena cava by entering between the two layers of the lesser omentum. It runs almost vertically upwards in the free edge, where the lesser omentum forms the anterior boundary of the epiploic foramen, lying behind the bile duct and the hepatic artery (Fig. 5.35), and reaches the porta hepatis. Here it divides into a right and left branch which enter the respective halves of the liver.

The portal vein receives the right and left gastric veins and the superior pancreaticoduodenal vein. The cystic vein or veins, when present, join the right branch of the portal vein, and the paraumbilical veins running with the ligamentum teres join the left branch. The ligamentum itself (the obliterated remains of the left umbilical vein) is often not completely fibrosed even in adults (50%), and can then be cannulated at the umbilicus, providing access to the portal venous system.

The portal vein is about 8 cm long. Although demonstrable during fetal life and a short postnatal period, thereafter no valves are present in the portal vein or its tributaries.

The five sites of portal/systemic anastomosis are considered with the appropriate territories: lower end of the oesophagus (see p. 216), upper end of the anal canal

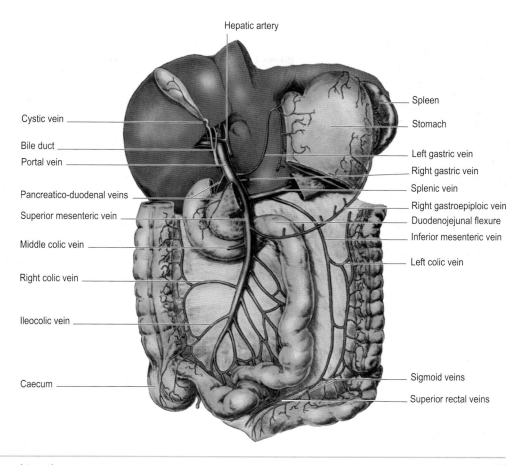

Fig. 5.38 Portal vein and its tributaries.

(see p. 326), bare area of the liver (see p. 272), peri-umbilical region (see p. 186) and retroperitoneal areas (see p. 267). In *portal hypertension* 80% of portal blood may be shunted into the collateral channels so that only 20% reaches the liver; however, the opening up of the collaterals does not decrease the level of hypertension.

PART EIGHT

Pancreas

The pancreas is a composite gland having exocrine acini which discharge their secretions into the duodenum to assist in digestion, and groups of endocrine cells, the islets of Langerhans, whose role is in carbohydrate metabolism. In shape the gland resembles the upper end of a thick walking-stick or hook, lying sideways with the handle or hook on the right and turned downwards (Fig. 5.26). Its length is about 15 cm.

The gland is of firm consistency, and its surface is finely lobulated. Its big head on the right is connected by a short neck to the body, which crosses the midline and tapers to a narrow tail on the left. The head and tail incline towards the paravertebral gutters, while the neck and body are curved boldly forward over the inferior vena cava and aorta in front of the first lumbar vertebra. The gland lies somewhat obliquely, sloping from the head upwards towards the tail behind the peritoneum of the posterior abdominal wall. The transpyloric plane (L1) is the guide to the *surface marking*; the neck lies on the plane, which passes across the head and body, and below the tail.

The **head**, the broadest part of the pancreas, is moulded to the C-shaped concavity of the duodenum, which it completely fills. It lies over the inferior vena cava and the right and left renal veins, mainly at the level of L2 vertebra. Its posterior surface is deeply indented, and sometimes tunnelled, by the terminal part of the bile duct. The lower part of the posterior surface has a hook-shaped extension upwards and to the left, behind the superior mesenteric vein and artery, in front of the aorta; this is the **uncinate process** of the head (Fig. 5.26). The transverse mesocolon is attached across the anterior surface of the head, which lies in both supracolic and infracolic compartments (Fig. 5.14).

The **neck** is best defined as the narrow band of pancreatic tissue that lies in front of the commencement of the portal vein, continuous to the right with the head and to the left with the body. At the lower margin of the neck the superior mesenteric vein is embraced between the neck and the uncinate process of the head, and behind the neck the splenic vein runs into its left side to form the portal vein. The transverse mesocolon is attached towards the lower border of the neck.

The **body** of the pancreas passes from the neck to the left, sloping upwards across the left renal vein and aorta, left crus of the diaphragm, left psoas muscle and lower part of left suprarenal gland, to the hilum of the left kidney. The body is triangular in cross-section with posterior, anterosuperior and anteroinferior surfaces separated by superior, anterior and inferior borders. The superior border crosses the aorta at the origin of the coeliac trunk (Fig. 5.39); the splenic artery passes to

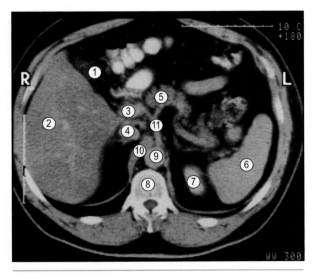

Fig. 5.39 CT scan of the upper abdomen, viewed from below. 1, gallbladder; 2, liver; 3, portal vein; 4, inferior vena cava; 5, pancreas; 6, spleen; 7, left kidney; 8, T12 vertebra; 9, abdominal aorta; 10, right crus of diaphragm; 11, coeliac trunk.

the left along the upper border of the body and tail, the crests of the waves showing above the pancreas, the troughs out of sight behind it (Fig. 5.26). The inferior border, alongside the neck, crosses the origin of the superior mesenteric artery. A slight convexity, the omental tuberosity, projects upwards from the right end of the superior border; above the lesser curvature of the stomach this touches the omental tuberosity of the left lobe of the liver, with the lesser omentum intervening. The splenic vein lies closely applied to the posterior surface and the inferior mesenteric vein joins the splenic vein behind the body of the pancreas in front of the left renal vein, where it lies over the left psoas muscle. The transverse mesocolon is attached along the anterior border; the body lies, therefore, behind the lesser sac, where it forms part of the stomach bed.

The **tail** of the pancreas passes forwards and to the left from the anterior surface of the left kidney. Accompanied by the splenic artery, vein and lymphatics it lies within the two layers of the splenorenal ligament and thus reaches the hilum of the spleen.

The **pancreatic duct** (of Wirsung) is a continuous tube leading from the tail to the head, gradually increasing in diameter as it receives tributaries. At the hepatopancreatic ampulla (Fig. 5.40D) it is joined at an angle of about 60° by the bile duct and the manner of their joint opening into the duodenum is described on page 275. In intubation of the ampulla for endoscopic retrograde cholangiopancreatography (ERCP), the catheter preferentially enters the pancreatic duct. It drains most of the pancreas except for the uncinate process and lower part of the head, which drains by the *accessory pancreatic duct* (of Santorini). This opens into the duodenum at the minor duodenal papilla situated about 2 cm proximal to the major papilla. The two ducts communicate with one another.

Blood supply

The main vessel is the splenic artery, which supplies the neck, body and tail. One large branch is named the *arteria pancreatica magna*. The head is supplied by the *superior* and the *inferior pancreaticoduodenal arteries*. Venous return is by numerous small veins into the splenic vein and, in the case of the head, by the superior pancreaticoduodenal vein into the portal vein and by the inferior pancreaticoduodenal vein into the superior mesenteric vein.

Lymph drainage

Lymphatics from the pancreas follow the course of the arteries. To the left of the neck the pancreas drains into the pancreaticosplenic nodes which accompany the splenic artery. The head drains from its upper part into the coeliac group and from its lower part and uncinate process into the superior mesenteric group of preaortic lymph nodes.

Nerve supply

Parasympathetic vagal fibres, which are capable of stimulating exocrine secretion, reach the gland mainly from the posterior vagal trunk and coeliac plexus, but, as with the gallbladder, hormonal control is more important than the neural. Sympathetic vasoconstrictor impulses are derived from spinal cord segments T6–10 via splanchnic nerves and the coeliac plexus, the post-ganglionic fibres running to the gland with its blood vessels. As with other viscera, pain fibres accompany the sympathetic supply, so that pancreatic pain may radiate in the distribution of thoracic dermatomes 6–10.

Structure

The pancreas is a lobulated gland composed of serous acini that produce the exocrine secretion, and the endocrine islets of Langerhans. The cells of the serous acini show the cytoplasmic basophilia typical of protein-secreting cells. Under the influence of secretin and CCK produced by neuroendocrine cells of the small intestine, the pancreatic acinar cells secrete various digestive enzymes, in particular trypsin and lipase, and some (the centroacinar cells) produce bicarbonate. The pale-staining islets are rounded groups of cells scattered among the acini. Special staining or electron microscopy is necessary to distinguish between the α-islet cells which secrete glucagon and the β-cells secreting insulin. There are also δ-cells that produce somatostatin.

Development

The pancreas develops as two separate buds, each an outgrowth of the endoderm at the junction of foregut and midgut (Fig. 5.40A). A *ventral bud* grows into the ventral mesogastrium in common with the outgrowth of the bile duct and a *dorsal bud* grows independently from a separate duct into the dorsal mesogastrium. The duodenal portion of the gut subsequently rotates and becomes adherent to the posterior abdominal wall, lying with the pancreatic outgrowths, behind the peritoneum. The duodenal wall grows asymmetrically; the openings of the two ducts, originally diametrically opposite, are thus carried around into line with each other (Fig. 5.40B, C), and the two parts of the gland fuse into the single adult pancreas. The duct systems of the two buds anastomose and there is eventually some interchange of drainage areas. The end result is that the duodenal end of the dorsal duct becomes the accessory pancreatic duct, and the duodenal end of the duct of the ventral bud joins with the remainder of the dorsal duct to form the main pancreatic duct (Fig. 5.40D). The tail, body, neck and part of the head of the pancreas develop from the dorsal bud; the rest of the head and the uncinate process develop from the ventral bud. Rarely the ventral bud may fail to rotate normally around the duodenum, resulting in a ring of pancreatic tissue encircling the second part of the duodenum.

The pancreatic acini develop by growth of cells from the terminal parts of the branching ducts. The islet cells appear to have an identical origin, but become separated from their parent ducts and undergo a complete change of secretory function.

Surgical approach

The head of the pancreas and the adjacent duodenum can be mobilized by incising the peritoneum along the right edge of the second part of the duodenum and turning the duodenum medially (Kocher's manoeuvre). This procedure gives access to the posterior surface of the duodenum and head of pancreas, and to the lower part of the bile duct. The inferior vena cava, ureter and gonadal vessels must not be damaged when peeling the duodenum and pancreatic head forwards. Resections of the head of the pancreas with the C-shaped duodenal loop involve restoring continuity by joining the bile duct to the end of the jejunum and the stomach and pancreas to the side of the jejunum. The portal vein, which must be free of pathological involvement, has to be safeguarded during this resection. Pseudocysts of the pancreas (fluid accumulations following pancreatitis) bulge into the lesser sac, usually behind the stomach, and can be drained intra-gastrically by incising the anterior wall of the stomach and then entering the cyst by incising the posterior gastric wall.

PART NINE

Spleen

The spleen, the largest of the lymphoid organs (see p. 10), lies under the diaphragm on the left side of the abdomen (Fig. 5.26), and although not part of the alimentary tract it drains to the portal venous system.

The odd numbers 1, 3, 5, 7, 9, 11 summarize some splenic statistics. It measures $1 \times 3 \times 5$ inches, weighs 7 oz and lies deep to the left 9th to 11th ribs (H. A.

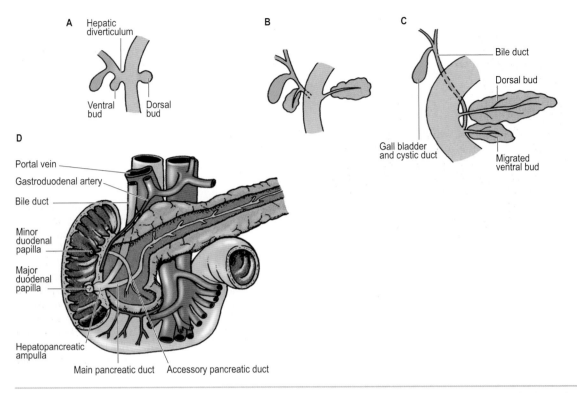

Fig. 5.40   Development of liver and pancreas. **A** The hepatic diverticulum and ventral and dorsal pancreatic buds. **B** The site of the original hepatic diverticulum and ventral pancreatic bud migrates dorsally, so that in **C** it comes to lie below the opening of the dorsal pancreatic bud. **D** The pancreatic duct systems anastomose and eventually the main pancreatic duct comes to be formed from the ventral bud duct and the distal part of the dorsal bud duct, and the proximal part of the dorsal duct becomes the accessory pancreatic duct.

Harris). These are average measurements; the size of the spleen varies considerably.

Being developed in the dorsal mesogastrium (see below), the spleen projects into the greater sac surrounded by peritoneum of the original left leaf of the dorsal mesogastrium. It lies at the left margin of the lesser sac (Fig. 5.49) below the diaphragm, and its diaphragmatic surface is moulded into a reciprocal convexity. Its *hilum* lies in the angle between the stomach and left kidney, each of which impresses a concavity alongside the attached splenic vessels (Fig. 5.41). Its long axis lies along the line of the tenth rib, and its lower pole does not normally project any further forward than the midaxillary line. A small colic area lies in contact with the splenic flexure and the phrenicocolic ligament. Its anterior border is notched, a relic of the fusion of the several 'splenules' from which the organ arises in the embryo.

Its visceral peritoneum, or serous coat, invests all surfaces (gastric, diaphragmatic, colic and renal). The

two leaves of the greater omentum pass from the hilum forwards to the greater curvature of the stomach (the gastrosplenic ligament) and backwards to the front of the left kidney (the splenorenal ligament) (Fig. 5.49). The hilum of the spleen makes contact with the tail of the pancreas, which lies within the splenorenal ligament.

If the spleen enlarges, its long axis extends down and forwards along the tenth rib in the direction of the umbilicus, and its anterior border approaches the costal margin to the left of the greater curvature of the stomach. (A kidney enlarging downwards does so in the direction of the iliac fossa.) The spleen must at least double its normal size before its anterior border passes beyond the left costal margin. A palpable spleen is identified by the notch in its anterior border. In some diseases the spleen is grossly enlarged and may extend across the upper abdomen beyond the umbilicus towards the right iliac fossa. Whatever the degree of enlargement the spleen glides in contact with the diaphragm and anterior

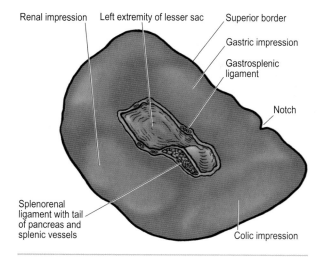

Renal impression   Left extremity of lesser sac   Superior border

Gastric impression

Gastrosplenic
ligament

Notch

Splenorenal
ligament with tail
of pancreas and
splenic vessels

Colic impression

Fig. 5.41 Visceral surface of the spleen, showing the impressions for adjacent viscera and the two layers of peritoneum that form the splenorenal and gastrosplenic ligaments.

abdominal wall in front of the splenic flexure, which remains anchored by the phrenicocolic ligament, and no colonic resonance is found on percussion over the organ. Retroperitoneal tumours (e.g. of the left kidney) do not displace the overlying colon and they are crossed by a band of colonic resonance.

The structures that are related to the surfaces of the spleen can be identified by holding the convexity (diaphragmatic surface) of the detached organ in the hollow of the left hand, and rotating it until the notched anterior border lies to the front, near the thumb (Fig. 5.41). The concavity between the notched anterior border and the hilum is the gastric impression. Behind the hilum is the concave renal surface, while at the lower pole (at the tip of the little finger of the left hand) is the small colic impression.

The *structure* of the spleen has been referred to on page 10.

Blood supply

The splenic artery passes between the layers of the splenorenal ligament and at the hilum divides into two or three main branches, from which five or more branches enter the spleen. Veins accompany the arteries and unite to form the splenic vein. Based on the vascular arrangement, it is possible that the spleen consists of two or three segments, with intersegmental vessels being small and scanty, but the evidence for such segmentation is not conclusive.

Lymph drainage

Lymph drains into several nodes lying at the hilum and thence, by way of the pancreaticosplenic nodes, to the coeliac nodes.

Nerve supply

The spleen is supplied from the coeliac plexus with sympathetic fibres only.

Development

The spleen begins to develop in the sixth week as several condensations of mesodermal cells in the dorsal mesogastrium which, because of the splenic presence, becomes divided into the splenorenal and gastrosplenic ligaments (Fig. 5.21B). The spleen thus comes to lie at the left margin of the lesser sac. The original condensations become aggregated into a single organ; the splenic notch may represent a region where there is incomplete fusion. 'Accessory spleens' are the result of lack of fusion; one or several may be found, usually along the splenic vessels or in the peritoneal attachments. They occur in up to 20% of the population and are rarely larger than 2 cm in diameter.

Surgical approach

Removal of the spleen (**splenectomy**) essentially involves cutting its two 'pedicles', the splenorenal and gastrosplenic ligaments. In an emergency after rupture with haemorrhage, the left or posterior layer of the splenorenal ligament is incised and the spleen turned medially so that the splenic vessels can be dissected away from the tail of the pancreas and ligated (arteries before veins). The short gastric vessels and the gastrosplenic ligament are then divided and removal completed. For an elective procedure it is usual to enter the lesser sac by dividing the gastrosplenic ligament and its vessels and then to deal with the splenic vessels and the splenorenal ligament. The stomach must not be perforated when ligating the short gastric vessels, and damage to the tail of the pancreas and splenic flexure of the colon must be avoided.

PART TEN

Posterior abdominal wall

The five lumbar vertebrae project forwards into the abdominal cavity as the lumbar spine has a normal lordosis (forward convexity). The midline forward projection is enhanced by the inferior vena cava and aorta, which lie in front of the bodies of the vertebrae (Fig. 5.42A). To each side of this convexity lie deep paravertebral gutters. They are floored in by the psoas and quadratus lumborum muscles and, below the iliac crest, by the iliacus muscle. The crura and adjacent parts of the diaphragm (see p. 191) are also part of the posterior abdominal wall. The kidneys lie high up in the paravertebral gutters.

The lumbar vertebrae are separated from each other by thick intervertebral discs, which unite them very strongly. A broad ribbon, the anterior longitudinal ligament, is attached anteriorly and crosses the lumbosacral prominence to become fused with the periosteum on the front of the upper sacrum.

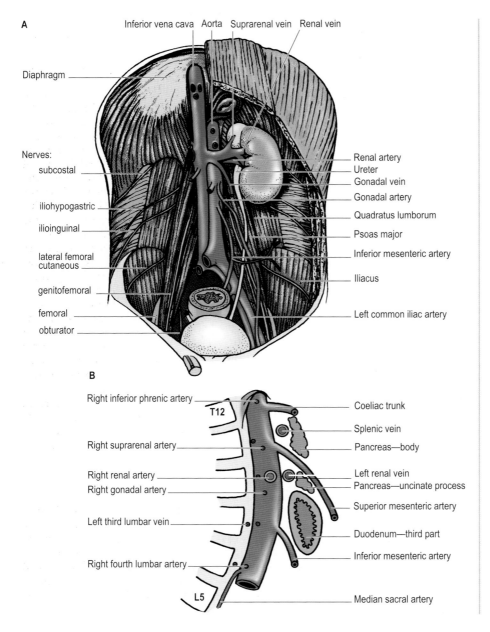

A

Inferior vena cava   Aorta   Suprarenal vein   Renal vein

Diaphragm

Nerves:

subcostal

iliohypogastric

ilioinguinal

lateral femoral cutaneous

genitofemoral

femoral

obturator

Renal artery
Ureter
Gonadal vein
Gonadal artery
Quadratus lumborum
Psoas major
Inferior mesenteric artery
Iliacus
Left common iliac artery

B

Right inferior phrenic artery

T12

Right suprarenal artery

Right renal artery
Right gonadal artery

Left third lumbar vein

Right fourth lumbar artery

L5

Coeliac trunk
Splenic vein
Pancreas—body
Left renal vein
Pancreas—uncinate process
Superior mesenteric artery
Duodenum—third part
Inferior mesenteric artery
Median sacral artery

Fig. 5.42 Posterior abdominal wall: **A** great vessels and nerves; **B** diagrammatic representation of the aorta as seen from the right side.

Muscles

Psoas major

This muscle lies in the gutter between the bodies and transverse processes of the lumbar vertebrae. Its vertebral attachment is to the discs above the five lumbar vertebrae, the adjoining parts of the bodies of the vertebrae, to fibrous arches that span the concavities of the sides of the upper four vertebral bodies and to the medial ends of all the lumbar transverse processes. Thus there is one continuous attachment from the lower border of T12 to the upper border of L5 vertebrae. The muscle passes downwards along the pelvic brim (Fig. 5.42A) and then beneath the inguinal ligament into the thigh, where its tendon is attached to the lesser trochanter of the femur. The lumbar plexus (see p. 288) is embedded within the muscle, and part of the external vertebral venous plexus is behind it (in front of the transverse processes). The genitofemoral nerve emerges from the front of the muscle, the iliohypogastric, ilioinguinal, lateral femoral cutaneous and femoral nerves from its lateral border, and the obturator nerve and the lumbosacral trunk from its medial border. The four lumbar arteries (see p. 286) and veins pass backwards medial to the four arches and run laterally behind the psoas muscle.

The strong *psoas fascia* (part of the iliac fascia) invests the surface of the muscle, attached to the vertebral bodies, the fibrous arches, and the transverse processes, and to the iliopubic eminence (see p. 171) as the muscle extends along the pelvic brim. It retains the pus of a psoas abscess, and spinal tuberculosis may present as a cold abscess in the groin. The sheath is not part of the lumbar fascia (see p. 284), but the lateral edge blends with the anterior layer of that fascia (over quadratus lumborum).

There is a thickening in the psoas fascia curving obliquely from the body of L1 (or L2) vertebra to the transverse process of L1 vertebra. This is the *medial arcuate ligament*, from which fibres of the diaphragm arise in continuity alongside the crus. The part of the psoas above this ligament is above the diaphragm, i.e. in the thorax. The sympathetic trunk passes from thorax to abdomen beneath this ligament.

Nerve supply. By the first three lumbar nerves, mainly L2.

Action. Its action on the hip joint is described on pages 122 and 133. Being attached to the sides of lumbar vertebrae it is a lateral flexor of the vertebral column. When acting from below with iliacus and their fellows of the opposite side, it assists in the flexion of the trunk produced by anterior abdominal wall muscles (especially rectus abdominis), psoas acting on the lumbar column and iliacus on the hip bone.

Psoas minor, present in only two out of every three individuals, is a slender muscle lying on the surface of psoas major. Its short belly arises from T12 and L1 vertebrae and its long tendon flattens out to blend with the psoas fascia and gain attachment to the iliopubic eminence. It is supplied by L1 nerve and is a weak flexor of the lumbar spine.

Quadratus lumborum

This is a flat sheet lying deep in the paravertebral gutter, edge to edge with psoas medially and transversus abdominis laterally (Fig. 5.42A). It lies in the anterior compartment of the lumbar fascia. It arises from the stout transverse process of L5 vertebra, from the strong iliolumbar ligament and from a short length of the adjoining iliac crest. Its fibres pass upwards to the transverse processes (lateral to psoas) of the upper four lumbar vertebrae and, more laterally, to the inferior border of the medial half of the twelfth rib. Its lateral border slopes upwards and medially and so crosses the lateral border of the iliocostalis component of erector spinae (see p. 446), which slopes upwards and laterally. Its anterior surface is covered by the anterior layer of the lumbar fascia. A thickening in front of this fascia passing from the first lumbar transverse process to the twelfth rib constitutes the *lateral arcuate ligament*. The fibres of the diaphragm arise in continuity from the ligament. The subcostal neurovascular bundle (vein, artery, nerve from above downwards) emerges from the thorax beneath the ligament and slopes down across the lumbar fascia. The muscle represents the innermost of the three muscular layers of the body wall and is in series with the diaphragm and the transversus thoracis muscle group.

Nerve supply. By T12 and the upper three or four lumbar nerves.

Action. Its chief action is to prevent the diaphragm from elevating the twelfth rib during inspiration. By depressing the twelfth rib it aids descent of the contracting diaphragm. Additionally it is a lateral flexor of the lumbar spine.

Iliacus

This muscle arises from the upper two-thirds of the iliac fossa up to the inner lip of the iliac crest and from the anterior sacroiliac ligament. It is triangular in shape and its fibres converge medially towards the lateral margin of psoas and pass out of the iliac fossa beneath the lateral part of the inguinal ligament. It is inserted into the psoas tendon and the adjacent part of the femur below the lesser trochanter.

The iliacus muscle is covered by the strong *iliac fascia*; this is attached to bone at the margins of the muscle, and to the inguinal ligament. The fascia is continuous with the psoas fascia, forms a floor to the abdominal cavity and serves for the attachment of parietal peritoneum. Apart from its prolongation into the femoral sheath (see p. 122) it does not extend into the thigh.

Nerve supply. By the femoral nerve (L2, 3) in the iliac fossa.

Action. It acts, with psoas, on the hip joint (see p. 122).

Fascia

Each muscle of the posterior abdominal wall (quadratus lumborum, psoas and iliacus) is covered with a dense and unyielding fascia. The fasciae over adjacent muscles blend at their margins. The psoas fascia and the iliac fascia have been described above.

Lumbar fascia. This is the lumbar part of the **thoraco-lumbar fascia**. In the lumbar part of the trunk of the body, three layers of fascia enclose two muscular compartments. The anterior and middle layers occupy only the lumbar region, but the posterior layer extends above this to the lower part of the neck and below to the dorsal surface of the sacrum. Quadratus lumborum occupies the anterior compartment, while erector spinae fills the posterior compartment. The *anterior layer* extends from the front of the iliolumbar ligament and adjoining iliac crest to the lower border of the twelfth rib. Medially it is attached to the front of each lumbar transverse process, adjoining the attachment of the psoas fascia. Laterally it blends with the middle layer along the lateral border of quadratus lumborum; here transversus abdominis and internal oblique take origin. The *middle layer* extends from the back of the iliolumbar ligament and adjoining iliac crest up to the twelfth rib. Medially it is attached to the tips of the lumbar transverse processes. Laterally it blends with both anterior and posterior layers. The latter line of fusion is along the lateral border of erector spinae. The *posterior layer* lies over the whole erector spinae mass of muscle. It is attached medially to the spinous processes and supraspinous ligaments of all the sacral, lumbar and thoracic vertebrae. Its lateral margin traced from below upwards extends along the transverse tubercles of the sacrum to the posterior part of the iliac crest, from where it slopes outwards to the twelfth rib. Above the twelfth rib its attachment is to the angles of all the ribs; its lateral border over the thoracic cage thus slopes up medially. In the thorax this single posterior layer constitutes the thoracic part of the thoracolumbar fascia; it is only below the thorax where there are no ribs that the thoracolumbar fascia is in three layers. The posterior layer is thick and strong over the lumbar region, being here reinforced by fusion of the aponeurotic origin of latissimus dorsi. Over the thorax it gradually becomes thinner and it fades out above the first rib over the extensor muscles of the neck, where it is replaced by the splenius muscle.

Vessels

The central vascular features of the posterior abdominal wall are the abdominal part of the aorta and the inferior vena cava, with the vein lying on the right side of the artery.

Abdominal aorta

The thoracic aorta becomes the abdominal aorta on passing behind the median arcuate ligament and between the crura of the diaphragm, on the front of the body of T12 vertebra (Fig. 5.43). It passes downwards behind the peritoneum on the bodies of the lumbar vertebrae, inclining slightly to the left, with the left sympathetic trunk at its left margin. On the body of L4 it divides into the two common iliac arteries.

Between the origins of the coeliac trunk and the superior mesenteric artery the aorta is crossed by the splenic vein and the body of the pancreas (Fig. 5.42B). Between the superior and inferior mesenteric origins lie the left renal vein, the uncinate process of the pancreas and the third part of the duodenum.

The *surface marking* of the abdominal aorta is from 2.5 cm above the transpyloric plane in the midline to a point 1 to 2 cm below and to the left of a normally situated umbilicus, level with the highest points of the iliac crests.

Branches

The main branches of the abdominal aorta fall into three groups: single ventral arteries to the gut and its derivatives (coeliac, superior and inferior mesenteric), paired branches to other viscera (suprarenal, renal and gonadal arteries) and paired branches to the abdominal wall (inferior phrenic and lumbar arteries). A small posterior branch, the **median sacral artery**, leaves the aorta a little above its bifurcation, and runs in the midline over the sacral promontory into the hollow of the sacrum. It anastomoses with the lateral sacral arteries and gives minute branches to the rectum. The gut branches have already been described (see p. 251 onwards); the remainder are considered below and where appropriate with the viscera concerned.

The **inferior phrenic arteries** are the first branches of the abdominal aorta, and may arise by a common stem

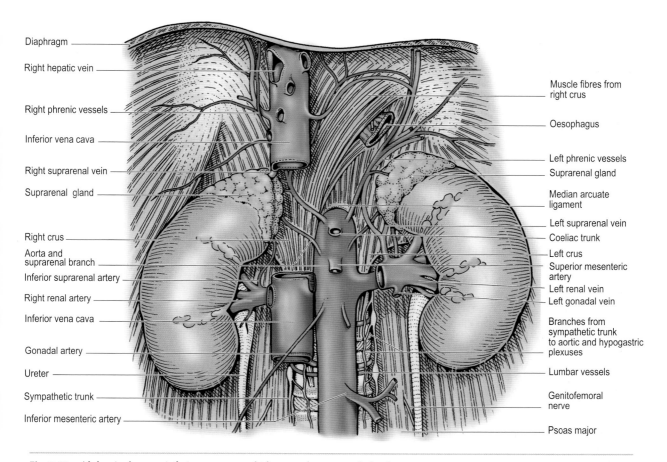

Diaphragm

Right hepatic vein

Right phrenic vessels

Inferior vena cava

Right suprarenal vein

Suprarenal gland

Right crus

Aorta and suprarenal branch

Inferior suprarenal artery

Right renal artery

Inferior vena cava

Gonadal artery

Ureter

Sympathetic trunk

Inferior mesenteric artery

Muscle fibres from right crus

Oesophagus

Left phrenic vessels

Suprarenal gland

Median arcuate ligament

Left suprarenal vein

Coeliac trunk

Left crus

Superior mesenteric artery

Left renal vein

Left gonadal vein

Branches from sympathetic trunk to aortic and hypogastric plexuses

Lumbar vessels

Genitofemoral nerve

Psoas major

Fig. 5.43   Abdominal aorta, inferior vena cava, kidneys and suprarenal glands.
(The sympathetic plexus on the front of the aorta has been omitted.)

just above the coeliac trunk. Each slopes upwards over the crus of the diaphragm, which they supply (Fig. 5.43). The left artery passes behind the oesophagus; the right passes behind the inferior vena cava. They give off small suprarenal branches.

The **suprarenal arteries** arise from the aorta between its inferior phrenic and renal branches (Fig. 5.43). They run laterally across the crus of the diaphragm. The right artery passes behind the inferior vena cava, and the left behind the posterior wall of the lesser sac, to reach the suprarenal glands.

The **renal arteries** are large vessels arising at right angles from the aorta at the level of L2 vertebra (Fig. 5.43). The left artery is shorter than the right; it crosses the left crus and psoas, behind the left renal vein, both being covered by the tail of the pancreas and the splenic vessels. The longer right artery crosses the right

crus and psoas behind the inferior vena cava and the short right renal vein; these structures separate the artery from the head of the pancreas and bile duct and from the second part of the duodenum. Each artery approaches the hilum of the kidney to supply the renal segments, as described on page 294 (Fig. 5.50).

Each renal artery gives off small suprarenal and ureteric branches. One or two accessory renal arteries arise frequently from the aorta, above or below the main artery.

The **gonadal arteries** have a similar origin and course in both sexes. The **testicular** or **ovarian arteries** arise from near the front of the aorta, below the renal arteries but well above the origin of the inferior mesenteric. They slope steeply downwards over psoas and genitofemoral nerve (the right artery first crossing the inferior vena cava, Fig. 5.43) crossing the ureter and supplying its middle portion, and being themselves crossed by the colic vessels. The right artery is also crossed by the third part of the duodenum and the root of the mesentery; the left artery is crossed by the inferior mesenteric vein. They reach the pelvic brim about halfway between the sacroiliac joint and the inguinal ligament, after which their course is different in the two sexes. The testicular artery runs along the pelvic brim above the external iliac artery, enters the deep inguinal ring and passes in the spermatic cord to the testis (Fig. 5.7). The ovarian artery crosses the pelvic brim and the external iliac vessels and enters the suspensory ligament to pass to the ovary and uterine tube (Fig. 5.62).

The **subcostal arteries** arise from the lowest part of the thoracic aorta and each enters the abdomen beneath the lateral arcuate ligament. It runs between the subcostal nerve and vein on the anterior surface of the lumbar fascia over quadratus lumborum behind the kidney, and passes laterally into the neurovascular plane of the anterior abdominal wall (between internal oblique and transversus).

The **lumbar arteries**, four in number, leave the abdominal aorta opposite the bodies of the upper four vertebrae. Hugging the bone they pass behind the lumbar sympathetic trunks and the fibrous arches in the psoas (Fig. 5.43). On the right side the inferior vena cava overlies the lower two and the right crus the upper two lumbar arteries; the left crus overlies the uppermost left artery. Each artery gives off posterior and spinal branches and passes laterally behind the psoas muscle. The three upper arteries pass laterally behind quadratus lumborum muscle into the neurovascular plane between transversus abdominis and internal oblique. The fourth lumbar artery, like the subcostal, passes across to the neurovascular plane in front of the lower border of quadratus lumborum, along the upper margin of the iliolumbar ligament. There is no fifth lumbar artery; its place is taken by the lumbar branch of the **iliolumbar artery** (from the internal iliac, see p. 318). It ascends from the pelvis in front of the lumbosacral trunk and passes laterally behind the obturator nerve and psoas muscle. The *lumbar branch* supplies psoas and quadratus lumborum and gives a spinal branch which enters the L5–S1 intervertebral foramen. The *iliac branch* runs into the iliac fossa, supplying iliacus and the ilium, and ends in the anastomosis at the anterior superior iliac spine.

The **common iliac arteries** are formed by the bifurcation of the aorta, on the body of L4 vertebra but to the left of the midline, so that the right artery is longer than the left (Fig. 5.47). Each passes to the front of the sacroiliac joint where the bifurcation into external and internal iliac arteries occurs; the ureter lies in front of this bifurcation or the very beginning of the external

iliac. The left common iliac is crossed by the inferior mesenteric (superior rectal) vessels lying beside the ureter behind the apex of the mesocolon (see p. 246). Each is also crossed by the sympathetic contributions to the superior hypogastric plexus, the sympathetic trunk itself passing behind the artery.

The **external iliac artery** continues in the line of the common iliac, along the pelvic brim on psoas, and passes beneath the inguinal ligament to enter the femoral sheath as the femoral artery. Its two branches are given off just above the ligament (Fig. 5.8). The *inferior epigastric artery* ascends along the medial margin of the deep inguinal ring, and the *deep circumflex iliac artery* runs above the inguinal ligament (see p. 233).

The *surface marking* of the common and external iliac arteries is along a line from the aortic bifurcation (see above) to the midpoint between the anterior superior iliac spine and the pubic symphysis. The common iliac artery corresponds to the upper third and the external iliac artery to the lower two-thirds of this line. The bifurcation of the common into the external and internal iliacs is 3 cm from the midline, level with the tubercles of the iliac crests (the intertubercular plane).

The **internal iliac arteries** enter the pelvis and are described on page 318.

Inferior vena cava

The inferior vena cava has a longer course than the aorta in the abdomen. It begins opposite L5 vertebra by the confluence of the two common iliac veins behind the right common iliac artery (Fig. 5.42A). It runs upwards on the right of the aorta, grooves the bare area of the liver, and pierces the central tendon of the diaphragm on a level with the body of T8 vertebra. It lies on the bodies of the lumbar vertebrae and the right crus of the diaphragm, overlapping the right sympathetic trunk, and crossing the right renal, suprarenal and inferior phrenic arteries (Fig. 5.43). It also partly overlaps the right suprarenal gland and the coeliac ganglion.

In the infracolic compartment the inferior vena cava lies behind the peritoneum of the posterior abdominal wall; it is crossed by the root of the mesentery, the right gonadal artery and the third part of the duodenum. In the supracolic compartment it lies at first behind the portal vein, head of the pancreas and bile duct, then behind the peritoneum that forms the posterior wall of the epiploic foramen. Above this it is behind the bare area of the liver, into which it excavates a deep groove (Fig. 5.32B).

With the exception of the gonadal (especially testicular) veins, the inferior vena cava and its tributaries do not have valves.

The *surface marking* of the inferior vena cava is a vertical line 2.5 cm to the right of the midline from the intertubercular plane to the sixth costal cartilage.

Tributaries

The vena caval tributaries are not identical with the branches of the abdominal aorta. In particular there is none corresponding to the three ventral branches to the gut. The blood from the alimentary tract, pancreas and spleen is collected by the portal venous system, and only after passing through the liver does it reach the vena cava via the hepatic veins, the vena cava's highest tributaries. Above its formation by the union of the two common iliac veins, the other tributaries (in ascending order) are the fourth and third lumbar veins of both sides, right gonadal, both renal, right suprarenal and both inferior phrenic veins.

Each **common iliac vein** is formed in front of the sacroiliac joint by the union of the internal iliac vein from the pelvis (see p. 320) and the external iliac vein, the continuation of the femoral vein, which enters the abdomen on the medial side of its corresponding artery and runs along the pelvic brim. The two common iliac veins continue upwards medial to their arteries to unite to form the vena cava behind the right common iliac artery (Fig. 5.42A). Because the vena cava is to the right of the midline, the left common iliac vein is longer than the right. It joins its fellow almost at a right angle after bulging forwards across the body of L5 vertebra, and may be compressed by the overlying artery. Each common iliac vein receives *iliolumbar* and perhaps *lateral sacral veins*, while the left usually receives the *median sacral vein* which lies on the right of the corresponding artery.

The **lumbar veins** accompany the lumbar arteries and drain the lateral and posterior abdominal walls, with anastomotic connections anteriorly with the epigastric veins and posteriorly with the vertebral venous plexuses. The fourth and third empty into the vena cava; those from the left pass behind the aorta, and all are expected to lie behind the sympathetic trunks but occasionally one or more may be in front. The second and first do not usually reach the vena cava but join the *ascending lumbar vein*, which connects common iliac, iliolumbar and lumbar veins and passes vertically upwards behind psoas and in front of the lumbar transverse processes; that on the right passes through the aortic opening and that on the left perforates the left crus. Before entering the thorax, each ascending lumbar vein joins the *subcostal vein* to form the **azygos** and **hemiazygos veins** respectively (see pp 217–219).

The **gonadal veins** accompany the arteries (testicular or ovarian) and each is usually paired. As they run up on psoas the two venae comitantes unite. On the right the vein usually enters the vena cava just below the renal vein at an acute angle; but the right testicular vein may occasionally join the renal vein. The left gonadal vein invariably joins the left renal vein at a right angle. The testicular veins usually have valves at their terminations; they may be present in the ovarian veins.

The **renal veins** lie in front of the renal arteries and behind the pancreas, and join the vena cava at right angles, at the level of L2 vertebra (Fig. 5.44). Each emerges from the hilum of the kidney as five or six tributaries which soon unite. The *left* renal vein is three times as long as the right (7.5 cm compared with 2.5 cm) and usually crosses in front of the aorta. It receives the left suprarenal vein and left gonadal vein and possibly a left inferior phrenic vein. In contrast the shorter *right* renal vein usually drains only its own kidney.

The left renal vein may have to be ligated and divided during surgery for aortic aneurysm. Provided that this is done to the right of the point of entry of the gonadal and suprarenal veins the kidney is not harmed. Rarely, the left renal vein may be double, with one vein passing anterior and one posterior to the aorta, or only a posterior vein may be present.

While the **left suprarenal vein** runs downwards and medially to the left renal vein, the **right suprarenal vein** is a very short vessel that passes horizontally to the posterior aspect of the inferior vena cava behind the bare area of the liver (Fig. 5.43)—an arrangement that complicates the surgery of the right gland.

The **inferior phrenic veins** accompany the arteries on the lower surface of the diaphragm and normally join the vena cava just below the liver, but the left vessel may join the left renal or suprarenal vein, or even be double with different destinations.

The three main **hepatic veins** (right, central and left) and several accessory hepatic veins enter the vena cava as it lies in its groove on the back of the liver; they are further described on page 272.

Lymph nodes and lymph trunks

From nodes which drain the alimentary tract, liver, biliary tract, spleen and pancreas (see p. 256), lymphatics pass back along the coeliac, superior and inferior mesenteric arteries to **preaortic nodes** situated around the origins of these three vessels. Similarly, lymphatics pass back along the paired branches of the aorta, both visceral and somatic, to **para-aortic nodes** which lie alongside the aorta at the origins of the paired vessels. The lymph drainage of any viscus follows its artery back to the aorta. Lymph from some pelvic viscera drains through nodes along the internal iliac arteries, to nodes along the

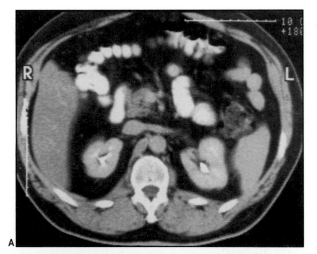

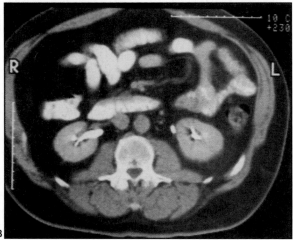

Fig. 5.44 CT scans of the upper abdomen (viewed by convention from below). In **A**, the left renal vein crosses in front of the aorta to enter the inferior vena cava. The right crus of the diaphragm is seen beside the aorta. In **B**, the pelvis of the right kidney is indicated by the white opacity (representing oral contrast medium which has been absorbed and excreted by the kidney), while on the left side the ureter, similarly outlined, lies immediately medial to the lower pole of the kidney. The psoas major and quadratus lumborum muscles are seen on either side of the lumbar vertebra.

common iliac arteries. These nodes also receive lymph from the lower limb via the inguinal (superficial and deep) nodes and external iliac nodes. The common iliac nodes drain up to the para-aortic nodes (Fig. 5.45).

From the highest of these aortic groups, a variable number of *intestinal* and *lumbar lymph trunks* (and

smaller lymphatics from the posterior ends of the lower intercostal spaces) join to form the elongated, sac-like **cisterna chyli** (though frequently the single cisterna is replaced by a confluence of lymph trunks). It is situated under cover of the right crus, in front of the bodies of L1 and L2 vertebrae, between the aorta and azygos vein. Its upper end becomes continuous with the thoracic duct (see p. 217).

Some of the fat absorbed by intestinal cells enters blood capillaries and so reaches the liver directly by the portal vein, but other processed lipid molecules enter the lacteals (lymph vessels) of the intestinal villi as chylomicrons, so producing the milky-looking lymph which enters the bloodstream via the cisterna chyli and thoracic duct.

Nerves

Somatic nerves

The anterior rami of the upper four lumbar spinal nerves at their emergence from the intervertebral foramina necessarily pass into the substance of psoas major. They give segmental branches of supply to psoas and quadratus lumborum and then break up into anterior and posterior divisions, which reunite to form the branches of the **lumbar plexus** within the substance of psoas. Most of the branches are for the supply of the lower limb; others innervate the lower anterior abdominal wall and give sensory branches to the parietal peritoneum. The branches of the lumbar plexus are summarized on page 336.

The segmental outflow from the spinal cord continues in series with the intercostal nerves of the thoracic wall. T12 (the subcostal nerve) and all five lumbar nerves emerge in series from the intervertebral foramina, but they do not all share in the supply of the anterior abdominal wall. Only T12 and L1 do so, in fact. L2, 3 and 4, after each giving a branch to the muscles of the posterior abdominal wall (psoas and quadratus lumborum) participate, through the lumbar plexus, in the formation of nerves for the flexor and extensor compartments of the thigh. The nerves to the thigh are the obturator (for the adductor compartment, a derivative of the flexor compartment of the thigh), and the femoral and lateral femoral cutaneous nerves (extensor compartment). A part of L4 and all L5 pass down as the lumbosacral trunk to the sacral plexus for distribution to the lower limb (see p. 321).

Nerves for the supply of the anterior abdominal wall cross the anterior surface of quadratus lumborum. They are the subcostal and the iliohypogastric and ilioinguinal nerves (Fig. 5.42A).

Fig. 5.45 Lymphangiogram showing lymph nodes on the pelvic brim and posterior abdominal wall.

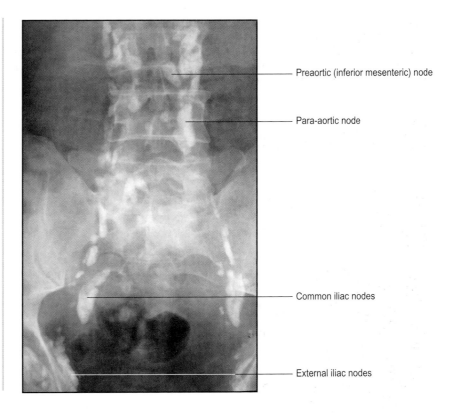

Preaortic (inferior mesenteric) node

Para-aortic node

Common iliac nodes

External iliac nodes

The **subcostal nerve** (T12) passes from the thorax behind the lateral arcuate ligament, where it lies below the vein and artery. The neurovascular bundle slopes down (parallel with the twelfth rib) across the front of the anterior layer of the lumbar fascia behind the kidney. The subcostal nerve passes through transversus abdominis to reach the neurovascular plane and continues around the anterior abdominal wall, whose muscles it supplies, ending by supplying the lower part of rectus abdominis, the pyramidalis muscle and the skin over them. It has a collateral (muscular) branch, and its lateral cutaneous branch pierces the oblique muscles and descends over the iliac crest to supply the skin of the anterior part of the buttock between the iliac crest and the greater trochanter.

The **iliohypogastric** and **ilioinguinal nerves** lie in front of quadratus lumborum at a lower level. They both arise from the anterior ramus of L1. The ilioinguinal nerve represents the collateral branch of the iliohypogastric. The nerves emerge from the lateral border of psoas major as a common stem (which then divides) or as separate nerves. As they slope across quadratus lumborum, behind the kidney, they pierce the anterior layer of the lumbar fascia and pass in front of it into transversus abdominis, to continue downwards and forwards, above the iliac crest, in the neurovascular plane.

The **iliohypogastric nerve** gives a lateral cutaneous branch which pierces the oblique muscles above the iliac crest to supply skin of the upper part of the buttock behind the area supplied by the subcostal nerve. The nerve then continues downwards in the neurovascular plane and pierces the internal oblique above the anterior superior iliac spine. It pierces the external oblique aponeurosis about 2.5 cm above the superficial inguinal ring and ends by supplying suprapubic skin.

The **ilioinguinal nerve** runs parallel with the iliohypogastric at a lower level. Piercing the lower border of internal oblique, it enters the inguinal canal and emerges through the superficial inguinal ring covered by the external spermatic fascia, which it pierces to become subcutaneous. It supplies the anterior one-third of the scrotum (mons pubis and labium majus), the root of the penis (clitoris), and the upper and medial part of the groin. Before it perforates the lower border of the internal oblique muscle it gives motor branches to those muscle fibres of internal oblique and transversus which are inserted into the conjoint tendon and are thereby of importance in maintaining the integrity of the inguinal canal.

The **lateral femoral cutaneous nerve** is formed by union of fibres from the posterior divisions of the anterior rami of L2 and L3. It emerges from the lateral border of psoas major and passes across the iliac fossa on the surface of the iliacus muscle (Fig. 5.42A) deep to the iliac fascia, posterior to the caecum on the right and the descending colon on the left. The nerve passes below or perforates the inguinal ligament a centimetre from the anterior superior iliac spine and so enters the thigh (see Fig. 3.2, p. 117). The nerve supplies the parietal peritoneum of the iliac fossa. Its distribution in the thigh is described on page 116.

The **femoral nerve** is formed in the substance of psoas major by union of branches from the posterior divisions of the anterior rami of L2–4. It emerges from the lateral border of psoas in the iliac fossa and runs down deep in the gutter between psoas and iliacus behind the iliac fascia. It gives branches to iliacus (L2 and 3) and leaves the iliac fossa by passing beneath the inguinal ligament to the lateral side of the femoral sheath, on the iliacus muscle (see Fig. 3.1, p. 116). Its course in the thigh is described on page 123.

The above nerves emerge from the lateral margin of psoas. The genitofemoral and obturator nerves have each a different pathway.

The **genitofemoral nerve** is formed in the substance of psoas major by union of branches from L1 and 2. It emerges from the anterior surface of psoas major and runs down on the muscle deep to the psoas fascia. In front of the fascia the left nerve is overlaid by the ureter, gonadal vessels, ascending branch of the left colic artery and the inferior mesenteric vein. The right nerve is overlaid by the ureter, gonadal vessels, the ileocolic artery and the root of the mesentery of the small intestine. Just above the inguinal ligament it perforates the psoas fascia and divides into genital and femoral branches (see Fig. 3.1, p. 116). The genital branch is composed of L2 and the femoral branch of L1 fibres.

The *genital branch* passes through the deep ring and enters the inguinal canal. It supplies motor fibres to the cremaster muscle, and sensory fibres to the spermatic fasciae, tunica vaginalis of the testis, and a small area of skin of the scrotum in males and the mons pubis and labium majus in females. The *femoral branch* passes down behind the inguinal ligament with the femoral artery, pierces the femoral sheath and the fascia lata, and supplies the skin over the upper part of the femoral triangle.

The **obturator nerve** and the lumbosacral trunk emerge from the medial border of psoas to enter the pelvis (see pp 320–321).

Autonomic nerves

The abdomen receives both sympathetic and parasympathetic nerves. The sympathetic supply is twofold, by the lumbar part of the sympathetic trunk and by the coeliac plexus which receives fibres from the thoracic part of the trunk. The coeliac plexus is wholly visceral; it supplies all the abdominal organs, including the gonads. The ganglionated lumbar trunk supplies somatic branches for the lower abdominal wall and the lower limb, but its visceral branches supply only the pelvic organs. The parasympathetic supply is provided by the vagus from above and the pelvic splanchnic nerves from below; it is wholly visceral. The vagus gives a branch to the coeliac plexus and the pelvic splanchnics join the inferior hypogastric plexus.

Sympathetic nerves

The **lumbar part of the sympathetic trunk** brings preganglionic fibres descending from the lower thoracic trunk, and it receives a further input of preganglionic fibres (white rami) from the first and second lumbar nerves. Its ganglia give off somatic and visceral branches, and the trunk passes down across the pelvic brim, behind the common iliac vessels, to become the sacral part of the trunk (see p. 322).

The lumbar part of the sympathetic trunk enters the abdomen by passing behind the medial arcuate ligament on the front of psoas major. It runs down behind the peritoneum on the vertebral bodies along the medial margin of the psoas muscle (Fig. 5.46). As elsewhere it lies in front of the segmental vessels, the lumbar arteries and veins, but some lumbar veins may pass in front of the trunk.

The left lumbar trunk lies beside the left margin of the aorta (Fig. 5.43) with para-aortic lymph nodes in front of it, while the right trunk lies behind the inferior vena cava.

The **lumbar ganglia** are usually four in number, but fusion of ganglia may reduce them. White rami communicantes from the first two lumbar nerves join the trunk and relay in the lumbar and sacral ganglia. Grey rami communicantes from the lumbar ganglia accompany the lumbar arteries around the sides of the vertebral bodies, medial to the fibrous arches, to join the anterior rami of lumbar nerves, for distribution to the body wall and lower limb, through the branches of the lumbar plexus. Vasoconstrictor fibres for the femoral artery and its branches travel in the femoral nerve.

Lumbar splanchnic nerves arise from all lumbar ganglia. Those from the first and second ganglia pass to plexuses in front of the aorta; those from the third and

Fig. 5.46 Sympathetic rami at L1 or L2 vertebral levels. An accessory ganglion in psoas major relays directly back to the segmental nerve; the remainder of L1 and L2 outflow passes into the sympathetic trunk for local or distant relay.

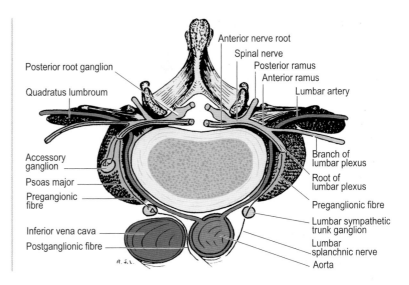

fourth ganglia pass respectively in front of and behind the common iliac arteries. They join with each other and with fibres from the aortic plexuses to form the **superior hypogastric plexus** (Fig. 5.47), which comprises both pre- and postganglionic sympathetic fibres. This plexus lies anterior to the aortic bifurcation and the left common iliac vein and between the common iliac arteries, in front of L5 vertebra and the sacral promontory. It was previously known as the presacral nerve—a misnomer as it is prelumbar and a plexus, not presacral and a single nerve. It lies behind the parietal peritoneum which can be stripped off its anterior aspect surgically, an avascular areolar tissue plane lying between them. The plexus often lies a little to the left of the midline, close to the apex of the attachment of the sigmoid mesocolon. The plexus divides in the manner of an inverted Y into the **right** and **left hypogastric nerves** (which may not be single but a bundle) which run down into the pelvis to join the inferior hypogastric plexuses (see p. 322). There are only a few ganglion cells in the superior hypogastric plexus; preganglionic white fibres in the hypogastric nerves pass through to relay in ganglia in the inferior hypogastric plexuses.

The **coeliac plexus** lies around the origin of the coeliac trunk above the upper border of the pancreas. The **greater** and **lesser splanchnic nerves** (see p. 219) pierce the crura of the diaphragm and enter the two large **coeliac ganglia** which lie in front of the crura, the right one behind the inferior vena cava and the left behind the splenic artery. The splanchnic nerves are almost all preganglionic (white) and many relay in the coeliac ganglia. The *least splanchnic nerve* relays in a small *renal ganglion* behind the renal artery. This is merely an offshoot of the main coeliac ganglion itself. Separated masses of ganglion may lie on the aorta at the superior and even the inferior mesenteric artery origins.

Postganglionic fibres from the coeliac ganglia and preganglionic splanchnic fibres form a network on the aorta, the relevant parts of which are the coeliac, superior mesenteric, intermesenteric (abdominal aortic) and inferior mesenteric plexuses, in accordance with their relation to the origin of the midline gut arteries. The fibres from these plexuses supply all the abdominal viscera, which they reach by streaming along the visceral branches of the aorta. Those passing to the kidney pick up the branches of the renal ganglion to form the renal plexus behind the renal artery. Testis and ovary are supplied by a sympathetic plexus that accompanies each gonadal artery.

The sympathetic fibres are vasomotor, motor to sphincters (e.g. pyloric), inhibitory to peristalsis, and carry sensory fibres from all the viscera supplied.

Pre-ganglionic fibres from the greater splanchnic nerve pass without relay to the cells of the suprarenal medulla (these cells share a common origin from neural crest ectoderm with the cell bodies of sympathetic ganglia). These preganglionic fibres cause the suprarenal medulla to pour forth adrenaline. The vasomotor supply to the suprarenal gland reaches it by postganglionic fibres which have relayed in the coeliac ganglion.

Lumbar sympathectomy

Surgical removal of the third and fourth lumbar ganglia employs an extraperitoneal approach through a transverse muscle-cutting incision in the anterior abdominal

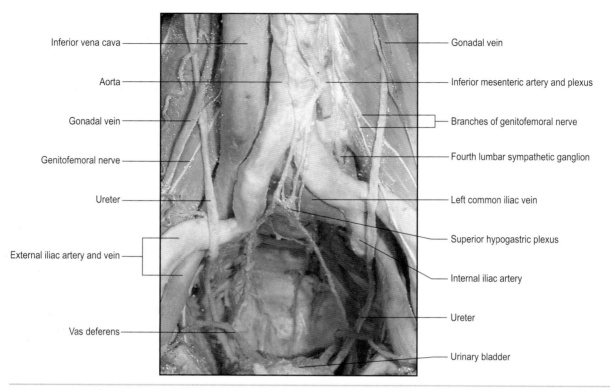

Fig. 5.47 Prosection of posterior abdominal wall and pelvis in the Anatomy Museum of the Royal College of Surgeons of England. The abdominal and pelvic viscera have been removed except for the urinary bladder. Red and blue resin has been injected into arteries and veins.

wall, or the flank, on the appropriate side. The intact peritoneum is stripped off the deep surface of transversus abdominis and the posterior abdominal wall as far as the vertebral column, carefully avoiding damage to the gonadal vessels, ureter and genitofemoral nerve overlying psoas major. Exposure of the right sympathetic trunk requires careful retraction of the inferior vena cava, which lies in front of it. On the left the trunk is beside the aorta and more easily accessed. Although the lumbar vessels usually lie behind the sympathetic trunks, some lumbar veins may pass in front of the trunks. Lumbar ganglia may also be destroyed by injecting them with phenol via a posterior paravertebral approach under radiographic or ultrasonic guidance.

Parasympathetic nerves

Both vagi, intermixed in the vagal trunks (see p. 259), contribute fibres to the coeliac plexus. Without relay they accompany postganglionic sympathetic fibres to the gut as far as the distal transverse colon. They also enter the renal plexus and pass into the kidney.

The **pelvic splanchnic nerves**, from cell bodies in the lateral horn of sacral segments 2 to 3 or 4 (see p. 22), arise from the anterior rami of those sacral nerves distal to the anterior sacral foramina. They join the inferior hypogastric plexus for distribution to pelvic viscera. Some fibres rise up out of the pelvis, usually passing to the left of the superior hypogastric plexus, occasionally through it, to ascend behind the peritoneum and supply the large intestine from the splenic flexure downwards.

The vagus is motor and secretomotor to the gut and its glands down to the transverse colon; the pelvic splanchnics fulfil this function from the splenic flexure distally. The vagus is inhibitory to the pyloric sphincter. Sensory fibres are present in the vagus and pelvic splanchnics.

PART ELEVEN

Kidneys, ureters and suprarenal glands

Kidneys

The kidneys lie high up on the posterior abdominal wall (Fig. 5.43) behind the peritoneum, largely under cover of the costal margin. At best only their lower poles can be palpated in the normal individual. Each kidney lies obliquely, with its long axis parallel with the lateral border of psoas major. It lies well back in the paravertebral gutter, so that the hilum, a vertical slit-like depression at the medial border transmitting the renal vessels and nerves and the renal pelvis (the beginning of the ureter), faces somewhat forwards as well as medially (Fig. 5.44). As a result of this slight 'rotation' of the kidney an anteroposterior radiograph gives a somewhat foreshortened picture of the width of the kidney. The normal kidney measures about $12 \times 6 \times 3$ cm and weighs about 130 g. The hilum of the right kidney lies just below, and of the left just above, the transpyloric plane 5 cm from the midline. The bulk of the right lobe of the liver accounts for the lower position of the right kidney. The upper pole of the left kidney overlies the eleventh rib, that of the right kidney the twelfth rib. Each kidney moves in a vertical range of 2 cm during the full respiratory excursion of the diaphragm.

The surfaces of the kidney, covered by its *capsule*, are usually smooth and convex though traces of lobulation, normal in the fetus, are often seen. The pelvis emerges from the hilum, behind the vessels, to pass down as the ureter.

Posteriorly the relations of both kidneys are similar, comprising mostly the diaphragm and quadratus lumborum muscles, with overlap medially on to psoas and laterally on to transversus abdominis. The upper pole lies on those fibres of the diaphragm which arise from the lateral and medial arcuate ligaments. A small triangular part of the **costodiaphragmatic recess of the pleura** lies behind the diaphragm and is an important posterior relation (Fig. 5.48), which is at risk in the lumbar approach to the kidney (see p. 296). The subcostal vein, artery and nerve, on emerging beneath the lateral arcuate ligament, lie behind the kidney, as do the iliohypogastric and ilioinguinal nerves as they emerge from the lateral border of psoas. The hilum of the kidney lies over psoas and the convexity of the lateral border lies on the aponeurosis of origin of transversus abdominis.

Fig. 5.48 Relationship of the pleural sacs to the upper poles of the kidneys, from behind. The ureters lie medial to the tips of the lumbar transverse processes.

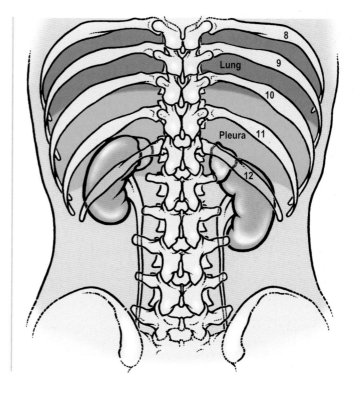

The suprarenal glands surmount the superior poles of both kidneys and overlap a small part of their anterior surfaces. The rest of the upper halves of each kidney lie in contact with peritoneum, which on the right kidney is the peritoneum of the hepatorenal pouch (part of the greater sac), and on the left is the peritoneum of the lesser sac (part of the stomach bed) medially, and the peritoneum of the greater sac laterally (between the kidney and the spleen), with the splenorenal ligament passing forwards between these areas (Fig. 5.49). The hilum is separated from the peritoneum, on the right side by the second part of the duodenum and on the left side by the body of the pancreas and splenic vessels (Fig. 5.26). The lateral part of the lower pole is separated from peritoneum by the hepatic and splenic flexures of the colon on the right and left sides respectively. The medial part of the lower pole, on each side, lies in contact with peritoneum which separates it from coils of jejunum; between peritoneum and kidney are ascending branches of the right and left colic arteries.

The **perinephric fat** lies outside the renal capsule (Fig. 5.49) and plays a part in retaining the kidney in position. Nephroptosis ('floating kidney') may develop after severe loss of weight. The **renal fascia** (of Gerota) surrounds the perinephric fat. It is not a very obvious

membrane in the living, but appears more convincingly in the embalmed cadavre. It is a condensation of the areolar tissue between the parietal peritoneum and the posterior abdominal wall and restrains the extension of a perinephric abscess. It ascends as a dome over the upper pole of the kidney and the suprarenal. However, a fascial septum separates the two organs, which explains why in nephrectomy the latter gland is not usually displaced (or even seen). At the lateral renal border the anterior and posterior layers fuse, while at the hilum the fascia is attached to the renal vessels and the ureter. When traced downwards, the fascia fades into the extra-peritoneal tissue around the ureter. Pus in the perinephric space and injections into it do not usually track down-wards, but increasing pressure may force the fascia to rupture and allow such contents to flow downwards retroperitoneally towards the pelvis.

The **renal pelvis** is the funnel-shaped commencement of the ureter, and is normally the most posterior of the three main structures in the hilum (though an arterial branch or venous tributary may lie behind it). The capacity of the average pelvis is less than 5 mL.

Blood supply and segments

The wide-bored **renal arteries** have a blood flow in excess of 1 litre per minute. They leave the abdominal aorta at right angles and lie behind the pancreas and renal veins.

Based on its blood supply, each kidney possesses five segments (Fig. 5.50). In the region of the hilum the artery typically gives rise to an anterior and a posterior division. The posterior division supplies the posterior segment, while the anterior division gives branches that supply the apical, upper, middle and lower segments. The pattern of branching of the vessels may vary, but there are always five segments with no collateral circula-tion between them. Abnormal or aberrant renal arteries, such as a vessel running from the aorta to the lower pole are, in fact, segmental vessels with an unusual origin (persistence of a fetal vessel, see below). They are not usually accompanied by veins.

Veins from the renal segments communicate with one another (unlike the arteries) and eventually form five or six vessels that unite at the hilum to form the single **renal vein** (see p. 287). The usual order of structures in the hilum of each kidney is vein, artery, ureter from front to back.

Lymph drainage

The lymphatics of the kidney drain to para-aortic nodes at the level of origin of the renal arteries (L2).

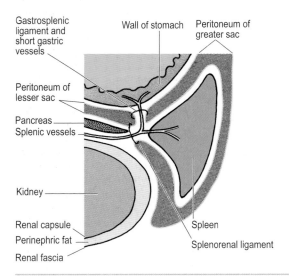

Gastrosplenic ligament and short gastric vessels

Wall of stomach

Peritoneum of greater sac

Peritoneum of lesser sac

Pancreas

Splenic vessels

Kidney

Renal capsule

Perinephric fat

Renal fascia

Spleen

Splenorenal ligament

Fig. 5.49 Diagrammatic transverse section through the left upper abdomen, viewed from below (like a CT scan), showing the peritoneal relationships of the spleen and renal fascia. The short gastric vessels run in the gastrosplenic ligament. The splenic vessels and the tail of the pancreas are in the splenorenal ligament. The kidney is surrounded by its own capsule, the perinephric fat and the renal fascia.

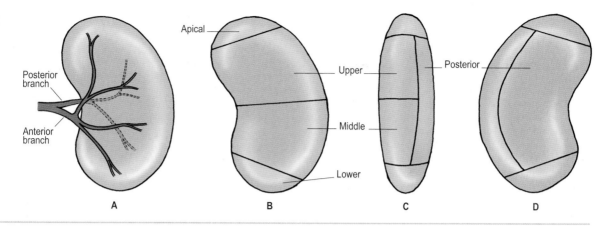

Fig. 5.50 Arterial segments of the left kidney. **A** shows branches of the renal artery; **B**, **C** and **D** indicate the segments as seen from the front, the lateral side and the back respectively. The posterior division of the artery supplies the posterior segment and the anterior division supplies the other four. There may be variations in the pattern of division but the segments are constant.

Nerve supply

Renal nerves are derived from both parts of the autonomic system. The sympathetic preganglionic cells lie in the spinal cord from T12 to L1 segments and they send preganglionic fibres to the thoracic and lumbar splanchnic nerves. These fibres synapse in the coeliac and renal ganglia. They are vasomotor in function. Afferent fibres, including those subserving pain, accompany the sympathetic nerves, as for most other viscera. The pathway for the pain of renal colic from a stone in the calyces or renal pelvis passes to the coeliac plexus and thence by the splanchnic nerves to the sympathetic trunk and via white rami communicantes to T12–L1 spinal nerves and so into the spinal cord by the posterior nerve roots. The pain may thus be referred to the back and lumbar region, and radiate to the anterior abdominal wall and down to the external genitalia. It is possible that some afferents run with the vagal fibres, and this could explain the nausea and vomiting that may accompany renal pain.

Structure

The internal structure of the kidney is displayed when the organ is split open longitudinally. A dark reddish **cortex** lies beneath the capsule and extends towards the pelvis as the *renal columns*, lying between a number of darker and triangular striated areas, the *pyramids* of the **medulla**. The apices of several pyramids open together into a *renal papilla*, each of which projects into a *minor calyx*. The minor calyces unite to form two or three *major calyces* which open into the renal pelvis.

The histological and functional unit of the kidney is the *nephron*, and there are about 1 million in each kidney. Each nephron consists of a glomerulus and a tubule system. The *glomerulus* is a tuft of capillaries surrounded by very thin epithelial cells (podocytes), the whole forming a mass which projects into a rounded capsule (of Bowman). The epithelium covering the capillaries is continuous with that forming the boundary of Bowman's capsule, which in turn continues into the epithelium of the tubule system. The part of the tubule adjacent to Bowman's capsule is the *proximal convoluted tubule*, and this leads into the thin-walled *loop of Henle* and so to the *distal convoluted tubule* and finally to the *collecting tubule* and *collecting duct*. The glomeruli and convoluted tubules are in the cortex, and the loops of Henle and collecting tubules and ducts in the medulla. The collecting ducts unite with one another, and the largest open at the tip of a renal papilla in a minor calyx. The glomerular capillaries are supplied by an afferent arteriole, and leaving them is an efferent arteriole which breaks up into peritubular capillaries surrounding the proximal and distal convoluted tubules. Urine is a glomerular filtrate (deproteinized plasma) which passes into the space of Bowman's capsule and so into the tubule system where it is modified by selective absorption and secretion. Certain arteriolar cells and distal convoluted tubule cells constitute the *juxtaglomerular apparatus* which secretes renin.

The pelvis, like the ureter, is lined by transitional epithelium and there is smooth muscle in its wall. Specialized muscle cells in the walls of the minor calyces act as 'pacemakers' that initiate contractile waves which pass down into the ureter.

Development

Three separate excretory organs appear in vertebrate evolution: the pronephros; mesonephros; and metanephros (see p. 25). The first two consist of excretory tubules arranged segmentally and they empty into the same duct. The third consists of a mass of tubules having no segmental arrangement and it drains into a new duct that develops specifically for the purpose (the ureter).

The *pronephros* is very evanescent, but its duct persists. *Mesonephric tubules* then develop and open into the pronephric duct which is henceforth called the *mesonephric* (Wolffian) *duct* (see p. 240). Caudal to the mesonephros the intermediate cell mass gives rise to about a million new tubules, forming the *metanephros*. The latter induces a bud, the ureter, to grow from the caudal end of the mesonephric duct. The *ureteric bud* separates from the mesonephric duct, leaving the latter to form part of the bladder (see p. 308) and in the male the ductus deferens and associated structures (see p. 311). The bud grows up and divides into the calyces of the pelvis (major and minor) and the collecting tubules of the medullary pyramids, into which the distal convoluted tubules of the metanephros come to drain. The fetal and neonatal kidney has a lobulated appearance, reflecting the way metanephric tissue overlies tubular budding from the calyces.

The definitive kidney (metanephros) develops in the pelvis and is supplied from the internal iliac artery. It subsequently migrates to its adult position, gaining successively new arteries of supply from the common iliac and then from the aorta. The older vessels degenerate as the new ones appear, until the (usually) single definitive artery forms. The hilum is at first anterior but the kidney rotates 90° medially.

Anomalies. Persistence of fetal lobulation is of no significance. Persistence of one of the fetal arteries is common (30% of individuals), especially a vessel from the aorta to the lower pole. Whether such vessels should be called accessory, abnormal, aberrant, supernumerary or whatever is debated. Fusion of the lower poles of the kidneys gives rise to *horseshoe kidney* (1 in 800); the ureters pass anterior to the isthmus of kidney substance, as does the inferior mesenteric artery which limits ascent of the horseshoe (Fig. 5.51). *Polycystic disease* (1 in 500) is a hereditary disorder which may be associated with cysts in the liver, pancreas and lungs. One person in 500 has only one kidney (*renal agenesis*), a situation which must be excluded before considering nephrectomy.

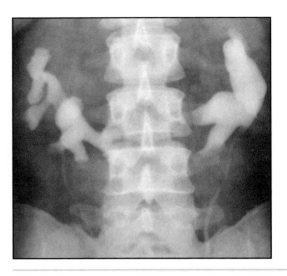

Fig. 5.51 Intravenous pyelogram showing a horseshoe kidney. The isthmus, which is not clearly seen, lies in front of the upper part of L4 vertebra, its further ascent being prevented by the origin of the inferior mesenteric artery from the front of the aorta. The calyces and pelvis on each side are generally rotated anteriorly causing the characteristic radiological appearance of calyces pointing medially.

Surgical approach

For many operations on the kidney including removal (*nephrectomy*) and removal of stones (*nephrolithotomy*) a lumbar approach is used (see p. 241). The renal fascia and perirenal fat are incised to expose the kidney, whose upper pole is freed leaving the suprarenal gland within its own compartment of the fascia. The overlying peritoneum is pushed away forwards and medially. The renal vessels can then be exposed, ligated and divided (the artery before the vein) to mobilize the organ further and transect the ureter. On the right a diseased kidney may adhere to the colon, duodenum, inferior vena cava or suprarenal gland, and on the left to the colon, spleen, pancreas or suprarenal. The right renal vein is only 2.5 cm long, so the inferior vena cava is very near the operation area.

For *percutaneous renal biopsy*, the lower pole of the kidney is entered by an approach 2.5 cm below the twelfth rib and at a distance from the midline determined radiologically. Damage to a renal vessel or calyx is a potential hazard, and the needle is only advanced while the patient is holding the breath so that the kidney is not torn by respiratory movement.

For *transplantation*, the donor kidney is placed retroperitoneally in the iliac fossa with the hilum parallel to the external iliac vessels. The renal artery is anastomosed to the internal or external iliac artery and the renal vein to the external iliac vein. The ureter is implanted into the bladder.

Ureters

The ureter is 25 cm long. Its points of narrowest calibre are at the pelviureteric junction, where it crosses the pelvic brim, and as it passes through the bladder wall.

The ureter passes down on psoas major under cover of the peritoneum and crosses in front of the genito-femoral nerve, being itself crossed anteriorly by the gonadal vessels. On the right the upper part is behind the third part of the duodenum, while lower down it is crossed anteriorly by the right colic and ileocolic vessels and by the root of the mesentery. On the left it is lateral to the inferior mesenteric vessels and is crossed anteriorly by the left colic vessels and, at the pelvic brim, by the apex of the sigmoid mesocolon. It leaves the psoas muscle at the bifurcation of the common iliac artery, over the sacroiliac joint, and passes into the pelvis (see p. 308). It adheres to the peritoneum of the posterior abdominal wall when that membrane is stripped off the posterior abdominal wall. It can be distinguished from vessels and nerves in the living body in that it is a whitish, non-pulsatile cord which shows peristaltic activity when gently pinched with forceps.

Its **surface markings** are of use in palpating it for tenderness and in identifying radiographic shadows. On the anterior abdominal wall it can be marked from the tip of the ninth costal cartilage (see p. 242) to the bifurcation of the common iliac artery (see p. 286).

More important is the line of projection of the ureter on a radiograph. It lies medial to the tips of the transverse processes of the lumbar vertebrae (Fig. 5.24 and 5.48) and crosses the pelvic brim at the sacroiliac joint. From here its pelvic shadow passes to the ischial spine and thence, foreshortened, to the pubic tubercle.

Blood supply

The upper end is supplied by the ureteric branch of the renal artery and the lower end by branches from the inferior and superior vesical and uterine arteries. The middle reaches of the ureter are supplied by branches from the abdominal aorta, the gonadal, common iliac and internal iliac arteries. All these vessels make a fairly good anastomosis with each other in the adventitia of the ureter, forming longitudinal channels. The blood supply is endangered if the ureter is stripped clean of its surrounding tissue.

Lymph drainage

The lymphatics run back alongside the arteries; the abdominal portion of the ureter drains into para-aortic nodes, the pelvic portion into common iliac and internal iliac nodes.

Nerve supply

Although sympathetic fibres from T10–L1 segments of the cord reach the ureter via the coeliac and hypogastric plexuses, together with parasympathetic fibres from the pelvic splanchnic nerves, their functional significance is not clear. Intact innervation of the renal pelvis or ureter is not necessary for the initiation or propagation of peristalsis from the calyceal pacemakers. There are no ganglion cells in or on the ureter. Pain fibres accompany sympathetic nerves, as from the kidney (see p. 295).

Structure

The ureter is a tube of smooth muscle lined internally by mucous membrane. The muscle often appears histologically to be arranged as a middle circular layer with inner and outer longitudinal layers. However, it is more accurate to consider the muscle as a single coat with fibres running in many different directions because they are parts of intertwining helices. The lax mucous membrane is lined by transitional epithelium; there is no muscularis mucosae.

Development

The ureter is of mesodermal origin; it is derived by a process of budding from the caudal end of the mesonephric duct (see p. 296). Its upper end divides into two or three (the major calyces of the renal pelvis) and further subdivisions produce the minor calyces and collecting tubules. Low division of the ureteric bud produces double ureter.

Suprarenal glands

These glands lie anterosuperior to the upper part of each kidney (Fig. 5.43). They are somewhat asymmetrical, yellowish in colour, and lie within their own compartment of the renal fascia. Adrenal gland is an alternative name.

The **right suprarenal gland** is pyramidal in shape and surmounts the upper pole of the right kidney. It lies on the diaphragm and encroaches on to the front of the right kidney. The anterior surface is overlapped medially by the inferior vena cava. The rest of the anterior surface is in contact above with the bare area of the liver, and is covered below by the peritoneum of the posterior wall of the hepatorenal pouch.

The **left suprarenal gland** is crescentic in shape and drapes over the medial border of the left kidney above the hilum. It lies on the left crus of the diaphragm and overlaps the front of the left kidney. The upper part of the anterior surface is covered by the peritoneum of the posterior wall of the lesser sac, forming part of the stomach bed; the lower part is in contact with the body of the pancreas and the splenic vessels.

Blood supply

Both glands receive blood from three sources: directly from the aorta and from the renal and inferior phrenic arteries, the last providing two or three small branches. In contrast there is usually a single vein. The right vein is only a few millimetres long and enters the vena cava; the left vein is longer and enters the left renal vein.

Lymph drainage

To para-aortic nodes.

Nerve supply

The main supply is by myelinated preganglionic sympathetic fibres from the splanchnic nerves via the coeliac plexus; the fibres synapse directly with medullary cells (see p. 20). Blood vessels receive the usual postganglionic sympathetic supply. Cortical control is not neural but by ACTH from the anterior pituitary.

Structure

The suprarenal gland has an outer yellow cortex completely enclosing a much thinner grey medulla. The **cortex**, whose principal products are cortisol, aldosterone, androgens and related hormones, consists of three layers or zones. They are, from the surface inwards, the zona glomerulosa (with small rounded cells), the zona fasciculata (parallel rows of pale-staining vacuolated cells) and the zona reticularis (a network of smaller and darker-staining cells). The rather small central **medulla** has larger cells secreting the catecholamines adrenaline (epinephrine) (80%) and noradrenaline (norepinephrine) (20%) and some dopamine. Many of the medullary cells exhibit the chromaffin reaction: they contain fine cytoplasmic granules (the catecholamine precursors) which are coloured brown by chromium salts. Dilated capillaries are usually prominent in the medulla but not in the cortex.

Development

The medulla is derived by migration of cells from the neural crest and is ectodermal in origin while the cortex is derived in situ from the mesoderm of the intermediate cell mass (see p. 25).

Surgical approach

For *bilateral adrenalectomy* the glands are usually approached from the front. A bilateral subcostal 'rooftop' incision provides appropriate transperitoneal access. For exposure of the right gland, after retraction of the right lobe of the liver, a Kocher manoeuvre (see p. 279) is employed to mobilize the second part of the duodenum and head of the pancreas from the upper pole of the kidney and inferior vena cava. For the left gland, after division of the phrenicocolic ligament to mobilize the splenic flexure of the colon, the posterior layer of the splenorenal ligament is incised and the spleen turned medially with the tail of the pancreas. On each side the suprarenal vein is ligated before the numerous small arteries; the right vein is particularly short and the vena cava is easily torn. The glands must be handled as little as possible before venous ligation to prevent surges of hormone release. The anterior, transperitoneal approach is also used for laparoscopic bilateral adrenalectomy.

A posterolateral extraperitoneal approach through the bed of the twelfth rib provides access for *unilateral adrenalectomy*. The removal of a large adrenal tumour may require a higher approach, through the bed of the eleventh or tenth ribs, and division of the diaphragm.

PART TWELVE

Pelvic cavity

Bony pelvis

The individual features of the hip bone (see p. 169), sacrum (see p. 453) and coccyx (see p. 455) are considered separately. When articulated the bones enclose a cavity; from the brim of the cavity the ala of each ilium projects up to form the iliac fossa, part of the posterior abdominal wall. The **pelvic brim** is formed in continuity by the pubic crest, pectineal line of the pubis, arcuate line of the ilium, and the ala and promontory of the sacrum. The plane of the brim is oblique, lying at 60° with the horizontal (Fig. 5.53); the vagina is in the same plane. From the brim the pelvic cavity projects back to the buttocks.

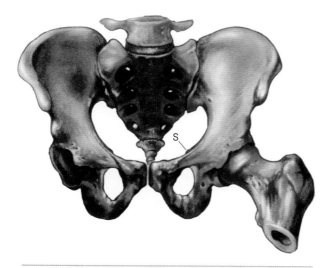

Fig. 5.52 Male pelvis, from the front. An imaginary horizontal plane through the top of the pubic symphysis traverses the tip of the coccyx, the ischial spine (S), the centre of the acetabulum and femoral head, and the tip of the greater trochanter.

The pelvic joints and ligaments are described on pages 335 onwards.

Sex differences are due to the two facts that the female pelvis is broader than that of the male for easier passage of the fetal head and that the female bones, including the head of the femur, are more slender than those of the male. In the male pelvis the sturdy bones make an acute subpubic angle (Fig. 5.52), pointed like a Gothic arch, while in the female the slender bones make a wide subpubic angle, rounded like a Roman arch. The outline of the pelvic brim differs. In the male the sacral promontory indents the outline, and the brim is widest towards the back (a 'heart-shaped' outline) while in the female there is less indentation of the outline by the sacral promontory and the brim is widest further forwards (a 'transversely oval' outline).

Position of the pelvis

In the erect individual the anterior superior iliac spines and the upper margin of the symphysis pubic lie in the same vertical plane. The upper border of the symphysis pubis, the spine of the ischium, the tip of the coccyx, the head of the femur and the apex of the greater trochanter lie in the same horizontal plane (Fig. 5.52). This plane passes through the pelvic cavity at a level with the tip of the finger of the clinician during rectal or vaginal examination. The ovaries in the female and the seminal vesicles in the male lie in this plane.

Pelvic walls

The word pelvis is Latin for a basin and, when tilted forwards into the anatomical position, the bony pelvis does bear some resemblance to a pudding basin but with much of the front wall missing. The deficiency is made good by the lower part of the anterior abdominal wall where the aponeuroses of all three anterolateral muscles lie in front of rectus abdominis.

The pelvic brim divides the 'false pelvis' (above the brim, and part of the general abdominal cavity) from the 'true pelvis' or pelvic cavity (below the brim).

The muscles of the pelvis are obturator internus and piriformis (which are also classified as lower limb muscles), and levator ani and coccygeus, (which, with their fellows of the opposite side, constitute the pelvic floor or pelvic diaphragm).

The side wall of the pelvis is formed by the hip bone, clad with obturator internus and its fascia. The curved posterior wall is formed by the sacrum with piriformis passing laterally into the greater sciatic foramen.

Piriformis

Piriformis arises from the middle three pieces of its own half of the sacrum, the muscle taking origin from the lateral mass and extending medially between the anterior sacral foramina (see Fig. 6.97, p. 454); thus the emerging sacral nerves and sacral plexus lie on the muscle (Fig. 5.56). It runs transversely to the greater sciatic foramen. The pelvic surface of the muscle and the sacral plexus are covered by pelvic fascia attached to the sacral periosteum at the margin of the muscle. The course of the muscle in the gluteal region, its nerve supply and action are described on page 130.

Obturator internus

The large obturator foramen contains in life a felted mass of fibrous tissue, the obturator membrane (Fig. 5.53), with a gap above that converts the obturator notch into a canal for the obturator nerve and vessels. The muscle arises from the whole membrane and from the bony margins of the foramen. The origin extends posteriorly as high as the pelvic brim and across the flat surface of the ischium to the margin of the greater sciatic notch (see Fig. 3.46, p. 172). On the ischial tuberosity the origin extends down to the falciform ridge. From this wide origin the muscle fibres converge fan-wise towards the lesser sciatic notch (Fig. 5.64). Tendinous fibres develop

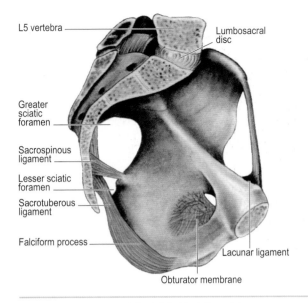

Fig. 5.53   Ligaments of the left half of the pelvis.

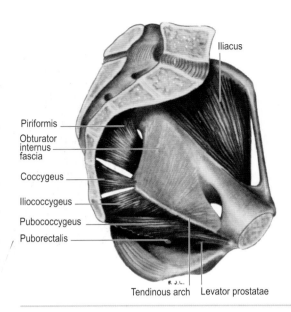

Fig. 5.54   Muscles of the left half of the pelvis.

on the muscle surface where it bears on the lesser sciatic notch and the bone often shows low ridges and grooves where the tendon takes a right-angled turn to pass into the buttock. The bone here is lined by hyaline cartilage and is separated from the tendon by a bursa. The muscle is described further on page 130.

The muscle is covered with a strong membrane, the obturator fascia (Fig. 5.54). This is attached to bone at the margins of the muscle and fuses below with the falciform process of the sacrotuberous ligament on the ischial tuberosity. The tendinous arch of origin of levator ani slopes across the obturator internus fascia (the pelvic cavity is above this line, the ischioanal fossa below it).

Pelvic floor

The pelvic floor consists of a gutter-shaped sheet of muscle, the pelvic diaphragm, slung around the midline body effluents (urethra and anal canal and, in the female, the vagina).

The muscles of the pelvic floor are the levator ani and the coccygeus. They arise in continuity from the body of the pubis, from the tendinous arch over the obturator fascia, and from the spine of the ischium, and are inserted into the coccyx and the postanal plate (see below). From their origin the muscle fibres slope downwards and backwards to the midline; the pelvic floor so produced is a gutter that slopes downwards and faces forwards.

Levator ani

Levator ani consists of two main parts, pubococcygeus and iliococcygeus (Fig. 5.55). Their fibres arise in continuity from the body of the pubis to the ischial spine across the obturator fascia, along a condensation of the fascia, the tendinous arch (Fig. 5.54). The levator ani originally arose from the pelvic brim (its present origin in most mammals) and in man has migrated down the side wall of the pelvis, bringing the tendinous arch with it. Residual aponeurotic fibres of levator ani contribute to the strength of the obturator fascia above the tendinous arch.

The **pubococcygeus** part is that part of levator ani which arises from the anterior half of the tendinous arch and from the posterior surface of the body of the pubis. The pubococcygeus fibres are in different functional sets. The bulk of its posterior fibres sweep backwards in a flat sheet on the pelvic surface of the iliococcygeus and are inserted by a tendinous plate to the front of the coccyx (Fig. 5.55). These constitute the pubococcygeus muscle proper. Fibres arising more anteriorly, from the body of the pubis, swing more medially and more inferiorly around the anorectal junction and join with fibres of the opposite side and the external anal sphincter. This part of the muscle is called **puborectalis** and forms a U-shaped sling which holds the anorectal junction angled forwards (Fig. 5.67). The most medial fibres pass backwards alongside the prostate and the sphincter

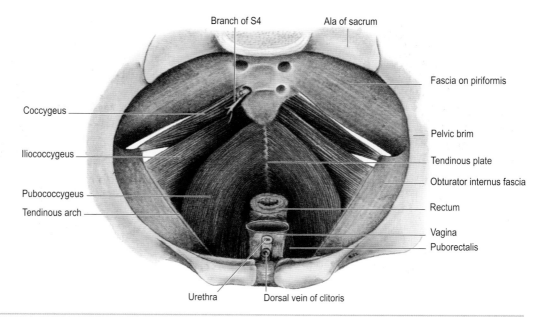

Fig. 5.55 Female pelvic floor from above. The pubococcygeus part of levator ani lies internal to the iliococcygeus part.

urethrae in the male and decussate across the midline behind the urethra; they are referred to as **pubourethralis**. In the female, these fibres sling around the posterior wall of the vagina and are referred to as **pubovaginalis**. In both sexes, fibres also attach to the perineal body. Some medial fibres pass backwards to blend with the longitudinal muscle of the rectum and fibroelastic strands to form the conjoint longitudinal coat of the anal canal (see p. 325).

The **iliococcygeus** part arises from the posterior half of the tendinous arch and the pelvic surface of the ischial spine and, overlapping the pelvic surface of coccygeus, its fibres are inserted into the side of the coccyx and the anococcygeal raphe (Fig. 5.67), which extends from the tip of the coccyx to the junction of rectum and anal canal. Although the iliococcygeus does not arise from the ilium, its name derives from its former origin on the iliac bone at the pelvic brim.

The *postanal plate*, also referred to as the anococcygeal ligament, is a layered musculotendinous structure between the anal canal and the caudal part of the vertebral column, on which the terminal rectum sits. From above downwards it consists of the presacral fascia (see p. 302), the tendinous plate of pubococcygeus, the muscular raphe of iliococcygeus, and the posterior parts of puborectalis and the external anal sphincter (see p. 324).

Coccygeus

The coccygeus is best thought of as ischiococcygeus. It arises from the tip of the ischial spine and its fibres fan out to be inserted into the side of the coccyx and the lowest piece of the sacrum; it lies edge to edge with the lower border of piriformis and is overlapped anteriorly by iliococcygeus (Fig. 5.55). Its gluteal surface is fibrous tissue, and is indeed the sacrospinous ligament (Figs 5.53 and 5.54).

Nerve supply. Levator ani is mainly supplied from the sacral plexus by branches of S3 and S4 which enter the upper (pelvic) surface of the muscle. Some of these somatic fibres may travel in or very close to the pelvic splanchnic nerves. Puborectalis, pubourethralis and pubovaginalis are supplied from below by the perineal branch of S4 and the inferior rectal branch of the pudendal nerve, in common with the external anal sphincter. Levator ani, like the external anal and urethral sphincter muscles, has a high proportion of slow twitch fibres. Coccygeus is supplied by branches of S3 and S4.

Actions. The pelvic floor helps to support the pelvic viscera and retain them in their normal positions. The floor contracts to counteract increased intra-abdominal pressure, which may be momentary, as in coughing and sneezing, or more prolonged as in muscular efforts like lifting. If an expulsive effort is required, the floor relaxes. Thus in defecation (see p. 326) when the abdominal wall and diaphragm contract, puborectalis relaxes to straighten out the anorectal junction and the floor descends to become more funnel-shaped, rising again as the process comes to an end. The pubovaginalis fibres of levator ani may be important in assisting the urethral sphincter at the end of micturition in the female. In parturition the floor initially directs the fetal head to the pelvic outlet, but the degree of stretching to which the muscular and fibrous parts of the floor are subjected may render it liable to damage by tearing.

Pelvic fascia

The parietal pelvic fascia on the pelvic surface of obturator internus is a strong membrane that fuses with the periosteum at the upper margin of the muscle. Below the tendinous arch that gives origin to levator ani, the fascia is thin where it covers obturator internus on the lateral wall of the ischioanal fossa (see p. 326). The fascia on the pelvic surface of piriformis fuses with the periosteum at the medial margins of the anterior sacral foramina. The sacral anterior primary rami emerging from these foramina thus lie behind this fascia. The internal iliac vessels are, however, in front of the fascia over piriformis. From the front of the lower sacrum a condensation of connective tissue, the *presacral* or *rectosacral fascia*, which varies in its thickness, passes downwards and forwards to fuse with the mesorectal fascia (see below) 3–5 cm proximal to the anorectal junction. The large (presacral) lateral sacral veins lie behind this fascia on the front of the sacrum. The fascia on the pelvic surface of levator ani and coccygeus is the *superior fascia of the pelvic diaphragm*. It is attached in front to the posterior surface of the body of the pubis and at the back to the ischial spine. In between these attachments it blends with the obturator fascia and a thickening of these two fused fasciae forms the tendinous arch of origin of levator ani. *The inferior fascia of the pelvic diaphragm* is the thin fascia that covers the undersurface of levator ani on the sloping medial wall of the ischioanal fossa; it blends with the obturator fascia laterally and with the fascia on the external anal and urethral sphincters medially.

PART THIRTEEN

Rectum

The Latin word 'rectus' means straight, and the **rectum** is straight in monkeys, but the human rectum follows the posterior concavity of the sacrum, and also shows three lateral curves or flexures that are most prominent when the viscus is distended (Fig. 5.56): upper and lower curves convex to the right and a middle curve convex to the left, the result being that the middle part appears to bulge to the left. The lowest part is slightly dilated as the rectal ampulla. Corresponding to the three curves seen externally, there are three sickle-shaped transverse rectal folds, formerly called rectal valves (of Houston), that project into the lumen from the wall on the concave side of these folds. They are produced by the circular muscle of the wall and are not confined merely to the mucous membrane, as is the case with the circular folds of the duodenum and jejunum. The middle fold, the largest, projects into the lumen from the right wall of the rectum just above the ampulla, at the level at which the peritoneum is reflected forwards off the rectum to form the floor of the rectovesical or rectouterine pouch (see below); it is about 8 cm from the anal orifice.

The rectum, which is about 12 cm long, is continuous with the sigmoid colon at the level of the third piece of the sacrum. The transition between the rectum and the sigmoid colon is a gradual one. At this junctional region the sigmoid mesocolon ends and the rectum has no mesentery. The taeniae of the sigmoid colon gradually broaden to form wide anterior and posterior muscular bands, which meet laterally to give the rectum a complete outer layer of longitudinal muscle; so the rectum has no sacculations. There are also no appendices epiploicae in the rectum.

The rectum turns downwards and backwards as the anal canal 2–3 cm in front of the tip of the coccyx. The anorectal junction is slung forwards by the U-loop of the puborectalis, which merges with the top of the external sphincter of the anal canal, forming a palpable ledge (the anorectal ring) on rectal examination. The posterior wall of the rectum appears to make a right-angled bend at the anorectal junction. This angle widens as the puborectalis muscle sling relaxes during defecation to allow faeces to enter the anal canal.

Although the rectum has no mesentery, the connective tissue and fat around the rectum is referred to by surgeons as the **mesorectum**. The visceral fascia surrounding it is the *mesorectal fascia* (Fig. 5.57). The mesorectum is bulkier posteriorly, where it tends to be grooved in the midline. It contains the superior rectal artery and its branches, the superior rectal vein and its tributaries, lymphatic vessels and nodes. A relatively avascular areolar tissue plane lies between the mesorectal fascia and the parietal pelvic fascia; this is the plane of surgical dissection in total mesorectal excision of the rectum for carcinoma. The plane is most evident posteriorly and is minimal laterally where the inferior hypogastric plexus (see p. 322) lies tangentially on the surface of the mesorectal fascia. Crossing this interface

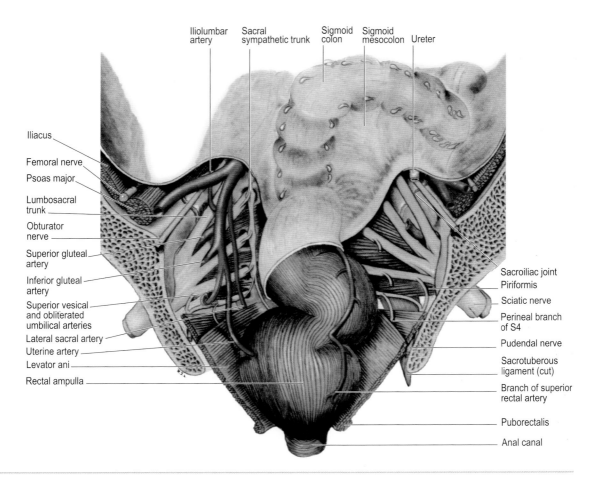

Fig. 5.56 Posterior half of a coronal section of the pelvis.
(The pelvic veins are not depicted. The rectum is shown in a distended state.)

are autonomic nerve fibres from the plexus to the rectum and occasional small middle rectal vessels. Surgical definition of surrounding connective tissue from the mesorectum comprises the iatrogenic 'lateral ligament' of the rectum; this is not seen on MRI or CT scanning.

Peritoneum covers the upper third of the rectum at the front and sides, and the middle third only at the front; the lower third is below the level of the peritoneum which is reflected forwards on to the upper part of the bladder (in the male) or upper vagina to form the **rectovesical pouch** or **rectouterine pouch** (of Douglas) (Fig. 5.63). These pouches form the lowest parts of the peritoneal cavity, and being 7.5 and 5.5 cm from the anal margins in the male and female respectively are within reach of the fingertip on rectal examination. They are normally occupied by coils of small intestine or sigmoid colon.

In front of the rectovesical pouch is the uppermost part of the base of the bladder and the tops of the seminal vesicles. Below the level of the pouch are the rest of the bladder base and seminal vesicles, the prostate, and the ends of each ureter and ductus deferens. Between these structures and the rectum, a thicker condensation of the mesorectal fascia forms a *rectogenital septum*—the *rectovesical fascia* of Denonvilliers (Fig. 5.58). It is connected to the floor of the rectovesical pouch above and to the apex of the prostate below. This fascia, which has a distinct whitish appearance in the living, is closer to the rectum than to the seminal vesicles and prostate and is removed in rectal excision for carcinoma.

In front of the rectouterine pouch is the uppermost part of the vagina (the fornix, with the cervix of the uterus projecting into it), while below the peritoneal

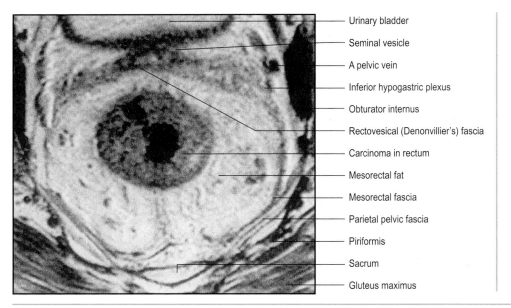

Fig. 5.57   Oblique axial MRI of the rectum. There is an annular carcinoma in the rectum.
(Provided by Dr G. Brown, The Royal Marsden Hospital, Sutton, Surrey.)

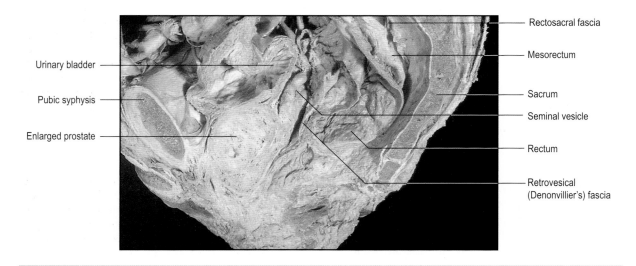

Fig. 5.58   Right half of a sagittal section of a male pelvis. The prostate is enlarged.

reflexion is more of the vagina, with the rectogenital septum intervening. This thin rectovaginal fascia fuses with the perineal body below.

Some slips from the longitudinal muscle of the rectal ampulla, the rectourethralis muscle, pass forwards to the perineal body and sphincter urethrae in the male; they must be cut at operations for excising the rectum and anal canal.

Blood supply

This is derived principally from the superior rectal artery, with contributions from the middle and inferior rectal and median sacral vessels. The lower end of the inferior mesenteric artery enters the sigmoid mesocolon and changes its name to superior rectal on crossing the pelvic brim. It crosses the left common iliac vessels medial to the ureter and descends in the base of the medial limb of the mesocolon. At the level of S3 vertebra (where the rectum begins) it divides into two branches which descend on each side of the rectum and subdivide into smaller branches. These vessels pierce the muscular wall and supply the whole thickness of the rectal wall including the mucous membrane. They continue submucosally into the anal canal, where they anastomose with branches of the inferior rectal artery. The middle rectal arteries are present in only one in five people; they are small and supply only the muscle of the mid and lower rectum. Experience in rectal surgery has shown that the inferior rectal arteries are capable of supplying the rectum from below to a level at least as high as the peritoneal reflexion from its anterior surface. The median sacral artery may make an unimportant contribution to the posterior wall in the region of the anorectal junction, but its main interest is that it may cause bleeding at operations in this region.

Veins correspond to the arteries, but anastomose freely with one another, forming an *internal rectal plexus* in the submucosa and an *external rectal plexus* outside the muscular wall. The lower end of the internal plexus is continuous with the vascular cushions of the anal canal (see p. 326). The main route of rectal venous drainage is via the superior rectal vein to the inferior mesenteric vein. The inferior rectal veins drain to the internal pudendal veins.

Lymph drainage

Lymphatic drainage from the rectum is mainly upwards. Lymphoid follicles in the mucous membrane drain to epicolic nodes on the surface of the rectum and to pararectal nodes in the mesorectum. The upward drainage is via nodes along the inferior mesenteric artery to preaortic nodes. Lymphatic drainage from the lower rectum to internal iliac nodes along middle rectal and inferior rectal vessels, and along the median sacral artery to nodes in the hollow of the sacrum, is minimal and unlikely to be a route for the metastatic spread of cancer that has not breached the mesorectal fascia.

Nerve supply

The *sympathetic* supply is by fibres that accompany the inferior mesenteric and superior rectal arteries from the inferior meseneteric plexus. The *parasympathetic* supply is from S2, 3 and 4 by the pelvic splanchnic nerves via the inferior hypogastric plexus; they are motor to rectal muscle. As from the bladder (see p. 307) pain

fibres appear to accompany both sympathetic and parasympathetic supplies. The sensation of distension is conveyed by parasympathetic afferents.

Rectal examination

The structures that can be palpated through the anal canal in either sex include the coccyx and sacrum behind, with the ischial spines at the sides. The anorectal ring (see p. 317) can be felt posteriorly at the anorectal junction as a shelf-like projection over which the tip of the finger can be hooked when the patient bears down. In the male at the front the prostate can be felt (but normal seminal vesicles are not usually palpable). In the female the cervix is felt through the vaginal wall, with the uterosacral ligaments laterally and sometimes the ovaries (compare with vaginal examination, p. 324).

Development

The rectum and the anal canal are derived from the anorectal canal (the dorsal part of the cloaca) and the proctodeum (see p. 31). The anal membrane breaks down, at a site probably represented by the pectinate line in the anal canal (see p. 325); the anal valves are said to indicate the remains of the membrane. The part of the anal canal continuous with the rectum above the pectinate line is endodermal, and the part below which is derived from the proctodeum is ectodermal, hence the difference in the blood and nerve supplies and lymph drainage of the upper and lower parts of the canal (see p. 326).

Surgical approach

In the surgical management of carcinoma of the rectum, depending on the site of the tumour, with access through the anterior abdominal wall most or all of the rectum and its surrounding mesorectum is removed, usually with the sigmoid colon and mesocolon, leaving the lower part and/or anal canal to which the mobilized descending colon is anastomosed. The procedure is termed *anterior resection* of the rectum. The rectovesical (rectovaginal) fascia is removed with the rectum after division of its attachment to the prostate (perineal body). The plane of dissection remains anterior to the presacral fascia and its attachment to the mesorectal fascia is divided. The ureter and the main neurovascular structures on the lateral wall of the pelvis are preserved. The superior hypogastric plexus and both inferior hypogastric plexuses are kept intact to safeguard sexual function and urinary voiding. The inferior mesenteric artery is divided close to its aortic origin to ensure removal of all lymph nodes along its courses, preserving the inferior mesenteric plexus on the aortic surface.

For complete excision of the rectum and anal canal, the freeing of the rectum as above is supplemented by a perineal approach (*abdominoperineal resection*), which includes dividing the pelvic floor (levator ani). Elliptical incisions either side of the anus allow the ischioanal fossae to be entered. The coccyx is dislocated or excised and the rectosacral fascia is divided from below. Anteriorly, the dissection extends up to the transverse perineal muscles and perineal body (see p. 327). The recto-urethralis muscle and rectogenital septum are divided and the plane between the septum and the prostate or vagina entered from below. A cylinder of tissue, including the freed bowel and a collar of levator ani and ischioanal fat, is removed through the perineum. The pelvic floor may be repaired by transferring a flap of muscle such as from gluteus maximus or rectus abdominis. A terminal colostomy is usually made in the left iliac fossa.

PART FOURTEEN

Urinary bladder and ureters in the pelvis

Urinary bladder

The empty bladder is situated entirely within the pelvic cavity. As the bladder distends it domes up into the abdominal cavity. The empty bladder is a flattened three-sided pyramid, with the sharp apex pointing forwards to the top of the pubic symphysis and a triangular base facing backwards in front of the rectum or vagina. There are two inferolateral surfaces cradled by the anterior parts of levator ani, a neck where the urethra opens, and a superior surface on which the small intestine and sigmoid colon or uterus lie.

The **apex** has the remains of the urachus attached to it, the latter forming the median umbilical ligament which runs up the midline of the anterior abdominal wall in the median umbilical fold of peritoneum (see p. 243).

Most of the **base**, or posterior surface, lies below the level of the rectovesical pouch and only the uppermost portion is covered by peritoneum between the ductus deferens on each side (Fig. 5.61). In addition to the latter the seminal vesicles are applied to this surface, and the ureters enter at the upper outer corner. In the female the base has a firm connective tissue union with the anterior vaginal wall and upper part of the uterine cervix with no peritoneum intervening (Fig. 5.63).

Each **inferolateral surface** slopes downwards and medially to meet its fellow, lying against the front part of the pelvic diaphragm and obturator internus. Where the surfaces meet below the apex there is a (retroperitoneal) space behind the pubic bones and symphysis, the *retropubic space* (of Retzius), containing loose fatty tissue and the fibromuscular *pubovesical ligaments* that extend from the bladder neck to the inferior aspect of the pubic bones.

The lowest part of the bladder is its **neck**, where the base and inferolateral surfaces meet and which is pierced by the urethra at the internal urethral orifice. In the male it lies against the upper surface or base of the prostate. In the female the neck is above the urethra in the connective tissue of the anterior vaginal wall.

The **superior surface** is covered by peritoneum which sweeps upwards on to the anterior abdominal wall. The distending bladder strips peritoneum from behind rectus abdominis, leaving the transversalis fascia on the back of the muscle; the distended bladder may thus be approached by cannula or scalpel in the midline above the pubic symphysis without entering the peritoneal cavity. At the posterior margin of this surface in the male the peritoneum continues on to the uppermost part of the base and is then continued backwards as the floor of the the rectovesical pouch, but in the female it is reflected from a little in front of the posterior margin of this surface on to the undersurface of the uterus.

The appearance of the interior of the bladder depends upon the state of distension of the organ. When collapsed the mucous membrane is thick and thrown into folds, when distended it is thin and smooth. The trabeculae of the muscle fibres can be seen through the mucous membrane. These remarks do not apply to the trigone, which varies but little with the state of distension of the organ.

The **trigone** is a triangular area at the base of the bladder lying between the two *ureteral orifices* (above and laterally) and the *internal uretheral orifice* (centrally and below) (Fig. 5.59). In the empty bladder these three openings are 2.5 cm apart from each other but when distended (as during cystoscopy) the ureteral orifices may be 5 cm apart. Being fixed on top of the prostate by the urethra, the trigone is the least mobile part of the bladder. In the female it is stabilized by the connective tissue surrounding the upper urethra at the front of the vagina. The trigone is smooth-walled and the mucous membrane is rather firmly adherent to the underlying muscle. The ureteric orifices are connected by a transverse ridge, the *interureteric bar*, prominent when viewed through the cystoscope; this is produced by continuity of the longitudinal muscle of the two ureters across the bladder wall. The orifices of the ureters lie at the ends of the bar; they are usually in the shape of an oblique slit,

Fig. 5.59 Trigone of bladder, prostate and prostatic urethra: coronal section.

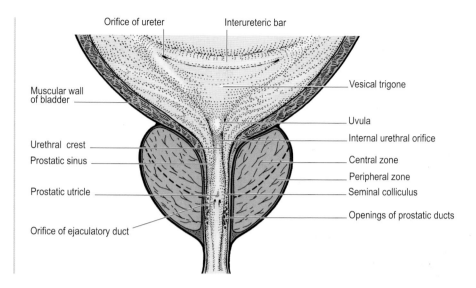

Orifice of ureter

Interureteric bar

Muscular wall of bladder

Vesical trigone

Uvula

Internal urethral orifice

Urethral crest

Prostatic sinus

Central zone

Peripheral zone

Prostatic utricle

Seminal colliculus

Openings of prostatic ducts

Orifice of ejaculatory duct

but considerable variations exist. The ureters pierce the muscle and mucosal walls very obliquely, an important factor in preventing reflux of urine when intravesical pressure rises. The ureteric orifices are closed by this pressure, except to open rhythmically in response to ureteric peristalsis each time a jet of urine is injected into the bladder (four or five times a minute normally).

In the male the trigone overlies the median part of the central zone of the prostate which, after middle age, may project above the internal urethral orifice as a rounded elevation, the *uvula* of the bladder.

Blood supply

The superior and inferior vesical arteries provide most of the arterial blood but there are small contributions to the lower part of the bladder from the obturator, inferior gluteal, uterine and vaginal arteries.

The veins of the bladder do not follow the arteries. They form a plexus that converges on the *vesicoprostatic plexus* in the groove between bladder and prostate and which drains backwards across the pelvic floor to the internal iliac veins. There is a similar plexus in the female, communicating with veins in the base of the broad ligament.

Lymph drainage

The lymphatics of the bladder drain mainly to external iliac nodes. Some lymph drains to internal iliac nodes including nodes in the obturator fossa.

Nerve supply

Parasympathetic fibres which provide the main motor innervation of the bladder reach it via the pelvic splanchnic nerves (see pp 22 and 322). Sympathetic fibres come from L1 and 2 segments of the cord via the superior and inferior hypogastric plexuses. For most of the bladder the sympathetic fibres are vasomotor and probably inhibitory to the detrusor muscle, but they are motor to the superficial trigonal muscle and (in the male) the muscle of the bladder neck (see below). The sensation of normal bladder distension travels with parasympathetic fibres and in the spinal cord is conveyed in the gracile tract, but it appears that bladder pain (e.g. from a stone) reaches the spinal cord (lateral spinothalamic tract) by both parasympathetic and sympathetic pathways.

Control of micturition

Normal emptying of the bladder occurs by contraction of the detrusor muscle and reciprocal relaxation of the external sphincter and pelvic floor (levator ani). The accumulation of urine distends the bladder wall with adjustment of tone (accommodation) so that tension does not at first increase. Later increased tension stimulates stretch receptors from which afferent impulses pass along the pelvic splanchnic nerves to sacral segments of the cord. Here the parasympathetic cell bodies are in turn stimulated and efferent impulses travel down the pelvic splanchnic nerves to synapse with the postganglionic cells within the bladder wall and so cause contraction. This autonomic stretch reflex giving bladder control at the spinal level is typical of the infant; with training, control by higher centres becomes superimposed on the spinal activity, and bladder evacuation is assisted by voluntary contraction of abdominal muscles. There is a *cortical inhibitory centre* in the inferior frontal gyrus (on the medial surface of the cerebral hemisphere, some distance in front of the motor 'perineal' area) with fibres passing to a *detrusor motor centre* in the medial part of the pontine reticular formation. From there reticulospinal fibres run down the cord mixed with those of the lateral corticospinal tract to the sacral segments.

The skeletal muscle of the sphincter urethrae (external urethral sphincter; p. 318 female, p. 328 male) is controlled by the perineal branch of the pudendal nerve (see p. 332), carrying fibres predominantly from anterior horn cells of S2 segment (Onuf's nucleus). A *storage centre* in the lateral part of the pontine reticular formation exerts central control on this nucleus. During micturition the sphincter relaxes as the detrusor contracts. In the female the pubovaginalis part of levator ani (see p. 302) assists the external sphincter at the end of micturition.

In spinal cord transection above the level of S2 segment, afferent impulses indicating distension cannot reach consciousness, cortical control of the sacral reflex is lost, and relaxation of the sphincter urethrae cannot be prevented. Because the 'sacral centre' itself is intact, the bladder automatically empties when distended, as in the infant (or as in the senile where cortical control has been lost through cerebral vascular disease). If the sacral segments themselves are destroyed, the detrusor muscle is paralysed and the bladder becomes abnormally distended until overflow incontinence occurs.

Structure

The smooth muscle of the bladder wall (*detrusor muscle*) is composed of an interlacing network of fibres running in various directions. Both externally and internally (beneath the mucous membrane) they produce a trabeculated appearance, which is exaggerated when muscular hypertrophy occurs as a result of progressive chronic obstruction to micturition, for example by prostatic enlargement or urethral stricture. They are well supplied by parasympathetic (cholinergic) nerve fibres. However, the trigone possesses a superficial triangular layer of muscle (*superficial trigonal muscle*) that is histologically and histochemically different from the rest of the bladder musculature (including the deep part of the trigone) and extends into the proximal urethra in both sexes. In further contrast to the detrusor muscle, the superficial trigonal muscle receives predominantly sympathetic (adrenergic) fibres. Contraction of this muscle may help to close the ureteral orifices.

At the bladder neck in the male, circular smooth muscle fibres form a collar around the internal urethral orifice, and extend distally to surround the proximal part of the prostatic urethra (the preprostatic part). This muscle, the preprostatic sphincter, too is profusely supplied with sympathetic (adrenergic) fibres. In the female the muscle in this region is arranged longitudinally and extends into the urethral wall. The muscle of the bladder neck has nothing to do with urinary continence; in the male it acts to prevent seminal regurgitation into the bladder during ejaculation.

The mucous membrane is thick and lax and lined by transitional epithelium. Glands are usually absent; mucus in shed urine has come from urethral glands. There is no muscularis mucosae.

Development

The endoderm of the vesicourethral part of the urogenital sinus (see p. 31) becomes the bladder epithelium, and the surrounding mesenchyme forms the muscle and connective tissue. Continued growth leads to the incorporation of the lower ends of the mesodermal mesonephric ducts into the posterior part of the bladder, so forming the trigone. These developmental differences may account for the structural differences in this region. The mesonephric ducts end up at a lower level as the ejaculatory ducts entering the urethra (see p. 311). The allantois regresses to form a fibrous cord, the urachus (median umbilical ligament).

Ureters in the pelvis

The **pelvic part of the ureter** forms about half of its 25 cm length (see p. 297). It crosses the pelvic brim in the region of the bifurcation of the common iliac artery. On the left it underlies the apex of the sigmoid mesocolon (Figs 5.56 and 5.63). It usually runs over the external iliac artery and vein and then down the side wall of the pelvis in front of the internal iliac artery (and behind the ovary). In order from above downwards, it crosses the obturator nerve, obliterated umbilical (superior vesical) artery, obturator artery and obturator vein (Fig. 5.64). On the right the appendix, if in a pelvic position, may lie adjacent. Reaching the level of the ischial spine, it turns forwards and medially above the pelvic floor to enter the base of the bladder at its upper lateral angle. Here *in the male* the ductus deferens crosses above the ureter and then runs down medial to the ureter. The upper end of the seminal vesicle usually lies just below the point where the ureter enters the bladder wall.

On the pelvic floor *in the female*, the ureter lies in the base of the broad ligament (see p. 314), where it is crossed above by the uterine artery (Fig. 5.62). Under the broad ligament the ureter penetrates the condensed tissue that forms the lateral cervical ligament (see p. 315), crossing the lateral vaginal fornix 1-2 cm from the cervix before entering the bladder in front of the fornix. The ureters are major hazards during hysterectomy, when ligating vessels and transecting ligaments.

In both sexes the ureters run obliquely through the bladder wall for 1–2 cm before reaching their orifices at the upper lateral angles of the trigone.

PART FIFTEEN

Male internal genital organs

Prostate

The prostate is a partly glandular, partly fibromuscular organ which lies beneath the bladder and above the urogenital diaphragm, and is penetrated by the proximal part of the urethra. It is normally broader than it is long, approximately $4 \times 3 \times 2$ cm. Its female homologue is the small group of paraurethral glands (of Skene; see p. 318). The prostate provides about 30% of the volume of seminal fluid (most comes from the seminal vesicle).

The prostate has a base and an apex, and anterior, posterior and inferolateral surfaces. The *base* is the upper surface, fused with the neck of the bladder and perforated by the urethra which traverses the whole length of the gland (Fig. 5.59). The blunt *apex* is the lowest part, and the prostatic urethra emerges from the front of the apex to become the membranous urethra which is surrounded by the sphincter urethrae (see p. 328). The *anterior surface* is at the back of the retropubic space and is connected to the bodies of the pubic bones by the puboprostatic ligaments. The *inferolateral surfaces* are clasped by the pubourethralis parts of levator ani. The *posterior surface* is in front of the lower rectum but separated from it by the rectovesical fascia (see p. 303). The ejaculatory ducts pierce the posterior surface just below the bladder and pass obliquely through the gland for about 2 cm to open into the prostatic urethra about halfway down. The prostate's own ducts also open into this part of the urethra (see below).

A thin strong layer of connective tissue at the periphery of the gland forms the 'true capsule' of the prostate, and outside this there is a condensation of pelvic fascia forming the 'false capsule'. Between these two capsules lies the prostatic plexus of veins. The gland consists of acini of varying shapes and sizes embedded in a fibromuscular stroma—a mixture of connective tissue and smooth muscle; this is the characteristic histological feature.

The **prostatic urethra**, 3–4 cm in length, passes through the substance of the prostate closer to the anterior than the posterior surface of the gland. It runs downwards and backwards from the internal meatus, then bends at the middle of its length and continues downwards and forwards to emerge from the anterior aspect of the apex. A midline ridge, the *urethral crest*, projects into the lumen from the posterior wall throughout most of the length of the prostatic urethra (Fig. 5.59). The shallow depression on either side of the crest is termed the *prostatic sinus*. At about the midlength of the crest the *seminal colliculus*, or *verumontanum*, forms a midline rounded eminence. The *prostatic utricle*, a small recess representing the fused ends of the paramesonephric (Müllerian) ducts, opens on to the middle of the verumontanum and the ejaculatory ducts open on either side of the utricle. The proximal part of the prostatic urethra, also termed the preprostatic part, is surrounded by a cylinder of smooth muscle, an extension of the circular muscle at the bladder neck; as has been noted above, this muscle contracts to prevent seminal regurgitation into the bladder during ejaculation.

The prostate is now considered to consist of a peripheral zone, a central zone and a transition zone, accounting for approximately 70%, 20% and 5% of the glandular substance, respectively, rather than being made up of lobes as previously described. The **central zone** is wedge-shaped and forms the base of the gland with its apex at the verumontanum (Fig. 5.59); it surrounds the ejaculatory ducts as they course through the gland. The **peripheral zone** surrounds the central zone from behind and below, but does not reach up to the base; it extends downwards to form the lower part of the gland. The transition zone lies around the distal part of the preprostatic urethra, just proximal to the apex of the central zone. The ducts of the transition zone open on the verumontanum, just above where the ducts of the peripheral zone open into the prostatic sinuses. Benign prostatic hyperplasia affects the transition zone which may increase markedly in size, compressing the peripheral zone (Fig. 5.60). The peripheral zone is almost exclusively the site of origin for carcinoma of the prostate. The central zone is rarely involved in any disease process.

There is very little glandular tissue anterior to the prostatic urethra, the anterior part of the prostate being mainly fibromuscular; it is overlapped from above by the detrusor muscle of the bladder and from below by the striated muscle of the urethral sphincter.

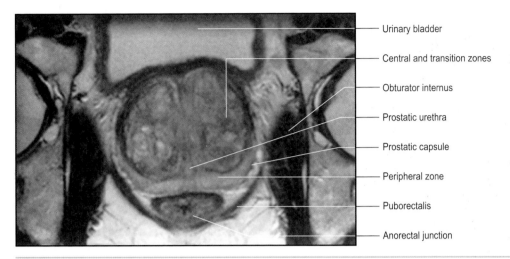

Urinary bladder

Central and transition zones

Obturator internus

Prostatic urethra

Prostatic capsule

Peripheral zone

Puborectalis

Anorectal junction

Fig. 5.60   Oblique axial MRI of the prostate. The transition zone is markedly enlarged by benign prostatic hyperplasia. (Provided by Dr G. Brown, The Royal Marsden Hospital, Sutton, Surrey.)

Blood supply

The main arterial supply is from the prostatic branch of the inferior vesical artery, with some small branches from the middle rectal and internal pudendal vessels. The veins run into a plexus between the true and false capsules and this joins the vesicoprostatic plexus situated at the groove between bladder and prostate. This plexus receives the deep dorsal vein of the penis, and drains backwards into the internal iliac veins.

Lymph drainage

The lymphatics of the prostate pass across the pelvic floor mainly to internal iliac nodes; a few may reach external iliac nodes.

Nerve supply

The acini receive parasympathetic (cholinergic) inner-vation from the pelvic splanchnic nerves (see p. 321) via the inferior hypogastric plexus. The muscle fibres of the stroma, which contract to empty the glands during ejac-ulation (see p. 333), are under sympathetic (adrenergic) control from the inferior hypogastric plexus (see p. 322).

Development

The pelvic part of the endodermal urogenital sinus (see p. 31) gives rise to lateral epithelial buds which become the prostatic acini of the peripheral and transition zones. Dorsal outgrowths from above the level of entry of the mesonephric ducts form the acini of the central zone. The fibromuscular stroma develops from the surrounding mesenchyme.

Surgical approach

Most operations for benign prostatic hyperplasia are now carried out by the transurethral route, with the resectoscope, the area of resection being restricted to above the verumontanum so that the external urethral sphincter, which is distal to it, is not damaged during the procedure. An approach through an abdominal supra-pubic incision into the retropubic space gives exposure for a total removal of the organ for prostatic carcinoma, which can also be achieved laparoscopically, or through a perineal approach. The bladder neck is anastomosed to the membranous urethra.

Ductus deferens and seminal vesicle

The origin of the **ductus (vas) deferens** as the continuation of the epididymis has been considered on page 239. It enters the abdomen at the deep inguinal ring and passes along the side wall and floor of the pelvis to reach the back of the bladder. In its course no other structure intervenes between it and the peritoneum.

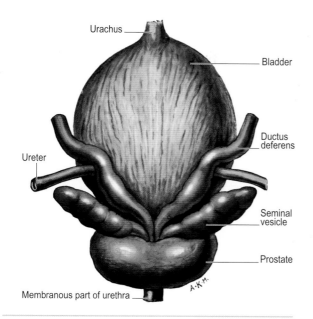

Urachus

Bladder

Ureter

Ductus deferens

Seminal vesicle

Prostate

Membranous part of urethra

A·K·M·

Fig. 5.61   Bladder, deferent ducts, seminal vesicles and prostate: posterosuperior aspect.

After hooking around the interfoveolar ligament and inferior epigastric artery at the deep inguinal ring, it crosses the external iliac artery and vein, obliterated umbilical artery and the obturator nerve, artery and vein, lying on the obturator fascia (Fig. 5.64). It curves medially and forwards, crosses above the ureter and approaches its opposite fellow. The two ducts now turn downwards side by side (Fig. 5.61) and each dilates in fusiform manner. This dilatation is the *ampulla*, the storehouse of spermatozoa. The proximal part of the ductus absorbs fluid produced by the seminiferous tubules of the testis, and the ductus itself makes only a small contribution to the volume of seminal fluid. The ampullae lie parallel and medial to the seminal vesicles; at their lower ends each loses its thick muscle wall and joins with the outlet of the seminal vesicle to form the **ejaculatory duct**. Each ejaculatory duct passes obliquely through the prostate to open on the verumontanum (Fig. 5.59).

The **seminal vesicle** is a thin-walled, elongated sac, like a lobulated, blind-ending tube much folded on itself. The pair produce about 60% of the seminal fluid, and are applied to the base of the bladder above the prostate (Fig. 5.61). The rectovesical fascia lies behind them and their tops are just covered by the peritoneum of the rectovesical pouch. Each lies lateral to the ampulla of the ductus deferens of its own side, and at the lower end of

the ampulla behind the prostate the duct of the seminal vesicle joins the ductus to form the ejaculatory duct.

Blood supplies. The artery to the ductus deferens is a branch of the superior vesical (or sometimes the inferior vesical) artery. It accompanies the ductus to the lower pole of the epididymis and anastomoses with the testicular artery (see p. 237). The seminal vesicles are supplied by branches from the inferior vesicle and middle rectal arteries.

Lymph drainage. Lymphatics accompany the blood vessels to the nearest iliac nodes.

Nerve supplies. The smooth muscle of the ductus and seminal vesicles receives fibres from the inferior hypogastric plexus. They are mainly sympathetic fibres from the first lumbar ganglion and are motor; their division produces sterility, for the paralysed muscle cannot contract to expel the stored secretion and spermatozoa, i.e. there is no emission or ejaculation (see p. 333).

Structure

The striking histological feature of the ductus deferens is the thickness of the muscular wall compared with the small size of the lumen. The smooth muscle of the ductus is arranged as inner and outer longitudinal and a middle circular layers. The mucous membrane is columnar with stereocilia (elongated microvilli).

The muscle coat of the seminal vesicle is thinner than that of the ductus. Although a single tube it is much convoluted and so appears in sections as a number of tubules, with mucosa that is very folded giving a glandular appearance. The epithelium is columnar.

Development

The ductus deferens is a main derivative of the mesonephric duct (see pp. 240 and 296), and at the back of the prostate a diverticulum from the duct forms the seminal vesicle.

PART SIXTEEN

Female internal genital organs and urethra

Uterus

The uterus is a muscular organ whose function is to provide a nidus for the developing embryo. In the virginal state it is the shape of a flattened pear. Its size is about $8 \times 5 \times 3$ cm. It possesses a fundus, body and cervix. It receives the uterine tubes, and the cervix protrudes into the vault of the vagina where it opens.

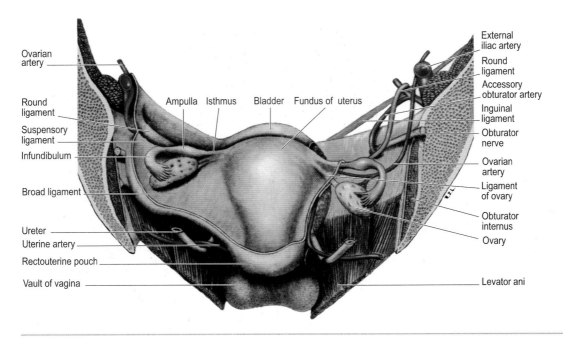

Ovarian artery

Round ligament

Ampulla Isthmus Bladder Fundus of uterus

External iliac artery

Round ligament

Accessory obturator artery

Inguinal ligament

Suspensory ligament

Infundibulum

Obturator nerve

Ovarian artery

Ligament of ovary

Broad ligament

Obturator internus

Ovary

Ureter

Uterine artery

Rectouterine pouch

Vault of vagina

Levator ani

Fig. 5.62   Anterior half of a coronal section of the female pelvis, from behind. The broad ligament and parietal peritoneum have been removed on the right side. The ovaries are displaced from their normal position in the parous female.

The **fundus** is the part above the entrance of the tubes (Fig. 5.62). It is convex and possesses a serous coat of pelvic peritoneum which continues downwards over the front and back of the body (Fig. 5.63).

The **body** of the uterus tapers downwards from the fundus and is flattened anteroposteriorly. Each upper angle (*cornu*), at the junction of fundus and body, receives the uterine tubes. The body is enclosed by peritoneum which laterally becomes the broad ligament. The intestinal surface of the body faces upwards with coils of intestine lying upon it, while the vesical surface faces downwards resting on the bladder with the peritoneum of the vesicouterine pouch intervening (Fig. 5.63). The cavity of the uterus occupies the body. A narrow slit in the virgin, it enlarges during pregnancy by growth of the uterine walls to accommodate the fetus.

The **cervix** of the uterus tapers below the body and its lower end is clasped by the vault of the vagina, into which it protrudes (Fig. 5.63). It thus has vaginal (lower) and supravaginal (upper) parts. The deep sulcus which surrounds the protruding cervix is the fornix of the vagina, and is deepest posteriorly. The posterior surface of the cervix is covered by peritoneum that continues from the body on to the upper part of the fornix, forming the anterior wall of the rectouterine pouch (of Douglas). The anterior surface has no peritoneal covering, being

deep to the vesicouterine pouch and attached to the bladder above the trigone by rather dense connective tissue. The ureter is about 2 cm from the cervix as it passes first lateral to and then in front of the fornix (Fig. 5.62). The body of the uterus is rarely exactly in the midline; when deviated to one side the cervix becomes deflected to the opposite side, so one ureter may be closer to the cervix than the other.

The *canal of the cervix* is continuous with the cavity of the body at what is commonly called the *internal os*. The lower opening into the vagina is the *external os*; this is circular in the nulliparous but usually a transverse slit after childbirth, with anterior and posterior lips, the anterior lying at a lower level than the posterior. The external os is normally on a level with the ischial spines.

Uterine tubes

Each tube is 10 cm long. The medial 1 cm (*intramural part*) is embedded in the uterine wall. Emerging from the cornu, the tube then lies in the upper edge of the broad ligament (Fig. 5.62), the peritoneal fold embracing it being the **mesosalpinx**. The part adjacent to the uterus (the *isthmus* of the tube) is straight and narrow. Next to it is the wider *ampulla*, forming more than half the length of the tube. The lateral end of the tube has

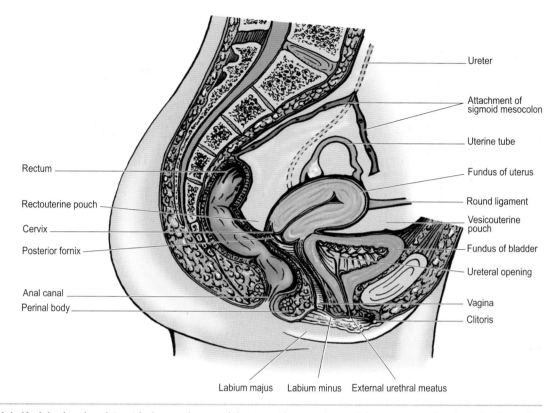

Ureter

Attachment of
sigmoid mesocolon

Uterine tube

Fundus of uterus

Round ligament

Vesicouterine
pouch

Fundus of bladder

Ureteral opening

Vagina

Clitoris

Rectum

Rectouterine pouch

Cervix

Posterior fornix

Anal canal

Perinal body

Labium majus   Labium minus   External urethral meatus

Fig. 5.63   Left half of the female pelvis with the attachment of the sigmoid mesocolon and the ureter entering the pelvis beneath its apex.

a trumpet-shaped expansion, the *infundibulum* or fimbriated end, with a number of finger-like processes, the *fimbriae*, one of which is longer and typically applied to the ovary. This open end lies behind the broad ligament adjacent to the lateral pelvic wall.

The tube, formed of two layers of smooth muscle (inner circular and outer longitudinal, like the gut), is lined by a mucous membrane thrown into folds. The surface epithelium is a mixture of ciliated and non-ciliated columnar cells. The cilia are most abundant at the fimbriated end, which is least muscular. The cilia beat towards the uterus.

Blood supply of uterus and uterine tubes

The uterus is supplied by the uterine artery, a branch of the internal iliac. It passes medially across the pelvic floor in the base of the broad ligament, above the ureter (Fig. 5.62), to reach the side of the supravaginal part of the cervix. Giving a branch to the cervix and vagina, the vessel turns upwards between the layers of the broad

ligament to run in a tortuous manner alongside the uterus as far as the cornu, giving off branches which penetrate the uterine walls and anastomose across the midline with corresponding branches of the opposite uterine artery. At the junction of uterus and uterine tube the artery turns laterally and ends by anastomosing with the tubal branch of the ovarian artery, which supplies the uterine tube.

The veins of the uterus course below the artery at the lower edge of the broad ligament where they form a wide plexus across the pelvic floor. This communicates with the vesical and rectal plexuses and drains to the internal iliac veins. The tubal veins join the ovarian veins (see p. 316).

Lymph drainage

Lymph from the cervix drains to external and internal iliac nodes, and also to sacral nodes via the uterosacral ligaments. The lower part of the uterine body drains to external iliac nodes. Lymphatics from the upper part of the body, the fundus and the uterine tube accompany those from the ovaries to para-aortic nodes; a few pass to external iliac nodes, and a few from the region of the uterine cornua accompany the round ligaments to reach the superficial inguinal nodes.

Nerve supply

The nerves of the uterus are branches from the inferior hypogastric plexus (see p. 322). The smooth muscle of the uterus is sensitive to hormonal influences. The sympathetic supply is vasoconstrictor, and also has a facilitating function in relation to uterine muscle, but division of all uterine nerves or high transection of the spinal cord does not affect uterine contractility, even in labour. Pain from the cervix is usually considered to be carried by the pelvic splanchnic nerves, although from the upper cervix it appears to run with sympathetic nerves as does pain from the body of the uterus (including labour pains). The cord segments concerned are T10–L1, and pain can be referred to the corresponding dermatomes. However, presacral neurectomy (cutting the hypogastric nerves from the superior hypogastric plexus) does not abolish labour pain, although it may improve dysmenorrhoea. The abolition of uterine sensation requires the division of all nerves, or transection of the cord, above T10 level. As with most hollow viscera, distension causes pain, but both the cervix and body are relatively insensitive to cutting and burning; in contrast, the uterine tube is sensitive to touching and cutting.

Structure

The bulk of the uterus is smooth muscle, the *myometrium*, whose fibres are often described as being in three layers, but these are ill-defined. The outer muscle fibres tend to be longitudinal and expulsive in function, while many of those more deeply placed are circular and act as sphincters round the larger blood vessels, the openings of the uterine tubes and the internal os. The mucous membrane or *endometrium* has a lining of columnar epithelium which dips down into the endometrial stroma to form the endometrial glands. The thickness of course varies with the different stages of the menstrual cycle; at menstruation the bases of the glands remain to provide the source for the new epithelial covering. The mucosa of the cervix does not take part in the cyclical changes and is not shed at menstruation; the surface cells are mucus-secreting and there are also mucous glands. Just inside the external os the epithelium changes to the stratified squamous variety of the vagina. The outer or serous covering of the uterus is the peritoneum.

Supports

The normal position of the uterus is one of *anteflexion* and *anteversion* i.e. the fundus and upper part of the body are bent forward in relation to the long axis of the cervix (angle of anteflexion), while the organ thus flexed leans forward as a whole from the vagina (angle of anteversion); the external os thus opens through the anterior wall of the vagina. As many as 20% of nulliparous females may have a retroverted uterus, without any ill effects. The most fixed part of the uterus is the cervix, because of its attachment to the back of the bladder and to the vaginal fornix, and a number of structures help directly or indirectly to maintain the normal position. These include the pelvic diaphragm, condensations of visceral pelvic fascia forming ligaments, and to a lesser extent peritoneal attachments.

The pubovaginalis part of levator ani and the perineal body with its inserted muscles (see p. 327) support the vagina and so assist indirectly in holding the cervix up. If these muscles are unduly stretched or damaged during childbirth the posterior vaginal wall sinks downwards (prolapses), and this is often followed by prolapse or retroversion of the uterus.

The **broad ligament** (Fig. 5.62) is not strictly speaking a ligament in the usual sense, as it consists of no more than a lax double fold of peritoneum lying lateral to the uterus, and it plays little part in uterine support. Its medial edge is attached to the side wall of the uterus and flows over its intestinal and vesical surfaces as its serous coat. The lateral edge is attached to the side wall of the pelvis. The two layers of its inferior edge, or base, pass forwards and backwards to line the pelvic cavity; as the posterior layer does so, it has the ureter adhering underneath it. The line of lateral attachment crosses the obturator nerve, superior vesical or obliterated umbilical vessels, and the obturator artery and vein. The upper border of the broad ligament is free, forming the mesosalpinx and containing the uterine tube. The upper lateral part of the broad ligament contains the ovarian vessels and lymphatics and is extended over the external iliac vessels as a fold, the *suspensory ligament of the ovary*.

The anterior layer of the broad ligament is bulged forwards by the round ligament of the uterus just below the uterine tube. The posterior layer has a fold projecting backwards suspending the ovary, the *mesovarium*. Between the two layers of the broad ligament is a mass of areolar tissue, the parametrium, in which lie the uterine vessels and lymphatics, the round ligament of the uterus, the ligament of the ovary (see p. 315), and vestigial remnants of mesonephric tubules (the epoöphoron and paroöphoron, see p. 316).

The **round ligament of the uterus** extends from the junction of the uterus and tube to the deep inguinal ring. It lies in the broad ligament below the uterine tube and bulges the anterior layer of the ligament forwards. Through its uterine attachment it is continuous with the ligament of the ovary, the two ligaments together representing the gubernaculum, the counterpart of the gubernaculum of the testis. The round ligament passes through the inguinal canal and is attached at its distal extremity to the fibrofatty tissue of the labium majus of the vulva. It is supplied by a branch of the ovarian artery in the broad ligament and by a branch from the inferior epigastric artery in the inguinal canal. It consists of smooth muscle and fibrous tissue, and it acts to hold the uterus forwards in anteflexion and ante-version, especially when forces tend to push the uterus backwards (e.g. distension of the bladder, gravity during recumbency).

The **transverse cervical ligament** (also known as the *lateral cervical*, *cardinal* or *Mackenrodt's ligament*) consists of thickenings of connective tissue in the base of each broad ligament, extending from the cervix and vaginal fornix laterally to the side wall of the pelvis. The ureter, uterine artery and inferior hypogastric plexus traverse the connective tissue of the ligament. It imparts lateral stability to the cervix and is an important support of the uterus. The **uterosacral ligaments**, comprising fibrous tissue and smooth muscle, extend backwards from the cervix below the peritoneum, embracing the rectouterine pouch and rectum and becoming attached to the front of the sacrum. They are palpable on rectal (not vaginal) examination. They keep the cervix braced backwards against the forward pull of the round ligaments on the fundus and so maintain the body of the uterus in anteversion.

Development

The paramesonephric (Müllerian) ducts develop as a linear invagination of the coelomic epithelium on the lateral aspect of the mesonephros (see p. 240). They grow caudally lateral to the mesonephric ducts, but then cross ventral to them, fuse at their caudal ends to make the uterus and continue to reach the dorsal wall of the urogenital sinus (see p. 31), thereby forming the upper part of the vagina. Their cranial ends persist as the uterine tubes. Incomplete fusion results in a median septum in the uterus or in a bicornuate uterus.

Surgical approach

An abdominal or vaginal approach may be used for total hysterectomy (removal of body and cervix). The broad, round and ovarian ligaments and the uterine tubes are divided on each side near the uterus. The lower ends of the ureters need to be safeguarded particularly when the uterine arteries are divided. The anterior and posterior vaginal walls are cut across below the cervix. For sub-total hysterectomy by the abdominal route, the cervix is cut across at the level of the lateral ligaments without opening into the vagina.

Ovary

The ovary is ovoid in shape, smaller than the testis. It is about 3 cm long, 2 cm wide and 1 cm thick, being smaller before menarche and postmenopausally. In the erect position, the ovary lies almost vertically. Its upper pole, the tubal extremity, is tilted laterally and is over-lapped by the fimbriated end of the uterine tube. Its lower pole is tilted towards the uterus to which it is attached by a fibromuscular band, the **ligament of the ovary**. This is continuous with the round ligament; both are attached to the cornu of the uterus, and are the remnants of the gubernaculum. The anterior border of the ovary is attached to the posterior leaf of the broad ligament by a double fold of peritoneum, the **mesovarium**. The peritoneum does not invest the rest of the surface of the ovary, which is covered with cuboidal epithelium and faces the peritoneal cavity.

The lateral surface of the ovary lies in the angle between the internal and external iliac vessels, against the parietal peritoneum which separates it from the obturator nerve laterally and the ureter posteriorly. A diseased ovary may therefore cause referred pain along the cutaneous distribution of this nerve on the inner side of the thigh. The medial surface is mainly related to the uterine tube.

The location and line of the ovary change during pregnancy and usually never return to their original state. The ovary in its normal position can just be reached through the vagina by the tip of the examining finger. It is overlaid by the coils of sigmoid colon and ileum that occupy the rectouterine pouch of Douglas.

Blood supply

The ovary is supplied by the ovarian artery, a branch of the abdominal aorta from just below the renal artery. The vessel runs down behind the peritoneum of the infracolic compartment and the colic vessels, crossing the ureter obliquely, on the psoas muscle. It crosses the brim of the pelvis and enters the *suspensory ligament* at the lateral extremity of the broad ligament. It gives off a branch to the uterine tube which runs medially between the layers of the broad ligament and anastomoses with the uterine artery, and it ends by entering the ovary (Fig. 5.62).

The ovarian veins form a plexus in the mesovarium and the suspensory ligament (the *pampiniform plexus*, as in the testis). The plexus drains into a pair of ovarian veins which accompany the ovarian artery. They usually combine as a single trunk before their termination. That on the right joins the inferior vena cava, that on the left the left renal vein.

Lymph drainage

The lymphatics of the ovary drain to para-aortic nodes alongside the origin of the ovarian artery (L2), just above the level of the umbilicus. Clinical observation shows that it is also possible for lymph to reach inguinal nodes via the round ligament and the inguinal canal, and to reach the opposite ovary by passing across the fundus of the uterus.

Nerve supply

Sympathetic (vasoconstrictor) fibres reach the ovary from the aortic plexus along its blood vessels; the pre-ganglionic cell bodies are in T10 and 11 segments of the cord. Some parasympathetic fibres may reach the ovary from the inferior hypogastric plexus via the uterine artery and are presumably vasodilator. Autonomic fibres do not reach the ovarian follicles; an intact nerve supply is not required for ovulation. Sensory fibres accompany the sympathetic nerves, so that ovarian pain may be periumbilical, like appendicular pain.

Structure

The ovary consists of an inner vascular medulla and an outer cortex (containing the ovarian follicles) encapsulated by a fibrous connective tissue layer, the tunica albuginea, covered by a layer of cubical cells, the superficial epithelium. During early fetal development primitive germ cells (oogonia) derived from endodermal cells of the yolk sac migrate into the developing ovarian cortex, where they multiply and grow to become primary oocytes, which are surrounded by a single layer of follicular cells to form primordial follicles. There are about 1 million primordial follicles at birth but this number is reduced to about 40 000 by puberty. After puberty, during each ovarian cycle a relatively small number of primordial follicles undergo a series of development changes and of these usually only one from either ovary comes to full maturity and releases its oocyte (ovulation) into the peritoneal cavity for transport into the uterine tube, potentially for fertilization. This development involves oocyte enlargement, follicle (granulosa) cell proliferation and fluid (liquor folliculi) accumulation as the primordial follicle is transformed successively into a primary, a secondary and a tertiary (Graafian) follicle, the surrounding stromal cells forming the theca of these follicles. Before ovulation the primary oocyte undergoes meiosis (cell division whereby the DNA amount and the chromosome number are halved), forming a secondary oocyte. At ovulation this is discharged, the liquor folliculi escapes and haemorrhage occurs into the collapsed follicle. The granulosa cells and some of the thecal cells now develop into a corpus luteum. This persists for 1 week if pregnancy does not occur, or for 9 months if it does. At the end of either time it atrophies and becomes replaced by a fibrous scar, the corpus albicans.

Since only about 400 ova can be shed in the course of reproductive life, most oocytes and follicles are destined never to reach maturity, and they can undergo degeneration at any stage of their development, becoming known as atretic follicles.

Development

The ovary develops from the paramesonephric ridge of the intermediate cell mass (see p. 25) in the same way as the testis. Its site of origin lies in the peritoneum of the posterior abdominal wall. It descends, preceded by the gubernaculum. The gubernaculum proceeds through the inguinal canal, as in the male, and becomes attached to the labium majus. The ovary does not follow its gubernaculum so far, and its descent is arrested in the pelvis as the gubernaculum becomes attached to the uterus and persists as the ligament of the ovary and the round ligament of the uterus.

The mesonephric tubules and mesonephric duct normally disappear in the female. Should they persist their remnants are to be found between the layers of the broad ligament. The *epoöphoron* consists of a number of tubules joining at right angles a persistent part of the mesonephric duct. It lies in the mesosalpinx between ovary and tube. The mesonephric duct may persist as a tube (duct of Gartner) opening into the lateral fornix of the vagina or even at the vestibule of the vulva alongside the vaginal orifice. The *paroöphoron* lies nearer the base of the broad ligament. It consists of a number of minute tubules, blind at each end. Distension of such a tubule produces a parovarian cyst.

Vagina

The vagina is a highly expandable fibromuscular tube, about 10 cm in length, that is directed upwards and backwards from its lower end, the **vaginal orifice**, or *introitus*. For much of its total length the anterior and posterior walls are in opposition and the lumen is an H-shaped slit, but the introitus is an anteroposterior cleft. It lies in front of the rectum, anal canal and perineal body, and behind the bladder and urethra (Fig. 5.63). Below the floor of the rectouterine pouch the vagina is separated from the rectum by the thin rectovaginal septum.

The upper end is slightly expanded and receives the uterine cervix which projects into it, forming round the margin of the cervix a circular groove or **vaginal fornix**, which for descriptive convenience is subdivided into anterior, posterior and lateral fornices. The posterior wall of the vagina is longer than the anterior wall and the posterior fornix is deeper than the other fornices. The posterior fornix is covered by peritoneum of the front of the rectouterine pouch (of Douglas); this is the only part of the vagina to have a peritoneal covering. The ureter is first adjacent to the lateral fornix and then passes across the front of the anterior fornix to enter the bladder.

Below the cervix the anterior wall of the vagina is in contact with the base (posterior surface) of the bladder, and below the bladder the urethra is embedded in the vaginal wall.

The vagina passes down between the pubovaginalis parts of levator ani, through the urogenital diaphragm and perineal membrane (i.e. through the deep perineal space) into the superficial perineal space where the vaginal orifice lies in the vestibule, the space between the labia minora (see p. 333). Here it may show internally the remains of the hymen, and the duct of the greater vestibular (Bartholin's) gland opens on each side just below the hymen in the posterolateral wall. The urethra opens immediately in front of the vaginal orifice, and the minute openings of the lesser vestibular glands are between the two orifices.

Blood supply

The vaginal branch of the internal iliac artery is supplemented by the uterine, inferior vesical and middle rectal vessels, whose branches all make good anastomotic connexions on the vaginal wall. Veins join the plexuses on the pelvic floor to drain into the internal iliac vein.

Lymph drainage

The lymphatics of the vagina, like those of the cervix, drain to external and internal iliac nodes, but the lowest part (below the hymen level) drains like other perineal structures to superficial inguinal nodes.

Nerve supply

The lower end of the vagina receives sensory fibres from the perineal and posterior labial branches of the pudendal nerve, and (with the anterior part of the vulva) from the ilioinguinal nerve. Autonomic nerve fibres from the inferior hypogastric plexuses supply blood vessels, the smooth muscle of the vaginal wall and the vestibular glands. The upper vagina is said to be sensitive only to stretch, the afferent fibres running with sympathetic nerves.

Structure

The vagina has a muscular layer of smooth muscle lined internally by mucous membrane and covered externally by fibrous tissue continuous with the pelvic fascia, except at the posterior fornix which has a peritoneal covering. The smooth muscle fibres consist of outer longitudinal and an inner circular layer which interlace. The mucous membrane has stratified squamous non-keratinizing epithelium overlying a connective tissue lamina propria in which there are large thin-walled veins as in erectile tissue. There are no muscularis mucosae and no glands. Before parturition, the mucous membrane of the anterior and posterior walls have median longitudinal ridges from which several transverse rugae extend bilaterally.

Vaginal examination

Using the index and middle fingers, the uterine cervix can be felt in the upper vagina, with the bladder, urethra and pubic symphysis at the front. Posteriorly, the contents of the rectouterine pouch are palpable. With pressure applied on the lower abdominal wall, the body of the uterus, ovaries and uterine tubes can be felt.

Development

Most of the vagina is formed (like the uterus, see p. 315) from the distal part of the fused paramesonephric (Müllerian) ducts, but the lower part is derived from the urogenital sinus (see p. 31), whose epithelium appears to replace that derived from the ducts. The labia minora that bound the vaginal orifice are formed from the urogenital folds (the labia majora are from the more laterally placed labioscrotal swellings).

Female urethra

The female urethra is about 4 cm long, passing from the neck of the bladder at the lower angle of the trigone to the external urethral meatus (Fig. 5.63), which is in front of the vaginal orifice and 2.5 cm behind the clitoris. Except its uppermost end, the urethra is embedded within the anterior vaginal wall. As it leaves the bladder, fibres of the pubovaginalis part of the levator ani lie adjacent to it, and they play some part in compressing it.

With the urethra being such a short straight tube, catheterization in the female is simple compared with the male, but it must be remembered that in the later stages of pregnancy the urethra may be considerably stretched so that the catheter may have to be passed for more than twice the normal distance. Vaginal stretching during birth can increase the urethral length to 10 cm. The pubic symphysis lies in front and the full-term fetal head can compress the urethra against it.

Blood supply

The upper part of the urethra is supplied by the inferior vesical and vaginal arteries, with the lower end receiving contributions from the internal pudendal artery. Veins drain to the vesical plexus and the internal pudendal vein.

Lymph drainage

Lymph vessels pass mainly to internal iliac nodes but some reach the external iliac group.

Nerve supply

Fibres reach the urethra from the inferior hypogastric plexuses and from the perineal branch of the pudendal nerve.

Structure

The mucous membrane is lined proximally by urothelium and distally by non-keratinized stratified squamous epithelium. There are a few mucous glands in the wall. The largest of these, the *paraurethral glands* (of Skene) open by a single duct on each side just inside the external meatus, and are the female homologue of the prostate. Superficial trigonal muscle fibres of the bladder extend into the upper urethra. The urethral smooth muscle is orientated mainly longitudinally; its contraction during micturition shortens the urethra and widens its lumen. Outside the smooth muscle is the striated circular muscle of the *sphincter urethrae* (external urethral sphincter). The sphincter is thickest near the middle of the urethra, and thicker in front than at the sides or back. It consists of small fibres of the slow twitch variety and is supplied by the pudendal nerve.

Development

The female urethra is developed from the urogenital sinus (see p. 31), and corresponds to the part of the male prostatic urethra that is proximal to the openings of the prostatic utricle and ejaculatory ducts (see p. 309).

PART SEVENTEEN

Pelvic vessels and nerves

Pelvic vessels

The pelvic walls and viscera are supplied by branches of the internal iliac artery and drain into tributaries of the internal iliac veins. Arteries and veins lie within the parietal pelvic fascia and only their branches that pass out of the pelvis (except the obturator vessels) need to pierce this fascia.

Internal iliac artery

The common iliac artery bifurcates at the pelvic brim opposite the sacroiliac joint (Fig. 5.64). From this point the **internal iliac artery** passes downwards and soon divides into a short posterior and a longer anterior division. The posterior division breaks up into three branches, all of which are parietal: iliolumbar; lateral sacral; and superior gluteal. The anterior division usually has nine branches, three associated with the bladder (superior vesical, obliterated umbilical and inferior vesical), three other visceral branches (middle rectal, uterine and vaginal), and three parietal branches (obturator, internal pudendal and inferior gluteal). The internal pudendal and inferior gluteal vessels are considered to be the terminal branches of the anterior division. The obliterated umbilical artery is a continuation of the superior vesical, which is usually the first (highest) branch to arise from this division. The remaining branches arise at variable levels and some may have common stems.

Branches of the posterior division

The **iliolumbar artery** (Fig. 5.56) passes upwards out of the pelvis in front of the lumbosacral trunk and behind the obturator nerve, running laterally deep to the psoas muscle. Its *lumbar branch* is really the fifth lumbar segmental artery. It passes laterally to supply psoas and quadratus lumborum and, by its posterior branch, erector spinae. This vessel gives a spinal branch into the foramen between L5 vertebra and the sacrum.

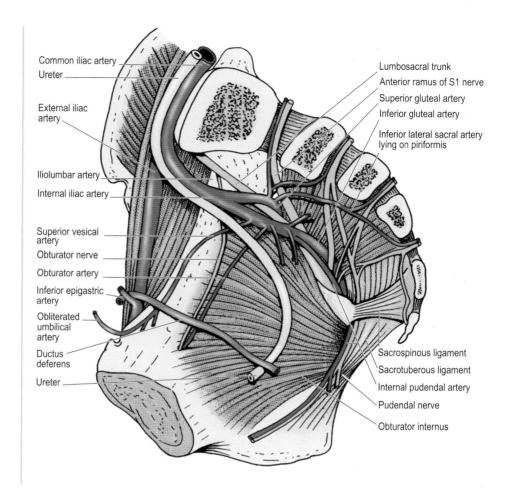

Fig. 5.64 Vessels and nerves of the right half of the pelvis, in a median sagittal section.

Common iliac artery

Ureter

External iliac artery

Iliolumbar artery

Internal iliac artery

Superior vesical artery

Obturator nerve

Obturator artery

Inferior epigastric artery

Obliterated umbilical artery

Ductus deferens

Ureter

Lumbosacral trunk

Anterior ramus of S1 nerve

Superior gluteal artery

Inferior gluteal artery

Inferior lateral sacral artery lying on piriformis

Sacrospinous ligament

Sacrotuberous ligament

Internal pudendal artery

Pudendal nerve

Obturator internus

The *iliac branch* supplies the iliac fossa, i.e. the iliacus muscle and the iliac bone. It extends to the anastomosis around the anterior superior iliac spine (deep and superficial circumflex iliac arteries, ascending branch of the lateral circumflex femoral artery and upper branch of deep division of superior gluteal artery).

The **lateral sacral artery** (frequently double) runs down lateral to the anterior sacral foramina, i.e. in front of the roots of the sacral plexus (Fig. 5.56). In the pelvis it supplies the roots and piriformis. Spinal branches enter the anterior sacral foramina, supply the spinal meninges and the roots of the spinal nerves and pass through the posterior sacral foramina to reach the muscles over the back of the sacrum. The artery takes over the segmental supply from the lumbar arteries; usually a superior sacral artery supplies the first two sacral segments and an inferior sacral artery supplies the remaining segments (Fig. 5.64).

The **superior gluteal artery**, the largest of all the branches of the internal iliac (Fig. 5.64), passes backwards by piercing the pelvic fascia usually between the lumbosacral trunk and S1 nerve, and leaves the pelvis through the greater sciatic foramen above the upper border of piriformis. Its course and distribution in the buttock are considered on page 130.

Branches of the anterior division

The **superior vesical artery** is the persistent patent proximal part of the fetal umbilical artery. The distal part becomes obliterated to form the medial umbilical ligament (see p. 243) which thus appears as the direct continuation of the vesical vessel. The superior vesical artery runs first along the side wall of the pelvis (Fig. 5.64) and then turns medially to reach the upper part of the bladder. It also supplies the adjacent ureter and ductus deferens.

The **inferior vesical artery** arises much lower than the superior and runs medially across the pelvic floor to supply the trigone and lower part of the bladder, the ureter, ductus deferens, seminal vesicle and prostate.

The **middle rectal artery** as a source of blood supply to the muscle of the rectum is frequently absent, and when present small. It may be repalced by a small branch from an artery that supplies other pelvic viscera, such as the prostate and seminal vesicles in the male and the vagina in the female.

The **uterine artery** crosses the pelvis in the base of the broad ligament, passing above the ureter. At the cervix it turns upwards closely applied to the muscle thereof and runs alongside the uterus in the broad ligament. At the entrance of the uterine tube it turns laterally to supply the tube and anastomose with the tubal branch of the ovarian artery.

The **vaginal artery** supplies the upper part of the vagina and corresponds to the inferior vesical artery in the male. It may be a branch of the uterine artery.

The **obturator artery** passes along the side wall of the pelvis below the nerve (Fig. 5.64) to enter the obturator foramen with the nerve and the vein and pass into the thigh. The artery gives off a small branch to the periosteum of the back of the pubis, and this vessel anastomoses with the pubic branch of the inferior epigastric artery. In about 30% of cases this anastomotic connection opens up to become the *accessory* or *abnormal obturator artery*, replacing the normal branch from the internal iliac in the latter instance. Such an artery in its passage from the inferior epigastric to the obturator foramen usually passes on the lateral side of the femoral ring, i.e. adjacent to the external iliac vein (Fig. 5.8). When it lies at the medial side of the ring, alongside the edge of the lacunar ligament, it is vulnerable to injury or division if the ligament has to be incised to release a strangulated femoral hernia.

The **inferior gluteal artery** runs backwards through the parietal pelvic fascia, passes below S1 nerve root (Fig. 5.64) (or sometimes S2) and leaves the pelvis through the greater sciatic foramen below piriformis, to continue its course in the buttock (see p. 131).

The **internal pudendal artery** lies in front of the inferior gluteal (Fig. 5.64), pierces the parietal pelvic fascia and passes out of the pelvis through the greater sciatic foramen below piriformis. It is distributed in the perineum to the anal region and the external genitalia (see p. 332).

Internal iliac vein

The internal iliac vein, a wide vessel about 3 cm long, begins above the greater sciatic notch by the confluence of gluteal veins with others that accompany branches of the internal iliac arteries. It passes upwards posteromedial to its artery to join the external iliac vein on the medial surface of psoas major and form the common iliac. Apart from tributaries that correspond to arteries, the internal iliac vein receives tributaries from the *rectal, vesical, prostatic, uterine* and *vaginal venous plexuses* in the appropriate sex. The presence of these venous plexuses and large draining veins below the pelvic peritoneum accounts for the severe retroperitoneal haemorrhage that may result from fracture of the pelvic bones. By the *lateral sacral veins* the internal iliac vein communicates with the vertebral venous plexuses. There are no valves in pelvic veins. Sudden increase in abdominal pressure (as in coughing) may be momentarily more than the inferior vena cava can accommodate, and this drives blood backwards up the internal vertebral plexus, into posterior intercostal veins and by azygos veins into the superior vena cava, bypassing the diaphragm. Emboli from disease of the pelvic viscera can thus find their way by reflux blood flow into the vertebrae. In this way secondary carcinomatous deposits may appear in the vertebrae from primary growths in any of the pelvic viscera.

Pelvic nerves

The **obturator nerve** is a branch of the lumbar plexus formed within the substance of psoas major from the anterior divisions of the second, third and fourth lumbar nerves (anterior rami). It is the nerve of the adductor compartment of the thigh, which it reaches by piercing the medial border of psoas and passing straight along the side wall of the pelvis to the obturator foramen. It crosses the pelvic brim medial to the sacroiliac joint (i.e. on the ala of the sacrum) and runs forward between the internal iliac vessels and the fascia on the obturator internus muscle. In front of the internal iliac vessels it is separated from the normally situated ovary only by the parietal peritoneum lining the pelvic wall. Pain from the ovary may be referred along the nerve to the skin on the medial side of the thigh. This may be less an irritation of the main nerve trunk than irritation or inflammation of the parietal peritoneum, which is here supplied by the obturator nerve.

The obturator artery and vein converge to the obturator foramen, in which the nerve lies highest, against the pubic bone (Fig. 5.64) with the artery and vein beneath it in that order. The nerve divides while in the foramen into *anterior* and *posterior divisions*; the former passes anterior to the upper border of obturator externus, while the posterior division pierces the obturator externus, after giving off a branch to supply the muscle. The distribution in the thigh is considered on page 127.

The **accessory obturator nerve**, which is occasionally present, also emerges from the medial border of psoas. But like the femoral nerve it passes over the superior pubic ramus to the thigh, where it supplies pectineus.

Sacral plexus

Not all the lumbar nerves are used up in the formation of the lumbar plexus. A part of L4 and all of L5 anterior rami enter the sacral plexus. After L4 has given off its branches to the lumbar plexus it emerges from the medial border of psoas and joins the anterior ramus of L5 to form the **lumbosacral trunk**. This large nerve passes over the ala of the sacrum and crosses the pelvic brim medial to the obturator nerve from which it is separated by the iliolumbar artery and veins. It descends to join the anterior rami of the upper four sacral nerves in the formation of the sacral plexus (Figs 5.56 and 5.75).

The **sacral plexus** is a broad triangular structure formed by the junction of the nerves lateral to the anterior sacral foramina (Fig. 5.56). It rests upon piriformis and is covered anteriorly by the parietal pelvic fascia which invests that muscle. Anterior to the fascia the lateral sacral arteries and veins lie in front of the sacral nerves. At a higher level the common iliac vessels lie over the lumbosacral trunk. The superior and inferior gluteal arteries usually pass backwards above and below S1 respectively; they may instead pass above and below S2. The ureter, lying in front of the internal iliac vessels, is well anterior to the upper part of the plexus and in front of all are the parietal pelvic peritoneum and pelvic viscera. The sacral nerves receive grey rami communicantes from the sacral sympathetic ganglia.

The sacral nerves give off certain branches and then divide, as does the lumbosacral trunk, into anterior and posterior divisions which thereupon branch and reunite to form nerves for supply of flexor and extensor compartments of the lower limb.

The **piriformis** is supplied by separate twigs from the posterior divisions of S1 and 2.

The **perforating cutaneous nerve** arises from the posterior divisions of S2 and 3. It pierces the sacrotuberous ligament and curves round the lower border of gluteus maximus to supply the skin of the buttock.

The **posterior femoral cutaneous nerve** is formed by branches from the posterior divisions of S1 and S2 and the anterior divisions of S2 and 3. It passes backwards below piriformis behind the sciatic nerve, which separates it from the ischium. It thus enters the gluteal region (see p. 131).

The **superior gluteal nerve** is formed from the posterior divisions of L4, 5 and S1. It passes out of the pelvis above the piriformis muscle (see p. 130).

The **inferior gluteal nerve** is formed from the posterior divisions of L5 and S1 and 2. It passes out of the pelvis below the lower border of piriformis (see p. 130).

The **coccygeal plexus** consists of a minor mingling of a branch from S4 and S5 and the coccygeal nerve. Branches supply the postanal skin over the coccyx.

The *tibial* part of the **sciatic nerve** is a big branch formed by union of branches from all five anterior divisions (L4, 5, S1–3). The *common peroneal* (*common fibular*) part of the **sciatic nerve** is formed by union of branches from the posterior divisions of L4, 5, S1, 2. They usually join in the pelvis, and the sciatic nerve so formed leaves the pelvis below the lower border of piriformis lying on the ischium, lateral to the ischial spine (see Fig. 3.13, p. 128). Its course in the gluteal region is considered on page 131. If the two components of the sciatic nerve do not join in the pelvis, the common peroneal part pierces the lower part of piriformis as it leaves the pelvis.

The **nerve to obturator internus** (anterior divisions of L5, S1, 2) also supplies the superior gemellus. It leaves the pelvis, lateral to the pudendal vessels, below the piriformis (see p. 131).

The **nerve to quadratus femoris** (anterior divisions of L4, 5, S1) also supplies the inferior gemellus and the hip joint. It leaves the pelvis in front of the sciatic nerve, which holds it down on the ischium (see p. 131).

The **pudendal nerve** arises from the anterior divisions of S2, 3 and 4 nerves. The nerve passes back between piriformis and coccygeus (Fig. 5.56), medial to the pudendal vessels. In the buttock (see Fig. 3.13, p. 128) it appears between piriformis and the sacrospinous ligament, and curls around the latter to run forward into the ischioanal fossa (see p. 327).

Muscular branches of S3 and S4 supply the pubococcygeus and iliococcygeus components of levator ani and coccygeus on their upper (pelvic) surfaces. The **perineal branch of S4** passes between coccygeus and levator ani to enter the ischioanal fossa and supply pubo rectalis, pubourethralis, pubovaginalis and perianal skin.

The parasympathetic **pelvic splanchnic nerves** (nervi erigentes) arise by several rootlets from the anterior surfaces of S2 and 3 and often 4; the contribution from S3 is usually the largest. They pass forward into the inferior hypogastric plexuses where they mix with the sympathetic nerves and are distributed to pelvic viscera and the distal colon (see below). The old term *nervi erigentes* is correct but incomplete; the nerves cause erection but much more (see below).

Sacral sympathetic trunks

The sympathetic trunks cross the pelvic brim behind the common iliac vessels and run down in the concavity of the sacrum along the medial margins of the anterior sacral foramina (Fig. 5.56). Each has usually four ganglia. The trunks converge at the front of the coccyx to unite at a small swelling, the *ganglion impar*.

Somatic branches are given off to all the sacral nerves (lower limb and perineum), and smaller vascular filaments to the lateral and median sacral vessels. Visceral branches join the inferior hypogastric plexuses.

Inferior hypogastric plexuses

The inferior hypogastric plexus is an autonomic plexus on the side wall of the pelvis on each side. In the male it is lateral to the rectum and posterolateral to the seminal vesicle, prostate and posterior part of bladder; the middle of the plexus is level with and just behind the top of the vesicle. In the female the plexus is lateral to the rectum, cervix, vaginal fornix and posterolateral to the bladder. The plexus is a rectangular, fenestrated plaque of nerves

and ganglia, measuring nearly 5 cm anteroposteriorly and 2 cm vertically (Fig. 5.65).

Its sympathetic components are derived from the superior hypogastric plexus (see p. 291), via the hypogastric nerve (Fig. 5.47) and from the sacral sympathetic ganglia. Preganglionic parasympathetic fibres join the plexus from S2, 3 and 4 nerves; these are the pelvic splanchnic nerves. About half the fibres in the hypogastric nerves are myelinated (preganglionic) and they relay in the ganglia of the inferior hypogastric plexus. The remaining sympathetic fibres and all the parasympathetic fibres pass through without relay. The parasympathetic motor and secretomotor fibres relay in the walls of the viscera.

Visceral branches of the inferior hypogastric plexus accompany visceral branches and tributaries of the internal iliac artery and vein as neurovascular bundles. In general it appears that the muscles of the bladder (detrusor muscle) and rectum are innervated by parasympathetic nerves from the pelvic splanchnics, the smooth muscle of the bladder neck, prostate, seminal vesicle and ductus deferens by sympathetic nerves from the superior hypogastric plexus, and the smooth muscle of the internal sphincter of the anal canal by branches

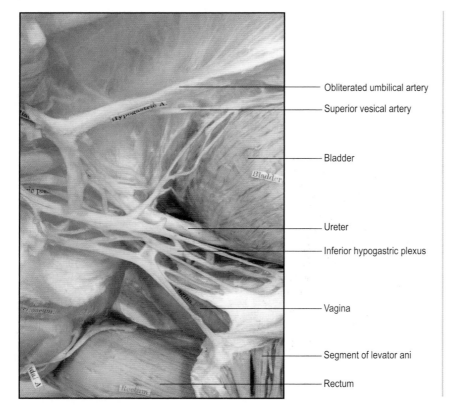

Fig. 5.65 Lateral aspect of the right inferior hypogastric plexus in an exhibit of the viscera and autonomic nerves from a female pelvis in the Anatomy Museum of the Royal College of Surgeons of England.

Obliterated umbilical artery

Superior vesical artery

Bladder

Ureter

Inferior hypogastric plexus

Vagina

Segment of levator ani

Rectum

from the sacral sympathetic ganglia; all these nerves emerge from the inferior hypogastric plexus. Normal sensations of distension of bladder and rectum probably pass through the pelvic splanchnic nerves; pain fibres are carried by both parasympathetic and sympathetic nerves.

As well as the pelvic viscera the pelvic splanchnic nerves supply the colon from the splenic flexure distally. These branches run up from the inferior hypogastric plexuses to the superior hypogastric plexus, or more often to its left, and then ascend with branches of the inferior mesenteric artery or as independent retroperitoneal nerves.

Thus the pelvic parasympathetics are motor to the emptying muscle of the bladder, and of the gut from splenic flexure to rectum. They are also secretomotor to the gut and vasodilator to the erectile tissue in the perineum. The sympathetics are motor to the visceral muscle of the bladder neck and internal anal sphincter. They are motor, too, to the ductus deferens, seminal vesicles and prostatic muscle. The sympathetics also have a facilitating function in relation to uterine muscle.

PART EIGHTEEN

Perineum

The perineum consists of that part of the trunk of the body caudal to the pelvic diaphragm (levator ani and coccygeus). A line joining the anterior parts of the ischial tuberosities divides this diamond-shaped area into a larger posterior anal region and a smaller anterior urogenital region (Fig. 5.66). The anal region contains the anal canal and the ischioanal fossae with their contents. Its sides are formed by the sacrotuberous ligaments (covered by the lower border of gluteus maximus) and its base is formed by the line between the anterior parts of the ischial tuberosities; its contents are the same in each sex. The urogenital region lies in front of the line and is bounded laterally by the conjoined ischiopubic rami; in each sex it contains the external genitalia.

Cutaneous nerves

The skin of each side of the anal region is supplied by the inferior rectal nerve (S3, 4), the perineal branch of S4 and some twigs from the coccygeal plexus (S5).

In the urogenital region, the ilioinguinal nerve (L1) supplies the anterior third of the scrotum (labium majus). The skin of the penis (clitoris) is mainly supplied by the dorsal nerve (S2), a branch of the pudendal nerve. The posterior two-thirds of the scrotum (labium majus) is supplied laterally by the perineal branch of the posterior femoral cutaneous nerve and medially (labium minus) by scrotal (labial) branches of the perineal branch of the pudendal nerve (S3). A pudendal nerve block will therefore not anaesthetize the whole vulva; the anterior and lateral parts must be locally infiltrated to supplement the main nerve block.

Fig. 5.66 Urogenital and anal regions of the pelvic outlet. The anterior urogenital region is triangular and contains the external genitalia. The anal region is a pentagon and contains the anal canal and ischioanal fossae.

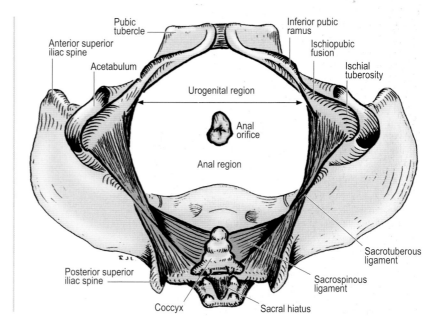

Pubic tubercle
Anterior superior iliac spine
Acetabulum
Inferior pubic ramus
Ischiopubic fusion
Ischial tuberosity
Urogenital region
Anal orifice
Anal region
Posterior superior iliac spine
Sacrotuberous ligament
Sacrospinous ligament
Coccyx
Sacral hiatus

Anal region

Anal canal

The anal canal is the last 4 cm of the alimentary tract; it is usually shorter in females. Like the rest of the gut it is a tube of muscle but the fibres are all circular, consisting of the internal and external anal sphincters, which are composed of visceral and skeletal muscle respectively. These sphincters, assisted by the configuration of the mucous membrane, hold it continually closed except for the temporary passage of flatus and faeces. The junction of rectum and anal canal is at the pelvic floor, i.e. at the level where the puborectalis part of levator ani clasps the gut and angles it forwards (Fig. 5.67). From this angled junction with the rectum, 2.5 cm in front of the tip of the coccyx, the anal canal passes downwards and somewhat backwards to the skin of the perineum.

The muscles of the anal canal can be regarded as forming 'a tube within a funnel' (Parks) (Fig. 5.68). The sides of the upper part of the funnel are the levator ani muscles, and the stem of the funnel is the external sphincter which is continuous with levator ani. The tube inside the stem of the funnel is the internal sphincter which is a thickened continuation of the inner circular layer of rectal muscle. Internally lies the submucosa and mucous membrane.

External anal sphincter

The sphincter has been described in the past as having deep, superficial and subcutaneous parts, based largely on the attachments of the middle (superficial) part, but the parts blend with one another to form a continuous tube.

At its upper (rectal) end, circular skeletal muscle fibres of this sphincter blend with the puborectalis part of levator ani (Fig. 5.68), except of course in the midline at the front where there are no levator ani fibres; here the sphincter fibres alone complete the ring. The region where puborectalis fuses with the external sphincter (which is also the level of the upper end of the internal sphincter) is termed the **anorectal ring**, and is palpable on rectal examination (see p. 305). Fibromuscular strands from the middle part of the external sphincter pass backwards to the posterior surface of the coccyx, contributing to an anococcygeal ligament. A retrosphincteric space occupied by fibrofatty tissue lies between these fibres and the muscular raphe formed by the iliococcygeal part of levator ani (Fig. 5.67). The multilayered fibromuscular anococcygeal ligament, with its external sphincter, iliococcygeus and pubococcygeus components, together with the overlying superior fascia of the pelvic diaphragm is also termed the postanal plate, on which lies the rectum (see p. 301). Anteriorly there is some intermingling of external sphincter muscle fibres with the transverse perinei and bulbospongiosus muscles at the perineal body; this is less evident in the male so that a surgical plane of cleavage can be established between the external sphincter and the perineal body. In the female, the external sphincter is shorter and the deep fibres are deficient anteriorly. The lowest part of the external sphincter curves inwards to lie below the lower end of the internal sphincter (Fig. 5.68). This submucosal apposition of the two sphincters is at the site of the palpable *intersphincteric groove* in the lower part of the anal canal. When operating on the anaesthetized patient, however, the internal sphincter is often found to extend to the anal orifice.

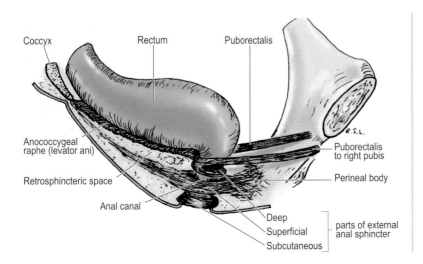

Coccyx — Rectum — Puborectalis

R.S.L.

Anococcygeal raphe (levator ani)

Retrosphincteric space

Anal canal

Puborectalis to right pubis

Perineal body

Deep
Superficial
Subcutaneous
} parts of external anal sphincter

Fig. 5.67 *Puborectalis and the external anal sphincter from the right. The three traditional parts of the sphincter are shown as though separate, but they merge with one another and the deep part is continuous with the puborectalis part of levator ani.*

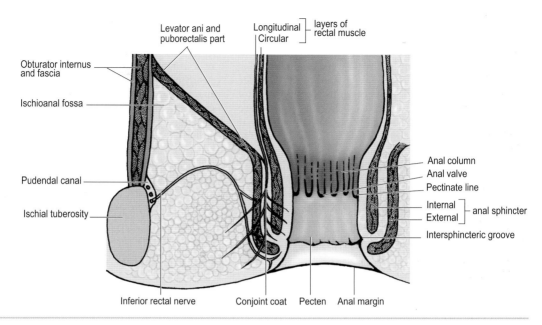

Fig. 5.68 Coronal section of the anal canal and the right ischioanal (ischiorectal) fossa. For clarity only the inferior rectal nerve is shown leaving the pudendal nerve in the pudendal canal; the corresponding vessels pursue a similar course across the fossa.

Internal anal sphincter

This is the thickened downward continuation of the inner circular muscle of the rectum which, in cadaveric prosections, is usually found to extend along three-quarters of the length of the anal canal. (Fig. 5.68). At the anorectal junction the outer longitudinal layer of rectal muscle becomes fibroelastic and, together with some striated muscle fibres of puborectalis, forms the *conjoint longitudinal coat* which runs down between the two sphincters. Strands from this sheet penetrate the internal sphincter and the lower part of the external sphincter; some reach the fat of the ischioanal fossa and the perianal skin; others pass through the internal sphincter to the mucosa of the anal canal, particularly at the pectinate line (see below), where strands tethering the mucous membrane were named the mucosal suspensory ligament by Parks. It is possible that the puckering of perianal skin is due to the attachment of these fibro-elastic strands to perianal skin, but some investigators describe separate smooth muscle fibres in this region, forming the so-called *corrugator cutis ani* muscle.

Mucous membrane

In the upper third of the anal canal the mucous membrane shows 6 to 10 longitudinal ridges, the *anal columns*. They are prominent in children. At their lower ends adjacent columns are joined together by small horizontal folds, the *anal valves*; the pockets so formed above the valves are the *anal sinuses*, into which open mucus-secreting *anal glands*. About half the anal glands are submucosal and the rest penetrate through the internal sphincter. Infection in these glands results in anal abscesses and fistulae. The level of the anal valves is the *pectinate line* (also called the dentate line) below which is a pale, smooth-surfaced area, the pecten, which extends down to the intersphincteric groove. Below the groove is a truly cutaneous area, continuous at the anus (anal margin) with the skin of the buttock. Histologically the lining below the groove is typical skin with keratinized stratified squamous epithelium, hair follicles, sebaceous glands and sweat glands. The lining of the pecten is non-keratinized stratified squamous epithelium, with no hair follicles, sebaceous glands or sweat glands. The anal column area, being continuous with rectal mucosa, has typical columnar intestinal cells and tubular glands. But immediately above and below the pectinate line there is a zone of variable often mixed epithelial structure, so that there is no abrupt line of change from the single-layered gut type to multilayered pecten type. (This contrasts with the gastro-oesophageal junction where there is an abrupt change from stratified squamous to columnar epithelium.)

Small submucous masses, comprising fibroelastic connective tissue, smooth muscle, dilated venous spaces and arteriovenous anastomoses, form *anal cushions* at left lateral (3), right posterior (7) and right anterior (11 o'clock) positions in the upper anal canal. Smaller cushions may be located in between. By their apposition these anal cushions assist the sphincter in maintaining watertight closure of the canal. Excessive straining at stool may cause enlargement of these cushions and the formation of haemorrhoids (piles).

The lining of the upper part of the anal canal is embryologically derived from the cloaca, i.e. it is endodermal; the lower part is from the proctodeum or anal pit and is ectodermal (see p. 31). The dividing line between these territories is usually considered to be at the pectinate line.

Blood supply

Branches of the superior rectal artery supply the upper end of the canal, their terminations lying within the anal columns. A small part of the muscular wall is supplied by the median sacral arteries, while the lower end, including its mucous membrane, receives the ends of the inferior rectal vessels which have crossed the ischioanal fossae. Within the walls there is good anastomosis between the various vessels.

The veins correspond to the above arteries and are continuous with the rectal venous plexuses (see p. 305). The upper part of the canal and plexus drains via the superior rectal and inferior mesenteric veins to the portal system, whereas the lower end drains to the internal iliac veins through the inferior and middle rectal veins. The anal canal is thus a site of portal–systemic anastomosis (see p. 276), the union being in the region of the anal columns.

Lymph drainage

The lymph drainage shows a watershed corresponding to the vascular pattern. The upper canal drains upwards to join the lymphatics of the rectum (see p. 305) whereas lymph from the lower end passes to the (palpable) superficial inguinal group.

Nerve supply

The inferior rectal branches of the pudendal nerves supply the external sphincter; they also provide the sensory supply from 1–2 cm above the pectinate line downwards, where the lining of the anal canal is highly sensitive. The motor fibres originate from Onuf's nucleus, situated mainly in the anterior horn of S2 segment, which also innervates the sphincter urethrae. The puborectalis and the deep part of the external anal sphincter have a high proportion of slow twitch fibres and function as tonic muscles, showing constant electromyographic activity even in sleep and under light anaesthesia. Autonomic nerves pass to the internal sphincter and the upper part of the canal. Sympathetic fibres from the pelvic plexus, with preganglionic cell bodies in the first two lumbar segments of the cord, cause contraction of the internal sphincter, and pelvic splanchnic (parasympathetic) nerves relax it. Afferent fibres from the upper end of the canal are carried by both sympathetic and parasympathetic nerves.

The *anal reflex* is described on page 18.

Defecation

Several factors contribute to normal anal continence: contraction of puborectalis and the external sphincter, maintenance of the angle between rectum and anal canal with abdominal pressure flattening the lower anterior rectal wall over the upper end of the canal, and the presence of mucosal cushions in the canal. The internal sphincter, although assisting closure, can only maintain continence if there is no distension (which causes relaxation of the sphincter). The rectum can accommodate itself to receive a certain amount of colonic content without any significant increase in pressure. There are no specialized receptors in the rectal wall, but they are present in the anal canal where gas, fluid and solid can be distinguished by the cerebral cortex, and there are also stretch receptors in levator ani and the perirectal tissues. When increasing rectal pressure causes faeces to enter the upper anal canal, the external sphincter contracts and forces the contents back into the rectum. If only gas enters, its presence can be tested by a slight conscious increase of abdominal pressure which will let it escape. Defecation is allowed to occur by release of the cortical inhibition that developed during childhood training. Abdominal pressure is increased, puborectalis relaxes and the anorectal angle straightens with relaxation of the external sphincter and contraction of the lower colon and rectum (via its parasympathetic supply).

Incontinence may follow damage to the external sphincter or pudendal nerve (e.g. in obstetrics and perineal operations). In cerebral or spinal cord lesions there may be loss of cortical control.

Ischioanal (ischiorectal) fossa

The ischioanal (ischiorectal) fossa is a wedge-shaped space filled with fat lateral to the anal canal (Figs 5.68 and 5.70A). The base of each fossa lies on the skin over the anal region of the perineum. The external sphincter of the anal canal and the sloping levator ani muscles form the medial wall of each fossa, while the lateral wall is formed by the ischial tuberosity below with obturator internus (covered by its fascia) above. The sharp apex of the wedge is where the medial and lateral walls meet (where levator ani is attached to its tendinous origin over the obturator fascia). At the base the anterior boundary is the posterior border of the perineal body and muscles of the urogenital diaphragm (see p. 328), and the posterior boundary is the sacrotuberous ligament overlapped by the lower border of gluteus maximus.

Each fossa has an anterior recess that passes forwards above the perineal membrane, potentially as far as the posterior surface of the body of the pubis. The recesses of the two sides do not communicate across the midline. Posteriorly, however, the two fossae communicate with one another, low down through the fibrofatty tissue of the retrosphincteric space within the anococcygeal ligament (see p. 324), providing a horseshoe-shaped path for the spread of infection from one fossa to the other.

The **pudendal canal** (of Alcock) is a connective tissue tunnel in the lower lateral wall of the fossa, overlying obturator internus and the medial side of the ischial tuberosity. The canal is formed by a splitting of the obturator fascia above the falciform process of the sacro-tuberous ligament. It contains the **pudendal nerve** and **internal pudendal vessels** (Fig. 5.69), which it conducts from the lesser sciatic notch to the deep perineal pouch above the perineal membrane (see p. 328).

The pudendal nerve and internal pudendal vessels leave the pelvis through the greater sciatic foramen, passing beneath the lower border of piriformis to reach the buttock. Their course in the buttock is short. They turn and enter the lesser sciatic foramen, the vessels

passing over the tip of the spine of the ischium, the nerve more medially over the sacrospinous ligament.

Running transversely across the ischioanal fossa from the pudendal canal towards the anal canal are the *inferior rectal branches* of the pudendal nerve and internal pudendal vessels. Their course is not straight across the base of the fossa, but arches convexly upwards through the fat towards the apex and then downwards to the anal canal. Incisions to drain ischioanal abscesses usually do not interfere with them. Accompanied by the vessels, the nerve breaks up into several branches which supply the external sphincter, mucous membrane of the lower anal canal and perianal skin.

At the front of the fossa the *posterior scrotal (labial) nerves* and *vessels* (from the pudendals) pass superficially into the urogenital region. At the back of the fossa the *perineal branch of S4 nerve* and the *perforating cutaneous nerve* traverse the fossa.

Perineal body

The perineal body, also called the *central tendon of the perineum*, is a midline fibromuscular mass to which a number of muscles gain attachment, and within which they decussate. It is attached to the posterior border of the perineal membrane (see p. 328). It lies between the anal canal and the vagina (Fig. 5.63) or bulb of the penis (Fig. 5.70A). The rectovaginal septum blends into it above. The muscles running into it include the external anal sphincter, pubovaginalis (pubourethralis) part of levator ani, bulbospongiosus, and the superficial and deep transverse perineal muscles. Its position and connections provide a stabilizing influence for pelvic and perineal structures. Injury to it during childbirth may weaken the pelvic floor and contribute to prolapse of the vagina and uterus.

Fig. 5.69 Lateral wall of the left ischioanal fossa from behind, with the connective tissue of the pudendal canal removed to show the pudendal nerve and vessels running forwards on the medial side of the ischial tuberosity. The middle part of the sacrotuberous ligament has been removed and the venae comitantes of the internal pudendal artery are not shown.

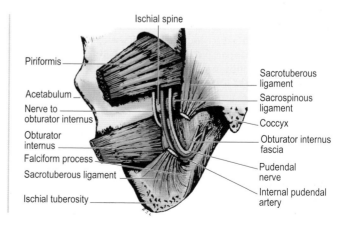

PART NINETEEN

Male urogenital region

In the male urogenital region two layers of fascia, the superior and inferior fasciae of the urogenital diaphragm, enclose the sphincter urethrae and the deep transverse perineal muscles; together these fasciae and muscles are referred to as the urogenital diaphragm. The superior fascia is thin and ill-defined; the inferior fascia is thicker and termed the perineal membrane. These fascia enclose between them a **deep perineal space** (pouch) which contains the membranous part of the urethra, the internal pudendal vessels, the dorsal nerve of penis and perineal nerve at the sides, and the paired bulbourethral glands, in addition to the sphincter urethrae and deep transverse perineal muscles.

The **perineal membrane** is an unyielding sheet of fibrous tissue which forms the basis upon which the penis and penile musculature are fixed (Fig. 5.70A). It is attached on either side to the ischiopubic rami from just behind the subpubic angle back to the level of the anterior part of the ischial tuberosities. Its anterior border forms the *transverse perineal ligament*, and there is a small gap between this and the arcuate pubic ligament through which the deep dorsal vein of the penis passes to reach the vesicoprostatic plexus. Its posterior border fuses centrally with the perineal body. When standing upright, the perineal membrane lies approximately horizontally. Above the membrane lies the membranous urethra surrounded by the urethral sphincter, below the apex of the prostate. The membrane is pierced by the urethra, the ducts of the bulbourethral glands, and by nerves and vessels.

After leaving the prostate just in front of the apex, the prostatic urethra (see p. 309) becomes the **membranous urethra** which passes down for about 1.5 cm and pierces the perineal membrane, 2.5 cm behind the pubic symphysis, to become the penile urethra. The membranous urethra is the shortest and least dilatable part of the urethra. In the upper part of its wall there are some smooth muscle fibres continuous with those of the prostatic urethra.

The **sphincter urethrae**, often called clinically the external urethral sphincter, is roughly pear-shaped. The thinner upper end of the 'pear' extends upwards out of the deep perineal pouch to surround the lower part of the prostatic urethra; the lower more bulbous part is below the apex of the prostate and above the perineal membrane. Some of its fibres arise from the pubic rami and pass as U-shaped loops in front of and behind the urethra, some run from the transverse perineal ligament to the perineal body, and some completely encircle the urethra. Although consisting of striated muscle, the sphincter fibres are of small diameter and are of the slow twitch variety. They are supplied by the perineal branch of the pudendal nerve (see p. 332). Above the posterior part of the perineal membrane the **deep transverse perineal muscle** extends from the ischial ramus to the perineal body, where its fibres decussate with those of the contralateral muscle and the external anal sphincter. It merges anteriorly with the sphincter urethrae and shares the same nerve supply.

The **bulbourethral glands** (of Cowper) lie one on each side of the membranous urethra in the deep perineal pouch, i.e. above (deep to) the perineal membrane, covered by the urethral sphincter. They are about 1 cm in diameter. The single duct from each, about 2.5 cm long, pierces the perineal membrane to open into the bulb of the penile urethra. The glands contribute a small amount to seminal fluid.

Deep to the skin of the urogenital region is the **superficial perineal fascia** (of Colles), a continuation into the perineum of the membranous fascia (of Scarpa) from the anterior abdominal wall (see p. 185). It is attached to the ischiopubic rami and the posterior margin of the perineal membrane, thus closing in a subfascial space, the **superficial perineal space** (pouch), that is in continuity with the space deep to the membranous (Scarpa's) fascia of the anterior abdominal wall (see Fig. 4.1, p. 185). From its marginal attachments in the urogenital region, this fascia is projected into a bulbous scrotal expansion and a cylindrical penile expansion (Fig. 5.70B), the distal end of the latter being attached round the corona of the glans penis. Rupture of the penile urethra permits extravasation of urine beneath Colles' fascia whence the collection distends the tissues of the scrotum and penis and can then pass upwards over the anterior abdominal wall beneath Scarpa's fascia. A *deep perineal fascia* intimately surrounds the cavernous bodies of the penis and clitoris and the superficial perineal muscles associated with them.

Penis

The penis has a root and a body. The **root** of the penis is attached to the inferior surface of the perineal membrane and consists of the (central) *bulb* of the penis with a *crus* on each side. Each crus is attached to the angle between the perineal membrane and the everted margin of the ischiopubic ramus, receives the *deep artery* of the penis near its anterior end, and continues forwards to become the **corpus cavernosum**. The bulb is the posterior end of the **corpus spongiosum**. At the front of the root area, below the subpubic angle, the two corpora

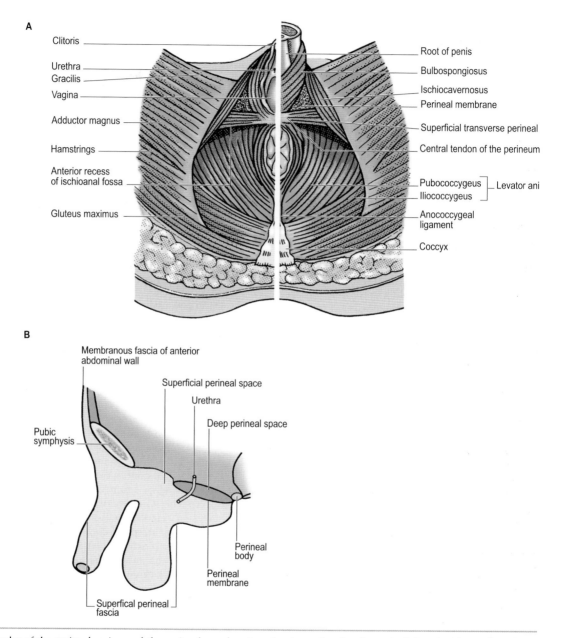

Fig. 5.70 Muscles of the perineal region and the perineal pouches: **A** perineal muscles, female on the left and male on the right of the picture; **B** diagrammatic representation of the perineal pouches in the male.

cavernosa are bound together side by side with the corpus spongiosum behind them (when the penis is dependent, but ventral to them when erect) to form the **body** of the penis. The penile urethra runs through the whole length of the corpus spongiosum from the bulb at the back to its expanded opposite end which is the **glans penis**. The glans forms the tip of the penis, overlapping the distal ends of the corpora cavernosa. The urethra enters the bulb from above near its front so that most of the bulge of the bulb is behind and below the urethra. The bulb

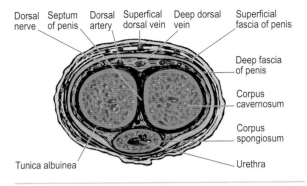

Dorsal nerve — Septum of penis — Dorsal artery — Superfical dorsal vein — Deep dorsal vein — Superficial fascia of penis

Deep fascia of penis

Corpus cavernosum

Corpus spongiosum

Tunica albuinea

Urethra

Fig. 5.71 Cross-section of the body of the penis.

has a slight (palpable) midline notch on its under surface and extends back towards the perineal body. The *arteries of the bulb* enter it near the urethra, which in this region receives the ducts of the bulbourethral glands.

The corpus spongiosum and the two corpora cavernosa (Fig. 5.71) are each surrounded by a tough fibrous sheath, the *tunica albuginea* of the corpus (not to be confused with the tunica albuginea of the testis); that of the corpus spongiosum enlarges distally to enclose the glans. From the tunica fibrous trabeculae pass into the corpora dividing their substance into numerous endothelial cell-lined cavernous spaces into which helicine arteries open (see p. 332). Between the corpora cavernosa there is a connective tissue *septum* which is partly divided into comb-like strands. The fibrous sheaths of the corpora are encircled by the *deep fascia of the penis*, an extension of the deep perineal fascia. This fascia is attached to the front surface of the pubic symphysis by a triangular sheet of fibrous tissue, the *suspensory ligament of the penis*. The midline *deep dorsal vein*, with a *dorsal artery* on each side and more laterally a *dorsal nerve*, lies deep to the deep fascia of the penis.

The skin is hairless and prolonged forwards in a fold, the **prepuce**, which partly overlaps the glans and doubles back to be attached to the neck of the glans. Beneath the skin is the *superficial fascia of the penis* (Buck's fascia), a cylindrical prolongation of Colles' fascia (see p. 328), and in the midline is the *superficial dorsal vein* which is accompanied by lymphatics from the skin and the anterior part of the urethra. On the inferior aspect of the glans, a fold of skin, the *frenulum*, passes from the prepuce to the posterior end of the urethral orifice.

Blood supply

The penis receives three pairs of arteries which are branches of the internal pudendals (see p. 320). The artery

to the bulb supplies the corpus spongiosum, including the glans. The deep artery of the penis supplies the corpus cavernosum. The dorsal artery supplies skin, fascia and glans. There is anastomosis, via the continuity of corpus spongiosum and glans, between the artery of the bulb and the dorsal artery; the deep arteries supply the corpora cavernosa only. The skin of the penis is also supplied by the superficial external pudendal branches of the femoral arteries.

Venous return from the corpora is partly by way of veins that accompany the arteries and join the internal pudendal veins, but mostly by the deep dorsal vein which pierces the suspensory ligament, passes above the perineal membrane and enters the vesicoprostatic venous plexus. The superficial dorsal vein drains the dorsal skin of the penis and divides to join the superficial external pudendal tributaries of the great saphenous veins.

Lymph drainage

Lymphatics from the penile skin pass to superficial inguinal nodes, but the glans and the corpora drain to deep inguinal nodes.

Nerve supply

The skin of the penis is supplied by the pudendal nerves (see p. 323) via the posterior scrotal and dorsal nerves; the latter supply the glans. The dermatome mainly involved is S2. A small area of skin on the dorsum of the proximal penis is supplied by the ilioinguinal nerve (L1). The bulbocavernosus and ischiocavernosus muscles (see below) which contract spasmodically during ejaculation are supplied by the perineal nerve (from the pudendal, S2, 3). The sympathetic nerves necessary for the initial stages of ejaculation (see p. 332) are derived from L1 segment of the spinal cord via the superior and inferior hypogastric plexuses. The pelvic splanchnic nerves (S2, 3) provide the parasympathetic supply to the cavernous tissue of all three corpora and allow increased blood flow for erection (see p. 332).

Circumcision

Ritual circumcision for religious or racial reasons is probably the oldest operation in the world. In children or adults circumcision may be required for a tightly constricting prepuce (*phimosis*). The prepuce is incised on the dorsum from the tip towards the base of the glans, dissecting away any adhesions, and then the incision is carried circumferentially, followed by suture of the skin edges. Bleeding from a vessel in the frenulum needs to be controlled.

Superficial perineal muscles

The bulb and each crus of the penis are provided with overlying muscles: bulbospongiosus and ischiocavernosus, respectively (Fig. 5.70A). In addition there is a transverse pair (superficial transverse perineal) along the posterior border of the perineal membrane. The three superficial perineal muscles of each side thus form a triangular pattern when viewed in the lithotomy position.

Bulbospongiosus arises from the perineal body and in front of that from a median raphe that joins the pair together. Its posterior fibres are directed forwards and laterally over the bulb to be inserted into the perineal membrane and a dorsal fibrous expansion on the penis; the more posterior of these fibres clasp the corpus spongiosum, while the more anterior extend on to the corpora cavernosa. Bulbospongiosus acts to empty the urethra at the end of micturition, assists in erection (by compressing the deep dorsal vein of the penis) and contracts during ejaculation.

Ischiocavernosus arises from the posterior part of the perineal membrane and from the ischial ramus and is inserted by an aponeurosis on to the surface of the corpus cavernosum. Their function is to assist in the support of, and move slightly, the erect penis.

The **superficial transverse perineal muscle** arises from the ischial tuberosity and is inserted into the perineal body. It helps to stabilize the perineal body.

Nerve supply. All three muscles are supplied by the perineal branch of the pudendal nerve (S2, 3).

Male urethra

The urethra consists of prostatic, membranous and spongy parts, with a total length of about 20 cm. The prostatic and membranous parts have already been described (see pp 309 and 328).

The spongy or **penile urethra**, about 15 cm long, is within the corpus spongiosum of the penis and can be divided into bulbous and pendulous parts. The posterior part of the corpus, attached to the undersurface of the perineal membrane, is enlarged as the bulb. After piercing the perineal membrane the urethra enters the bulb and at once takes a right-angled curve forwards within the bulb. The urethra continues through the corpus spongiosum beyond the root of the penis into its body. Just proximal to the **external urethral meatus** at the tip of the glans there is a short dilated region, the *navicular fossa*. The lining here is stratified squamous epithelium, in contrast to the whole of the rest of the urethra which possesses the transitional epithelium typical of the urinary tract. The urethral mucosa displays some very small blind-ending pockets (lacunae) and there are numerous mucous urethral glands (of Littre). The empty urethra is horizontal in cross-section but the meatus is a vertical slit, hence the spiral stream of urine.

The urethra is narrowest at the external meatus, and shows dilatations in the prostatic part, bulb and navicular fossa. When passing a catheter the 90° change of direction in the bulbar part before the membranous urethra is entered has to be kept in mind. On account of a particularly large lacuna on the roof of the navicular fossa, any instruments being passed through the external meatus should initially be pointed towards the floor of the fossa.

Blood supply

As with many tubular structures, there is no single 'artery to the urethra'; the blood supply is from any adjacent vessels as it passes through the prostate, sphincter urethrae and corpus spongiosum.

Nerve supply

The mucous membrane of the penile part receives a branch from the perineal nerve, with filaments from the inferior hypogastric plexuses reaching more proximal parts. The urethral sphincters and the control of micturition have been described on page 307.

Development

The part of the urethra proximal to the openings of the ejaculatory ducts and prostatic utricle is formed, like the trigone of the bladder, from the lower ends of the mesonephric ducts and ureters that are absorbed into the bladder wall (see p. 31). The rest is from the pelvic and phallic parts of the urogenital sinus and the genital tubercle, supplemented ventrally in the penile part by the fusion of the urogenital folds (see p. 31). The epithelium of the navicular fossa (ectoderm from the genital tubercle) is a solid column that becomes canalized; if it fails to do so, and there is accompanying failure of complete fusion of the urogenital folds, the result is hypospadias—a midline opening on the ventral surface.

Scrotum

The scrotum is a pouch of skin containing the testes and spermatic cords. The subcutaneous tissue has no fat, but contains the **dartos muscle** which sends a sheet into the midline fibrous *septum* of the scrotum (Fig. 5.12). The rugosity of the skin is due to contraction of the dartos. The dartos is smooth muscle, and is supplied by sympathetic fibres probably carried by the genital branch of the genitofemoral nerve.

Blood supply

The blood supply of the skin is from the superficial and deep external pudendal arteries (from the femoral) and from scrotal branches of the perineal artery (from the internal pudendal). Venous drainage is mainly by external pudendal veins, superficial and deep, to the great saphenous vein (see Fig. 3.3, p. 118).

Lymph drainage

Lymph drainage is to the superficial inguinal nodes.

Nerve supply

The anterior axial line (see p. 15) crosses the scrotum. The anterior one-third of the scrotal skin is supplied by the ilioinguinal nerve (L1) and the genital branch of the genitofemoral nerve (L1). The posterior two-thirds is supplied by scrotal branches of the perineal nerve (S3), reinforced laterally by the perineal branch of the posterior femoral cutaneous nerve (S2).

Development

The scrotum develops from the labioscrotal swellings and the urogenital folds (see p. 31). Where the urogenital folds meet is marked by a midline cutaneous raphe on the scrotum, which continues on to the inferior surface of the penis. (In the female, the labioscrotal folds form the labia majora, and the urogenital folds remain separate as the labia minora.)

Perineal vessels and nerves

The **internal pudendal artery** (see p. 320) enters the deep perineal pouch from the anterior end of the pudendal canal and passes forwards along the ischiopubic ramus above the perineal membrane, with the dorsal nerve of penis above it and the perineal nerve below it. The *perineal branch* of the artery pierces the posterior angle of the perineal membrane and gives origin to *posterior scrotal* and *transverse perineal* branches. Further forward another branch, *artery to the bulb*, pierces the membrane alongside the urethra to enter the corpus spongiosum. It gives branches to the cavernous tissue of this corpus and passes forwards to supply the glans penis.

Near the anterior margin of the perineal membrane the internal pudendal artery divides into its terminal branches, the deep and dorsal arteries of the penis.

The *deep artery* pierces the membrane to enter the crus of the penis and supplies, by its helicine branches, the erectile cavernous tissue of the corpus cavernosum. The *dorsal artery* pierces the membrane and passes between the crus and the pubic symphysis to pierce the suspensory ligament and run forward, alongside the median deep dorsal vein and with the dorsal nerves laterally, between the deep fascia of the penis and the fibrous sheaths of the corpora cavernosa. The arteries pass to the glans where they anastomose with the terminal branches of the arteries to the bulb.

The **deep dorsal vein** of the penis drains most of the blood from the corpora. It runs proximally in the midline, pierces the suspensory ligament and passes upwards in the gap between the pubic symphysis (arcuate pubic ligament) and the perineal membrane to enter the pelvis and join the vesicoprostatic plexus.

The **pudendal nerve** (see p. 321) divides within the pudendal canal into its terminal branches, the dorsal nerve of the penis and the perineal nerve. Both enter the deep perineal pouch, running forwards respectively above and below the internal pudendal artery. The *dorsal nerve of the penis* appears to be the direct continuation of the pudendal nerve. It pierces the anterior angle of the perineal membrane and then accompanies the dorsal artery on its lateral side. It supplies the skin of the penis and glans and gives branches to the corpus cavernosum. It has no branches in the deep perineal pouch.

The *perineal nerve*, which is the larger terminal branch of the pudendal, gives muscular branches to the superficial and deep perineal muscles and to the sphincter urethrae. The branch to bulbospongiosus supplies sensory fibres to the mucous membrane of the urethra. Either before or just after entering the deep perineal pouch the perineal nerve gives off the *posterior scrotal* branches which run forwards superficial to the perineal membrane to supply scrotal skin.

Erection and ejaculation

The neural controls of erection and ejaculation are different; **erection** is *parasympathetic* and **ejaculation** is *sympathetic* and *somatic*. Impulses in the genital branches of the pelvic splanchnic nerves (parasympathetic) lead to vasodilatation of the helicine arteries of the erectile tissue of the corpora cavernosa (hence the old name of nervi erigentes). As the spongy tissue becomes engorged there may be some compression of the draining veins, but erection (whether reflex from physical stimulation or psychogenic) occurs mainly by increased arterial flow following relaxation of smooth muscle in the trabeculae of the corpora, which is dependent on the production of nitrous oxide and cyclic GMP.

The sympathetic outflow from segments T11 to L2 to the epididymis, ductus deferens, seminal vesicle, ejaculatory duct, prostate, superficial trigonal muscle of the bladder and circular muscle of the bladder neck causes contraction of the smooth muscle of those structures, so causing the flow of seminal fluid into the prostatic urethra (*emission*). The internal urethral opening of the bladder neck becomes constricted so that there is no retrograde flow into the bladder. Rhythmic contraction of bulbospongiosus (supplied by the perineal nerve) compresses the penile urethra and expels the fluid. Orgasmic sensations run in the spinothalamic tract and are abolished by cord transection, but in transections above the lower thoracic segments ejaculation can still occur.

PART TWENTY

Female urogenital region

The female external genitalia include the mons pubis, labia majora, labia minora, clitoris, vestibule, bulbs of the vestibule and the greater vestibular glands. Collectively they form the **vulva**. All the formations and structures seen in the male are present in the female, but greatly modified for functional reasons. The essential difference is the failure in the female of the midline fusion of the genital folds. The scrotum is represented by the labia majora and the corpus spongiosum by the labia minora and the bulb of the vestibule, with corresponding vessels and nerves.

The **mons pubis** is the mound of hairy skin and subcutaneous fat in front of the pubic symphysis and pubic bones. It extends backwards on either side as the **labia majora** which are fatty cutaneous folds forming the boundary of the pudendal cleft. The round ligaments of the uterus end in the anterior part of each labium. A persistent processus vaginalis, and consequently an inguinal hernia, may reach a labium. The labia are joined in front as the *anterior commissure*; at the back they fade away behind the vagina, the connecting skin between them forming a low ridge, the *posterior commissure*, which overlies the perineal body.

The **labia minora** are cutaneous folds without fat lying internal to the labia majora and forming the boundaries of the vestibule. Their front ends split to form the (dorsal) *prepuce* and (ventral) *frenulum* of the clitoris, while at the back they unite by a small skin fold, the frenulum of the labia.

The **clitoris** lies at the front ends of the labia minora. It is formed by two miniature *corpora cavernosa* and

the anterior ends of the bulbs of the vestibule. Its free extremity, the *glans*, is highly sensitive to sexual stimulation and is usually overlapped by the prepuce.

The **vestibule** is bounded by the labia minora and contains the external urethral meatus, the vaginal orifice and the ducts of the greater vestibular glands.

The **perineal membrane** is wider but weaker than in the male, being pierced by the vagina. It gives attachment to the *crura of the clitoris*, each of which is covered by an *ischiocavernosus* muscle. Medial to each crus, attached to the perineal membrane at the side of the vagina, is a mass of erectile tissue, the *bulb of the vestibule*, one on each side of the orifices of the vagina and urethra. They join in front of the urethral orifice and pass forwards to the glans of the clitoris. Each bulb is covered by a *bulbospongiosus* muscle, whose fibres extend from the perineal body round the vagina and urethra to the clitoris. They form a perineal sphincter for the vagina in addition to its pelvic sphincter (the pubovaginalis parts of levator ani).

The **greater vestibular glands** (of Bartholin) form pea-shaped masses less than 1 cm in diameter lying at the side of the vaginal opening, one behind the posterior end of each bulb and deep to bulbospongiosus. Each opens by a single duct 2 cm long into the posterolateral part of the vaginal orifice, in the groove between the labium minus and the hymen or its remains. The duct may be subject to cyst formation, and the gland to infection (bartholinitis). The glands may play a minor role in lubricating the lower vagina. They are homologous with the bulbourethral (Cowper's) glands of the male, but unlike in the male they are superficial to the membrane.

The *lesser vestibular glands* are very small mucous glands with minute openings between the urethral and vaginal openings.

The **hymen** is a mucosal fold of variable extent and thickness at the margins of the vaginal opening. It may be absent or may even completely close the opening, in which case it must be incised at the age when menstruation begins. Its remains after rupture by the first sexual intercourse may form small tags (*hymenal carunculae*).

The **deep perineal space** is traversed by both the urethra and vagina. As in the male it contains the sphincter urethrae, deep transverse perineal muscles, nerves and vessels. The pudendal nerve and internal pudendal vessels have a corresponding course and distribution in the female deep perineal space and vulval region to that in the male deep and superficial perineal spaces, but the neurovascular branches are generally smaller. The pudendal nerve can be infiltrated with a local anaesthetic (*pudendal nerve block*) via a needle passed through the vaginal wall, directed towards the ischial spine and sacrospinous ligament which are palpable per vaginam.

Female orgasm

Sexual excitement induces vascular dilatation and engorgement in the vulva, especially the bulbs of the vestibule and glans clitoris, and is due, as in the male, to parasympathetic activity. There is dilatation of the thin-walled submucous veins of the vagina, which becomes moistened by a transudation of fluid through the mucous membrane. The vestibular glands probably make a negligible contribution. At the climax there is some vaginal smooth muscle and perineal skeletal muscle contraction.

PART TWENTY-ONE

Pelvic joints and ligaments

The joints of the pelvis are the sacroiliac and sacrococcygeal joints and the pubic symphysis, while the chief ligaments of the pelvis (vertebropelvic ligaments) are the sacrotuberous, sacrospinous and iliolumbar.

Sacroiliac joint

The sacroiliac joint is a synovial joint between the auricular surfaces of the ilium (see Fig. 3.46, p. 172) and sacrum (see Fig. 6.98, p. 455). The articulating surfaces are jagged and there is very little movement. With increasing age fibrous adhesions and gradual obliteration of the joint cavity occur; earlier in males, after the menopause in females.

The capsule is attached to the articular margins. Ligamentous bands surround the capsule. The **anterior sacroiliac ligament** is a flat band which joins the bones above and below the pelvic brim (Fig. 5.72); stronger in the female, it indents a preauricular groove on the female ilium just below the pelvic brim. A mass of ligaments attaches the sacrum to the ilium behind the joint. Most of them constitute the very strong **interosseous sacroiliac ligament**, whose fibres are attached to deep pits on the posterior surface of the lateral mass of the sacrum. The most superficial fibres form the **posterior sacroiliac ligament** (Fig. 5.73). The posterior rami of the spinal nerves and vessels pass between the interosseous and posterior ligaments.

The stability of the sacroiliac articulation depends entirely upon ligaments. Body weight transmitted through L5 vertebra tends to push the sacrum downwards and forwards towards the symphysis. Opposing any gliding movement of the joint surfaces are the interosseous sacroiliac ligament and the iliolumbar ligament, while opposing forward rotation of the sacral promontory around the joint are the sacrotuberous and sacrospinous ligaments (see below). The sacroiliac ligaments soften

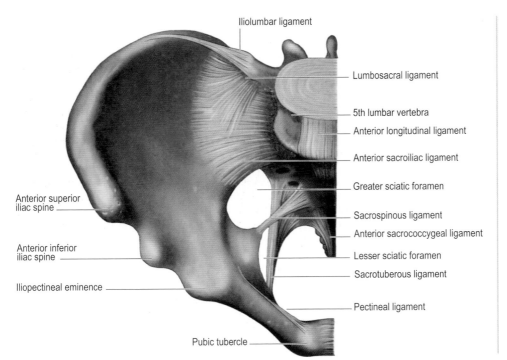

Iliolumbar ligament

Lumbosacral ligament

5th lumbar vertebra

Anterior longitudinal ligament

Anterior sacroiliac ligament

Greater sciatic foramen

Sacrospinous ligament

Anterior sacrococcygeal ligament

Lesser sciatic foramen

Sacrotuberous ligament

Pectineal ligament

Anterior superior iliac spine

Anterior inferior iliac spine

Iliopectineal eminence

Pubic tubercle

Fig. 5.72 Ligaments of the right half of the pelvis: anterior aspect.

Fig. 5.73 Ligaments of the right half of the pelvis: posterior aspect.

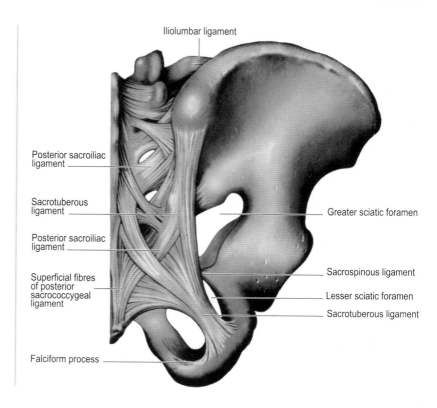

Iliolumbar ligament

Posterior sacroiliac ligament

Sacrotuberous ligament

Posterior sacroiliac ligament

Superficial fibres of posterior sacrococcygeal ligament

Falciform process

Greater sciatic foramen

Sacrospinous ligament

Lesser sciatic foramen

Sacrotuberous ligament

towards the later months of pregnancy and permit some slight rotation of the sacrum during parturition.

Sacrotuberous ligament

The sacrotuberous ligament is a flat band of great strength. It is blended with the posterior sacroiliac ligament and is attached to the posterior border of the ilium and the posterior superior and posterior inferior iliac spines, to the transverse tubercles of the sacrum below the auricular surface, and to the upper part of the coccyx (Fig. 5.73). From this wide area the ligament slopes down to the medial surface of the ischial tuberosity. The lower edge of the ischial attachment is prolonged forwards and attached to a curved ridge of bone. This prolongation is the *falciform process*; it lies just below the pudendal canal. The sacrotuberous ligament is narrower in the middle than at either end. Its gluteal surface gives origin to gluteus maximus. The ligament is said to be the phylogenetically degenerated tendon of origin of the long head of biceps femoris. It is pierced by the perforating cutaneous nerve and branches of the inferior gluteal vessels and coccygeal nerves.

Sacrospinous ligament

The sacrospinous ligament lies on the pelvic aspect of the sacrotuberous ligament (Fig. 5.72). It has a broad base which is attached to the side of the lower part of the sacrum and the upper part of the coccyx. It narrows as it passes laterally, where its apex is attached to the spine of the ischium. The coccygeus muscle lies on the pelvic surface of the ligament. The ligament is the phylogenetically degenerated posterior surface of the coccygeus muscle.

The sacrotuberous and sacrospinous ligaments, with the lesser sciatic notch of the ischium, enclose the lesser sciatic foramen, whose lateral part is occupied by the emerging obturator internus muscle and whose medial part leads forwards into the pudendal canal above the falciform process of the sacrotuberous ligament (Fig. 5.69).

Iliolumbar ligament

The iliolumbar ligament is shaped like a V lying sideways, the apex of the V being attached to the transverse process of L5 vertebra, from which upper and lower bands fan outwards. The upper band passes to the iliac crest, giving partial origin to quadratus lumborum and becoming continuous with the anterior layer of the lumbar fascia. The lower band runs laterally and downwards to blend with the front of the anterior sacroiliac ligament.

Sacrococcygeal joint

The sacrococcygeal joint is a symphysis between the apex of the sacrum and the base of the coccyx, with an intervening disc of fibrocartilage. A short *anterior sacrococcygeal ligament* unites the bones at the front. Behind, there are two *posterior sacrococcygeal ligaments*: a short deep one uniting the adjacent bones and a superficial which closes over the sacral hiatus at the lower end of the sacral canal. At each side there is a *lateral sacrococcygeal ligament* running from the transverse process of the coccyx to the inferolateral angle of the sacrum, completing a foramen for the anterior ramus of the fifth sacral nerve. This ligament may become ossified. Slight flexion and extension are possible at this joint.

Pubic symphysis

The pubic symphysis as its name implies, is a secondary cartilaginous joint. The body surfaces of the pubes are each covered with a thin plate of hyaline cartilage and the two sides are connected by fibrocartilage forming an interpubic disc. Centrally a tissue-fluid space may develop, but it is never lined with synovial membrane. Ligamentous fibres forming the **superior pubic ligament** reinforce the symphysis above, and below it is strengthened by the **arcuate pubic ligament**. No perceptible movement occurs at the symphysis; some separation of the pubes may occur during parturition.

PART **TWENTY-TWO**

Summary of lumbar and sacral plexuses

The two plexuses have already been described, and accounts of their branches are found in the descriptions of the appropriate regions; the branches are summarized below.

Lumbar plexus

After the anterior rami of the upper four lumbar nerves have supplied psoas and quadratus lumborum segmentally,

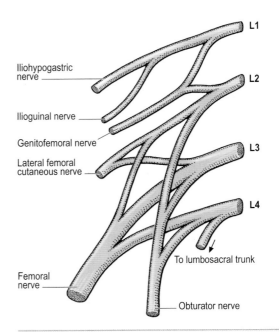

Fig. 5.74 Right lumbar plexus.

they form the plexus in the substance of psoas major. The plexus (Fig. 5.74) innervates part of the lower abdominal wall, but is chiefly concerned in supplying skin and muscle in the lower limb. It reinforces the sacral plexus, which is the true plexus of the lower limb.

Branches of the lumbar plexus

L1 Iliohypogastric and ilioinguinal
L1, 2 Genitofemoral
L2, 3 (posterior divisions) Lateral femoral cutaneous
L2, 3, 4 (posterior divisions) Femoral
L2, 3, 4 (anterior divisions) Obturator.

Iliohypogastric and ilioinguinal nerves (L1)

These are only by convention included in the lumbar plexus. They are really just the first lumbar segmental body–wall nerve and its collateral branch, in series with the thoracic nerves (see p. 13). Apart from supplying skin over the inguinal region and the front of the scrotum, they provide the important motor supply for the fibres of internal oblique and transversus that form the roof of the inguinal canal and reach the conjoint tendon.

Genitofemoral nerve (L1, 2)

The *femoral* part supplies an area of skin below the middle of the inguinal ligament. The *genital* part supplies that part of the abdominal wall herniated into the scrotum for the descent of the testis (i.e. the spermatic cord). It is sensory to tunica vaginalis and the spermatic fasciae, and motor to cremaster muscle. It supplies a small area of anterior scrotal and labial skin.

Lateral femoral cutaneous nerve (L2, 3—posterior divisions)

The nerve is wholly sensory, to the iliac fascia and peritoneum of the iliac fossa, and to the lateral side of the thigh down to the knee. It emerges from the lateral border of psoas and enters the thigh by passing through or under the lateral part of the inguinal ligament.

Femoral nerve (L2, 3, 4—posterior divisions)

This nerve issues from the lateral border of psoas and crosses the iliac fossa in the gutter between psoas and iliacus, deep to the iliac fascia. It supplies iliacus in the abdomen and passes beneath the inguinal ligament lateral to the femoral sheath. As it enters the femoral triangle it supplies pectineus and breaks up at once into several branches.

The *nerve* to *pectineus* runs behind the femoral sheath to reach the muscle. Of two *nerves to sartorius* one often pierces the muscle and continues on as an *intermediate femoral cutaneous nerve* which supplies skin and fascia lata over the front of the thigh down to the knee. The *medial femoral cutaneous nerve* supplies the medial side of the thigh, and an anterior branch reaches the front of the knee.

The nerve to *rectus femoris* is usually double, and the upper branch supplies also the *hip joint*. The nerve to *vastus lateralis* runs down with the descending branch of the lateral femoral circumflex artery between rectus femoris and vastus intermedius. The nerve to *vastus intermedius* sinks into the anterior surface of that muscle. The nerve to *vastus medialis* enters the upper part of the subsartorial canal and sinks into the muscle. The nerves to all three vasti also supply the knee joint.

The *saphenous nerve* crosses in front of the femoral artery in the subsartorial canal, and emerges from behind the posterior border of sartorius. Its *infrapatellar branch* pierces sartorius to run into the patellar plexus. The saphenous nerve pierces the fascia lata between the tendons of sartorius and gracilis and descends to supply skin and periosteum over the subcutaneous surface of the tibia. It runs with the great saphenous vein in front of the medial malleolus and ends on the medial side of the foot just short of the big toe.

Obturator nerve (L2, 3, 4—anterior divisions)

Emerging from the medial side of psoas the nerve lies on the ala of the sacrum lateral to the lumbosacral trunk. It slants down to the side wall of the pelvis between the origin of the internal iliac artery and the ilium. From the angle between external and internal iliac vessels it runs straight to the obturator foramen, supplying the parietal peritoneum of the side wall of the pelvis (in the female the ovary lies here). In the obturator canal it splits into anterior and posterior divisions.

The *posterior division* supplies obturator externus, then pierces the upper border of that muscle and runs into the thigh deep to adductor brevis. It runs down on adductor magnus, whose pubic part it supplies. A slender branch accompanies the femoral artery into the popliteal fossa to supply the knee joint.

The *anterior division* passes over obturator externus and, emerging into the thigh, it supplies the hip joint. It runs down over adductor brevis, deep to pectineus and adductor longus. It supplies these two adductors and may supply pectineus. It also supplies gracilis. It supplies the medial side of the thigh by a cutaneous branch which runs through the subsartorial plexus.

The *accessory obturator nerve*, when occasionally present, passes over the superior pubic ramus to supply pectineus.

Sacral plexus

This is a flat, triangular formation on the front of piriformis muscle. It is formed out of the lumbosacral trunk (L4, 5) and the upper four anterior sacral rami (Fig. 5.75). These rami divide and unite as they converge to the greater sciatic foramen, forming the branches of the sacral plexus.

The **nerves to piriformis** (S1, 2) are twigs that pass back from the upper sacral nerves into the muscle.

The **perforating cutaneous nerve** (S2, 3) pierces the sacrotuberous ligament and the fibres of gluteus maximus that arise there, and supplies a small area of skin on the lower medial side of the buttock.

The **posterior femoral cutaneous nerve** (S1, 2, 3) has a wide distribution. It runs down below piriformis on the sciatic nerve. From the lower border of gluteus maximus it runs down the posterior midline beneath the fascia as far as the lower ends of the gastrocnemius bellies. It supplies a strip of deep fascia and skin, between anterior

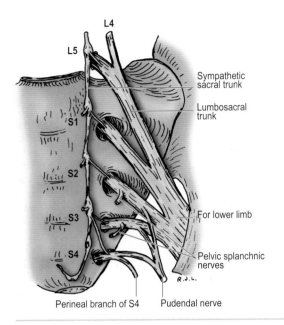

Fig. 5.75 Left sacral plexus. The branches from its anterior surface (three Ps) are shown.

and posterior axial lines, from the buttock to the midcalf by a series of branches which pierce the deep fascia.

Gluteal branches wind around gluteus maximus to supply skin over the convexity of the buttock. The long *perineal branch* winds around the hamstrings and gracilis origins and pierces the fascia lata at the medial convexity of the upper thigh. It supplies the lateral part of the posterior two-thirds of the scrotum (labium majus).

The **pelvic splanchnic nerves** (S2, 3, 4) constitute the sacral parasympathetic outflow and the fibres join the inferior hypogastric plexus. They are motor to the bladder and to the large intestine from the splenic flexure downwards, and cause penile (clitoral) erection. Their afferent fibres include those for distension and pain from the bladder, lower cervix, lower colon and rectum. Referred pain may be felt in the distribution of the posterior femoral cutaneous nerve.

The **pudendal nerve** (S2, 3, 4) runs down and curls around the gluteal surface of the sacrospinous ligament to enter the pudendal canal. It is the nerve of the pelvic floor and perineum.

At the posterior end of the canal it gives the *inferior rectal nerve* which arches through the fat of the ischioanal fossa; its branches supply the external anal sphincter, anal canal and perianal skin.

The *perineal nerve* emerges from the anterior end of the canal as a terminal branch of the pudendal. It runs

forward and breaks up to supply skin of the posterior two-thirds of the scrotum and vulva, and the mucous membrane of the urethra and vagina. It is motor to the perineal muscles, namely, ischiocavernosus, bulbo-spongiosus, superficial and deep transversus perinei and the sphincter urethrae.

The *dorsal nerve* of the penis (clitoris) is the other terminal branch of the pudendal. It runs forward deep to the perineal membrane, which it pierces just below the symphysis pubis to supply the skin of the penis (clitoris).

Muscular branches of S3 and S4 supply levator ani and coccygeus on their upper (pelvic) surfaces.

The **perineal branch of S4** passes between levator ani and coccygeus to supply the puborectalis, pubourethralis and pubovaginalis parts of levator ani from below, and the skin over the ischioanal fossa.

The **nerve to quadratus femoris** (L4, 5, S1) lies on the ischium deep to the sciatic nerve and runs down deep to obturator internus to sink into the deep surface of quadratus femoris. It also supplies the inferior gemellus and gives a branch to the hip joint.

The **nerve to obturator internus** (L5, S1, 2) passes below piriformis, curls around the base of the ischial spine and sinks into obturator internus. It also supplies the superior gemellus.

The **superior gluteal nerve** (L4, 5, S1) passes back through the greater sciatic notch above piriformis, runs in the plane between glutei medius and minimus, supplies both, and ends in the tensor fasciae latae.

The **inferior gluteal nerve** (L5, S1, 2) passes back below piriformis and sinks into the deep surface of gluteus maximus.

Sciatic nerve

The sciatic nerve is the largest branch of the sacral plexus from which it is formed at the lower margin of piriformis by union of its tibial and common peroneal parts. It passes into the buttock lying on the posterior surface of the ischium. Here the nerve to quadratus femoris is deep to it and the posterior femoral cutaneous nerve lies superficial. From midway between the greater trochanter and the ischial tuberosity, the sciatic nerve passes vertically downwards into the hamstring compartment. It lies on obturator internus and gemelli, quadratus femoris and then on adductor magnus. It is overlaid by the long head of biceps. The main trunk of the sciatic nerve supplies all the hamstrings and the ischial fibres of adductor magnus and it then divides, usually at the upper angle of the popliteal fossa, into the tibial and common peroneal nerves. The branches for the long head of biceps, the two 'semi-' muscles and adductor magnus are from the tibial part, but the branch to the short head of biceps comes from the common peroneal part.

Common peroneal (fibular) nerve (L4, 5, S1, 2)

The common peroneal nerve supplies the extensor and peroneal compartments of the leg and the dorsum of the foot. It enters the apex of the popliteal fossa and runs medial to the biceps tendon just beneath the deep fascia. It crosses plantaris, lateral head of gastrocnemius and curves around the neck of the fibula, through peroneus longus, where it divides into two terminal branches, the deep and superficial peroneal (fibular) nerves. It can be palpated on the neck of the fibula, where it can be rolled on the bone. It is the nerve most commonly injured in the lower limb.

The common peroneal nerve itself supplies no muscles. Three articular branches, the *upper* and *lower lateral* and *recurrent genicular nerves*, supply the knee joint; the lateral genicular nerves accompany arteries, the recurrent supplies the superior tibiofibular joint as well.

There are two cutaneous branches. The *sural communicating nerve* joins the sural nerve below the gastrocnemius heads. The *lateral cutaneous nerve of the calf* supplies skin and deep fascia over the upper half of the peroneal compartment.

The **deep peroneal nerve** is formed in the substance of peroneus longus, spirals down over the fibula deep to extensor digitorum longus and reaches the interosseous membrane. It runs down lateral to the vessels, crosses the lower end of the tibia and the dorsum of the foot, and ends by supplying the skin of the first interdigital cleft.

It supplies the muscles of the extensor compartment of the leg: extensor digitorum longus, tibialis anterior, extensor hallucis longus and peroneus tertius. On the dorsum of the foot it gives a lateral branch which supplies extensor digitorum brevis.

The **superficial peroneal nerve** is formed in the substance of peroneus longus and runs down in the muscle, emerging from its anterior border about a third of the way down the leg. It supplies peroneus longus and brevis, then perforates the fascia to supply the skin over the peronei and extensor muscles in the lower third of the leg. Above the ankle it divides into a medial and a lateral branch which supply skin and deep fascia on the dorsum of the foot. The medial branch breaks up to supply the medial side of the big toe and the second interdigital cleft, while the lateral branch breaks up to supply the third and fourth clefts.

Tibial nerve (L4, 5, S1, 2, 3)

The tibial nerve supplies the calf and the sole of the foot around to the toenails. The nerve enters the apex of the popliteal fossa and, in the midline of the limb, passes vertically down deep to the heads of gastrocnemius behind the knee joint and across the popliteus muscle, to run beneath the fibrous arch in soleus.

Branches in the popliteal fossa. Three *genicular nerves*, upper and lower medial and a middle, accompany the arteries and supply the knee joint. *Five muscular branches* supply the muscles of the fossa: plantaris, both heads of gastrocnemius, soleus and popliteus. The last-named branch recurves around the lower border of the muscle to enter its deep (anterior) surface. A single cutaneous branch, the *sural nerve*, lies in the groove between the two heads of gastrocnemius and pierces the deep fascia halfway down the leg. Here it is joined by the sural communicating nerve. The sural nerve runs down alongside the small saphenous vein behind the lateral malleolus and ends on the lateral side of the little toe.

From the fibrous arch the nerve runs down with the posterior tibial vessels deep to the soleus muscle. The neurovascular bundle lies in the groove between the bellies of flexor hallucis longus and flexor digitorum longus. Behind the medial malleolus, beneath the flexor retinaculum, the nerve divides into its terminal medial and lateral plantar branches.

Branches in the calf. Four muscular branches supply soleus, tibialis posterior and the flexors hallucis and digitorum longus. *Medial calcanean* branches pierce the flexor retinaculum and supply the weight-bearing skin of the heel.

The *medial* and *lateral plantar nerves* correspond approximately to the median and ulnar nerves in the hand as far as skin and muscle supplies are concerned. The medial plantar supplies the medial part of the sole and plantar surface of the medial three and a half digits, and innervates flexor digitorum brevis, abductor hallucis, flexor hallucis brevis and the first lumbrical, with the lateral plantar supplying the rest of the sole and the other small muscles of the foot.

Head and neck and spine

6

PART ONE

General topography of the neck

The first thoracic vertebra lies at the highest part of the sloping thoracic inlet. From its upper border rises the cervical spinal column, gently convex forwards, and supporting the skull. A mass of *extensor musculature* lies behind the vertebrae, supplied segmentally by posterior rami of cervical nerves that emerge from intervertebral foramina. A much smaller amount of prevertebral *flexor musculature*, covered by prevertebral fascia, lies in front of the vertebrae and behind the pharynx, supplied segmentally by anterior rami.

Projecting forwards and downwards from the base of the skull in front of the upper part of the pharynx is the face. The hard palate lies on a level with the anterior arch of the atlas (C1 vertebra); the lower border of the mandible lies between C2 and 3 vertebrae. The pharynx extends from the base of the skull to the level of the cricoid cartilage (C6) and then continues on as the oesophagus.

In front of the lower pharynx and upper oesophagus lie the larynx and trachea. Lying above the larynx is the hyoid bone at C3 vertebra level. It is connected to the mandible by the mylohyoid muscles, which are at the upper limit of the anterior part of the neck and form the floor of the mouth. The hyoid bone is suspended by muscles from the skull and the larynx is suspended from the hyoid by a membrane and muscles. Inferiorly they are connected by muscles to the sternum and the scapula. Deep to these muscles the thyroid gland, enclosed in the pretracheal fascia, lies alongside the larynx and trachea.

On each side of the pharynx is the carotid sheath, containing the common and internal carotid arteries and the internal jugular vein, with the cervical sympathetic trunk behind it. Descending into the neck are the ninth, tenth, eleventh and twelfth cranial nerves; the ninth and twelfth pass forwards to the oropharynx and tongue, the eleventh runs backwards to the sternocleidomastoid and trapezius muscles, the vagus continues down in the carotid sheath.

Surrounding the whole neck is a collar of fascia, the investing layer of deep cervical fascia, which encloses the trapezius and sternocleidomastoid muscles; the fascia and the muscles are attached above to the base of the skull and below to the clavicle at the root of the neck.

Superficial structures

The **platysma** is a broad flat sheet of muscle that lies superficial to the investing layer of deep cervical fascia. It extends from the fascia over the upper parts of pectoralis major and deltoid to the lower border of the mandible; some fibres continue on to the face, blending with the muscles of facial expression. The muscle covers the external and anterior jugular veins. The two muscles are separated below, but converge above towards the midline just beneath the chin.

Nerve supply. By the cervical branch of the facial nerve; afferent (proprioceptive) fibres run with the transverse cervical nerve.

Action. It plays a part in facial expression and may assist in opening the mouth.

The **anterior jugular veins** commence beneath the chin and pass downwards, side by side beneath the platysma, to the suprasternal region (Fig. 6.3). Here they pierce the deep fascia and come to lie in the suprasternal space,

341

where they are often connected by a short anastomotic vein. Each now angles laterally and passes deep to sternocleidomastoid, but superficial to the strap muscles, to open into the external jugular vein near its termination.

Deep cervical fascia

The deep cervical fascia consists of four parts: the investing layer, pretracheal fascia, prevertebral fascia, and the carotid sheath.

Investing layer

This fascia, comparable in every way to the deep fascia that underlies the subcutaneous fat in the limbs and elsewhere, surrounds the neck like a collar (Fig. 6.1). It splits around sternocleidomastoid and trapezius and posteriorly it blends with the ligamentum nuchae, which is attached to the spines of the cervical vertebrae. Anteriorly it is attached to the hyoid bone; and above to the lower border of the mandible and to the mastoid process, superior nuchal line and external occipital protuberance at the base of the skull.

Between the angle of the mandible and the tip of the mastoid process the investing layer is strong and splits to enclose the parotid gland. The superficial part extends superiorly as the *parotidomasseteric fascia* and reaches up to the zygomatic arch. The deep part extends to the base of the skull; between the styloid process and the angle of the mandible it is thickened as the *stylomandibular ligament.*

Below, the investing layer is attached to the spine and acromion of the scapula and the clavicle with the trapezius, and to the clavicle and the manubrium of the sternum with the sternocleidomastoid. In the intervals between these muscles, it is attached to both clavicles and to the jugular (suprasternal) notch by two layers into which it splits a short distance above them. The layers are attached to the anterior and posterior borders of the jugular notch, enclosing between them the **suprasternal space** which contains the lower parts of the anterior jugular veins, an anastomotic arch between them, the sternal heads of the sternocleidomastoids and sometimes a lymph node. Of the two layers that adhere to the middle third of the clavicle, the deeper splits around the inferior belly of the omohyoid, forming a fascial sling

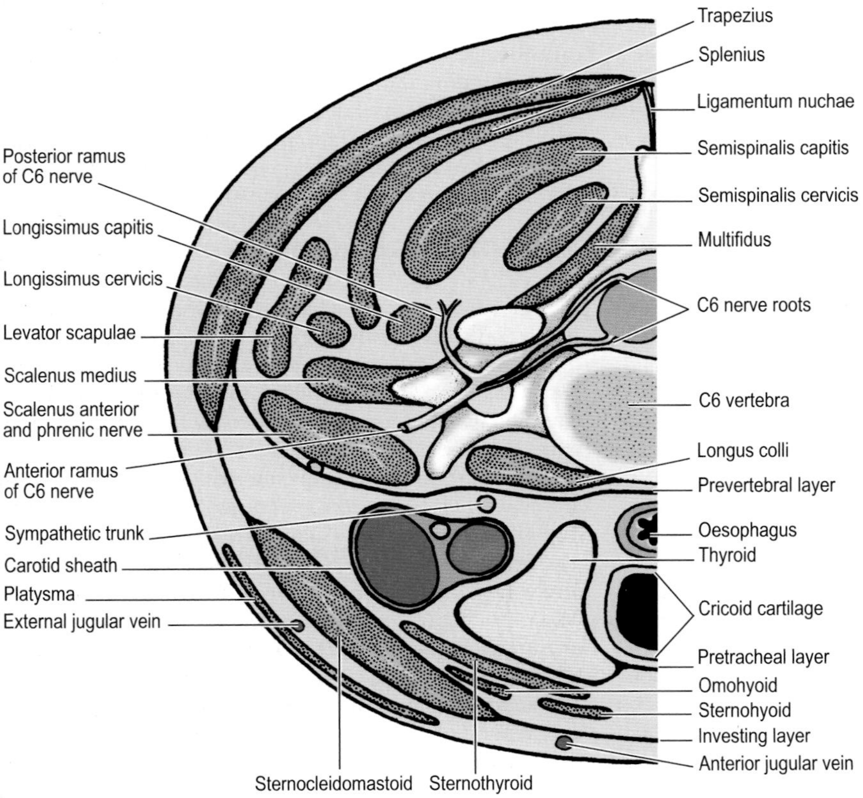
Trapezius
Splenius
Ligamentum nuchae
Semispinalis capitis
Semispinalis cervicis
Multifidus
C6 nerve roots
C6 vertebra
Longus colli
Prevertebral layer
Oesophagus
Thyroid
Cricoid cartilage
Pretracheal layer
Omohyoid
Sternohyoid
Investing layer
Anterior jugular vein
Posterior ramus of C6 nerve
Longissimus capitis
Longissimus cervicis
Levator scapulae
Scalenus medius
Scalenus anterior and phrenic nerve
Anterior ramus of C6 nerve
Sympathetic trunk
Carotid sheath
Platysma
External jugular vein
Sternocleidomastoid
Sternothyroid

Fig. 6.1 Deep cervical fascia of one half of the neck, showing its four components: the investing, pretracheal and prevertebral layers and the carotid sheath.

which keeps this muscle belly low down in the neck (see Fig. 2.2, p. 41). The two layers are pierced by the external jugular vein.

Prevertebral fascia

This is a firm, tough membrane that lies in front of the prevertebral muscles (Fig. 6.1). It extends from the base of the skull, in front of the longus capitis, rectus capitis lateralis and longus colli muscles, downwards to blend with the anterior longitudinal ligament on the body of T4 vertebra. It extends sideways across the scalenus anterior, scalenus medius and levator scapulae muscles (Fig. 6.8), getting thinner further out and fading under cover of the anterior border of trapezius. It covers the muscles that form the floor of the posterior triangle of the neck and all the cervical nerve roots (thus the cervical plexus and trunks of the brachial plexus lie deep to it). The lymph nodes of the posterior triangle and the accessory nerve lie superficial to it. The third part of the subclavian artery lies deep to the fascia, which becomes prolonged over the artery and the brachial plexus below the clavicle as the *axillary sheath* to a varying extent in the axilla. It does not invest the subclavian or axillary vein; these lie in loose areolar tissue anterior to it, free to dilate during times of increased venous return from the upper limb. The fasica is pierced by the four cutaneous branches of the cervical plexus (great auricular, lesser occipital, transverse cervical and supraclavicular nerves).

Pretracheal fascia

This thin fascia lies deep to the infrahyoid strap muscles (sternothyroid, sternohyoid and omohyoid) so that its upward attachment is limited by the respective attachments of those muscles, namely, the body of the hyoid bone and the oblique line of the thyroid cartilage. It splits to enclose the thyroid gland, to which it is not adherent except between the isthmus and second, third and fourth rings of the trachea. Laterally, it fuses with the front of the carotid sheath on the deep surface of the sternocleidomastoid and inferiorly it passes behind the brachiocephalic veins to blend with the adventitia of the arch of the aorta and the fibrous pericardium. The pretracheal fascia is also described in some accounts as being part of a cervical visceral fascia that surrounds the pharynx, oesophagus, larynx and trachea.

Carotid sheath

This is not a fascia in the sense of a demonstrable membranous layer, but consists of a feltwork of areolar tissue that surrounds the common and internal carotid arteries, internal jugular vein, vagus nerve and some deep cervical lymph nodes (Fig. 6.1). It is thin where it overlies the internal jugular vein, allowing the vein to dilate during increased blood flow. The sheath is attached to the base of the skull at the margins of the carotid canal and jugular fossa, and is continued downwards along the vessels to blend with the adventitia of the aortic arch. In front the lower part of the sheath fuses with the fascia on the deep surface of the sternocleidomastoid. Where they lie alongside, the sheath blends with the pretracheal fascia. Behind the carotid sheath there is a minimum of loose areolar tissue between it and the prevertebral fascia; the cervical sympathetic trunk lies here in front of the prevertebral fascia (Fig. 6.8). The carotid sheath is described further on page 379.

Tissue spaces of the neck

Behind the prevertebral fascia is the closed **prevertebral space** from which an anterior escape can only be made by a perforation in the fascia. Hence pus from an abscess in a cervical vertebra can lift the prevertebral fascia as far down as the superior mediastinum.

Immediately in front of the prevertebral fascia is a space that extends from the base of the skull to the diaphragm passing through the superior into the posterior mediastinum as it does so (see Fig. 4.9, p. 196). Its upper part is the **retropharyngeal space**, which is continuous laterally with a **parapharyngeal space** at the side of the pharynx; the upper part of this space is in the infratemporal fossa (see p. 373), bounded laterally by the pterygoid muscles and the parotid sheath.

In the upper part of the neck is the **submandibular space** below the mylohyoid muscle and deep to the investing layer of fascia between the hyoid bone and the mandible. This space communicates around the posterior border of mylohyoid with a sublingual space under the mucous membrane of the floor of the mouth. Ludwig's angina is a rare but severe form of cellulitis that involves these spaces and spreads backwards into the parapharyngeal space.

Three or four small **submental lymph nodes** lie beneath the chin, some superficial and others deep to the investing layer of deep cervical fascia (Fig. 6.6). They drain, across the midline, a wedge of tissue in the floor of the mouth opposite the four lower incisor teeth, including those teeth, gums and lip, and the tip of the tongue (Fig. 6.34). In their turn they drain to submandibular nodes or directly to the upper deep cervical group.

About half a dozen **submandibular lymph nodes** lie on the surface of the submandibular gland, some embedded within the gland (Fig. 6.6). They drain the submental nodes, the lateral parts of the lower lips, all the upper lip and external nose, and the anterior part of the tongue, mainly but not exclusively from their own side. They also receive lymph from the anterior half of the nasal walls and the paranasal sinuses that drain there (frontal, anterior and middle ethmoidal, and maxillary), and from all the teeth (except lower incisors).

PART **TWO**

Triangles of the neck

To assist the description of the topographical anatomy of the neck and the location of pathological lesions, each side is divided into anterior and posterior triangles by the obliquely placed sternocleidomastoid muscle (Fig. 6.2). The **posterior triangle** lies between the posterior border of sternocleidomastoid, the anterior border of trapezius and the clavicle, and the anterior triangle between the anterior border of sternocleidomastoid, the lower border of the mandible and the midline. The **anterior triangle** can be subdivided into submental, digastric, carotid and muscular triangles (see p. 357).

Sternocleidomastoid

This prominent neck landmark has two heads of origin below: that from the sternal manubrium is a rounded tendon, that from the clavicle a flat, fleshy mass (Fig. 6.2). A triangular interval exists between the two above the sternoclavicular joint, and the lower end of the internal jugular vein lies here, where it can be entered by needle or catheter. The manubrial tendon is attached to the

front of the bone below the jugular notch; the clavicular head arises from the superior surface of the medial third of the clavicle. The muscle is attached by a tendon to the lateral surface of the mastoid process and by a thin aponeurosis to the lateral half of the superior nuchal line of the occipital bone. The clavicular fibres spiral behind the sternal fibres with the deep aspect of which they blend. The clavicular fibres are directed mainly to the mastoid process, while the sternal fibres run more obliquely chiefly to the occipital bone. The spinal accessory nerve enters the muscle under cover of the lobule of the ear, about 3 cm below the tip of the mastoid process, accompanied by a branch to the muscle from the occipital artery. It runs through the deep part of the muscle to emerge from between a third and a half of the way down the posterior border of the muscle.

Sternocleidomastoid is enclosed within a sheath of the investing layer of deep cervical fascia, which splits to surround it (Fig. 6.1). The muscle is crossed superficially by the great auricular nerve, the external jugular vein and the transverse cervical nerve, in that order from above downwards. Deep to the upper half of the muscle lies the cervical plexus; deep to its lower part lies the carotid sheath and its contents, overlying scalenus anterior.

The blood supply of the muscle is from branches of the occipital and superior thyroid arteries.

Nerve supply. By the spinal part of the accessory nerve, from a branch which leaves the nerve proximal to its point of entry into the muscle. The pathway for innervation by the cerebral cortex of the anterior horn cells of the segments concerned (mostly C2 and 3) is disputed; projection to the muscle from either or both hemispheres has been described. Branches from the

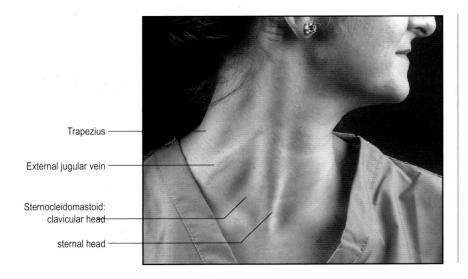

Fig. 6.2 The position of underlying structures in the right side of the neck have been indicated. The subject is turning her face to the left by contracting her right sternocleidomastoid.

Trapezius

External jugular vein

Sternocleidomastoid:
clavicular head

sternal head

cervical plexus (C2, 3) carrying proprioceptive fibres enter the muscle directly or by joining the accessory nerve.

Action. Contraction of one muscle tilts the head towards the ipsilateral shoulder, and rotates the head and face to the opposite side. Both muscles acting together from below draw the head forwards. With the head fixed, the muscles can assist in raising the roof of the thorax in forced inspiration.

Test. The face is turned to the opposite side against resistance and the muscle palpated.

Posterior triangle

This is an area enclosed between the sternocleidomastoid and trapezius muscles. Its *apex* lies high up at the back of the skull on the superior nuchal line, where there is a small gap between the attachments of the two muscles. Its *base* is the middle third of the clavicle at the side of the root of the neck. Its *roof* is formed by the investing layer of deep cervical fascia. Its *floor* consists of the prevertebral fascia lying on, from above downwards, splenius, levator scapulae and scalenus medius. Depending on the size of the sternocleidomastoid and the degree of depression of the shoulder, scalenus anterior and the first digitation of serratus anterior may contribute to the floor, and at the apex of the triangle, splenius may be low enough to expose a little of semispinalis capitis.

Although the subclavian artery, the three trunks of the brachial plexus and branches of the cervical plexus are deep to the prevertebral fascia, they are listed as contents of the posterior triangle; in operations on the triangle all these structures are safe provided the prevertebral fascia is left intact. The *pulsation* of the subclavian artery can be felt by pressing downwards behind the clavicle at the posterior border of sternocleidomastoid.

The cutaneous branches of the **cervical plexus** pierce the investing fascia at the posterior border of sternocleidomastoid. The cervical branches to trapezius pass across the floor of the triangle deep to the prevertebral fascia.

Lying between the roof and floor are the **lymph nodes** of the posterior triangle. Two or three occipital nodes lie in the subcutaneous tissue at the apex and several supraclavicular nodes lie above the clavicle; the latter are really outlying members of the lower group of deep cervical nodes (see p. 426).

The **accessory nerve** emerges from sternocleidomastoid, about a third of the way or a little lower down its posterior border. It passes downwards and backwards, with a characteristic wavy course adherent to the inner surface of the fascia of the roof of the triangle, to disappear beneath the anterior border of trapezius, about a third of the way from its lower end and 3–5 cm above

the clavicle. These points of reference to the borders of sternocleidomastoid and trapezius enable the *surface marking* of the accessory nerve in the posterior triangle, where it is particularly liable to injury in operations involving the removal of lymph nodes, one or two of which may lie in contact with the nerve. More proximally, the nerve lies in front of the transverse process of the atlas (palpable between the mastoid process and mandibular ramus) and it enters the substance of sternocleidomastoid between the upper two quarters of the muscle.

The **inferior belly of omohyoid** crosses the lower medial part of the triangle and is kept in place by its sling of investing fascia. Deep to the omohyoid are the **transverse cervical** and **suprascapular** vessels, just above the clavicle. The external jugular vein pierces both split layers of the lower part of investing fascia to enter the posterior triangle on its way to the subclavian vein, which itself is too low to be a content of the triangle; the wall of the vein is adherent to the fascia as it passes through.

Cervical plexus

The cervical plexus (Fig. 6.3) is formed by loops between the anterior rami of the upper four cervical nerves, after each has received a grey ramus communicans from the superior cervical ganglion. It lies in series with the brachial plexus, on the scalenus medius, behind the prevertebral fascia. It is covered by the upper part of sternocleidomastoid, and does not lie in the posterior triangle.

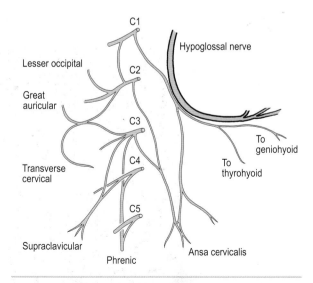

Fig. 6.3 Right cervical plexus.

The upper three cervical nerves have meningeal branches for the posterior cranial fossa. C1 fibres ascend with the hypoglossal nerve, C1 and 2 fibres ascend with the vagus nerve and C2 and 3 fibres ascend through the foramen magnum.

Muscular branches. Muscular branches are given off segmentally to the prevertebral muscles (longus capitis, longus colli and the scalenes). Other muscular branches are:

- A branch from C1 to the hypoglossal nerve, by which the fibres are carried to the superior root of the ansa cervicalis and the nerves to thyrohyoid and geniohyoid.
- Branches from C2 and 3 to sternocleidomastoid, and from C3 and 4 to trapezius. These fibres are mainly proprioceptive, but occasionally the whole of trapezius is not paralysed when the accessory nerve is damaged, as some of the cervical fibres may be motor.
- The **inferior root of the ansa cervicalis** is formed by union of a branch each from C2 and C3. The nerve spirals around the lateral side of the internal jugular vein and descends to join the superior root (C1) at the ansa (see p. 356).
- The **phrenic nerve** is formed mainly from C4 with contributions from C3 and C5 and runs down vertically over the obliquity of the scalenus anterior muscle, passing from lateral to medial borders, beneath the prevertebral fascia, lateral to the ascending cervical branch of the inferior thyroid artery. It passes behind the subclavian vein into the mediastinum (see p. 202). It may be joined below the vein by a branch (the **accessory phrenic nerve**) from the nerve to subclavius; this branch may descend in front of the subclavian vein. The phrenic nerve is one of the most important in the body, being the sole motor supply to its own half of the diaphragm (see p. 193), and it also has an extensive afferent distribution, not only to the diaphragm but to the pericardium, pleura and peritoneum (see pp 204, 219 and 247).

Cutaneous branches. Cutaneous branches of the plexus (Fig. 6.4) supply the front and sides of the neck and contribute to the supply of the scalp, face and chest.

The **lesser occipital nerve** (C2) is a slender branch that hooks around the accessory nerve and runs up along the posterior border of sternocleidomastoid to supply the posterior part of the upper neck and adjacent scalp behind the auricle. It may contribute to the supply of the auricle.

The **great auricular nerve** (C2, 3, mostly 2) is a large trunk passing almost vertically upwards over sternocleidomastoid; it is distributed to an area of skin on the face over the angle of the mandible and the parotid gland and to the parotid fascia. It also supplies the skin of the auricle over the whole of its cranial surface and on the lower part of its lateral surface below the external

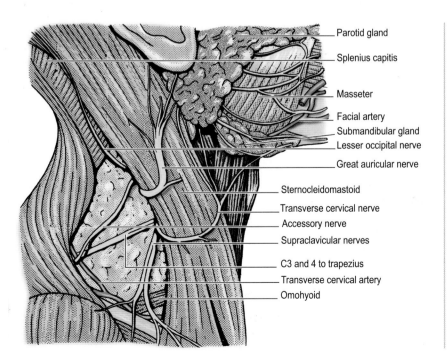

Parotid gland

Splenius capitis

Masseter

Facial artery
Submandibular gland
Lesser occipital nerve

Great auricular nerve

Sternocleidomastoid

Transverse cervical nerve

Accessory nerve

Supraclavicular nerves

C3 and 4 to trapezius

Transverse cervical artery

Omohyoid

Fig. 6.4 Right lower face and posterior triangle of neck. The fat in the lower part of the triangle overlies deeper structures. The accessory nerve has been depicted taking a lower than usual course through the posterior triangle. The transverse cervical and suprascapular arteries are usually deep to the inferior belly of omohyoid.

acoustic meatus, and skin over the mastoid region. Branches passing deep to the parotid gland supply the deep layer of the parotid fascia.

The **transverse cervical** nerve (C2, 3) curves round the posterior border of sternocleidomastoid, perforates the investing fascia and divides into ascending and descending branches that innervate the skin of the front of the neck from chin to sternum. The ascending branch communicates with the cervical branch of the facial nerve.

The **supraclavicular nerve** (C3, 4, but mostly 4) emerges with the other three nerves at the posterior border of sternomastoid and soon divides into several branches. They are distributed in three main groups (see Fig. 1.8, p. 13). The medial group supply the skin as far down as the sternal angle. The intermediate group proper pass anterior to the clavicle and supply skin as far down as the second rib. The lateral group cross the acromion to supply skin halfway down the deltoid muscle, and pass posteriorly to supply skin as far down as the spine of the scapula.

Dermatomes of the neck

In addition to the cutaneous branches of the cervical plexus described above, which supply the anterior and lateral skin of the neck, the greater occipital and third occipital nerves from posterior rami of C2 and C3 respectively provide sensory fibres for the back of the neck (Fig. 6.15). The first cervical nerve does not supply any skin. C2 supplies most of the superior part of the neck, extending into the occipital region of the scalp and forwards to the auricle and the face over the parotid gland. C3 supplies the cylindrical part of the neck, C4 extends over the clavicle to the sternal angle, across the top of the shoulder and down to the scapular spine at the back. There is much overlap across dermatome boundary lines.

Anterior triangle

Beneath the investing layer of deep cervical fascia, between the mandible and the manubrium of the sternum, are longitudinal muscles supplied by the anterior rami of the upper three cervical nerves. They lie above or below the hyoid bone and there are four muscles in each group. The *suprahyoid muscles* comprise digastric, stylohyoid, mylohyoid and geniohyoid; the mylohyoids of each side unite to form the floor of the mouth, with the digastrics and stylohyoids superficial (below) and geniohyoids deep (above) to them. The *infrahyoid muscles* are sternohyoid and omohyoid, lying side by side in the same plane, and more deeply a wider sheet of muscle attached to the thyroid cartilage, namely thyrohyoid and sternothyroid. The last four are called the 'strap muscles' from their flat shape.

Suprahyoid muscles

Digastric

This arises as the posterior belly, from the digastric notch on the medial surface of the base of the mastoid process. The triangular fleshy belly tapers down to the intermediate tendon, which is held beneath a fibrous sling attached to the junction of the body and the greater horn of the hyoid bone. The tendon is lubricated by a synovial sheath within the fibrous sling. The bifurcated tendon of insertion of stylohyoid which embraces the tendon plays no part in holding it down. The anterior belly lies on the inferior surface of mylohyoid, and connects the intermediate tendon to the digastric fossa on the inner surface of the mandible near the midline.

Nerve supply. The posterior belly is supplied by the facial nerve, by a branch arising between the stylomastoid foramen and the parotid gland, and the anterior belly by the nerve to mylohyoid.

Action. To depress and retract the chin, and to assist the lateral pterygoid in opening the mouth.

Stylohyoid

This arises from the back of the styloid process, high up near the base of the skull, and slopes down along the upper border of digastric. Its lower end divides to embrace the digastric tendon and is inserted by two slips into the junction of the greater horn and body of the hyoid bone.

Nerve supply. By the facial nerve, by a branch from that to the posterior belly of digastric.

Action. To retract and elevate the hyoid bone when swallowing.

Mylohyoid

The muscles of each side unite to make a thin sheet forming the 'diaphragm' of the floor of the mouth (Fig. 6.6). Each arises from the whole length of the mylohyoid line of its own side on the inner aspect of the mandible from as far back as medial to the third molar tooth to below the mental spines (see Fig. 8.5B, p. 533). The two muscles slope downwards towards each other, and the posterior quarter of each is inserted into the anterior surface of the body of the hyoid bone. In front of this the anterior three-quarters of each interdigitate in a midline raphe which extends from the chin to the hyoid bone.

Nerve supply. By its own nerve, a branch of the inferior alveolar (from the mandibular division of the trigeminal nerve), which arises just before the parent nerve enters the mandibular foramen, pierces the sphenomandibular ligament and runs forward on the inferior surface of the mylohyoid, supplying it and the anterior belly of the digastric.

Action. It forms a mobile but stable floor of the mouth. The two muscles together form a gutter; contraction makes the gutter more shallow, thus elevating the tongue and the hyoid bone as when swallowing or protruding the tongue.

Geniohyoid

This slender muscle extends from the inferior mental spine (genial tubercle) of the mandible (see Fig. 8.5B, p. 533) to the upper border of the body of the hyoid bone (see Fig. 8.6, p. 535). The two muscles lie side by side between the mylohyoids and the base of the tongue (genioglossus), on the floor of the mouth.

Nerve supply. By a branch from the hypoglossal nerve, consisting of fibres from the C1 nerve and not from the hypoglossal nucleus.

Action. To protract and elevate the hyoid bone in swallowing, or if the hyoid is fixed, to depress the mandible.

Infrahyoid muscles

Sternohyoid

This flat strap of muscle is attached to the back of the upper part of the manubrium and the adjoining sternoclavicular joint and clavicle. Its upper attachment is to the lower border of the body of the hyoid bone. The two muscles lie edge to edge at the hyoid bone, but diverge from each other below.

Nerve supply. By a branch from the ansa cervicalis which enters the lower part of the muscle.

Omohyoid

This flat strap of muscle lies edge to edge with sternohyoid at its attachment to the lateral part of the inferior border of the hyoid bone (Fig. 6.5). As it descends it diverges somewhat from the sternohyoid and, passing deep to sternocleidomastoid, it comes to lie over the carotid sheath. Where it lies over the internal jugular vein, the muscle fibres are replaced by a flat tendon, a useful guide at operation to the underlying vein. A change of direction now occurs, and the inferior belly runs almost horizontally just above the level of the clavicle to pass back to its attachment to the upper border of the scapula and the transverse scapular ligament. The intermediate tendon and supraclavicular portion of the muscle are bound down close to the clavicle in a fascial sling derived from the deep layer of the investing layer of deep cervical fascia (see Fig. 2.2, p. 41), which results in the angulated course of the muscle.

Nerve supply. The superior root of the ansa cervicalis supplies the superior belly and the ansa supplies the inferior belly.

Thyrohyoid

This is a broader and shorter muscle that lies under cover of the upper ends of sternohyoid and omohyoid. It arises from the greater horn of the hyoid bone, and is inserted into the oblique line of the thyroid cartilage alongside sternothyroid.

Nerve supply. By a branch of the hypoglossal nerve, but the fibres are all 'hitch-hiking' from C1.

Sternothyroid

Broader than sternohyoid and lying deep to it, this muscle is attached lower down than sternohyoid to the posterior surface of the manubrium and the adjacent first costal cartilage. Its upper attachment is to the oblique line of the thyroid cartilage.

Nerve supply. By the ansa cervicalis, which gives a branch to the lower part of the muscle.

Actions of the infrahyoid muscles

They are all depressors of the larynx. Sternothyroid acts directly on the thyroid cartilage, the others act indirectly via the hyoid bone. Depression of the larynx increases the volume of the resonating chambers during phonation and thus affects the quality of the voice. The infrahyoid muscles also oppose the elevators of the larynx (mylohyoid, palatopharyngeus, stylopharyngeus, salpingopharyngeus), enabling them to act progressively and gradually. The infrahyoid muscles prevent ascent of the hyoid bone when the digastric and geniohyoid lower the mandible.

Submandibular gland

The submandibular gland, mixed mucous and serous in type, consists of a large superficial part and a small deep part which are continuous with one another round the free posterior margin of mylohyoid (Fig 6.24).

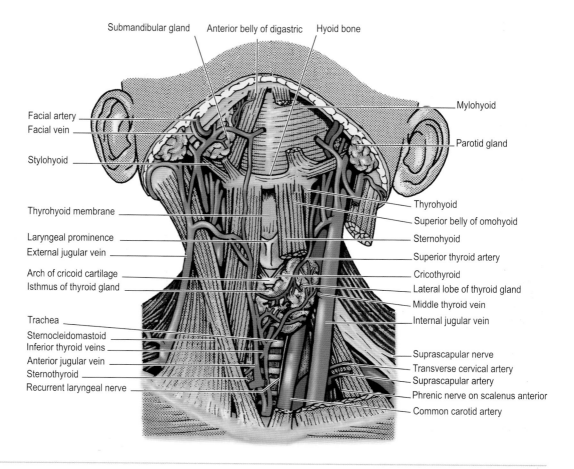

Fig. 6.5 Thyroid gland and the front of the neck.

The *superficial part* (Fig. 6.6) has three surfaces: lateral, inferior and medial. The lateral surface lies against the submandibular fossa of the mandible (see Fig. 8.5, p. 533), overlapping the front of the medial pterygoid insertion and being deeply grooved posteriorly by the facial artery which hooks under the mandible to reach the face at the front of the masseter muscle. The inferior or superficial surface is covered by skin, platysma and the investing fascia and is crossed by the facial vein and the cervical branch of the facial nerve, and sometimes by the marginal mandibular branch of the facial nerve (see p. 366), the nerves lying outside the investing fascia. Submandibular lymph nodes lie in contact with the surface of the gland and within its substance, hence the need to remove the gland as well as nodes in the operation of radical neck dissection. The medial surface lies against the mylohyoid, and behind it

on the hyoglossus, lingual nerve, hypoglossal nerve and its accompanying veins. The facial artery is at first deep to the gland, and then grooves the posterosuperior part as it hooks over the top of the gland on to its lateral surface.

The *deep part* of the gland extends forwards for a variable distance, between mylohyoid and hyoglossus, below the lingual nerve and above the hypoglossal nerve.

The **submandibular duct** (of Wharton) is 5 cm long (the same length as the parotid duct) and emerges from the medial surface of the superficial part of the gland near the posterior border of mylohyoid. It runs with the deep part, forwards and slightly upwards, first between mylohyoid and hyoglossus, and then between the sublingual gland and genioglossus, to open into the floor of the mouth on the sublingual papilla beside the frenulum

349

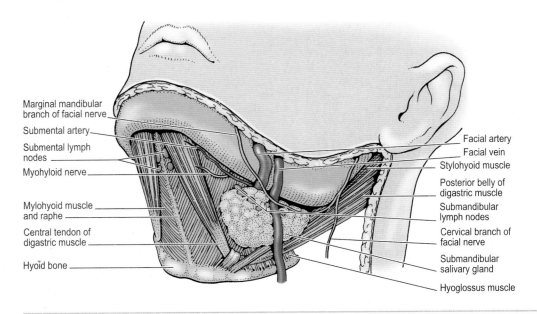

Marginal mandibular branch of facial nerve

Submental artery

Submental lymph nodes

Myohyloid nerve

Mylohyoid muscle and raphe

Central tendon of digastric muscle

Hyoid bone

Facial artery

Facial vein

Stylohyoid muscle

Posterior belly of digastric muscle

Submandibular lymph nodes

Cervical branch of facial nerve

Submandibular salivary gland

Hyoglossus muscle

Fig. 6.6   Left submandibular region.

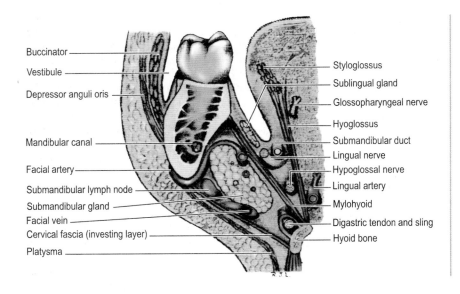

Buccinator

Vestibule

Depressor anguli oris

Mandibular canal

Facial artery

Submandibular lymph node

Submandibular gland

Facial vein

Cervical fascia (investing layer)

Platysma

Styloglossus

Sublingual gland

Glossopharyngeal nerve

Hyoglossus

Submandibular duct

Lingual nerve

Hypoglossal nerve

Lingual artery

Mylohyoid

Digastric tendon and sling

Hyoid bone

Fig. 6.7   Coronal section of the left side of the mandible and adjacent structures, just behind the first molar tooth, viewed from behind.

of the tongue. As it lies on hyoglossus, the duct is crossed laterally by the lingual nerve which then turns under the duct to pass medially to the tongue (Fig. 6.7).

Blood supply

From the facial artery, with veins draining into the facial vein.

Lymph drainage

To the submandibular lymph nodes.

Nerve supply

Secretomotor fibres to the gland have their cell bodies in the *submandibular ganglion* (see p. 23), which hangs suspended from the lingual nerve on the surface of hyo-glossus. The preganglionic fibres pass from cell bodies in the superior salivary nucleus in the pons by way of the nervus intermedius, chorda tympani and the lingual nerve (see p. 379). Postganglionic fibres pass to the submandibular gland and also to the lingual nerve for transmission to the sublingual gland. Sympathetic (vaso-constrictor) fibres come from the plexus around the facial artery.

Development

An ectodermal groove in the floor of the mouth becomes converted into a tunnel whose blind end proliferates to form the secreting acini.

Surgical approach

The gland is exposed by a skin crease incision about 4 cm below the mandible, which continues through platysma and investing fascia on to the gland, to avoid the marginal mandibular branch of the facial nerve which may lie over the gland (see p. 366). Removal of the gland requires ligation of the facial vein which lies on the gland surface. The facial artery needs to be separated from its groove on the posterosuperior part of the gland, or a segment of the artery removed with the gland. The hypo-glossal nerve and lingual nerve need to be safeguarded, the latter particularly when the duct is ligated and divided. The removal of a stone from the duct is carried out from within the mouth by incising the mucous membrane and duct over the stone; the mucosal and duct incisions are not sutured.

Thyroid gland

The thyroid gland is situated low down at the front of the neck. It consists of two symmetrical lobes united by an isthmus that lies in front of the second, third and fourth tracheal rings (Fig. 6.5). The lobes lie on either side of the larynx and trachea, extending from the oblique line of the thyroid cartilage to the sixth tracheal ring. It weighs about 25 g. In addition to its own capsule, the gland is enclosed by an envelope of pretracheal fascia.

Each **lateral lobe** is pear-shaped with a narrow upper pole and a broader lower pole, and appears approxi-mately triangular on cross-section with lateral, medial and posterior surfaces. The *lateral (superficial) surface* is under cover of sternothyroid and sternohyoid. The *medial surface* lies against the lateral side of the larynx and upper trachea, with the lower pharynx and upper

oesophagus immediately behind. This surface is related to the cricothyroid muscle of the larynx and the inferior constrictor of the pharynx, as well as to the external and recurrent laryngeal nerves. The *posterior surface* overlaps the medial part of the carotid sheath, i.e. the part containing the common carotid artery; if enlarged, the lobe may extend across the more laterally placed internal jugular vein. The parathyroid glands usually lie in contact with this surface, between it and the fascial sheath.

The relationship of the **recurrent laryngeal nerves** (see p. 381) to the thyroid lobes has importance in thyroid surgery. As they approach the medial surface of the gland from below, the nerves lie in or in front of the groove be-tween the trachea and oesophagus. The left nerve, which recurves around the arch of the aorta in the superior mediastinum, is more likely to have entered the groove and lies posterior (though occasionally anterior) to the inferior thyroid artery. The right nerve recurves around the right subclavian artery at the root of the neck and may be more lateral to the trachea, passing anterior or posterior to the inferior thyroid artery or in between its branches. Each nerve is behind the pretracheal fascia, and runs medial or lateral or through a thickening of the fascia attached to the cricoid cartilage and upper tracheal rings (the *suspensory ligament* of Berry). The nerve runs behind the cricothyroid joint and passes upwards under cover of the inferior constrictor. At the level of the upper border of the isthmus the nerve often divides into two. If so, the anterior (larger) branch is the motor branch to laryngeal muscles, and the posterior branch is sensory only. The rare non-recurrent right laryngeal nerve (see p. 30) may be a hazard during thyroid surgery.

The smaller *external laryngeal nerve* lies on the inferior constrictor, close behind the superior thyroid artery, as it runs down medial to the upper pole to supply cricothyroid.

The **isthmus** joins the anterior surfaces of the lobes, towards their lower poles. The posterior surface of the isthmus is firmly adherent to the second, third and fourth rings of the trachea, and the pretracheal fascia is here fixed between them. This fixation and the investment of the whole gland by pretracheal fascia are responsible for the gland moving up and down with the larynx during swallowing. An anastomosis between the two superior thyroid arteries runs across the upper border of the isthmus, and tributaries of the inferior thyroid veins emerge from its lower border.

A small portion of gland substance often projects upwards from the isthmus, generally to the left of the midline, as the **pyramidal lobe** and represents a devel-opment of glandular tissue from the caudal end of the thyroglossal duct (see p. 28). It may be attached to the inferior border of the hyoid bone by fibrous tissue; muscle fibres sometimes present in it are named *levator glandulae thyroideae* and are innervated by a branch of the external laryngeal nerve. Separate masses of thyroid tissue (*accessory thyroid glands*) are not uncommonly found near the hyoid bone, in the tongue, in the superior mediastinum, or anywhere along the path of descent of the thyroglossal duct, though their presence may only be revealed by histological study.

Blood supply

The **superior thyroid artery**, the first branch from the anterior aspect of the external carotid (see p. 355), after giving off its sternocleidomastoid and superior laryngeal branches, pierces the pretracheal fascia as a single vessel to reach the summit of the upper pole. The external laryngeal nerve is immediately behind the artery as the vessel approaches the pole. The artery divides on the gland into an anterior branch that runs down to the isthmus and a posterior branch that runs down the back of the lobe and anastomoses with an ascending branch of the inferior thyroid artery from the lower pole. In thyroidectomies the artery is ligated close to the upper pole, or its anterior and posterior branches are ligated instead, to avoid damage to the external laryngeal nerve.

The **inferior thyroid artery**, from the thyrocervical trunk (see p. 361), arches upwards and medially behind the carotid sheath and then loops downwards to the lower pole. It divides outside the pretracheal fascia into branches that pierce the fascia separately to reach the lower part of the gland. As described above, the recurrent laryngeal nerve has a variable relationship to the artery but always lies behind the pretracheal fascia. Ligating the inferior thyroid artery well lateral to the gland, or carefully ligating its small branches on the surface of the gland, helps to safeguard the nerve. The inferior thyroid artery gives off the ascending cervical artery and small pharyngeal, oesophageal, laryngeal and tracheal branches before its terminal distribution to the thyroid gland; the small inferior laryngeal artery ascends with the recurrent nerve.

The *thyroidea ima artery* enters the lower part of the isthmus in 3% of individuals. It arises from the brachiocephalic trunk, arch of the aorta or right common carotid artery.

From a venous plexus on the surface of the gland the **superior thyroid vein** follows the superior thyroid artery and enters either the internal jugular or facial vein in about equal proportions. The **middle thyroid vein** crosses anterior to the common carotid artery to drain into the internal jugular vein. The **inferior thyroid veins** are multiple and drain downwards mainly into the left brachiocephalic vein; one may enter the right brachiocephalic vein.

Lymph drainage

The lymphatics from the thyroid gland drain mainly to deep cervical nodes. A few pass into prelaryngeal, pre- and paratracheal nodes, and a few drain directly into the thoracic duct.

Nerve supply

Sympathetic (vasoconstrictor) nerves from the superior, middle and inferior cervical ganglia accompany the thyroid arteries.

Structure

The thyroid consists essentially of a mass of more or less rounded *follicles* containing varying amounts of *colloid* produced by the single layer of *epithelial (follicular) cells* that form the walls of the follicles. The thyroid is unique in being the only endocrine gland to store its secretion outside the cells. The colloid is iodinated when in the follicle and reabsorbed by the cells before being discharged into blood capillaries. The main hormonal products are thyroxine (T_4) and triiodothyronine (T_3). Less than 2% of the epithelial cells are the C or *parafollicular cells* which secrete calcitonin. The C cells are scattered on the outer aspects of the follicles and do not reach the lumina of the follicles. The thyroid gland is highly vascular.

Development

The gland develops as a proliferation of cells from the caudal end of the thyroglossal duct (see p. 28). The parafollicular calcitonin-producing cells develop from the ultimobranchial body (fifth pharyngeal pouch), under the influence of neural crest cells.

Surgical approach

The thyroid gland is approached surgically through a transverse incision in a low skin crease on the front of the neck. The investing fascia is divided vertically and the sternohyoid and the sternothyroid muscles retraced, or divided at a high level, to safeguard their nerve supply and to prevent adherence of their subsequent suture line to the closure of the skin incision. The pretracheal fascia needs to be divided to expose the gland proper.

Parathyroid glands

The small parathyroid glands normally lie behind the lobes of the thyroid gland. There are usually four glands (in 90% of subjects), two on each side. Each weighs about 50 mg.

The *superior gland* is the more constant in position; it is usually within the thyroid's pretracheal fascial capsule, at the middle of the back of the thyroid lobe, level with the first tracheal ring and above the inferior thyroid artery. The *inferior gland* is less constant in position. It is usually within the pretracheal fascial sheath behind the lower pole; but it may be in the gland itself, or outside the fascial sheath in a variable position in the neck, or in the superior or posterior mediastinum. The glands are not necessarily on the same level on each side. They are brownish-yellow, which helps to distinguish them from the deep red of the thyroid gland. They are easily subject to subcapsular haematoma formation on handling.

Blood supply

Both upper and lower parathyroids are usually supplied by the inferior thyroid artery, otherwise by an anastomosis between the superior and inferior arteries. Their minute veins join thyroid veins.

Lymph drainage

As for the thyroid gland (above) and thymus (see p. 203).

Nerve supply

Sympathetic vasoconstrictor fibres enter with the arteries.

Structure

The gland is a mass of small closely packed chief or *principal cells* which secrete the parathyroid hormone (PTH). The mass of cells bears a superficial resemblance to lymphoid tissue, but the number of blood capillaries in the gland provides a clear distinction. Scattered among the chief cells are small groups of slightly larger *oxyphil cells*.

Development

The superior gland is termed *parathyroid IV* because it develops from the fourth pharyngeal pouch. The inferior gland is *parathyroid III*, developed from the third pouch, but displaced caudally by the descent of the thymus from the same pouch (see p. 28); hence its liability to end up in unusual positions.

Surgical approach

For *parathyroidectomy* the lobes of the thyroid gland are exposed as for thyroidectomy, and then retracted forwards and medially so that the posterior surfaces can be inspected for the parathyroids. If not obvious, branches of the inferior thyroid artery are followed and should lead to the glands. Exposure of the thymus through a median sternotomy may be necessary.

Trachea

The trachea (Fig. 6.5) begins at the level of C6 vertebra in continuity with the larynx, being attached to the lower margin of the cricoid cartilage by the cricotracheal ligament. Of the total length of 10 cm, 5 cm are in the neck from the cricoid cartilage to the jugular notch. From the neck the trachea passes into the thorax.

The cervical part lies in the midline of the neck, in contact with the front of the oesophagus. In the groove between trachea and oesophagus runs the recurrent laryngeal nerve. To the side of the trachea is the carotid sheath. The isthmus of the thyroid gland is adherent to the second, third and fourth tracheal rings and the lobes of the gland lie against the lateral side of the trachea as far down as the sixth ring. The inferior thyroid veins and anterior jugular venous arch lie in front, and also (if present) the thyroidea ima artery, the levator glandulae thyroideae and the upper end of a persistently large thymus. On account of the shape of the lower cervical and upper thoracic parts of the vertebral column, the trachea passes downwards and backwards as it enters the thorax. Although close to the skin at the upper end, it is 2 cm or more deep to the front of the jugular notch.

The thoracic part of the trachea and other features are described on page 200.

Tracheotomy and tracheostomy

Tracheotomy implies making an incision in the trachea; tracheostomy involves removing a small part of the wall (making a stoma), but the strict distinction between these terms is often ignored. In an emergency, laryngotomy (incising the cricothyroid ligament, see p. 408) provides a subglottic airway; the procedure also gives access to the trachea for sucking out excess secretions. Depending on the speed with which tracheostomy needs to be performed, the skin incision is vertical from the lower border of the thyroid cartilage to the jugular notch, or (preferably) transverse 2 cm below the cricoid cartilage.

The sternohyoid and sternothyroid muscles are retracted laterally. The isthmus of the thyroid gland is usually divided and an opening made by removing part of the second and third tracheal rings so that a tracheostomy tube can be inserted. In the narrow trachea of children only a vertical incision is made in the trachea (tracheotomy), as removal of any segment of tracheal wall tends to lead to tracheal stenosis.

Oesophagus

The oesophagus commences in continuity with the pharynx at the level of the lower border of the cricoid cartilage (C6 vertebra). It lies in front of the prevertebral fascia behind the trachea. It is overlapped on either side by the lower poles of the thyroid gland, beyond which, on the left side, its edge is visible posterolateral to the trachea. The thoracic duct runs upwards behind the lower part of its left border. The recurrent laryngeal nerves are on each side in the groove between trachea and oesophagus.

The oesophagus continues into the thorax and is further described on page 215.

Great vessels of the neck

Common carotid artery

The common carotid artery arises on the *left* side from the arch of the aorta, where it lies in front of the subclavian artery up to the sternoclavicular joint. Here the two arteries diverge. On the *right* the brachiocephalic trunk bifurcates behind the sternoclavicular joint into common carotid and subclavian arteries. The common carotid gives off no branches proximal to its bifurcation. It lies within the medial part of the carotid sheath, with the internal jugular vein lateral to it and the vagus nerve deeply placed between the two vessels. The sympathetic trunk is behind the artery and outside the sheath, which is overlapped superficially by the infrahyoid muscles and sternocleidomastoid. Medial to the sheath is the trachea and oesophagus and, at a higher level, the larynx and pharynx. The thyroid gland overlaps the sheath anteromedially and the inferior thyroid artery crosses from the thyrocervical trunk to the gland behind the sheath.

The common carotid artery usually bifurcates at the level of the upper border of the lamina of the thyroid cartilage (upper border of C4 vertebra) into the external and internal carotids; it may do so higher near the tip of the greater horn of the hyoid bone (C3 vertebra). The terminal portion of the artery is often dilated into the carotid sinus, which includes the commencement of the internal carotid artery.

The *carotid pulse* can be felt by pressing backwards between the trachea and lower larynx medially and sternocleidomastoid laterally, pressing the artery against the anterior tubercle of the transverse process of C6 vertebra (carotid tubercle of Chassaignac). The *surface marking* of the common carotid artery is along a vertical line from the sternoclavicular joint to the level of the upper border of the thyroid cartilage. The vessel can be *surgically exposed* by retracting the lower part of sternocleidomastoid backwards and incising the carotid sheath. The middle thyroid vein is divided between ligatures.

External carotid artery

The external carotid artery at its commencement lies against the side wall of the pharynx somewhat anteromedial to the internal carotid artery. It then ascends in front of the internal carotid deep to the posterior belly of digastric and stylohyoid, above which it pierces the deep lamina of the parotid fascia and enters the gland. It divides within the gland behind the neck of the mandible into the maxillary and superficial temporal arteries. As the external carotid artery lies in the parotid gland it is separated from the internal carotid by the deep part of the gland and its fascia, styloid process and its continuation the stylohyoid ligament, styloglossus and the 'pharyngeal' structures: stylopharyngeus muscle, glossopharyngeal nerve and pharyngeal branch of the vagus (and, if present, the track of a branchial fistula, see p. 28). At the commencement of the artery the internal jugular vein lies lateral, but higher up it is posterior and deep to the artery. The facial vein crosses the artery, with the hypoglossal nerve lying between. Except at its commencement the vessel lies in front of the anterior border of sternocleidomastoid.

The *surface marking* of the external carotid is along a line from the bifurcation of the common carotid passing up behind the angle of the mandible to a point immediately in front of the tragus of the ear.

Surgical approach. The vessel can be exposed in front of the upper part of sternocleidomastoid before entering the parotid gland by ligating the facial vein. The hypoglossal nerve which crosses the external and internal carotids superficially must not be damaged.

Branches. Before it divides into its two terminal branches the external carotid artery gives off six branches, three from in front, two from behind and one deep (medial). The three from in front are the superior thyroid, lingual and facial, and they diverge widely. The two from behind are the occipital and posterior auricular, which pass up deep to and above the posterior belly of digastric respectively. The branch from the medial side is the ascending pharyngeal, which ascends to the base of the skull on the side wall of the pharynx, alongside the internal carotid artery.

The **superior thyroid artery** arises at the commencement of the external carotid. It runs almost vertically downwards, with the vein, to the upper pole of the thyroid gland (see p. 352), with the external laryngeal nerve close behind it, alongside the larynx (Fig. 6.24). Before reaching the thyroid gland it gives off infrahyoid, sternocleidomastoid, superior laryngeal and cricothyroid branches. The *superior laryngeal artery* pierces the thyrohyoid membrane with the internal laryngeal nerve. The cricothyroid artery crosses the upper part of the cricothyroid membrane to anastomose with the contralateral artery.

The **lingual artery** arises from the front of the external carotid above the superior thyroid, near the tip of the greater horn of the hyoid bone. It forms a short loop (Fig. 6.22), then passes forwards along the upper border of the greater horn, deep to hyoglossus (p. 396). It is accompanied by the lingual vein. The loop of the artery is crossed laterally by the hypoglossal nerve and its companion vein, the latter opening into the facial vein.

The **facial artery** arises from the front of the external carotid above the lingual artery (sometimes by a common *linguofacial trunk* with the lingual) and runs upwards on the superior constrictor, deep to the digastric and stylohyoid muscles, then deep to the submandibular salivary gland. It grooves the posterosuperior part of the gland. As the artery lies on the superior constrictor muscle it gives off a *tonsillar* and an *ascending palatine branch* to the tonsil and soft palate. The facial artery then makes an S bend, curling over the submandibular gland (Fig. 6.7) and crosses the inferior border of the mandible, where its pulsation can be felt, at the anterior border of masseter. Before passing to the face it gives off the *submental artery*, which accompanies the mylohyoid nerve into the submandibular fossa and sends perforating branches through the mylohyoid to anastomose with a sublingual branch of the lingual artery.

The **occipital artery** arises from the back of the external carotid on a level with the facial artery. It courses backwards deep to the lower border of the posterior belly of digastric. It grooves the base of the skull at the occipitomastoid suture, deep to the digastric notch on the mastoid process, and passes through the apex of the posterior triangle to supply the back of the scalp (see p. 369). The artery gives off two branches to sternocleidomastoid. The upper branch is a guide to the accessory nerve in front of the upper border of the muscle. At its origin the occipital artery crosses lateral to the hypoglossal nerve, which hooks around it from behind

(Fig. 6.24), the nerve being held down here by the lower sternocleidomastoid branch of the artery (Fig. 6.23).

The **posterior auricular artery** arises above the level of the digastric muscle, often within the substance of the parotid gland. It runs up superficial to the styloid process above the digastric posterior belly and crosses the surface of the mastoid process to supply the scalp. Auricular branches supply the pinna of the ear. Its *stylomastoid branch* enters the stylomastoid foramen and supplies the facial nerve; this branch may arise instead from the occipital artery.

The **ascending pharyngeal artery** arises just above the commencement of the external carotid, from its deep aspect. It runs up along the side wall of the pharynx in front of the prevertebral fascia, deep to the internal carotid artery. It supplies the pharyngeal wall and the soft palate and sends meningeal branches through the nearby foramina in the base of the skull (foramen lacerum, jugular foramen, hypoglossal canal).

Internal carotid artery

The internal carotid artery arises at the bifurcation of the common carotid (see p. 354) and continues upwards within the carotid sheath (see p. 379). At its commencement it shows a slight bulge, the **carotid sinus**. Here the arterial wall is thin and its contained *baroreceptors* are supplied by the glossopharyngeal and vagus nerves, which mediate blood pressure impulses to medullary centres. The **carotid body** is a small structure lying behind the bifurcation of the common carotid artery, or between its branches, from which it receives two or three very small glomic arteries. Its cells are *chemoreceptors* concerned (like the aortic bodies, see p. 198) with respiratory reflexes, and are innervated by the glossopharyngeal and vagus nerves. Carotid body tumours form a swelling at the anterior border of sternocleidomastoid at the level of the carotid bifurcation, and exhibit transmitted pulsation from the arteries.

The internal carotid artery is lateral to the external carotid at its origin, but soon passes up posteriorly to a medial and deeper level. It has no branches and passes straight up in the carotid sheath, beside the pharynx, to the carotid canal in the base of the skull; its intracranial course is considered on pages 463 and 466.

Behind the internal carotid artery in the neck is the sympathetic trunk (outside the carotid sheath), pharyngeal veins and the superior laryngeal branch of the vagus. The ascending pharyngeal artery is medial to it. The internal jugular vein is lateral, with the vagus nerve deeply placed between artery and vein. Superficially near its origin it is crossed by the lingual and facial veins, the occipital artery and hypoglossal nerve; the superior root of the ansa cervicalis runs downwards along it, embedded in the carotid sheath. At a higher level it is overlapped by sternocleidomastoid and crossed by the posterior belly of digastric and stylohyoid and the posterior auricular artery, and by the structures that separate it from the external carotid (see above).

The *surface marking* of the internal carotid artery in the neck is along a line from the bifurcation of the common carotid artery to the head of the mandible.

Surgical approach. The internal carotid is exposed in the neck by an incision along the anterior border of sternocleidomastoid. The muscle is retracted backwards, the facial and lingual veins divided between ligatures, and the carotid sheath is incised. The hypoglossal nerve must be safeguarded and this may require division of the lower sternocleidomastoid branch of the occipital artery. The emergence of branches from the external carotid artery ensures its differentiation from the internal carotid.

Internal jugular vein

The internal jugular vein emerges from the jugular bulb at the posterior compartment of the jugular foramen. At first behind the internal carotid artery, it lies on the transverse process of the atlas, crossed by the accessory nerve. It receives the inferior petrosal sinus as its first tributary, just below the base of the skull; the sinus passes back lateral or medial to the glossopharyngeal, vagus and accessory nerves. The vein passes down to gain the lateral side of the internal carotid artery, within the loose lateral part of the carotid sheath, with the vagus nerve deeply placed between the vein and artery. In the lower part of their course the vessels are overlaid by the sloping sternocleidomastoid. Deep cervical lymph nodes are closely adjacent to the vein throughout its course. Its posterior relations include the cervical plexus lying on levator scapulae and scalenus medius, and the phrenic nerve on scalenus anterior. The thoracic duct crosses behind the left vein at the level of C7 vertebra. The inferior root of the ansa cervicalis curls round its lateral border, to unite with the superior root (from the hypoglossal nerve) at a variable level in front of the vein. Low down the tendon of omohyoid crosses the vein, providing a useful guide to its position. The terminal part of the vein lies deep to the triangular interval between the sternal and clavicular heads of sternocleidomastoid (Fig. 6.2). It joins the subclavian to form the brachiocephalic vein behind the sternal end of the clavicle.

The tributaries of the internal jugular vein below the inferior petrosal sinus are the pharyngeal, lingual, facial and superior and middle thyroid veins. The lingual and superior thyroid veins may join the facial vein and other variations are possible.

At its commencement and termination the vein is slightly dilated to form superior and inferior bulbs. There is a pair of valves above the inferior bulb.

The *surface marking* of the internal jugular vein is along a line from the lobule of the ear to the sternal end of the clavicle, between the two heads of sternocleidomastoid. The jugular venous pulse is a guide to jugular venous pressure, which is the same as right atrial or central venous pressure and thus an indicator of cardiovascular function. With a patient reclining at 45° the jugular venous pulse should be visible just above the clavicle.

Catheterization. The right internal jugular vein (on a direct path to the right atrium) can be cannulated for the insertion of a central venous line, for measurements of central venous pressure, or the rapid administration of drugs when a peripheral approach would be too slow. The vein is usually approached through the centre of the triangle formed by the two heads of sternocleidomastoid and the clavicle. The needle is directed caudally, parallel to the sagittal plane at a 30° posterior angle with the coronal plane, entering the vein at about 4–5 cm depth. (The subclavian vein is an alternative, see p. 360). The most common complication is haematoma formation; others include common carotid artery puncture, vagus nerve injury and pneumothorax due to pleural perforation.

The **ansa cervicalis** lies on the front of the internal jugular vein and gives branches to the infrahyoid muscles. It is usually embedded within the anterior wall of the carotid sheath and classified as one of its contents. It is formed by union of superior and inferior roots. The *superior root* is a branch of the hypoglossal nerve containing only C1 fibres, which have hitch-hiked along the hypoglossal nerve. It runs down on the front of the internal and common carotid arteries, giving a branch to the superior belly of omohyoid.

The *inferior root* is formed by union of a branch each from C2 and C3 anterior rami in the cervical plexus. The single nerve so formed spirals from behind around the internal jugular vein and runs down to join the superior root in a wide loop over the lower part of the vein, from which branches arise for the infrahyoid muscles (sternohyoid, sternothyroid and inferior belly of omohyoid). Sometimes the inferior root passes forwards between internal jugular vein and internal carotid artery.

The uppermost part of the **hypoglossal nerve** in the neck is described on page 382. It emerges between the internal carotid artery and internal jugular vein deep to the posterior belly of digastric. Hooking round the occipital artery, which runs backwards lateral to the nerve, it curves forwards lateral to the internal and external carotids and the loop of the lingual artery (Fig. 6.23). As it crosses these arteries it lies just below the posterior belly of the digastric, behind its tendon and just above the tip of the greater horn of the hyoid bone. It gives off the superior root of the ansa cervicalis as it crosses the internal carotid and the branch to thyrohyoid (C1 fibres) as it crosses the lingual artery. It passes forwards on the lateral surface of hyoglossus deep to mylohyoid to enter the mouth, giving off the branch to geniohyoid (C1 fibres) as it does so (Fig. 6.24).

Summary of triangles of the neck

Posterior triangle

Boundaries. Sternocleidomastoid, trapezius, clavicle.

   Contents. Occipital, transverse cervical, suprascapular and subclavian arteries; transverse cervical, suprascapular and external jugular veins; accessory nerve, cervical plexus branches and brachial plexus trunks; inferior belly of omohyoid; lymph nodes.

Anterior triangle

Boundaries. Sternocleidomastoid, mandible, midline. Subdivided into:

Carotid triangle

Boundaries. Sternocleidomastoid, posterior belly of digastric, superior belly of omohyoid.

   Contents. Bifurcation of common carotid artery and branches of external carotid (except posterior auricular); lingual, facial and superior thyroid veins; hypoglossal, internal and external laryngeal nerves, and superior root of ansa cervicalis; lymph nodes.

Digastric triangle

Boundaries. Mandible, anterior and posterior bellies of digastric.

   Contents. Submandibular gland and lymph nodes; facial, submental and mylohyoid vessels; hypoglossal and mylohyoid nerves.

Submental triangle

Boundaries. Anterior bellies of digastric, body of hyoid bone. (Triangle crosses midline.)

   Contents. Anterior jugular veins; lymph nodes.

Muscular triangle

Boundaries. Sternocleidomastoid, superior belly of omohyoid, midline from hyoid bone to jugular notch.

   Contents. Parts of larynx, trachea, pharynx, oesophagus, thyroid and parathyroid glands; their vessels and nerves; lymph nodes.

PART THREE

Prevertebral region

Prevertebral muscles of the neck

Some relatively weak flexor muscles extend in front of the vertebral column from skull to superior mediastinum. They are covered anteriorly by the strong prevertebral fascia (Fig. 6.8).

   Rectus capitis anterior extends from just in front of the occipital condyle to the lateral mass of the atlas.

   Rectus capitis lateralis lies edge to edge with the former muscle; it extends from the jugular process of the occipital bone to the transverse process of the atlas. The **anterior ramus of C1**, passing forwards lateral to the atlanto-occipital joint, supplies each muscle and then passes between them to sink into the overlying longus capitis muscle. It gives a branch to the hypoglossal nerve, which is distributed in the meningeal branch, the superior root of the ansa cervicalis and the branches to thyrohyoid and geniohyoid. These two small rectus muscles assist in flexion and lateral flexion of the head.

   Longus capitis is attached to the basiocciput, in front of rectus capitis anterior and behind the wall of the nasopharynx (pharyngobasilar fascia, see p. 398), which it bulges forwards slightly. It is attached below by four tendons, in line with those of scalenus anterior, to the anterior tubercles of the transverse processes of the four 'typical' cervical vertebrae (C3–6). It is supplied by anterior rami of the upper four cervical nerves. It flexes the head.

   Longus colli extends from the atlas into the superior mediastinum. It consists of upper, lower and central fibres, which together give the muscle a triangular shape, the elongated base of the triangle being close to the midline (Fig. 6.8). It is attached to the anterior tubercle of the altas, the front of the bodies of vertebrae C2–7 and T1–3, and to the anterior tubercles of the transverse processes of vertebrae C3–6.

   Longus colli is supplied segmentally by the anterior rami of the spinal nerves. It is a flexor of the neck.

   The *prevertebral fascia* is described on page 343.

Cervical sympathetic trunk

The **cervical part** of the **sympathetic trunk** (Fig. 6.8) ascends from the thorax across the neck of the first rib,

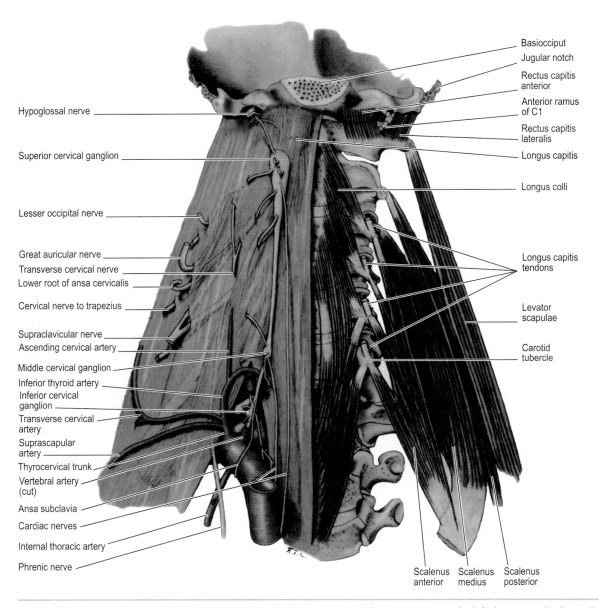

Fig. 6.8   Prevertebral region of the neck. The right half of the prevertebral fascia is intact; on the left the prevertebral muscles are exposed.

medial to the highest intercostal vein. It runs up medial to the vertebral artery and lies in front of the prevertebral fascia, behind the carotid sheath and medial to the vagus nerve. It ends at the superior cervical ganglion.

The **superior cervical ganglion**, containing about 1 million cell bodies, is about 3 cm long and lies in front of C2 and C3 vertebrae. The **middle cervical ganglion** is a small, inconstant ganglion lying medial to the carotid tubercle (C6 vertebra) and in front of the inferior thyroid artery. The **inferior cervical ganglion** lies behind the commencement of the vertebral artery. A small mass when separate, it is often fused with the first thoracic ganglion to form the **cervicothoracic (stellate) ganglion**, in front of the neck of the first rib. The middle ganglion is connected to the inferior (or stellate) ganglion by two or more strands, one of which loops down in front of and under the subclavian artery, the *ansa subclavia* (Fig. 6.8).

No white rami enter the ganglia from the cervical nerves: all the preganglionic fibres ascend from the thoracic part of the trunk. As elsewhere, the branches of the ganglia are somatic and visceral in their distribution.

Grey rami pass to all eight cervical nerves. The superior ganglion gives grey rami to the first four (i.e. to the cervical plexus), the middle ganglion to the next two (5 and 6) and the inferior ganglion to the last two (7 and 8) anterior rami (i.e. to the brachial plexus for distribution to the upper limb).

Each ganglion gives a *cardiac branch*. The branch from the upper left ganglion runs down to the superficial cardiac plexus, the others all pass to the deep plexus. All six cardiac branches pass down behind the common carotid and subclavian arteries to reach the superior mediastinum.

Vascular branches 'hitch-hike' their way along arteries. The superior ganglion gives branches to the internal carotid and external carotid arteries. The internal carotid nerve accompanies the internal carotid artery into the skull and forms the *internal carotid plexus*, from which fibres are distributed to all branches of the artery, the pterygopalatine ganglion and the eyeball, the latter including the motor supply of the dilator pupillae of the iris. The plexus on the external carotid artery accompanies all branches of the vessel and in addition supplies sympathetic fibres to the pharyngeal plexus and the submandibular and otic ganglia.

The *middle cervical ganglion* gives branches to the inferior thyroid artery.

The *inferior cervical ganglion* gives branches to the subclavian artery and a large branch to the vertebral artery, which forms the vertebral plexus.

Interruption of the cervical sympathetic pathway gives rise to *Horner's syndrome*, described on page 423.

PART **FOUR**

Root of the neck

The **root of the neck** (thoracic outlet) is bounded by the first thoracic vertebra, the first pair of ribs and their cartilages and the manubrium of the sternum. The key to the root of the neck is the scalenus anterior muscle and its relations (Figs 6.8, 6.9A and 6.10).

Scalenus anterior

This flat muscle arises from the anterior tubercles of the four 'typical' cervical vertebrae (3–6) by four slender tendons of origin which lie end to end with those of longus capitis (Fig. 6.8). The muscle passes forwards, laterally and downwards to end in a narrow tendon attached to the scalene tubercle and adjacent ridge on the inner border and upper surface of the first rib (see Fig. 4.34, p. 227).

Nerve supply. By separate branches from the anterior rami of C4–6 nerves.

Action. It is more important as a landmark than an active muscle. It assists in flexion and rotation of the neck, and helps to stabilize the first rib. Even in quiet respiration it shows some electromyographic activity.

Anterior relations

The *phrenic nerve* passes vertically down across the obliquity of the muscle, plastered thereto by the prevertebral fascia (Fig. 6.10) and a pad of fat lies in front of the prevertebral fascia. The nerve leaves the medial border of the muscle low down and crosses in front of the subclavian artery and its internal thoracic branch, behind the subclavian vein. (Occasionally the phrenic nerve may pass in front of the subclavian vein or posterior to the internal thoracic artery.) Lying on the suprapleural membrane it passes medial to the apex of the lung, crossing in front of the vagus nerve as it enters the superior mediastinum. The *ascending cervical artery*, a branch of the inferior thyroid artery or the thyrocervical trunk, runs up on the prevertebral fascia medial to the phrenic nerve.

In front of the prevertebral fascia the *transverse cervical* and *suprascapular arteries* lie between the scalenus anterior and the carotid sheath (internal jugular vein). The *vagus nerve* in the carotid sheath passes down in front of the subclavian artery, on the right side giving off its *recurrent laryngeal* branch. The latter hooks under the artery and passes upwards (Fig. 6.9A). The vagus nerve inclines posteriorly and runs on the medial surface of the apex of the lung to enter the superior mediastinum. The *internal jugular vein* is surrounded by inferior *deep cervical lymph nodes*.

The **subclavian vein** lies in a groove on the first rib and, due to the slope of the rib, lies at a lower level than the insertion of scalenus anterior. Running medially it joins the internal jugular vein at the medial border of scalenus anterior to form the brachiocephalic vein; the thoracic duct on the left and the right lymph duct on the right enter the angle of confluence of the two veins.

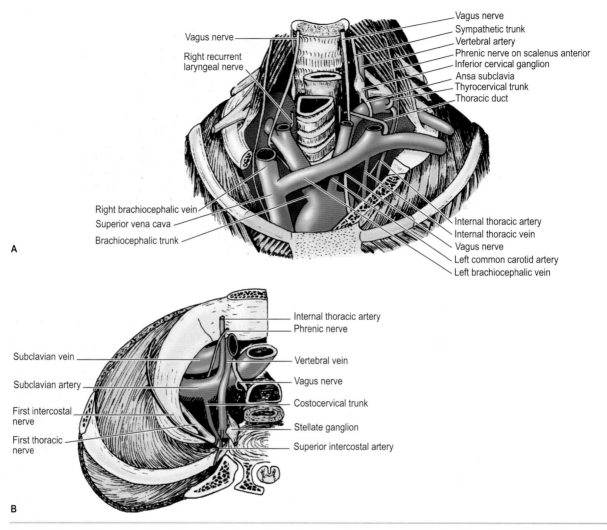

Fig. 6.9 Root of the neck and superior mediastinum: **A** from the front after removal of the clavicles and manubrium; **B** root of the neck on the right side, from below. In both **A** and **B**, the phrenic nerve is shown crossing the internal thoracic artery on its posterior aspect; usually the nerve crosses the artery anteriorly. In **A**, a segment of the vertebral artery has been removed to show the inferior cervical ganglion, which lies behind it. In **B**, the first costal cartilage has ossified.

Catheterization. The right subclavian vein can be used for the placement of a central venous line, instead of the internal jugular (see p. 356); it is preferred by many operators and is more comfortable for the patient. The usual approach is infraclavicular, from a point 2 cm below the midpoint of the clavicle along a line that passes behind the clavicle towards the jugular notch of the sternum. The needle pierces the clavipectoral fascia and enters the vein just behind the fascia. The most common complications are pneumothorax due to puncture of the pleura and lung, and puncture of the subclavian artery. The vein is also used for the placement of wires from cardiac pacemakers, which are usually implanted in connective tissue over the upper lateral part of pectoralis major.

Medial relations

The medial edge of scalenus anterior makes a pyramidal space with the lateral border of the lower part of longus

Fig. 6.10   Prevertebral fascia and the scalene muscles.

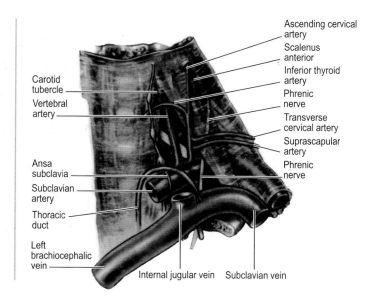

colli. The prevertebral fascia in front of these muscles is attached to bone at their opposing margins and there is no fascial roof across the pyramidal space between the muscles. The base of the space is formed by the subclavian artery, lying on the suprapleural membrane. The apex of the space is the carotid (Chassaignac's) tubercle on the transverse process of C6 vertebra (Figs 6.8 and 6.10).

The common carotid artery, medial to the internal jugular vein, lies deep to sternocleidomastoid immediately in front of the pyramidal space. Behind the artery and the carotid sheath, the space contains the inferior cervical sympathetic (or stellate) ganglion, with the vertebral artery and vein(s) in front of it. The *inferior thyroid artery* arches medially in a bold curve whose upper convexity lies in front of the apex of the pyramidal space (C6 level), with the sympathetic chain, usually the middle ganglion, in front of the artery. At a lower level, and further forward, the *thoracic duct* (or right lymphatic duct) makes a similar convexity behind the carotid sheath as it arches over the lung apex and subclavian artery to enter the confluence of the subclavian and internal jugular veins (Fig. 6.10).

The relationship of the scalenus anterior to the subclavian artery is used to descriptively divide the subclavian artery into three parts. The **first part of the subclavian artery** is medial to scalenus anterior. It arches over the suprapleural membrane and impresses a groove upon the apex of the lung. It has three branches. The *vertebral artery* is the first; this arises from the upper convexity of the subclavian and passes up to disappear, at the apex of the pyramidal space, into the foramen of

the transverse process of C6 vertebra. The accompanying sympathetic nerve runs up behind the artery. Rarely this first part of the vertebral artery may initially enter the foramen of the transverse process of a higher vertebra than C6. A connecting loop between middle and inferior cervical ganglia passes in front of the subclavian artery and turns up behind it, forming the *ansa subclavia*. The recurrent laryngeal nerve recurves under the right subclavian artery, while the thoracic duct loops over the left artery. The *thyrocervical trunk* arises lateral to the vertebral artery from the upper surface of the subclavian. It divides immediately into transverse cervical, suprascapular and inferior thyroid arteries, which have already been noted. The *internal thoracic artery* arises from the lower surface of the subclavian and passes downwards over the lung apex, crossed anteriorly by the phrenic nerve.

The *vertebral vein* emerges from the foramen in the transverse process of C6 vertebra and runs forward in front of the vertebral and subclavian arteries to empty into the brachiocephalic vein. It may be accompanied by a companion vein that passes through the foramen of the transverse process of C7 vertebra and passes behind the subclavian artery to the same destination.

Posterior relations

Scalenus anterior is separated from scalenus medius by the subclavian artery and the anterior rami of the lower cervical and first thoracic nerves. The **second part of the subclavian artery** lies behind scalenus anterior. Its only branch is the *costocervical trunk*. It passes back across the suprapleural membrane towards the neck of the first rib and there divides into a descending branch, the *superior intercostal artery*, which enters the thorax across the neck of the first rib, and an ascending branch, the *deep cervical artery*, which passes backwards between the transverse process of C7 vertebra and the neck of the first rib to run upwards behind the cervical transverse processes.

Lateral relations

The *trunks* of the **brachial plexus** and the **third part of the subclavian artery** emerge from the lateral border of scalenus anterior. They lie behind the prevertebral fascia on the floor of the posterior triangle (Fig. 6.10). The *dorsal scapular* usually arises from the third part. It runs laterally through the brachial plexus in front of scalenus medius and then deep to levator scapulae to take part in the scapular anastomosis (see p. 49). It is frequently replaced by the deep branch of the transverse cervical artery, and this branch then takes the name of dorsal scapular.

The *surface marking* of the subclavian artery in the neck is along a line arching upwards from the sterno-clavicular joint to the middle of the clavicle and about 2 cm above it.

Surgical approach. The artery can be exposed by dividing the clavicular head of sternocleidomastoid from the clavicle and then detaching scalenus anterior from the first rib, taking particular care not to damage the phrenic nerve.

Pressure on the subclavian artery and lowest root (T1) of the brachial plexus as they cross over a cervical rib or fibrous band, when present at the root of the neck, is described on page 439. Elevation of the first rib by scalenus anterior may also cause or aggravate such a *thoracic outlet syndrome*, and the muscle is usually divided close to its insertion when the syndrome is treated surgically.

Scalenus medius and scalenus posterior

Scalenus medius arises from the lateral ends of the transverse processes of atlas and axis and from the posterior tubercles of all the other cervical vertebrae and is inserted into the quadrangular area between the neck and subclavian groove of the first rib (see Fig. 4.34, p. 227).

Scalenus posterior is a small unimportant muscle that arises from the posterior tubercles of the lower cervical vertebrae, passes across the outer border of the first rib deep to the upper digitation of serratus anterior, and is inserted into the second rib.

Nerve supplies. Both muscles are supplied segmentally by the anterior rami of cervical nerves, scalenus medius by C3–8.

Actions. Scalenus medius, mainly a lateral flexor of the neck, can elevate the first rib as an accessory muscle of respiration.

PART FIVE

Face

The face is the part of the front of the head between the ears and from the chin to the hairline (or where it ought to be).

Skin of the face

The skin of the face has numerous sweat and sebaceous glands. It varies in thickness and is very thin on the eyelids. The muscles underlying the skin of the face are attached to the dermis in places. Senile facial wrinkles lie at right angles to the line of pull of the underlying muscles (horizontal wrinkles on the brow, 'crow's foot' wrinkles at the lateral canthus, vertical wrinkles on both lips). There is no deep fascia on the face.

Muscles of the face

The muscles of 'facial expression' are developed from the mesoderm of the second pharyngeal arch, from which they migrate widely to their adult positions. They are supplied by the nerve of the second arch, the seventh cranial (facial) nerve. Functionally the muscles are differentiated to form groups around the orifices (Fig. 6.11). The orifices of orbit, nose and mouth are guarded by eyelids, nostrils and lips and there is a sphincter and an opposing dilator arrangement peculiar to each. The purpose of the facial muscles is to control these orifices. The varying expressions so produced on the face are side effects.

Some of the muscles of the face participate in a superficial muscular aponeurotic system (SMAS). This is described on page 372.

Muscles of the eyelids

The palpebral fissure is surrounded by a sphincter, the orbicularis oculi, and has a dilator mechanism consisting of levator palpebrae superioris (considered with the orbital muscles, see p. 415) and occipitofrontalis which is part of the scalp (p. 369).

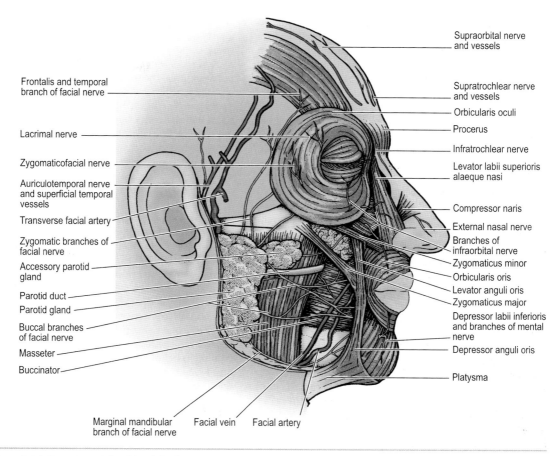

Fig. 6.11   Superficial dissection of the side of the face.

Orbicularis oculi has a palpebral part, confined to the lids, and an orbital part, extending beyond the bony orbital margins on to the face. The *palpebral part* consists of fibres that arise from the medial palpebral ligament (see p. 413), arch across both lids, anterior to the tarsal plates, and interdigitate laterally to form the lateral palpebral raphe. Fibres of a deeper *lacrimal part* are attached medially to the posterior lacrimal crest and lacrimal sac; laterally they join the upper and lower palpebral fibres. The *orbital part*, much the larger, arises from the nasal part of the frontal bone, the anterior lacrimal crest and the frontal process of the maxilla, whence the fibres circumscribe the orbital margin in a series of concentric loops.

Nerve supply. By temporal and zygomatic (mainly) branches of the facial nerve.

Action. Contraction of the palpebral fibres closes the lids gently without burying the eyelashes. Orbital and palpebral parts contracting together close the eyelids forcibly so that the eyelashes are buried and only their tips are visible. In normal closing of the eye, the lateral part of the upper lid comes down before the medial part, so helping to spread lacrimal secretion from the gland side (lateral) towards the nose.

Levator palpebrae superioris is the opponent of the upper palpebral fibres of orbicularis oculi; occipitofrontalis opposes the orbital part.

Muscles of the nostrils

The sphincter muscle of the nostril is the transverse part of *nasalis* (**compressor naris**), which forms an aponeurosis over the bridge of the nose with its fellow of the opposite side. Its opponent is the alar part of nasalis (**dilator naris**), which is inserted into the lateral part of the ala. Each arises from the maxilla. In addition, levator labii superioris alaeque nasi (see p. 365) and depressor septi contribute to widening the nostril. Depressor septi arises from the maxilla above the central incisor and is attached to the nasal septum. All these muscles are supplied by buccal branches of the facial nerve.

Muscles of the lips and cheeks

The sphincter is the orbicularis oris; the dilator mechanism consists of the remainder of the facial muscles, which radiate outwards from the lips like the spokes of a wheel.

Orbicularis oris consists of fibres proper to itself and fibres that are added to these from the dilators. The muscle is made up of four quadrants (upper, lower, right and left) each of which has a larger peripheral part and a smaller marginal part in the red zone of the lips. The bulk of the orbicularis muscle is formed of extrinsic fibres; most of these come from the buccinator. The fibres of buccinator converge towards the modiolus (see below). At the modiolus they form a chiasma; the uppermost and lowermost fibres pass straight on into their respective lips, while the middle fibres decussate, the upper fibres of buccinator passing into the lower lip, the lower into the upper lip (Fig. 6.12).

Incisivus labii superioris and *incisivus labii inferioris* are attached to the incisive fossa of the maxilla and mandible, respectively, from where they arch laterally, interlacing with fibres of the peripheral part of orbicularis oris as they approach the modiolus. They are the deepest fibres in the lips and are attached to the mucous membrane.

Nerve supply. By buccal and marginal mandibular branches of the facial nerve. Damage to the latter branch (such as in the surgical approach to the submandibular gland) causes asymmetry of the mouth when speaking or smiling.

Action. Contraction of the orbicularis oris causes a narrowing of the mouth, the lips becoming pursed up into the smallest possible circle (the whistling expression).

Buccinator has a bony origin from both jaws opposite the molar teeth, horizontally on the maxilla and from the oblique line of the mandible. Between the tuberosity of the maxilla and the hamulus at the bottom of the medial pterygoid plate (of the sphenoid), the muscle arises from a fibrous band (the *pterygomaxillary ligament*), above which the tendon of tensor palati hooks around the base of the hamulus (Fig. 6.13).

From the tip of the hamulus the *pterygomandibular raphe* extends to the mandible just above the posterior end of the mylohyoid line; between them the lingual nerve is in contact with the mandible where the bone is often thinned by a shallow groove (Fig. 6.22). The buccinator arises from the whole length of the raphe, along which it interdigitates with the fibres of the superior constrictor (see p. 396). The muscle converges on the modiolus, where its fibres of origin from the raphe decussate; the maxillary and mandibular fibres pass medially without decussation into the upper and lower lips respectively. The muscle is pierced by the parotid duct opposite the third upper molar tooth. The duct also passes through the buccal fat pad which lies on the outer surface of buccinator and is particularly prominent in infants, giving them their chubby cheeks. Beneath the fat lie a few small *molar glands*; their ducts pierce the muscle to open on the mucous membrane of the cheek, which lines the muscle's inner surface and to which muscle fibres are attached.

Nerve supply. By the buccal branches of the facial nerve. The buccal branch of the mandibular nerve supplies proprioceptive fibres.

Action. It is essentially an accessory muscle of mastication, being indispensable to the return of the bolus from the cheek pouch to the grinding mill of the molars. It is, however, classified as a muscle of facial expression on account of being supplied by the facial nerve. When the cheeks are puffed out the muscle is relaxed, and the muscle contracts in forcible expulsion of air from the mouth, as in blowing a trumpet. (Buccinator is the Latin name for a trumpeter.)

Dilator muscles of the lips

Radiating from orbicularis oris like the spokes of a wheel is a series of dilator muscles, some inserted into the lips, some into the modiolus. All contracting together open the lips into the widest possible circle, an action

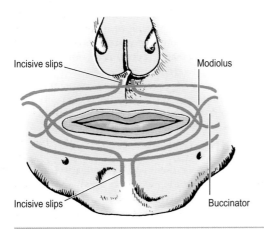

Fig. 6.12 Fibres of orbicularis oris.

Fig. 6.13 Left pterygoid hamulus and related structures.

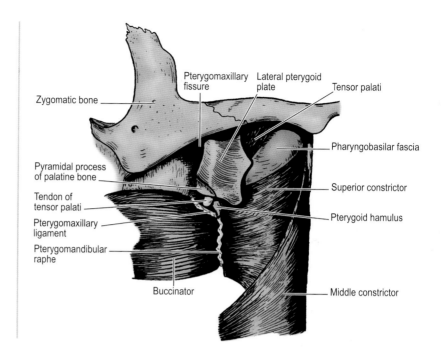

that is usually accompanied by simultaneous opening of the jaws. Upper and lower lips have flat sheets of elevator and depressor muscles. Other muscles converge towards the angle of the mouth, where their decussating fibres form a knot of muscle with the chiasma in the buccinator fibres, bound together by fibrous tissue; this is termed the **modiolus** and is situated about 1 cm lateral to the angle of the mouth, opposite the second upper premolar tooth. Its position and movements are of importance in prosthetic dentistry.

Levator labii superioris alaeque nasi arises from the frontal process of the maxilla and is inserted into the ala of the nose and the upper lip; it elevates both. **Levator labii superioris** arises from the inferior orbital margin and is inserted into the remainder of the upper lip, which it elevates. The muscle overlies the exit of the infraorbital nerve. From the canine fossa below the infraorbital foramen arises **levator anguli oris**; the infraorbital nerve lies sandwiched between it and the overlying levator labii superioris. The fibres of this muscle, deep to the superficial sheet of muscle, converge to the modiolus and pass through it to become superficial. They merge into the fibres of depressor anguli oris. **Zygomaticus minor** from the zygomaticomaxillary suture and **zygomaticus major** further out on the surface of the zygomatic bone converge to the modiolus. **Risorius** is a variable muscle that converges on the modiolus from the parotid fascia.

All these muscles are supplied by buccal branches of the facial nerve.

Depressor anguli oris arises from the mandible below the mental foramen. It lies superficial but its fibres pass through the modiolus to the deeper stratum (levator anguli oris). **Depressor labii inferioris** arises from the mandible in front of the mental foramen, deep to the former muscle; its fibres are inserted into the lower lip. **Mentalis** is a muscle that arises near the midline of the mandible. Its fibres pass downwards to reach the skin. It is an elevator of the skin of the chin (which it sometimes dimples) and its contraction may disturb a lower denture. These muscles are supplied by the marginal mandibular branch of the facial nerve.

Nerve supply of face muscles

The supply from the facial nerve to the muscles described above is motor. Proprioceptive impulses from the facial muscles are conveyed centrally by the *trigeminal* nerve, whose cutaneous branches connect freely with branches of the facial nerve.

The **facial nerve** emerges from the base of the skull through the stylomastoid foramen, near the origin of the posterior belly of digastric. It immediately gives off the **posterior auricular nerve** which passes upwards behind the ear to supply auricularis posterior and the occipital

365

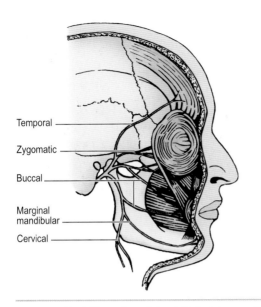

Temporal

Zygomatic

Buccal

Marginal
mandibular

Cervical

Fig. 6.14   Facial branches of the right facial nerve. The marginal mandibular branch frequently has a lower course partly below the ramus of the mandible.

belly of occipitofrontalis. A **muscular branch** is next given off which divides to supply the posterior belly of digastric and stylohyoid. The nerve now approaches the posteromedial surface of the parotid gland. Just before entering or within the gland it divides into an upper *temporofacial* and a lower *cervicofacial* division. Within the substance of the parotid gland each divides and re-joins to divide again and finally emerge from the parotid gland in five main groups of branches (Fig. 6.14). This plexiform arrangement, the *pes anserinus*, lies in the gland superficial to the retromandibular vein and the external carotid artery.

The **temporal branches** emerge from the upper border of the gland, cross the zygomatic arch, and supply auricularis anterior and superior, and part of frontalis. They are only important for wrinkling the forehead. (The most posterior temporal branch is also termed the frontal branch.)

The **zygomatic branches** cross the zygomatic arch and zygomatic bone, lying directly on the periosteum. They may be damaged in fractures or operations in this region. These branches supply orbicularis oculi. Paralysis of this muscle prevents blinking and the precorneal film of tears is no longer spread. The dry cornea easily ulcerates. The resultant scar impairs vision and this is the most serious consequence of impaired facial nerve function.

The **buccal branches** run forwards close to the parotid duct, often one above and one below the duct. They supply buccinator and the muscle fibres of the nose and the upper lip. Paralysis of the buccinator prevents emptying of the cheek pouch; the bolus lodges there and cannot be returned to the molar teeth. Chewing has to be performed on the other side.

The **marginal mandibular branch** is frequently single and runs forwards above, along, or below the lower border of the mandible. From below the mandible it crosses the inferior border of the bone to reach the face just beyond the anterior border of the masseter muscle, passing superficial to the facial artery and vein. A small lymph node lies here (Fig. 6.62). The nerve is in danger when an incision is made at or near the lower border of the mandible. This nerve does not communicate with a buccal branch and damage to the nerve invariably causes detectable paralysis of the depressors of the lower lip and mouth angle, there being no alternate pathway for motor fibres to these muscles.

The **cervical branch** passes downwards from the lower border of the parotid gland and supplies platysma.

The details of the pattern of branching of the facial nerve differs in different individuals and even on the two sides of the face of the same person.

Sensory nerve supply of the face

The trigeminal nerve has three divisions (officially called branches): ophthalmic, maxillary and mandibular. The skin of the face is supplied in three zones by the branches of the three divisions of the trigeminal nerve (Fig. 6.15A). These zones meet at the margins of the eyelids and the angle of the mouth, and the junctional lines of the zones curve outwards and upwards from there. The pattern of a facial haemangioma (port wine stain, as in Sturge–Weber syndrome), and the distribution of the vesicles when herpes zoster affects the trigeminal ganglion, is often in accordance with this arrangement of the sensory supply of facial skin. However, the spatial representation of the face in the spinal nucleus of the trigeminal nerve in the brainstem, particularly with regard to pain sensation, is probably different and more akin to an 'onion skin' pattern, with fibres from the central area of the face reaching the highest (cranial) part of the nucleus and fibres from the more posterior part of the face passing to progressively lower (caudal) levels of the nucleus (Fig. 6.15B).

The great auricular nerve supplies the skin over the parotid gland and part of the auricle of the ear (see p. 346); the fibres reach the C2 segment of the spinal cord.

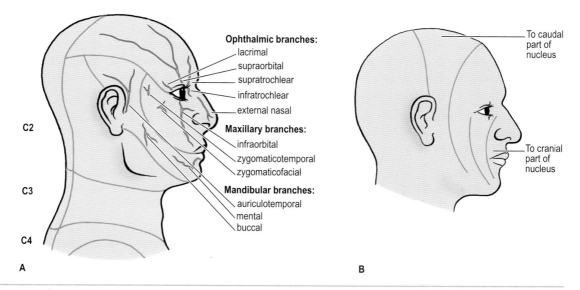

Fig. 6.15   Dermatomes and cutaneous nerves of the right side of the head and neck: **A** dermatomes and trigeminal nerve branches; **B** 'onion-skin' representation of the facial areas in the spinal nucleus of the trigeminal nerve. Fibres from the most anterior part of the face synapse with cells of the most cranial part of the nucleus.

Ophthalmic nerve

Five cutaneous branches:

The **lacrimal nerve** supplies a small area of skin over the lateral part of the upper lid.

A third of the way lateral to the medial end of the upper margin of the orbit, the **supraorbital nerve** indents the bone into a notch or a foramen. The nerve passes up, breaking into several branches which radiate out and supply the forehead and scalp up to the vertex.

The smaller **supratrochlear nerve** passes up on the medial side of the supraorbital nerve to supply the middle of the forehead up to the hairline.

The **infratrochlear nerve** supplies skin on the medial part of the upper lid and, passing above the medial palpebral ligament, descends along the side of the external nose, supplying skin over the bridge of the nose.

These four branches of the ophthalmic nerve also supply upper lid conjunctiva.

The **external nasal nerve** supplies the middle of the external nose down to the tip. It emerges between the nasal bone and the upper nasal cartilage.

The supraorbital and supratrochlear nerves are branches of the frontal nerve. The infratrochlear and external nasal nerves are derived from the nasociliary, the former directly and the latter via the anterior ethmoidal branch; when these nerves are involved in herpes zoster infection, the cornea (supplied by the ciliary branches of

the nasociliary) may also become affected and lead to dangerous corneal ulceration.

Maxillary nerve

Three cutaneous branches:

The **infraorbital nerve** emerges through its foramen and lies between levator labii superioris and the deeper placed levator anguli oris. It is a large nerve that immediately breaks up into a tuft of branches; these radiate away from the foramen to supply the lower eyelid (including conjunctiva), cheek, nose, upper lip and labial gum.

The **zygomaticofacial nerve** emerges from a foramen on the outer surface of the zygomatic bone; its branches supply the overlying skin.

The **zygomaticotemporal nerve** emerges in the temporal fossa through a foramen in the temporal (posterior) surface of the zygomatic bone. It supplies a small area of temporal skin.

Mandibular nerve

Three cutaneous branches:

The **auriculotemporal nerve** passes around the neck of the mandible and ascends over the posterior root of the zygomatic arch behind the superficial temporal vessels. The *auricular* part of the nerve supplies the

367

external acoustic meatus, surface of the tympanic membrane and skin of the auricle above this level. The *temporal* part supplies the hairy skin over the temple.

The **buccal nerve** gives off cutaneous twigs before it pierces the buccinator muscle. They supply a small area over the cheek just below the zygomatic bone, between the areas of the infraorbital nerve and the great auricular nerve (see p. 346).

The **mental nerve** is a cutaneous branch of the inferior alveolar nerve. Like the infraorbital nerve it breaks up into a tuft of branches that radiate away from the mental foramen to supply the skin and mucous membrane of the lower lip and labial gum from the midline to about the second premolar tooth.

Blood supply of the face

The **facial artery** hooks upwards over the inferior border of the mandible at the anterior border of the masseter muscle. It pursues a tortuous course towards the medial angle of the eye, lying on the buccinator deep to the sheet of dilator muscles that radiate out from the lips. Its labial branches are sizeable. Each **superior** and **inferior labial artery** runs across the lip beneath the red margin and anastomoses end to end with the corresponding artery of the opposite side. The larger superior labial artery gives a septal branch to the nasal septum. The **transverse facial artery**, a branch of the superficial temporal artery, runs across the cheek just above the parotid duct. The forehead is supplied from the orbit by the **supraorbital** and **supratrochlear** branches of the ophthalmic artery. The bigger supraorbital artery anastomoses with the superficial temporal artery, establishing communication between internal and external carotid systems. The dorsal nasal artery, a small terminal branch of the ophthalmic artery, supplies skin at the root of the nose.

The **venous return** from the face is normally entirely superficial. From the forehead the **supraorbital** and **supratrochlear veins** pass to the medial canthus, where they unite to form the *angular vein*. This becomes the **facial vein** which pursues a straight course behind the tortuous facial artery to a point just below the border of the mandible. Here in the neck it pierces the investing layer of the deep fascia and is joined by the anterior branch of the retromandibular vein, and sometimes by the superior thyroid vein. Blood from the temple is collected into the tributaries of the **superficial temporal vein**. The latter is joined by the **maxillary vein** from the pterygoid plexus to form the **retromandibular vein**. This passes downwards in the substance of the parotid gland and on emerging from its lower border divides into anterior and posterior branches. The *anterior branch*

joins the facial vein which empties into the internal jugular. The *posterior branch* pierces the investing layer of deep cervical fascia and is joined by the posterior auricular vein to form the **external jugular vein**. This courses down in the subcutaneous tissue over sternocleidomastoid and pierces the investing layer of deep cervical fascia to enter the posterior triangle and empty into the subclavian vein. It has valves about 4 cm above the clavicle and at its termination.

Deep venous anastomoses

At the medial angle of the eyelids there is a communication with the *ophthalmic veins*, which drain directly into the *cavernous sinus*. Blood from the forehead normally flows via the facial vein; if the latter is blocked by thrombosis, blood above the obstruction will flow through the orbit into the cavernous sinus. Hence the 'danger area' of infection of the upper lip and nearby cheek. A further communication is the **deep facial vein**. This passes backwards from the facial vein, between the masseter and buccinator muscles, to the *pterygoid plexus*. The plexus connects with the cavernous sinus by emissary veins that pass through the foramen ovale and the foramen lacerum. The danger area of the face lies between the angular and deep facial veins.

Lymph drainage of the face

The face drains into three superficial groups of nodes (see p. 426) from three wedge-shaped blocks of tissue. Centrally a small triangular area that includes the chin and tip of the tongue drains into *submental nodes*. A wedge of tissue above this, which extends laterally as far as the facial vessels, drains to *submandibular nodes*; this wedge extends from central forehead and frontal sinuses through the anterior half of the nose and maxillary sinuses to the upper lip and lower part of the face, and includes the tongue and the floor of the mouth. Beyond this wedge, forehead, temple, orbital contents and cheek drain to *preauricular* (parotid) *nodes*. Eventually all lymph from the face reaches deep cervical nodes.

PART SIX

Scalp

The scalp extends from the supraorbital margins anteriorly to the highest nuchal lines at the back of the skull and down to the ears and zygomatic arches at the sides. The forehead, from eyebrows to hairline (or where it should be), is common to the face and scalp. The composition of the scalp is traditionally recalled from the five letters of the words that indicate its five layers: Skin; Connective tissue; Aponeurosis with muscle at the front and back; Loose areolar tissue; and Pericranium.

The **skin** of the scalp is the thickest in the body and is thickest of all in the occipital region. Apart from being usually the hairiest part of the body it also contains a high concentration of sebaceous glands. Many of the fibres of the scalp muscle are inserted into it. Elsewhere it is firmly attached by *dense connective tissue* (the second layer) to the underlying *muscle and aponeurosis*. The vessels and nerves run within this firm tissue which unites the first and third layers.

Occipitofrontalis consists of occipitalis and frontalis muscular parts with an intervening *epicranial aponeurosis (galea aponeurotica)* into which they are inserted at the back and front respectively. *Occipitalis* arises from the highest nuchal line and passes forwards into the aponeurosis which lies over the top of the skull. The muscle bellies are separated across the midline by the aponeurosis which extends backwards to be attached to the external occipital protuberance and the most medial part of the highest nuchal line. Laterally the aponeurosis blends with the *temporoparietal fascia* (superficial temporal fascia) and comes down over the deep temporal fascia (see p. 370) to the zygomatic arch. *Frontalis* arises from the front of the aponeurosis and passes forwards to become attached to the upper part of orbicularis oculi and the overlying skin of the eyebrow. The right and left frontalis muscles meet in the midline. The midline fibres blend with procerus, a small muscle that arises from the nasal bone and cartilage and inserts into the skin of the lower forehead; its contraction produces transverse wrinkles over the bridge of the nose.

Nerve supply. By the facial nerve; the posterior auricular branch to occipitalis, and temporal branches to frontalis.

Action. While occipitalis can pull the scalp back in certain individuals, usually it merely anchors the aponeurosis while frontalis elevates the eyebrows and produces wrinkles in the skin of the forehead.

Beneath the muscles and aponeurosis is a small amount of *loose areolar tissue* providing a plane above which the rest of the scalp can be moved and through which avulsion can occur (scalping). Through this plane a flap of the overlying scalp can be rotated on a vascular pedicle as a surgical procedure. This subaponeurotic space extends down beneath orbicularis oculi into the eyelids. Bleeding anywhere beneath the aponeurosis may appear as a 'black eye' by the blood tracking down through the space.

The *pericranium* is the periosteum of the vault of the skull. This is rather loosely attached to the bone and is easily stripped up by a subperiosteal haematoma. Such a haematoma outlines the bone concerned, since the pericranium is very firmly attached at the sutures.

Blood supply

The arteries of the scalp are derived from the external carotid artery by the occipital, posterior auricular and superficial temporal branches, and from the internal carotid artery by the supraorbital and supratrochlear branches. All these arteries anastomose very freely with each other. The arterial walls are attached to the dense connective tissue of the second layer of the scalp and tend to be held open and bleed profusely when cut. Scalping does not cause necrosis of the bones of the vault, most of whose blood comes from the middle meningeal artery.

The **occipital artery** emerges from the apex of the posterior triangle and runs with the greater occipital nerve to supply the back of the scalp up to the vertex. The *posterior auricular artery* runs with the lesser occipital nerve to supply the scalp behind the ear.

The **superficial temporal artery** is a terminal branch of the external carotid. Running up behind the temporomandibular joint and in front of the ear and the auriculotemporal nerve, it crosses the zygomatic arch, where its pulsation can be felt, and branches out widely into the skin that overlies the temporalis fascia. One branch, the *middle temporal artery*, pierces the fascia, supplies temporalis and anastomoses with the deep temporal branches of the maxillary artery.

The **supraorbital** and **supratrochlear arteries** (from the ophthalmic) run with the corresponding nerves. The supraorbital is the larger and supplies the front of the scalp up to the vertex. Its anastomosis with the superficial temporal artery connects the internal and external carotid systems.

The **veins** of the scalp run back with the arteries. In forehead, temple and occipital regions they receive diploic veins from frontal, parietal and occipital bones.

The supraorbital and supratrochlear veins drain by the angular vein into the facial vein. The superficial temporal veins run into the retromandibular vein, and occipital veins reach the plexus around the suboccipital muscles which drains into the vertebral vein. The posterior auricular vein drains the scalp behind the ear to the external jugular vein; it also receives the mastoid emissary vein from the sigmoid sinus. Spread of infection to this emissary vein from mastoid air cells can be dangerous or fatal, from retrograde thrombosis of cerebellar and medullary veins. At the vertex a parietal emissary vein on either side of the midline connects scalp veins with the superior sagittal sinus.

Lymph drainage

There are no lymph nodes within the scalp; lymphatic channels from the posterior half of the scalp drain to occipital and mastoid nodes, and from the anterior half to preauricular (parotid) nodes. The lymph eventually reaches the nodes of the deep cervical chain.

Nerve supply

The main sensory nerves run with the arteries. Posteriorly the greater occipital and third occipital nerves (posterior rami of C2 and C3 respectively) extend to the vertex and the posterior scalp respectively. The lesser occipital (anterior ramus of C2) supplies skin behind the ear. The temple is supplied by the auriculotemporal and the zygomaticotemporal nerves, and the forehead and front of the scalp by the supratrochlear and supraorbital nerves.

Temporal fossa and zygomatic arch

The **temporal fossa** is the area bounded by the temporal lines above and the zygomatic arch below (see Fig. 8.1, p. 525). Its roof (lateral wall) is the temporalis fascia and its floor (medial wall) is the part of the side of the skull that includes the pterion, where the frontal, the parietal and the squamous part of the temporal bones articulate with the greater wing of the sphenoid. (It lies on the course of the anterior branch of the middle meningeal artery and marks the position of the stem of the lateral cerebral fissure.) The zygomatic processes of the frontal bone, the zygomatic bone, and the maxilla are in the anterior wall. The fossa is filled by the temporalis muscle which arises from the floor and the overlying fascia. Deep to the arch, at the level of the infratemporal crest of the greater wing of the sphenoid (Fig. 6.19), the fossa becomes continuous with the lateral part of the infratemporal fossa (see p. 373).

The **zygomatic arch** is formed by processes of the squamous temporal and zygomatic bones, which meet at a suture sloping downwards and backwards. The arch is completed anteriorly by the zygomatic process of the maxilla.

Nerves crossing the arch are vulnerable in incisions or in fractures. The auriculotemporal nerve crosses well back, just in front of the ear, and temporal and zygomatic branches of the facial nerve cross the arch, to reach the frontalis and orbicularis oculi muscles.

The **temporal fascia** (deep temporal fascia) is attached to the superior temporal line and passes down to the upper border of the zygomatic arch. Above the arch it splits into two layers, one attached to the lateral and the other to the medial margin of the upper border of the arch. The space between these two layers is occupied by fat, which is traversed by a branch of the superficial temporal artery and the zygomaticotemporal branch of the maxillary nerve. The temporal and zygomatic branches of the facial nerve, the superficial temporal vessels and the auriculotemporal nerve lie in or just deep to the overlying temporoparietal fascia (superficial temporal fascia, see p. 369). In surgical procedures in this region, the temporal fascia is divided at a high level and the space between its two layers entered from above to access the zygomatic arch, thereby safeguarding the overlying neurovascular structures.

Temporalis

This muscle (one of the muscles of mastication) arises from the temporal fossa over the whole area between the inferior temporal line and the infratemporal crest, and from the deep surface of the temporalis fascia. The most anterior fibres are vertical and the most posterior are horizontal, turning downwards in front of the temporomandibular joint. The fan-shaped muscle converges towards the coronoid process of the mandible, becomes tendinous, and is inserted into a bevelled surface on the medial aspect of the coronoid process adjacent to its posterior border, apex and anterior border. From the anterior part of this insertion, two tendinous bands extend downwards and forwards to the posterior end of the alveolar process enclosing the retromolar fossa between them. The deep, larger tendinous band is attached to a slight (temporal) crest on the mandible, and is palpable through the vestibule of the mouth; a useful guide when performing an inferior alveolar nerve block.

The blood supply of the muscle is derived from the temporal branches of the maxillary and superficial temporal arteries.

Nerve supply. Two or three deep temporal branches of the mandibular nerve enter the deep surface of the muscle.

Action. Temporalis elevates the mandible when the open mouth is closed, and it retracts the protruded mandible.

PART SEVEN

Parotid region

The part of the face in front of the ear and below the zygomatic arch is the parotid region. The principal features are the parotid gland and the masseter muscle.

Masseter

This quadrilateral muscle of mastication arises from the lower border of the zygomatic arch and is inserted into almost the whole of the lateral surface of the mandibular ramus. Most of its fibres slope downwards and backwards at 45°. The posteriormost fibres arise from the deep surface of the arch and pass vertically downwards to be inserted into the upper part of the ramus; these fibres blend with the lower fibres of temporalis. The upper anterior part of the muscle is covered by an aponeurosis on which the parotid duct and the accessory parotid gland lie.

The muscle receives blood supply from branches of the facial artery, maxillary artery and superficial temporal artery, particularly its transverse facial artery. These vessels form an anastomotic network on the surface of and within the muscle.

Nerve supply. By the masseteric branch of the mandibular nerve, which passes through the mandibular notch to enter the deep surface of the gland.

Action. Masseter elevates and draws forwards the angle of the mandible when the jaws are approximated.

The deep fibres assist temporalis in retracting the mandible.

Parotid gland

The parotid gland is the largest of the major salivary glands, i.e. glands that drain saliva into the mouth through ducts. It is a mainly serous gland, with only a few scattered mucous acini. It is a large, irregular, lobulated gland which extends from the zygomatic arch to the upper part of the neck, where it overlaps the posterior belly of digastric and the anterior border of sternocleidomastoid (Fig. 6.16). Anteriorly the gland overlaps masseter and a small, usually detached accessory parotid lies above the parotid duct on the aponeurotic part of masseter. The gland extends below the external acoustic meatus posteriorly onto the mastoid process. In transverse section the gland is wedge-shaped, occupying the gap between the ramus of the mandible and the mastoid and styloid processes of the temporal bone, and reaching close to the lateral wall of the oropharynx; hence the need to look at the region of the fauces when examining a patient with a parotid mass.

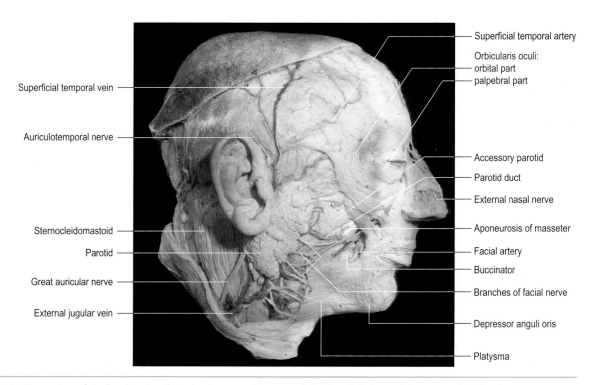

Fig. 6.16 Prosection of the head and neck in the Anatomy Museum of the Royal College of Surgeons of England.

The *lateral* (superficial) *surface* of the gland is covered by skin and superficial fascia. The investing layer of deep cervical fascia splits to envelope the gland and the inner leaf passes up to the base of the skull (see p. 342). The outer leaf extends superiorly as the *parotidomasseteric fascia* and reaches up to the zygomatic arch. On the gland, the fascia tends to be termed the parotid capsule and, more anteriorly, the masseteric fascia. Overlying the gland is a *superficial muscular aponeurotic system* (SMAS), which is continuous above with the temporo-parietal fascia (see p. 369) and frontalis, below with platysma and over the gland with risorius. SMAS is adherent to the parotidomasseteric fascia in the pretragal area and becomes separate from it as the fascia enters the cheek where it overlies the parotid duct, facial nerve branches and buccal fat pad. The nerve branches penetrate the parotidomasseteric fascia as they proceed peripherally to inervate overlying facial muscles. The great auricular nerve supplies the fascia superficial and deep to the parotid gland, and transmits the pain caused by stretching of the fascial envelope when acute enlargement of the gland occurs as in mumps.

The *anteromedial surface* is grooved by the posterior border of the mandibular ramus, and is related to the masseter and medial pterygoid muscles which are attached to the ramus. The gland is also wrapped around the capsule of the temporomandibular joint. The anterior edge of this surface meets the lateral surface over, as well as below, the masseter forming the irregularly convex anterior border of the gland. The parotid duct and the facial nerve branches emerge from the anteromedial surface and run forwards deep to the anterior border. The terminal branches of the external carotid artery (superficial temporal and maxillary) leave this surface further back.

The *posteromedial surface* is in contact with the mastoid process with its attached sternocleidomastoid and posterior belly of digastric muscles. More medially, the styloid process and its attached muscles (stylohoid, stylopharyngeus and styloglossus) separate the gland from the carotid sheath and its contained internal jugular vein and internal carotid artery. The external carotid artery enters the gland through the lower part of this surface. The facial nerve trunk, or its temporofacial and cervicofacial divisions, enter the gland between the mastoid and styloid processes.

Within the gland the branches of the facial nerve run in different directions corresponding with their destinations, i.e. scalp, eyelids, mid-face, lower face and neck, and they do so in different (superficial to deep) planes. There is no specific, developmentally determined plane in which the facial nerve branches pass between superficial and deep lobes of the gland; the parotid is an integral gland, not divided into lobes. Within the gland the nerve branches communicate with each other, forming a plexiform arrangement that lies superficial to the retromandibular vein, which in turn is superficial to the external carotid artery. The retromandibular vein is formed within the parotid by the confluence of the superficial temporal and maxillary veins. The retro-mandibular vein emerges from the lower part (pole) of the gland and divides into an anterior branch which joins the facial vein and a posterior branch which joins the posterior auricular vein to form the external jugular vein; however, the division may occur within the gland and the two branches emerge from the lower pole. Lymph nodes of the preauricular (parotid) group lie on or deep to the fascial capsule of the parotid, as well as within the gland.

The **parotid duct** (of Stensen), about 5 cm long, passes forwards across the masseter and turns around its anterior border to pass through the buccal fat pad and pierce the buccinator. It lies on the middle third of a line between the intertragic notch of the auricle and the midpoint of the philtrum (the vertical midline groove between the nasal septum and the upper lip) and is palpable on the clenched masseter muscle. The duct opens on the mucous membrane of the cheek opposite the second upper molar tooth (Fig. 6.17); it pierces the buccinator further back and runs forwards beneath the mucous membrane to its orifice. When intraoral pressure is raised this submucous part of the duct is compressed between the buccinator and the mucous membrane, preventing inflation of the gland.

An **accessory parotid gland** usually lies on the masseter between the duct and the zygomatic arch. Several ducts open from it into the parotid duct. It and the duct lie on the aponeurotic part of the surface of the masseter muscle.

Blood supply

Branches from the external carotid artery supply the gland. Venous return is to the retromandibular vein.

Lymph drainage

Lymph drains to the preauricular (parotid) nodes and thence to nodes of the upper group of deep cervical nodes.

Nerve supply

Secretomotor fibres arise from cell bodies in the otic ganglion (see p. 24) and reach the gland by 'hitch-hiking' along the auriculotemporal nerve. As it passes backwards

Surgical approach

The most common neoplasm of the parotid gland is a pleomorphic adenoma (mixed parotid tumour) which requires removal with a margin of normal parotid tissue, conserving the facial nerve and its branches. On account of the wide extent of the gland, it is approached through an S-shaped incision made from in front of the ear, backwards to the mastoid process and then downwards and forwards below the angle of the mandible. The gland is retracted forwards from the sternocleidomastoid to expose the posterior belly of digastric and stylohyoid and the cartilage of the external meatus. The facial nerve is approached along a plane in front of the anterior margin of the cartilage. The trunk emerges from the stylomastoid foramen, just deep to the junction of the cartilaginous and bony parts of the external meatus, about 1 cm above and medial to the upper end of the posterior belly of digastric (Fig. 6.18). The cartilage in this region has a slight arrow-headed projection that points downwards to the emerging nerve trunk. The stylomastoid branch of the posterior auricular artery is superficial to the facial nerve and is a guide to its proximity. Once identified, the facial nerve is followed forwards into the gland and the required amount of parotid tissue removed with preservation of facial nerve branches. An alternative approach to facial nerve conservation is to first find a facial nerve branch as it leaves the gland and to follow this in a centripetal manner back to the trunk and other branches. The marginal mandibular branch may be identified as it lies superficial to the retromandibular vein or its anterior branch, aided by the colour contrast between the white nerve and the dark vein; occasionally this branch may pass behind the vein. Alternatively, the cervical branch may be followed up from its communication with the ascending branch of the transverse cervical nerve.

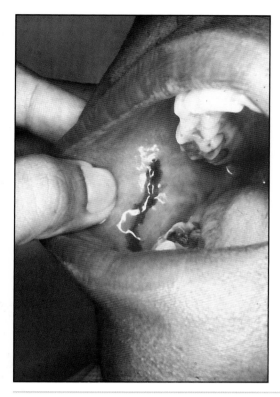

Fig. 6.17 The site of the orifice of the right parotid duct is indicated by the bloody discharge emanating from it in a patient with a malignant parotid tumour. In the absence of a discharge, the tiny orifice is barely visible.

along the mandibular neck and ascends behind the temporomandibular joint, the auriculotemporal nerve is in contact with the anteromedial surface of the gland, which is penetrated by filaments from the nerve. The preganglionic fibres arise from cell bodies in the inferior salivary nucleus in the medulla, and travel by way of the glossopharyngeal nerve, its tympanic branch, the tympanic plexus and the lesser petrosal nerve to the otic ganglion. Sympathetic (vasoconstrictor) fibres reach the gland from the superior cervical ganglion by way of the plexus on the external carotid and middle meningeal arteries.

Development

A groove that appears in the ectoderm of the mouth pit (stomodeum, see p. 30) becomes converted into a tunnel, from the blind end of which cells proliferate to form the gland.

PART EIGHT

Infratemporal region

Infratemporal fossa

This is a space lying beneath the base of the skull between the side wall of the pharynx and the ramus of the mandible. It is also referred to as the parapharyngeal or lateral pharyngeal space.

Boundaries

Its *medial boundary* is the lateral surface of the lateral pterygoid plate with, behind it, the tensor palati muscle

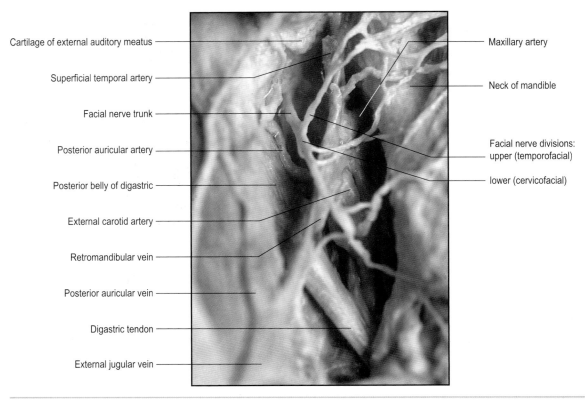

Cartilage of external auditory meatus

Superficial temporal artery

Facial nerve trunk

Posterior auricular artery

Posterior belly of digastric

External carotid artery

Retromandibular vein

Posterior auricular vein

Digastric tendon

External jugular vein

Maxillary artery

Neck of mandible

Facial nerve divisions:
upper (temporofacial)

lower (cervicofacial)

Fig. 6.18   Prosection demonstrating the trunk and proximal branches of the facial nerve, following removal of the parotid gland.

and the superior constrictor. In front of the lateral pterygoid plate, between it and the maxilla, is the pterygo-maxillary fissure through which the infratemporal fossa communicates with the pterygopalatine fossa (see p. 383). The *lateral wall* is the ramus of the mandible and its coronoid process. The *anterior wall* is the posterior surface of the maxilla, at the upper margin of which is a gap between it and the greater wing of sphenoid—the inferior orbital fissure. The *roof* of the fossa is formed medially by the infratemporal surface of the greater wing of the sphenoid (perforated by the foramen ovale and foramen spinosum) and the adjacent squamous part of the temporal bone in front of the articular eminence (Fig. 6.19). This infratemporal surface of the sphenoid is bounded laterally by the infratemporal crest, where the bone takes an almost right-angled turn upwards to become part of the side of the skull, deep to the zygomatic arch and part of the temporal fossa. Thus the roof of the infratemporal fossa lateral to the infratemporal crest is not bony, but is the space deep to the zygomatic arch where the temporal and infratemporal fossae

communicate. The *posterior boundary* is the styloid process with the carotid sheath behind it.

Contents

The fossa contains the deep part of the parotid gland, the medial and lateral pterygoid muscles, the insertion of temporalis into the coronoid process, the maxillary artery and its branches, the pterygoid venous plexus, the mandibular nerve and its branches together with the otic ganglion, the chorda tympani, and the posterior superior alveolar branches of the maxillary nerve.

Lateral pterygoid

This muscle arises by two heads: the upper from the roof of the infratemporal fossa and the lower from the lateral surface of the lateral pterygoid plate. The two heads, lying edge to edge, converge and fuse into a short thick tendon that is inserted into the pterygoid fovea on the front of the neck of the mandible. The upper fibres of

Fig. 6.19 Right infratemporal and palatal regions of the base of the skull. The petrosquamous and petrotympanic fissures lie in front of and behind the tegmen tympani.

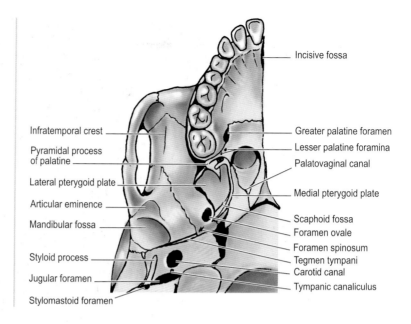

Labels: Incisive fossa; Infratemporal crest; Pyramidal process of palatine; Lateral pterygoid plate; Articular eminence; Mandibular fossa; Styloid process; Jugular foramen; Stylomastoid foramen; Greater palatine foramen; Lesser palatine foramina; Palatovaginal canal; Medial pterygoid plate; Scaphoid fossa; Foramen ovale; Foramen spinosum; Tegmen tympani; Carotid canal; Tympanic canaliculus

the tendon pass back into the capsule and the articular disc of the temporomandibular joint (Fig. 6.20).

Nerve supply. By a branch from the anterior division of the mandibular nerve.

Action. When the muscle contracts it draws condyle and disc forwards from the mandibular fossa down the slope of the articular eminence (Fig. 6.35). It is indispensable to active opening of the mouth. It participates with medial pterygoid in chewing movements.

Medial pterygoid

This muscle also arises by two heads. The larger *deep head* arises from the medial (deep) surface of the lateral pterygoid plate. The muscle diverges down from the lateral pterygoid muscle at nearly a right angle from their common origin on either side of the lateral pterygoid plate (Fig. 6.20). A small slip of muscle, the *superficial head*, arises from the tuberosity of the maxilla and the pyramidal process of the palatine bone which insinuates itself between the tuberosity and the lower end of the lateral pterygoid plate (Fig. 6.13). Passing over the lower margin of the lateral pterygoid muscle, the superficial head fuses with the main muscle mass. In this way the two heads, very unequal in size, embrace the lower edge of the lateral pterygoid. The muscle passes down and back at 45°, and laterally to reach the angle of the mandible. It is inserted into the rough area on the medial surface of the angle as far as the groove for the mylohyoid vessels and nerve (see Fig. 8.5B, p. 533). The muscle is characterized by tendinous intersections on its surface, which account for the roughness of the area of insertion on the mandible.

Nerve supply. By a branch from the main trunk of the mandibular nerve (Fig. 6.21).

Action. The pull of the muscle on the angle of the mandible is upwards, forwards and medially (i.e. it closes the mouth) and it moves the mandible towards the opposite side in chewing. Contracting with its opposite fellow and the two lateral pterygoids, it helps to protrude the mandible.

Maxillary artery

The maxillary artery is, with the superficial temporal artery, a terminal division of the external carotid. It enters the infratemporal fossa by passing forwards deep to the neck of the mandible, between the neck and the sphenomandibular ligament. Here the auriculotemporal nerve lies above it, and the maxillary vein below it. It usually runs deep (sometimes superficial) to the lower head and passes forward between the two heads of the lateral pterygoid muscle (Fig. 6.20). It then passes deeply into the pterygomaxillary fissure and so into the pterygopalatine fossa.

It is described conventionally in three parts, before, on and beyond the lateral pterygoid muscle and this is useful, since five branches come from each part. From first and third parts the five branches all enter foramina in bones, from the second part the branches are mainly muscular.

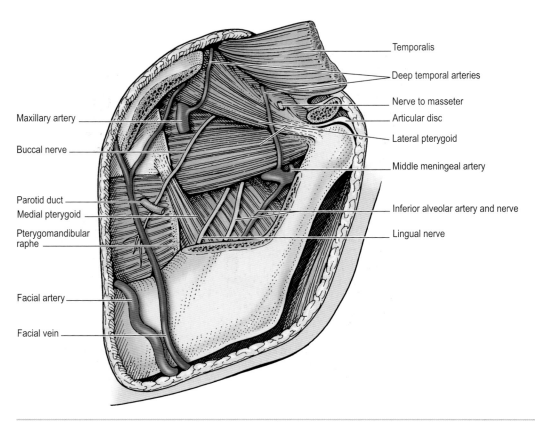

Fig. 6.20 Left pterygoid muscles and related structures.

The five branches from the **first part** are the inferior alveolar, middle meningeal, accessory meningeal and two branches to the ear.

The **inferior alveolar artery** passes downwards and forwards (vein behind it) towards the inferior alveolar nerve, which it meets at the mandibular foramen, into which all three enter. It passes forwards in the mandible, supplying the pulps of the mandibular molar and premolar teeth and the body of the mandible. Its *mental branch* emerges from the mental foramen and supplies the nearby lip and skin.

The **middle meningeal artery** passes vertically upwards to the foramen spinosum. It is embraced by the two roots of the auriculotemporal nerve (Fig. 6.21). Its course and distribution are described on page 459. From the sympathetic plexus on the artery a branch enters the otic ganglion.

The **accessory meningeal artery** passes upwards through the foramen ovale and supplies the dura mater of the floor of the middle fossa and of the trigeminal

(Meckel's) cave. It is the chief source of blood supply to the trigeminal ganglion.

The remaining two arteries pass upwards to enter the ear and run superficial and deep to the tympanic membrane. The **deep auricular artery** is the more superficial of the two and supplies the external acoustic meatus, passing between the cartilage and bone. The deeper is the **anterior tympanic artery** which passes through the petrotympanic fissure to the middle ear to join the circular anastomosis around the tympanic membrane.

The **second part** of the maxillary artery gives off branches to the pterygoid muscles and masseter, and *deep temporal* branches to temporalis which ascend between the muscle and the temporal fossa. A small branch accompanies the buccal nerve.

The **third part** of the maxillary artery, in the pterygopalatine fossa, gives five branches which accompany nerves including branches of the pterygopalatine ganglion (see p. 384). The artery then passes forwards, with the maxillary nerve, through the inferior orbital fissure

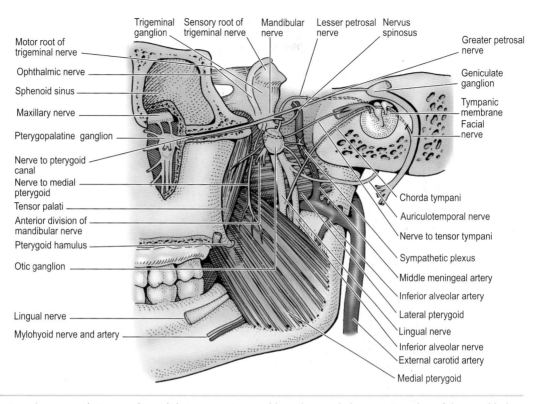

Fig. 6.21 Right otic and pterygopalatine ganglia and their connections and branches: medial aspect. Branches of the mandibular nerve and maxillary artery (first part) are also displayed.

into the orbit as the small **infraorbital artery**, which continues along the floor of the orbit and infraorbital canal to emerge with the infraorbital nerve on the face; its middle (occasional) and anterior superior alveolar branches supply maxillary incisor and canine teeth.

The **sphenopalatine artery** passes through the sphenopalatine foramen to enter the nasal cavity as its main artery of supply (see p. 389). The **posterior superior alveolar artery** gives branches that accompany the corresponding nerves through foramina in the posterior wall of the maxilla. The **greater palatine artery** gives off *lesser palatine branches* to the soft palate and passes through the greater palatine foramen to supply the hard palate (see p. 394). The very small *pharyngeal artery* enters the palatovaginal canal, and the *artery of the pterygoid canal* runs into its own canal.

The **posterior superior alveolar nerve** is a branch of the maxillary, given off in the pterygopalatine fossa and soon dividing into two or three branches which pierce the posterior wall of the maxilla separately. They are distributed to the molar teeth and the mucous membrane of the maxillary sinus. Another branch does

not pierce the bone but runs along the alveolar margin of the maxilla as far forward as the first molar tooth, to supply the gingiva of the vestibule alongside the molar teeth. The posterior superior alveolar nerves can be blocked here by an injection through the vestibule of the mouth; on account of the proximity of the posterior superior alveolar vessels and the pterygoid venous plexus, a haematoma of some size may be a complication.

The **pterygoid plexus** is a network of very small veins that lie around and within the lateral pterygoid muscle. The veins draining into the pterygoid plexus correspond with the branches of the maxillary artery, but they do not return all the arterial blood, much of which returns from the periphery of the area by other routes (facial veins, pharyngeal veins, diploic veins). On the other hand the pterygoid plexus receives the drainage of the *inferior ophthalmic vein* (see p. 419), via the inferior orbital fissure, and the *deep facial vein*. The pterygoid plexus drains into a short **maxillary vein** which lies deep to the neck of the mandible. It runs back to join the superficial temporal vein and form the retromandibular vein. The plexus is valved and acts as a 'peripheral heart', aiding venous return by the pumping action of the lateral pterygoid muscle. Emissary veins connect the pterygoid plexus with the cavernous sinus through the foramen ovale and the foramen lacerum.

The **sphenomandibular ligament** is a flat band of tough fibrous tissue extending from a narrow attachment on the spine of the sphenoid. It broadens as it passes downwards to be attached to the lingula and inferior margin of the mandibular foramen (see Fig. 8.5, p. 533). It is derived from the perichondrium of Meckel's cartilage (see Fig. 1.21, p. 27). Between it and the neck of the mandible pass the auriculotemporal nerve and the maxillary artery and vein. Between it and the ramus of the mandible the inferior alveolar vessels and nerve converge to the mandibular foramen. Any remaining space between the ligament and the mandible is occupied by parotid gland tissue. The ligament is pierced by the mylohyoid nerve, a branch from the inferior alveolar nerve, and the accompanying small mylohyoid artery and vein.

Mandibular nerve

The mandibular branch from the trigeminal ganglion lies in the dura mater of the middle cranial fossa lateral to the cavernous sinus. With the motor root of the trigeminal nerve it enters the foramen ovale, where the two join and emerge as the mandibular nerve (like spinal nerve roots in intervertebral foramina). The nerve lies deep to the upper (infratemporal) head of the lateral pterygoid, between it and the tensor palati muscle, with the otic ganglion applied to the deep surface of the nerve (Fig. 6.21). This point is 4 cm deep to the articular tubercle through the mandibular notch. After a short course the nerve divides into a small anterior (mainly motor) and a large posterior (mainly sensory) branch.

Branches from the main trunk

One sensory and one motor. The **meningeal branch**, or *nervus spinosus*, re-enters the middle cranial fossa via the foramen spinosum, or the foramen ovale, supplying the meninges of the middle cranial fossa, and the mastoid air cells.

The **nerve to the medial pterygoid** runs forwards to the muscle, and gives a branch which passes through the otic ganglion without synapse to supply the two tensor muscles, tensor palati and tensor tympani.

Branches from the anterior division

This division is motor, except for one branch (the buccal nerve).

Two **deep temporal branches** to temporalis pass above the upper border of the lateral pterygoid muscle; one may be a branch of the buccal nerve.

The **masseteric nerve**, passing above the upper border of the lateral pterygoid, emerges through the mandibular notch to enter the deep surface of the masseter. It gives an articular branch to the temporomandibular joint.

The **nerve to the lateral pterygoid** runs with the buccal nerve and supplies both heads of the muscle.

The **buccal nerve** contains all the fibres of common sensation in the anterior division of the mandibular nerve. It emerges between the two heads of the lateral pterygoid (Fig. 6.20) and courses downwards and forwards on the buccinator, giving branches to the skin over the cheek. It then pierces the buccinator (giving proprioceptive fibres to it) and supplies the mucous membrane of the cheek and the gum of the lower jaw opposite the lower molars and second premolar (i.e. up to the mental foramen).

Branches from the posterior division

This division is sensory except for the motor fibres which are distributed via the mylohyoid nerve. There are three branches.

The **auriculotemporal nerve** is derived by two roots from the posterior division; they embrace the middle meningeal artery (Fig. 6.21). The nerve passes backwards between the neck of the mandible and the sphenomandibular ligament, lying above the maxillary vessels. It gives a branch to the temporomandibular joint, and ascends over the lateral aspect of the zygomatic arch behind the superficial temporal vessels (Fig. 6.11). The *auricular* part innervates the skin of the tragus and upper part of the lateral surface of the pinna, the external acoustic meatus and the outer surface of the tympanic membrane. The *temporal* part is distributed to the skin of the temple. The auriculotemporal nerve is in contact with the anteromedial surface of the parotid gland, and supplies it with postganglionic secretomotor fibres from the otic ganglion.

The **inferior alveolar (dental) nerve** emerges below the lower head of the lateral pterygoid and curves down on the medial pterygoid (Fig. 6.20). The nerve lies anterior to its vessels between the sphenomandibular ligament and the ramus of the mandible, and enters the mandibular foramen. It is into this region, just above the foramen, that anaesthetic solution is introduced for inferior alveolar nerve block (see p. 393). The inferior alveolar nerve lies midway between the anterior and posterior borders of the mandibular ramus at the level of the midpoint of the posterior border of the ramus. The *mylohyoid nerve* leaves the inferior alveolar at the

Fig. 6.22   Course of the right lingual nerve from outside the pharynx to within the mouth. In **A**, viewed from within the mouth, the nerve is seen passing under the free lower border of the superior constrictor, which interdigitates with buccinator at the pterygomandibular raphe. In **B**, the nerve is viewed from above, entering the mouth in contact with the periosteum below and behind the third molar tooth.

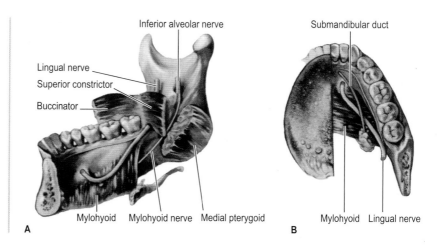

foramen. It pierces the sphenomandibular ligament and lies on a groove on the mandible in front of the insertion of the medial pterygoid (see Fig. 8.5B, p. 533), accompanied by small branches of the inferior alveolar artery and vein. The mylohyoid nerve then runs forward on the superficial (cervical) surface of the mylohyoid supplying it and the anterior belly of the digastric (Fig. 6.6); the nerve often carries sensory fibres from a small area of submental skin and may participate in the sensory supply to lower incisors.

The inferior alveolar nerve runs with its vessels in the mandibular canal. It supplies the three molar and two premolar teeth. Then it divides into the *mental nerve* (see p. 368) and the *incisive nerve*. The latter nerve supplies the pulps and periodontal membranes of the canine and both incisors, with some overlap into the opposite central incisor.

The **lingual nerve** appears below the lateral pterygoid and passes forwards and downwards on the medial pterygoid (Fig. 6.20). It then comes into contact with the mandible, where the bone is thinned to form a shallow groove below and medial to the third molar, just above the posterior end of the mylohyoid line (see Fig. 8.5B, p. 533). This groove separates the attachments of the pterygomandibular raphe above and mylohyoid muscle below (Fig. 6.22). The nerve is characteristically flattened here, rather than round, and it enters the mouth on the superior surface of the mylohyoid. It gives off a gingival branch which supplies all the lingual gum and mucous membrane of the floor of the mouth. The lingual nerve then crosses the submandibular duct (see p. 350) and runs forwards and medially to the tongue.

The **chorda tympani** (from the facial nerve, see p. 434) emerges through the petrotympanic fissure (Fig. 6.35), grooves the medial surface of the spine of the sphenoid, and joins the lingual nerve at an acute angle (Fig. 6.21), 2 cm below the base of the skull, and is distributed with it to the anterior two-thirds of the tongue. It carries all the parasympathetic secretomotor fibres to the submandibular ganglion and all the taste fibres from the anterior two-thirds of the tongue (see p. 397).

Otic ganglion

This small body lies between the tensor palati and the mandibular nerve, just below the foramen ovale. It is a flat plaque, about 2–3 mm in diameter, closely applied to the medial surface of the nerve (Fig. 6.21). It is a relay station for parasympathetic secretomotor fibres to the parotid gland; the lesser petrosal branch of the glossopharyngeal nerve brings these fibres. Postganglionic sympathetic fibres from the plexus around the middle meningeal artery, sensory fibres from the auriculotemporal nerve and a branch from the nerve to the medial pterygoid (to tensor tympani and palati) pass through the ganglion without relay.

Carotid sheath and cranial nerves

Carotid sheath

The carotid sheath extends from the base of the skull to the arch of the aorta. In its upper part it is attached to the margins of the carotid canal and the jugular fossa. It contains here the internal carotid artery and internal jugular vein (see p. 356) and the last four (ninth to twelfth) cranial nerves. Medial to it lies the pharynx; laterally the deepest part of the parotid gland touches the sheath, partly separated by the styloid process and its three muscles. Anteriorly is the infratemporal fossa.

Behind the carotid sheath lies the cervical sympathetic trunk on the prevertebral fascia.

The carotid canal lies immediately in front of the jugular foramen (which lies deep to the external acoustic meatus) with the hypoglossal canal more medially between them. The internal jugular vein lies behind the internal carotid artery at the base of the skull, but slopes as it descends, and at a lower level lies lateral to the common carotid artery as the vessels lie on scalenus anterior. At all levels the vagus nerve lies deep in the groove between the two, within the carotid sheath. The glossopharyngeal and accessory nerves emerge at the base of the skull between artery and vein and immediately curve away from each other superficial to the vessels (Fig. 6.23). The hypoglossal nerve emerges from the hypoglossal canal medial to the sheath. It passes through the sheath behind the inferior vagal ganglion and turns forwards to emerge between the artery and vein.

Glossopharyngeal nerve

The glossopharyngeal nerve emerges from the anterior part of the jugular foramen on the lateral side of the inferior petrosal sinus (see p. 464). It makes a deep notch in the inferior border of the petrous bone and here its inferior ganglion bulges the nerve. The ganglion contains the cell bodies of most sensory fibres in the nerve. The nerve passes down on the lateral aspect of the internal carotid artery and curves forward around the lateral side of stylopharyngeus (Figs 6.23 and 6.41). It passes deep to the external carotid artery and continues forward deep to the hyoglossus and to reach the tongue (see p. 397).

The **tympanic branch** (Jacobson's nerve) leaves the nerve at the jugular fossa and passes through a canaliculus on the ridge of petrous bone between the carotid and jugular foramina (Fig. 6.19) to enter the temporal bone and supply the middle ear, mastoid air cells and

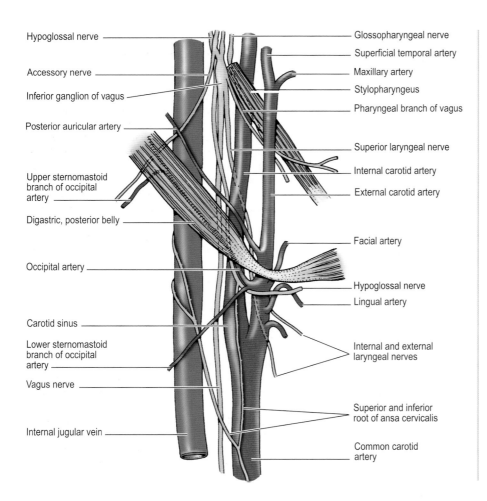

Hypoglossal nerve

Accessory nerve

Inferior ganglion of vagus

Posterior auricular artery

Upper sternomastoid branch of occipital artery

Digastric, posterior belly

Occipital artery

Carotid sinus

Lower sternomastoid branch of occipital artery

Vagus nerve

Internal jugular vein

Glossopharyngeal nerve

Superficial temporal artery

Maxillary artery

Stylopharyngeus

Pharyngeal branch of vagus

Superior laryngeal nerve

Internal carotid artery

External carotid artery

Facial artery

Hypoglossal nerve

Lingual artery

Internal and external laryngeal nerves

Superior and inferior root of ansa cervicalis

Common carotid artery

Fig. 6.23   Right internal jugular vein, carotid arteries and related cranial nerves.

bony part of the auditory tube with sensory fibres. In this branch are also parasympathetic fibres from the inferior salivary nucleus. They run through the tympanic plexus on the promontory and continue in the *lesser petrosal nerve*. This nerve leaves the middle ear through its roof and runs along the floor of the middle cranial fossa to the foramen ovale, through which it passes to reach the otic ganglion (Fig. 6.27). The parasympathetic fibres relay in the otic ganglion for the secretomotor supply of the parotid gland and the other small glands of the vestibule of the mouth.

The **motor branch** to stylopharyngeus is given off as the nerve spirals around the posterior border of that muscle.

The **carotid sinus nerve** is the main supply to the carotid sinus and carotid body (baroreceptors and chemoreceptors.

One or more **pharyngeal branches** join the pharyngeal plexus on the middle constrictor muscle (see p. 400). They pierce the muscle and supply the mucous membrane of the oropharynx with common sensation and (a few) taste fibres.

The **tonsillar branch** supplies the mucous membrane over most of the (palatine) tonsil.

The **lingual** branch supplies the posterior one-third of the tongue with sensory fibres (common sensation and taste) and secretomotor fibres to the glands of the posterior third. These last relay in small ganglia in the mucous membrane.

Vagus nerve

The vagus nerve emerges through the middle compartment of the jugular foramen, in which a small enlargement constitutes the *superior ganglion*. Just below the base of the skull the elongated **inferior ganglion** dilates the trunk. The ganglia contain cell bodies of the afferent fibres of the vagus; the superior ganglion for the meningeal and auricular branches, the inferior ganglion for all the other sensory fibres. Just above the inferior ganglion the vagus is joined by a large branch from the accessory nerve (cranial part), comprising nucleus ambiguus fibres for the skeletal muscle of the soft palate and larynx.

The nerve runs straight down the neck, within the carotid sheath, between and behind carotid (internal and common) artery and jugular vein. In the root of the neck it passes in front of the subclavian artery and so enters the mediastinum (see p. 202) to supply thoracic and abdominal viscera.

Meningeal branches pass up from the superior ganglion to supply the dura mater of the posterior fossa below the tentorium.

The **auricular branch** (Arnold's nerve) runs laterally through a canaliculus in the lateral wall of the jugular fossa. It supplies the posteroinferior quadrant of the outer surface of the tympanic membrane and a small adjacent area of skin of the external acoustic meatus and a little area of skin on the cranial auricular surface.

The very fine **carotid body branch** forms a plexus with the carotid sinus branch of the glossopharyngeal for the supply of those structures.

The **pharyngeal branch** of the vagus passes forward between the internal and external carotid arteries (Fig. 6.23) and joins the pharyngeal plexus on the middle constrictor muscle. The fibres supply the muscles of the pharynx (except stylopharyngeus) and the muscles of the soft palate (except tensor palate, see p. 404).

The **superior laryngeal nerve** slopes downwards on the side wall of the pharynx deep to the internal carotid artery (Fig. 6.23). It divides into a large *internal laryngeal nerve* which pierces the thyrohyoid membrane to reach the piriform recess (see p. 402), carrying sensory fibres for the pharynx and larynx, and a small *external laryngeal nerve* which runs down close to the superior thyroid vessels, outside the larynx, to supply cricothyroid and contribute to the supply of the inferior constrictor.

The **cervical cardiac branches** are two on each side. They all pass down to the deep part of the cardiac plexus (see p. 200), except for the lower left branch which goes to the superficial part of the plexus.

The **recurrent laryngeal nerve** on the right hooks around the subclavian artery at the root of the neck (Fig. 6.9). Thence it runs up to ascend along the posterior border of the trachea and pass under the lower border of the inferior constrictor. On the left side the recurrent laryngeal nerve is given off in the superior mediastinum and recurves around the ligamentum arteriosum under the arch of the aorta (see Fig. 4.13, p. 199). Both nerves have cardiac branches, and also supply the trachea, oesophagus and the cricopharyngeus part of the inferior constrictor, before entering the pharynx and larynx to supply the laryngeal muscles (except cricothyroid) and the laryngeal mucosa from the vocal folds downwards (see p. 411).

Accessory nerve

The accessory nerve is formed in the posterior cranial fossa by union of *cranial* and *spinal* (cervical) *roots*. The nerve occupies the middle compartment in the jugular foramen, just lateral to the vagus, with which it shares a meningeal sleeve. All the fibres of its cranial root leave the nerve in a branch which joins the vagus. The nerve, now consisting of cervical fibres only, runs downwards and backwards on the internal jugular vein (Fig. 6.23), where the latter lies on the transverse process of the atlas; the nerve crosses lateral (usually) or medial to the vein.

It passes deep to the styloid process and posterior belly of the digastric, where it is crossed by the occipital artery. With the upper sternocleidomastoid branch of the occipital artery it reaches the sternocleidomastoid, supplies it and enters its deep surface. Emerging from the posterior border of the muscle it crosses the posterior triangle (see p. 345) to supply trapezius.

Hypoglossal nerve

The hypoglossal nerve emerges from the hypoglossal canal. It picks up a branch from the anterior ramus of C1 and then spirals behind the inferior ganglion of the vagus to emerge between the internal carotid artery and internal jugular vein, passing through the carotid sheath. It then descends on the carotid sheath, deep to the styloid muscles and the posterior belly of digastric. It is crossed by the occipital artery and its lower sterno-cleidomastoid branch and then turns forwards, superficial to both carotid arteries and the loop of the lingual artery (Fig. 6.23), just above the tip of the greater horn of the hyoid bone. It continues forwards on the hyoglossus (Fig. 6.24), accompanied by veins draining the tip of the tongue, to supply tongue muscles.

The C1 fibres that join the hypoglossal nerve leave it progressively in the superior root of the ansa cervicalis and in the branches to thyrohyoid and geniohyoid. The small meningeal branch which enters the posterior fossa through the hypoglossal canal also comprises C1 fibres.

Styloid apparatus

The **styloid process** is a part of the temporal bone. From its tip the *stylohyoid ligament* passes to the lesser horn of the hyoid bone (Fig. 6.24). Both process and ligament are remnants of the second pharyngeal arch cartilage (see p. 27). Hence the styloid process is very variable in length, the ligament varying likewise, inversely with it.

Three muscles diverge from the styloid process and are described elsewhere. The **stylopharyngeus** (see p. 400) arises highest from the medial side of the base of the process and passes downwards to the larynx. The **stylohyoid** (see p. 347) arises from the posterior surface near the base, and the **styloglossus** (see p. 396) from in front low down and from the upper end of the stylohyoid ligament; they diverge as they pass downwards and forwards to the hyoid bone and side of the tongue respectively. Each of the three muscles has a different nerve supply. They all act significantly during swallowing.

The styloid apparatus (process and muscles) lies lateral to the carotid sheath. The external carotid artery passes between the muscles of the stylohyoid apparatus. It runs up deep to digastric and stylohyoid, but superficial to stylopharyngeus (Fig. 6.23), to enter the parotid gland. The retromandibular vein, on the other hand, passes down from the parotid gland superficial to stylohyoid and digastric.

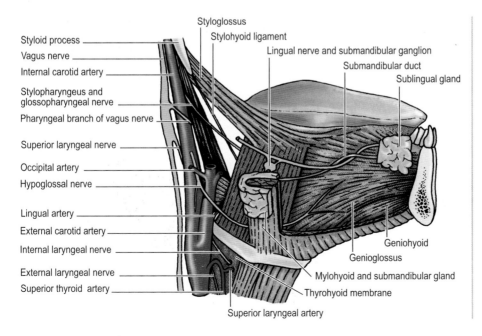

Styloglossus
Stylohyoid ligament
Lingual nerve and submandibular ganglion
Submandibular duct
Sublingual gland

Styloid process
Vagus nerve
Internal carotid artery
Stylopharyngeus and glossopharyngeal nerve
Pharyngeal branch of vagus nerve
Superior laryngeal nerve
Occipital artery
Hypoglossal nerve
Lingual artery
External carotid artery
Internal laryngeal nerve
External laryngeal nerve
Superior thyroid artery

Geniohyoid
Genioglossus
Mylohyoid and submandibular gland
Thyrohyoid membrane
Superior laryngeal artery

Fig. 6.24 Right styloid process and submandibular region. The right half of the mandible and part of the submandibular and sublingual glands have been removed. The glossopharyngeal nerve, stylohyoid ligament and lingual artery pass deep to the posterior border of hyoglossus; the lingual nerve, submandibular duct and hypoglossal nerve are superficial to hyoglossus.

PART NINE

Pterygopalatine fossa

At the anterior end of the medial wall of the infratemporal fossa the lateral pterygoid plate is separated from the maxilla by the *pterygomaxillary fissure*, which leads into the small pterygopalatine fossa. At the bottom of the fissure, the pyramidal process of the palatine bone articulates with the lateral pterygoid plate and maxilla closing off the fissure and forming the narrow floor of the pterygopalatine fossa (Fig. 6.13). The roof is the body of the sphenoid. Medially the fossa is walled in by the perpendicular plate of the palatine bone (Fig. 6.25), part of the lateral wall of the nose (Fig. 6.31A). This plate splits at the top into an orbital process and a sphenoidal process which, with the roof of the fossa, bound the sphenopalatine foramen that communicates with the nasal cavity. The perpendicular plate articulates with the maxilla and between the two lies the greater palatine canal which opens below at a foramen on the hard palate. The posterior wall of the maxilla forms the anterior wall of the fossa, which is interrupted at the top by the medial end of the inferior orbital fissure that opens into the orbit. The pterygopalatine fossa is bounded posteriorly by the sphenoid bone (root of the pterygoid process containing the pterygoid canal and greater wing containing the foramen rotundum; Fig. 6.26).

The fossa contains the maxillary vessels and nerve and the pterygopalatine ganglion and fat (Figs 6.20 and 6.26). The ganglion sends branches into the nose, palate and nasopharynx. The maxillary nerve supplies the posterior, upper teeth and passes forwards into the orbit. Branches of the maxillary vessels accompany all these nerves.

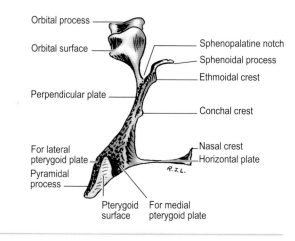

Fig. 6.25   Left palatine bone, from behind.

Maxillary nerve

The maxillary nerve, giving a meningeal branch to the front of the middle cranial fossa, passes through the foramen rotundum in the greater wing of the sphenoid bone into the pterygopalatine fossa. Deviating laterally in the inferior orbital fissure for about 1 cm, it turns forwards to enter the infraorbital groove and canal in the floor of the orbit, changing its name to the **infra-orbital nerve** and eventually emerging from the front end of the canal at the infraorbital foramen to supply skin on the face (see p. 367). The **zygomatic nerve** arises from the maxillary in the fossa and runs above the maxillary in the inferior orbital fissure to enter the orbit (see p. 417). The **posterior superior alveolar nerve** is also given off in the fossa. It passes through the pterygomaxillary fissure on to the posterior wall of the maxilla (see p. 377).

Fig. 6.26   Sphenoid bone, from the front.

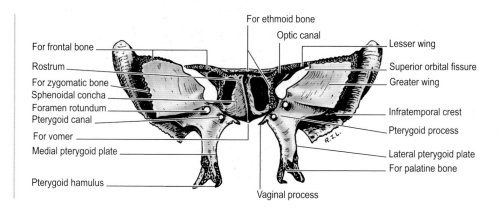

In the fossa the maxillary nerve is connected to the pterygopalatine ganglion by two branches that carry fibres going both to and from the ganglion.

Pterygopalatine ganglion

The pterygopalatine ganglion is a relay station between the superior salivary nucleus in the pons and the lacrimal gland and mucous and serous glands of the palate, nose and paranasal sinuses. It is the ganglion of hay fever ('running nose and eyes'). Its connections are summarized on page 23.

The ganglion lies immediately in front of the opening of the pterygoid canal and the nerve of that canal runs straight into the back of the ganglion. The canal is below and medial to the foramen rotundum (Fig. 6.26), and so is the ganglion in relation to the maxillary nerve.

The autonomic root is the **nerve of the pterygoid canal** (Vidian nerve). This nerve is formed in the foramen lacerum by union of the *greater petrosal nerve* (see p. 434), containing mainly parasympathetic secretomotor fibres, with the *deep petrosal nerve*, containing sympathetic vasoconstrictor fibres. The former is a branch of the facial nerve and the latter is a branch from the internal carotid sympathetic plexus. The combined nerve passes forward in the pterygoid canal and joins the ganglion.

The postganglionic secretomotor fibres to the lacrimal gland leave the ganglion and join the maxillary nerve, pass in its zygomatic branch into the orbit, join the lacrimal branch of the ophthalmic nerve and so reach the lacrimal gland.

The rest of the fibres in the connections between the maxillary nerve and the ganglion are sensory and, like the sympathetic fibres in the deep petrosal nerve, they pass through the ganglion without relay. The only cell bodies in the ganglion are parasympathetic (secretomotor). The branches of the pterygopalatine ganglion are distributed to the nose, palate and nasopharynx. Every branch carries a mixture of all three kinds of fibres: sensory, secretomotor and sympathetic.

Medial posterior superior nasal nerves pass through the sphenopalatine foramen, cross the roof of the nose, and are distributed to the septum. The largest of these is termed the **nasopalatine nerve**, as it continues beyond the septum through the incisive canal to supply the anterior part of the hard palate.

The **lateral posterior superior nasal nerves** pass through the sphenopalatine foramen and turn forward to supply the posterosuperior part of the lateral wall of the nose.

The **greater palatine nerve** passes down through the greater palatine canal, between the perpendicular plate of the palatine bone and the maxilla (Fig. 6.27). At the greater palatine foramen it turns forward to supply the mucous membrane of the hard palate. As it descends it also supplies the posteroinferior part of the lateral wall of the nose and the medial wall of the maxillary sinus.

The **lesser palatine nerves**, two in number, pass down behind the greater palatine nerve and emerge through the lesser palatine foramina. They pass back to the soft palate and the mucous membrane of the palatine tonsil. They carry the only non-secretomotor fibres transmitted in the greater petrosal nerve; these are sensory (taste) fibres that have their cell bodies in the genicular ganglion of the facial nerve.

The **pharyngeal nerve** passes back through the palato-vaginal canal (a little canal between the vaginal process of the medial pterygoid plate and the sphenoidal process of the palatine bone) and supplies the mucous membrane of the nasopharynx. A few fine **orbital branches** enter the orbit via the inferior orbital fissure and supply periosteum of the orbital floor and the mucous membrane of the sphenoidal and ethmoidal sinuses.

Maxillary vessels

The **maxillary artery** passes through the pterygomaxillary fissure, enters the pterygopalatine fossa in front of the ganglion and gives off five branches. These and the artery's further course into the orbit are described on page 376. The branches of the maxillary artery in the pterygopalatine fossa may be ligated by an approach through the maxillary sinus (see p. 390), the fossa being entered instrumentally through the posterior wall of the sinus. An alternative endoscopic approach is via the sphenopalatine foramen.

Veins accompany the above arteries and, passing through the fossa, emerge at the pterygomaxillary fissure to drain into the pterygoid plexus. In general, vessels in the fossa lie anterior to the nerves.

PART TEN

Nose and paranasal sinuses

The nose is for breathing; the design of its cavity results in warming and moistening the inspired air, and in cleaning it too. Since odours are airborne, the olfactory receptors are placed in the nose. The floor of the nose is the hard palate. Hence chewing can go on in the mouth cavity without interfering with breathing; the flap valve of the soft palate, in the dependent position, meanwhile shuts off the mouth cavity from the airway through the oropharynx. Breathing is arrested during swallowing; the soft palate is elevated and shuts off the nose (i.e. the nasopharynx) from the foodway through the oropharynx.

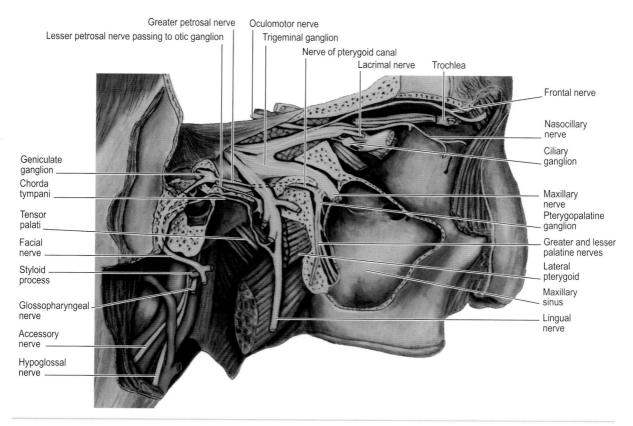

Fig. 6.27 Right trigeminal and geniculate ganglia, petrosal nerves and pterygopalatine and otic ganglia, from the right. Much of the right side of the skull has been removed, including most of the maxillary sinus, leaving only its medial wall.

Thus the oropharynx is the crossroads of airway and foodway; collisions between air stream and food are avoided by the control mechanism of the soft palate acting as the policeman on point duty.

The **nose** consists of the *external nose* and the *nasal cavity,* which is divided into right and left halves by the midline *nasal septum.*

External nose

The external nose projects forwards from the face. Its upper end or *root* is continuous with the forehead. At its lower end (base) are the *nares* (nostrils). The sides of the nose meet in the midline anteriorly to form the *dorsum.* The upper part of the dorsum is the *bridge* and at the lower end of the dorsum is the *tip* of the nose. The lower flared part of the side of the nose is the *ala.*

The supporting framework of the nose consists of bone and cartilage. The upper part is supported by the pair of **nasal bones** articulating posteriorly with the

maxillae and above with the frontal bones. Inferiorly the nasal bones overlap the superior margins of the (upper) **lateral cartilages**, with fusion of their periosteum and perichondrium. In their lower parts the lateral cartilages are separated by a cleft in which the septal cartilage extends to the dorsum of the nose. The lateral cartilages are connected to the maxillae posteriorly and to the **major alar** (lower lateral) **cartilages** inferiorly by fibrous tissue. The latter cartilages are markedly curved, being bent upon themselves towards the nasal cavity, each having a lateral crus that supports the ala and a medial crus which, with its fellow of the opposite side, forms the *columella* that separates the nares in the midline. The lateral crus does not reach the margin of the naris, the rim being formed by fibrofatty tissue. The same tissue connects the posterior end of the lateral crus to the maxilla and two or three **minor alar cartilages** lie here.

The **skin** of the nose is thinnest at its upper part where it is loosely attached to the nasal bones and the upper lateral cartilages. The skin is thickest at the lower part where it has an abundance of sebaceous glands and is tightly bound down to the alar cartilages. The muscles of the nose are described with the muscles of the face on page 363.

The skin is supplied by the external nasal nerve (the terminal part of the anterior ethmoidal, which notches the inner surface of the nasal bone); this nerve emerges at the lower margin of the nasal bone and passes down on the upper and lower nasal cartilages to the tip of the nose. The infratrochlear branch of the nasociliary nerve and nasal branches of the infraorbital nerve also contribute to the supply of nasal skin (Fig. 6.15A).

The blood supply is by the dorsal nasal artery (a terminal branch of the ophthalmic) at the root, and lower down by the external nasal artery (from the anterior ethmoidal) and by lateral nasal and septal branches of the facial artery and its superior labial branch.

Nasal cavity

The **nasal cavity** extends from the nares, through the external nose and between the bones of the face, as far back as the posterior nasal apertures or choanae (between the posterior borders of the medial pterygoid plates of the sphenoid and the vomer), where the nasal cavity communicates with the nasopharynx (see p. 401).

The **lateral wall** is formed mainly by the *maxilla*. But the maxilla has a large defect on its medial aspect (Fig. 6.28). Several bones contribute towards closing this defect and thereby form part of the lateral wall of the nose. The *perpendicular plate of the palatine bone* does so posteriorly and beyond this the *medial pterygoid plate*, with which it articulates, extends as far back as the choana (Fig. 6.31A). The sphenopalatine foramen at the top of the perpendicular plate provides a portal for neurovascular communication between the nasal cavity and the pterygopalatine fossa (see p. 383). The *labyrinth (lateral mass) of the ethmoid bone* occupies much of the upper part of the maxillary hiatus. The *inferior concha* lies below it, articulating anteriorly with the maxilla and posteriorly with the palatine bone. The superior and middle conchae are part of the ethmoidal labyrinth. These conchae (traditionally, and often clinically, termed turbinates) are curved shelves of bone which project into the nasal cavity from their attachments on the lateral wall. Each partly encloses a passage, the meatus, under its concave inferior surface (Figs 6.29 and 6.30). A depression in front of the middle concha, the atrium,

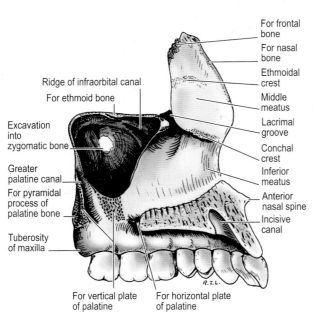

Fig. 6.28 Left maxilla, from the medial side.

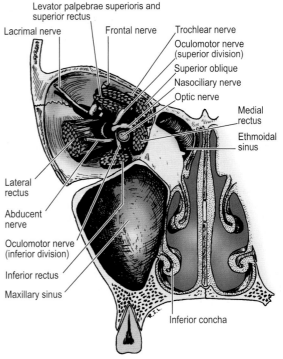

Fig. 6.29 Coronal section of the nasal cavity, right orbit and maxillary sinus, from the front at the level of the second premolar tooth.

Fig. 6.30 Lateral wall of the left half of the nasal cavity and nasopharynx. In the lower figure parts of the conchae have been removed to show the openings of the sinuses and the nasolacrimal duct.

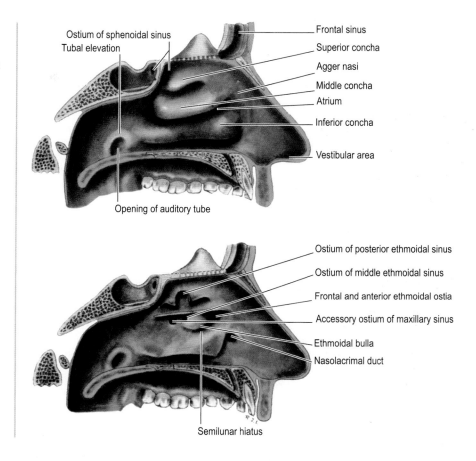

Ostium of sphenoidal sinus
Tubal elevation
Frontal sinus
Superior concha
Agger nasi
Middle concha
Atrium
Inferior concha
Vestibular area
Opening of auditory tube

Ostium of posterior ethmoidal sinus
Ostium of middle ethmoidal sinus
Frontal and anterior ethmoidal ostia
Accessory ostium of maxillary sinus
Ethmoidal bulla
Nasolacrimal duct
Semilunar hiatus

leads upwards into the meatus behind it. The atrium is bounded anteriorly and above by a ridge, the agger nasi, which may contain a few ethmoidal air cells. The antero-superior part of the lateral wall is formed by the *nasal bone* and the frontal process of the maxilla. The *lacrimal bone* articulates with the latter and with the inferior concha, enclosing between them the canal for the naso-lacrimal duct, which opens into the upper part of the inferior meatus about 1 cm behind the anterior end of the concha.

The medial wall, or **nasal septum**, consists of bone and cartilage. The triangular *vomer*, articulating above with the sphenoid body, forms the posterior border of the septum (Fig. 6.31B). Inferiorly it is slotted into a grooved ridge on the hard palate and extends beyond the incisive canal. The vomer is grooved on each side by the nasopalatine nerves. The *perpendicular plate of the ethmoid* articulates with the upper margin of the vomer but not throughout its length. The *septal cartilage*, the unossified part of the ethmoid's perpendicular plate, forms the anterosuperior part of the septum. Inferiorly

it is slotted into a bony groove at its vomerine and maxillary articulations. The nasal septum is frequently deviated from the midline and small bony spurs may project from the septal surface into the nasal cavity. The anteroinferior corner of the septum is mobile, being formed by the medial crura of the paired major alar cartilages.

The **floor** of the nose is the upper surface of the hard palate, which forms the roof of the mouth, and comprises the palatal process of the *maxilla* and the horizontal plate of the *palatine bone*. Anteriorly on either side of the septum a small opening leads to an incisive canal traversed by the nasopalatine nerve and the greater palatine artery.

The central part of the **roof** is the *cribriform plate of the ethmoid*. At the front, sloping downwards, are the nasal spine of the *frontal bone* and the *nasal bones*. At the back is the sloping anterior aspect of the *sphenoid body*.

The **nasal cavity** is piriform, or pear-shaped, broader below and narrow at the top. Nasal intubation for

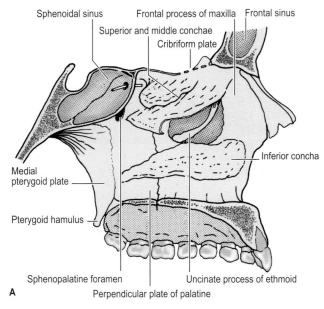

A

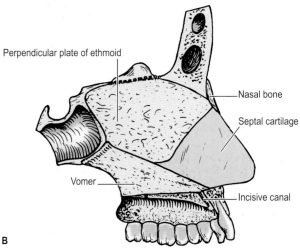

B

Fig. 6.31 Skeleton of the nose: **A** the lateral wall of the left side of the nasal cavity. Part of the middle concha and the ethmoidal bulla have been removed to show the uncinate process of the ethmoid. There is a marker in the ostium of the sphenoidal sinus; **B** the nasal septum from the right.

anaesthetic purposes is therefore more easily performed along an inferior meatus. The conchae project into the nasal cavity with increasing prominence from above downwards, so that the distances between conchae and septum are about equal. The lateral walls are roughly

semicircular in shape and the nasal cavity is correspondingly tallest halfway along, where the cribiform plate forms the roof. The surface marking of the cribiform plate is the horizontal plane on which the pupils lie as the eyes gaze directly forwards.

The *skin* of the external nose is reflected around the naris to line the vestibule, the part of the nasal cavity bounded by the ala. The skin here bears stiff hairs. The mucocutaneous junction is marked by a crescentic infolding, the limen nasi, which coincides with the upper margin of the major alar cartilage. The mucous membrane lining the roof and the upper part of the septum and lateral wall (covering the superior concha but not below it) is *olfactory epithelium*. This is neuroepithelium containing the bipolar cells of the primary receptor neurons of the olfactory pathway; their dendrites are directed towards the nasal cavity and their axons pass up through the cribiform plate, gathered together in about 20 bundles. Olfactory mucous membrane also has supporting cells and subepithelial mucus-secreting glands. It is thicker and of a lighter (yellowish-brown) colour than the rest of the (pink) nasal mucous membrane which is respiratory in type, i.e. pseudostratified ciliated columnar epithelial cells interpersed with goblet cells. In addition there are subepithelial mucous and serous glands. Mucous secretion traps particulate matter and ciliary action wafts the mucous film back into the nasopharynx. The watery secretion of serous glands evaporates to moisten the inspired air. The mucous membrane is very vascular, with large venous sinusoids and arteriovenous shunts, especially over the inferior concha and the lower part of the septum; this helps to warm the inspired air. The mucous membrane of the nose is adherent to the underlying periosteum or perichondrium of the nasal walls, and when a submucous resection is performed surgically mucoperichondrium and mucoperiosteum are elevated before resection of septal cartilage and bone.

The **sphenoethmoidal recess** lies above and behind the superior concha. It receives the ostium of the sphenoidal air sinus.

The **superior concha** is small. It extends posteriorly from its junction with the middle concha. Its lower edge is free and overlies the **superior meatus**, into which drain the posterior ethmoidal air cells.

The **middle concha** is midway in size and position between superior and inferior. It extends back from its junction with the superior concha. It overhangs the middle meatus, which can be seen only when the concha is displaced (Fig. 6.30). Immediately behind the posterior end of the middle concha beneath the mucous membrane is the sphenopalatine foramen. The flat area in front of the concha is the atrium of the nose.

The **middle meatus** presents a convex bulge beneath the concha. This is the *ethmoidal bulla* of the ethmoid, produced by the bulging of middle ethmoidal air cells, which open on or above the bulla (Fig. 6.30). Anterior to the bulla is a curved two-dimensional slit, the *hiatus semilunaris*, between the anterior surface of the bulla and the posterior edge of the uncinate process (a thin, hook-like bony leaflet which projects posteroinferiorly from the ethmoidal labyrinth; Fig. 6.31A). The hiatus semilunaris leads into the ethmoidal *infundibulum*, a curved cleft bordered medially by the uncinate process and laterally by the orbital plate of the ethmoid. The infundibulum extends upwards and forwards and is frequently continuous with the *frontonasal recess* into which the frontal sinus often opens (Fig. 6.32). The anterior ethmoidal cells open into the infundibulum or the frontonasal recess. The maxillary sinus ostium is usually on the lateral aspect of the infundibulum between its middle and posterior third; an accessory ostium may be present anterior or posterior to the lower part of the uncinate process.

The attachment of the middle concha, referred to by rhinologists as the ground (basal) lamella of the middle turbinate, is considered to divide the ethmoidal air cells into anterior and posterior ethmoidal systems (Fig. 6.32). The anterior part of the attachment lies sagittally at the lateral edge of the cribriform plate. The middle part turns laterally across the skull base to the orbital plate where it turns inferiorly and the posterior part is attached horizontally. The area under the middle turbinate into which

the maxillary sinus, frontal sinus and anterior ethmoidal system open is termed the ostiomeatal complex.

Blood supply

The main artery of the nasal cavity is the **sphenopalatine** branch of the maxillary artery, which enters the nose through the sphenopalatine foramen. It supplies the mucosa over the conchae and the meatuses, and also much of the septum. It anastomoses with the septal branch of the superior labial (entering through the nostril) and the ascending branch of the greater palatine (entering through the incisive canal) so forming Kieselbach's plexus, on the lower anterior part of the septum (Little's area), a common site for epistaxis (nosebleed). Anterior and posterior ethmoidal branches of the ophthalmic artery enter the nose from the orbit and supply the roof and upper parts of the lateral wall and septum. Thus both external and internal carotid artery systems supply the nose.

Veins accompany the arteries and drain in various directions to the pterygoid plexus, facial vein and ophthalmic veins. Rarely (1%) an emissary vein may traverse the foramen caecum in front of the cribriform plate and connect nasal veins with the superior sagittal sinus.

Lymph drainage

Lymphatics drain to submandibular, retropharyngeal and deep cervical nodes.

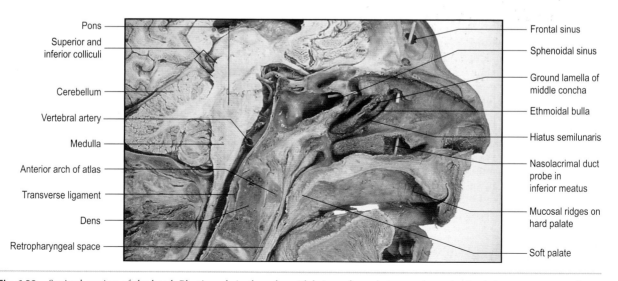

Fig. 6.32 Sagittal section of the head. Plastic rods in the sphenoidal sinus, frontal sinus and nasolacrimal duct are seen entering the sphenoethmoidal recess, middle meatus and inferior meatus. The soft palate is elevated, as in the act of swallowing.

Nerve supply

The *olfactory area* of the roof, and upper parts of the lateral walls and septum are supplied by the olfactory nerves.

The *vestibular area* is supplied by the infraorbital nerve from the face. The *respiratory area* of the lateral wall is supplied at the front by the anterior ethmoidal nerve (from the orbit) in the upper part, and in the lower part by filaments from the anterior superior alveolar nerve (through the wall of the maxillary sinus); at the upper back part by the lateral posterior superior nasal branches from the pterygopalatine ganglion (through the sphenopalatine foramen); and at the lower back part by the posterior inferior nasal branches of the greater palatine nerve (through foramina in the perpendicular plate of the ethmoid bone).

The nerves supplying the *septum* are the olfactory in the upper part, anterior ethmoidal at the front and medial posterior superior nasal, including the nasopalatine, at the back.

Paranasal sinuses

Certain bones that form the boundaries of the nasal cavities are hollowed out. The cavities so produced, the paranasal sinuses, are lined with respiratory mucous membrane, and they communicate by small apertures (ostia) with the nasal cavity. They may thus contribute to warming and humidifying inspired air. They may also allow enlargement of certain areas of the skull, thereby determining the position of the eyes and nose, while minimizing corresponding increase of bone mass.

All the sinuses are lined with respiratory mucous membrane, incorporating a sensory nerve supply; the region of the ostium is the most sensitive part, with the main part of each sinus being relatively insensitive. The glands produce a film of mucus which is moved by the cilia in spiral fashion towards the ostium. The mucous membrane is thinner, less vascular and less adherent to adjacent periosteum than in the nasal cavity.

There are four (bilateral) sinuses. The maxillary and ethmoidal sinuses are beside the lateral walls of the nose. The frontal and sphenoidal sinuses are above and behind the nose; they abut at the midline, separated by a bony septum that is almost always off centre, causing asymmetry of these sinuses.

Maxillary sinus

The maxillary sinus is the space within the body of the maxilla, previously known as the maxillary antrum (of Highmore). The sinus is pyramidal in shape, with the apex in the zygomatic process of the maxilla and the base at the lateral wall of the nose. The roof of the sinus is the floor of the orbit. The floor of the sinus is the alveolar part (tooth-bearing area) of the maxilla; in adults it lies at a lower level than the floor of the nose. Behind the posterior wall are the infratemporal and pterygopalatine fossae. In front of the maxilla is the cheek. A ridge projecting into the cavity at the junction of roof and anterior wall is produced by the downward passage of the infraorbital nerve within its canal (Fig. 6.28).

The maxillary sinus is present at birth, but is no more than a shallow slit just beneath the medial side of the floor of the orbit. The body of the neonatal maxilla lateral to this is full of developing teeth. The sinus increases in size and after the second dentition, about the age of 8 years, the floor of the sinus is level with the floor of the nose. Rapid growth of the sinus occurs after puberty and the adult sinus varies in size; a large one may extend into the zygomatic process of the maxilla and into the alveolar process so that the roots of the molar teeth (and possibly of the premolars also) lie immediately beneath the floor or project into it. The roots are usually enclosed in a thin layer of bone; when this is absent the apex of the root is in contact with the mucous membrane. This is more likely to occur in old age, when 'growth' of a sinus is due to resorption of surrounding bone. Extraction of such a tooth leaves a fistula by rupture of the mucous membrane. These fistulae mostly heal spontaneously.

The *ostium* of the sinus is high up and well back on its nasal wall (Fig. 6.27). It is 2–4 mm in diameter. It opens at the posterior part of the infundibulum in the middle meatus of the lateral wall of the nose. An accessory ostium may open anterior or posterior to the lower part of the uncinate process (Fig. 6.30). The wall of the sinus adjacent to the ostia may only consist of mucosa and periosteum; these areas are called fontanelles.

Blood supply is by small arteries that pierce the bone from the facial, maxillary, infraorbital and greater palatine arteries; veins accompany these vessels to the facial vein and to the pterygoid plexus. *Lymph drainage* is to submandibular nodes. *Nerve supply* is from the infraorbital and superior alveolar (posterior, middle and anterior) branches of the maxillary nerve. These alveolar nerves run down to the teeth in the walls of the sinus, and as they do so minute branches pierce the bone to supply the mucous membrane of the sinus.

The *surgical approaches* for drainage of the maxillary sinus include access through the lateral wall of the nose at the inferior meatus, and through the vestibule of the mouth at the canine fossa of the maxilla. Using flexible endoscopes drainage can also be effected by increasing the size of a natural ostium. This is functionally more effective as the cilia waft secretions towards the ostium; the procedure is a part of functional endoscopic sinus surgery (FESS).

Ethmoidal sinus

Each ethmoidal sinus lies between the orbit and the nose (Fig. 6.29), in the ethmoidal labyrinth (lateral part of the ethmoid bone). The sinus is not a single cavity, being divided by bony septa into a variable number of *ethmoidal air cells* (sometimes themselves called sinuses). There may be only three or as many as 18, each with their own ostium, and they are called anterior, middle or posterior according to where they drain. The lateral wall of the labyrinth, in the medial wall of the orbit, is paper-thin (the lamina papyracea). The superior and middle nasal conchae project from its medial (nasal) wall. The labyrinth does not have its own roof but is closed in by the orbital part of the frontal bone (Fig. 6.39), whose medial edge articulates with the cribriform plate of the ethmoid. The anterior and posterior ethmoidal nerves pass between the roof of frontal bone and the ethmoid itself.

The *anterior ethmoidal air cells* occupy the anterior part of the sinus. Roofed in by the frontal bone, the bony walls are completed by the lacrimal bone. The *ostia* usually open into the infundibulum in the middle meatus; or else may open into the frontonasal recess that drains the frontal sinus. One or more cells may lie further forwards in the agger nasi.

The *middle ethmoidal air cells* also drain into the middle meatus. One or more project as a convexity into the lateral wall of the nose under cover of the middle concha, forming the *ethmoidal bulla*. Ostia on or above the bulla open into the middle meatus.

The anterior and middle ethmoidal air cells, situated in front of the ground lamella, of the middle turbinate are considered to constitute an anterior ethmoidal system.

At the back of the labyrinth the wall of the *posterior ethmoidal air cells* are completed by fusion of the orbital process of the palatine bone and the sphenoidal concha (Figs 6.25 and 6.26). The *ostia* of the posterior air cells open into the superior meatus. The most posterior air cell may extend far enough back to lie immediately adjacent to the optic nerve in its canal (a surgically important relationship).

Blood supply is by branches from the supraorbital, anterior and posterior ethmoidal and sphenopalatine arteries. *Lymph drainage* is to submandibular and retropharyngeal nodes. *Nerve supply* is from the supraorbital, anterior and posterior ethmoidal, lateral posterior superior nasal nerves and orbital twigs from the pterygopalatine ganglion. Hence both ophthalmic and maxillary branches of the trigeminal receive fibres from the ethmoidal sinus, with the possibility of referred pain to either branch.

Sphenoidal sinus

The pair of sphenoidal sinuses occupy the body of the sphenoid bone (Figs 6.30 and 6.26). The two are separated by a septum which is usually not in the midline, and they can vary greatly in size. When small the sinus lies in front of the pituitary fossa; as it enlarges it lies beneath the fossa and may extend back into the basiocciput. A large sinus may also extend into the greater wing of sphenoid and pterygoid process. At birth the sinuses are minute and their main development occurs after puberty.

A typical sinus is related above to the pituitary fossa and middle cranial fossa, and laterally to the cavernous sinus and internal carotid artery. Behind lie the posterior cranial fossa and pons, while below is the roof of the nasopharynx. One or both sinuses may be closely related to and even indented superolaterally by the optic canal with the optic nerve; laterally by the internal carotid artery; and inferiorly by the pterygoid canal with its nerve.

The *ostium* is in the anterior wall of the sinus about 1 cm above the choana, and opens into the sphenoethmoidal recess behind the superior concha (Fig. 6.32).

Blood and nerve supply is from the posterior ethmoidal artery and nerve. *Lymph drainage* is to retropharyngeal nodes.

Frontal sinus

The frontal sinuses are the only sinuses not present at birth; they appear during the second year as excavations into the diploë between the outer and inner tables of the frontal bone. Each extends above the medial end of the eyebrow into the squamous part of the frontal bone and backwards into the orbital part and so into the medial part of the roof of the orbit (Fig. 6.30). The two sinuses are unequal in extent and are separated by a bony septum in the midline region. They vary much in size and rarely may be absent. The important relations are the anterior cranial fossa and the orbit. The sinus drains through an *ostium* at its lower medial corner into the frontonasal recess, which opens into the middle meatus at the front end of the infundibulum (Fig. 6.32) or through anterior ethmoidal air cells.

Blood supply is by supraorbital and anterior ethmoidal arteries. Venous drainage is into superior ophthalmic veins. *Lymph drainage* is to submandibular nodes. *Nerve supply* is from the supraorbital nerves.

PART ELEVEN

Mouth and hard palate

The mouth is for eating and talking through, and its structure is adapted accordingly. It also serves as an emergency airway in dyspnoea but its structure has nothing to do with this function; it merely provides a bigger airhole than the narrow nostrils. The tongue is for grasping food, for moving it during mastication, and for helping to swallow it. The delicate movements of the tongue turn laryngeal noise into articulate speech. In addition its mucous membrane is highly sensitive, even more than fingertips, and it also possesses the sense of taste.

The **mouth** extends from the lips to the palatoglossal arches (anterior pillars of the fauces). It is enclosed by the lips and cheeks; the slit-like space between lips/cheeks and teeth/gingivae (gums) is the *vestibule of the mouth*. The space inside the teeth and gums is the *mouth (oral) cavity* proper. The floor is the mylohyoid muscle, and the roof is the hard palate. Rising from the floor of the mouth, the tongue occupies much of the oral cavity.

The lips and cheeks are covered with hairy skin, except for the *red margin* of the lips, which is devoid of hair, and has a rich capillary blood supply, hence the colour. The red margin is highly sensitive and is represented by a large area in the sensory cortex. It is the main exploratory sensory area in babies, before they learn to use their hands for stereognosis.

The oral cavity is lined with stratified squamous epithelium, which is keratinized on the gums, hard palate and much of the dorsum of the tongue, but not elsewhere. The *mucous membrane* is adherent on lips and cheek to the face muscles, on tongue to the muscles thereof, and on the hard palate to the periosteum of the bone. It is therefore seldom caught between the teeth when chewing.

On the mucous membrane of the cheek the parotid duct opens opposite the second upper molar tooth (Fig. 6.17). Nearby are the tiny openings of the ducts of the molar glands which lie on the outer surface of the buccinator. There are many other mucous glands (buccal and labial) scattered in the mucous membrane of the vestibule.

Nerve supply. Much of the mucous membrane of the inside of the cheeks and lips is supplied by the *buccal* branch of the *mandibular nerve*, with contributions from the *mental* branch of the *inferior alveolar* (also mandibular) and the *infraorbital* branch of the *maxillary nerve*; the last two also supply the red margin of the lower and upper lips respectively.

The **gingivae** (gums) are firmly attached to the alveolar margins of the jaws and surround the necks of the teeth. They consist of dense vascular fibrous tissue covered by epithelium. At the gingival crest, the epithelium dips down to line a sulcus, at the floor of which the epithelium is attached to the surface of the tooth. The change from alveolar mucosa (continuous with that of the cheek) to gingival mucosa is marked by an abrupt change of colour, from red shiny alveolar to pink opaque gingival.

The upper gums are supplied by the *superior alveolar*, *greater palatine* and *nasopalatine nerves* (maxillary), while the lower receive their innervation from the *inferior alveolar*, *buccal* and *lingual nerves* (mandibular). The buccal nerve does not usually innervate the upper gums.

Teeth

The bulk of a tooth consists of **dentine**, a hard avascular calcified tissue penetrated by minute canals, the *dentinal tubules*. The part of the tooth that projects into the mouth is the **crown** which is covered by **enamel**, the hardest tissue in the body, and the part held in the jaw is the *root* which is covered by **cementum**, a calcified tissue rather like bone. The junction between enamel and cementum is the cervical margin or *neck*. Because enamel and cementum meet, dentine is not normally exposed on the surface. Inside the dentine is the *pulp cavity*. The cavity is filled by **dental pulp**, loose connective tissue, with nerves (below), blood vessels (see p. 376) and lymphatics (see p. 343), all of which gain access to the pulp through the apical foramen. The pulp is covered with a single layer of tall columnar cells, the *odontoblasts*, lying in contact with the inner surface of the dentine. Throughout life they retain the power to produce dentine within the pulp cavity if the surface of the dentine is breached. The odontoblasts give off fine cytoplasmic processes that occupy the dentinal tubules.

The tooth is slung in its bony socket by the **periodontal ligament**, consisting of collagen fibres passing obliquely from the alveolar bone towards the apex of the tooth. It is really the modified periosteum of the alveolar bone and is radiolucent; it shows as a clear interval between tooth and bone shadows in a radiograph.

Permanent dentition

The human adult has from the midline 2 incisors, 1 canine, 2 premolars and 3 molars; that is, 8 teeth in each half-jaw, or 32 teeth in all. The shape of a tooth is adapted to its function. The incisors are for biting and cutting, the canines for holding and tearing, the premolars and molars for chewing and grinding. In clinical dentistry it is common to refer to teeth by number (1 to 8 starting from the midline) rather than by name.

The teeth can be distinguished from one another by the characteristics of their roots and crowns. The upper molars have three roots each; two are lateral and one is medial. The lower molars have two roots each, one anterior and one posterior. All the other teeth have a single root, except for the first upper premolar which usually has a bifid root.

The incisor crowns are chisel-shaped. Upper and lower incisors do not meet edge to edge, but by a sliding overlap, like the blades of a pair of scissors. The canine crowns are pyramidal or conical, The premolar (bicuspid teeth) crowns have two cusps (lingual and buccal). Upper molars have four, lower molars five, cusps on their crowns.

Nerve supply

The term nerve supply of a tooth really means the nerve supply of the pulp; some fine nerve filaments may enter some dentinal tubules, but most of the dentine and all the enamel and cementum have no innervation. The pulp and periodontal ligament share the same nerve.

The upper teeth are supplied by the superior alveolar nerves, anterior, middle and posterior, which form a plexus above the apices of the teeth. The middle nerve may be absent.

In the lower jaw the molars and premolars are supplied by the main trunk of the inferior alveolar nerve, whose terminal incisor branch supplies the canine and incisors, overlapping to the opposite central incisor.

Dental anaesthesia

The alveolar bone of the maxilla is relatively porous, so anaesthetic solution deposited in the gingivae opposite the apex of a tooth root will readily penetrate the bone to anaesthetize the tooth for dental procedures. Infiltration of the buccal aspect of the jaw will allow painless drilling of the tooth, but for extraction the palatal aspect must be infiltrated as well.

For the teeth of the lower jaw **infiltration anaesthesia** is usually effective only for the incisors. The other mandibular teeth are embedded in bone that is denser and does not allow sufficient penetration of the anaesthetic agent. For these teeth, **inferior alveolar nerve block** is required; for extraction it is necessary to include block of the nearby lingual and buccal nerves as well in order to anaesthetize the adjacent soft tissues.

For *infiltration anaesthesia* on the buccal (outer) aspect of the jaw, the needle is inserted opposite the appropriate tooth just below or into the buccal fold (where the mucosa is reflected between jaw and cheek), with the tip of the needle directed to the level of the apex of the tooth. On the palatal side, the point of insertion of the needle is midway between the gingival margin and the midline of the palate.

For *inferior alveolar and lingual nerve block*, the needle is inserted orally through the buccinator above the level of the occlusal surface of the molar teeth and in front of the pterygomandibular raphe, which raises a visible and palpable ridge in the opened mouth; the needle passes behind the (palpable) deep tendinous band of the temporalis muscle (see p. 370). The line of approach is from the premolar teeth of the opposite side, and a small injection is made 0.5 cm from the mucosal surface, when the needle is above the lingual nerve; the main injection is made another 1 cm deeper above the lingula, where the inferior alveolar nerve enters the mandibular foramen, which is situated midway between the anterior and posterior borders of the mandibular ramus. Entry of the anaesthetic agent within the parotid fascia around the deep part of the parotid, and its diffusion through the gland substance, may cause a transient facial paralysis.

Tooth position

The teeth of the upper jaw lie in a continuous curve, like a horseshoe. In the alveolar bone the outer (buccal) plate is thinner than the inner (palatal) plate. In the lower jaw the curve of the anterior teeth straightens out in the molar region. In the alveolar bone of the mandible the labial (outer) plate is thinner than the lingual (inner) plate over incisors, canines and premolars, but in the posterior molar region the lingual plate is thinner than the buccal; the lingual nerve lies here beside the third molar tooth and is at risk when the tooth is extracted.

The attachment of mylohyoid is below the apices of most of the mandibular teeth—an apical abscess thus points in the mouth. The apices of the second and third molars lie below the mylohyoid line and an apical abscess bursting through the inner plate points in the neck.

Deciduous dentition

The deciduous, or milk, teeth begin to erupt at about the sixth month and are completely erupted at the end of the second year. They consist of 5 teeth in each half-jaw, 20 in all. There are 2 incisors, 1 canine and 2 molars. They are shed as the permanent teeth erupt. The deciduous molars are replaced by the permanent premolars, not by permanent molars which have no counterpart in the deciduous dentition.

Development and eruption of teeth

Teeth are derived by budding of the epithelium (ectoderm) lining the mouth. The buds of *ectoderm* produce only the *enamel*; they evoke a reaction in the surrounding *mesoderm*, which differentiates to produce the *dentine* and *cementum* under the influence of *neural crest cells*.

In the mouth cavity (stomodeum) of the 5-week embryo (12 mm long) an ingrowth of ectoderm occurs over the site of the future gums. A curved sheet of ectoderm grows into the adjacent mesoderm, tilting medially. This is the *primary dental lamina*. From its outer surface a series of buds grow into the mesoderm, one for each deciduous tooth. At a later stage a similar series of buds grow (more medially) from the depths of the primary dental lamina, one bud for each permanent tooth. When these epithelial buds are well formed the primary dental lamina becomes absorbed. Remnants of this epithelium may later grow into cysts or tumours.

The developed tooth erupts by a combination of elongation of the root and absorption of the overlying bone. The elongating root remains ensheathed in an upgrowth of alveolar bone.

The approximate normal times of eruption are:

Deciduous teeth

6 months	Lower central incisors
7 months	Upper central incisors
8–9 months	Lateral incisors
1 year	First molars
18 months	Canines
2 years	Second molars.

Permanent teeth

6 years	First permanent molars
7 years	Central incisors
8 years	Lateral incisors
9 years	First premolars
10 years	Second premolars
11 years	Canines
12 years	Second permanent molars
17–21 years	Third permanent molars (wisdom teeth).

A lower tooth usually precedes its opposite number in the upper jaw. The first permanent molar (the 6-year molar) erupts before any deciduous teeth have been shed. The second permanent molar does not erupt until 12 years of age. In the intervening period the five deciduous teeth in each half-jaw are replaced. The order of replacement is first the incisors, central and lateral, then the milk molars, first and second and, last of all, the long-rooted canine.

Hard palate

The palate is the roof of the mouth. Between the teeth it lies on a basis of bone, the hard palate. Behind the teeth and hard palate the soft palate projects down.

The hard palate is made up of the palatal process of the maxilla and the horizontal plate of the palatine bone, meeting at a cruciform suture formed of intermaxillary, interpalatine and palatomaxillary sutures. In the midline at the front of the hard palate lies the incisive fossa, into which open the incisive canals, each ascending into its half of the nasal cavity. The greater palatine foramen lies between the palatine bone and maxilla, medial to the last molar tooth; just behind it the lesser palatine foramina perforate the palatine bone.

The *mucous membrane* of the front of the hard palate is strongly united with the periosteum and the attachment of the periosteum to the bone is secured by multiple fibrous tissue pegs (Sharpey's fibres) that leave a finely pitted bone surface on the dried skull. This fixation is for mastication; the moving bolus does not displace the mucous membrane. There are transverse masticatory ridges in this part of the mucoperiosteum. From a little papilla overlying the incisive fossa a narrow low ridge, the palatine raphe, runs anteroposteriorly; the submucosa is absent here. Over the horizontal plate of the palatine bone mucous membrane and periosteum are separated by a mass of mucous gland tissue; Sharpey's fibres are few here, and the bone surface is smooth. From the hard palate the mucous membrane curves down to the undersurface of the soft palate. The stratified squamous epithelium is keratinized on the hard palate, and non-keratinized on the soft palate.

Blood supply is by the greater palatine artery (from the third part of the maxillary artery), which emerges from the greater palatine foramen and passes forwards around the palate (lateral to the nerve) to enter the incisive canal and pass up into the nose. Veins accompany the artery back to the pterygoid plexus. Other veins pass back to the supratonsillar region and join the pharyngeal plexus.

Lymph drainage is to retropharyngeal and deep cervical lymph nodes.

Nerve supply is by the greater palatine nerve (from the maxillary via the pterygopalatine ganglion) as far forward as the incisive fossa. The anterior part of the palate, behind the incisor teeth (the area of the premaxilla) is supplied by the two nasopalatine nerves, from the same source.

Tongue

The tongue is essentially a mass of skeletal muscle covered by mucous membrane, and with a midline fibrous septum separating the two muscular halves. It has a dorsum, tip, inferior surface and root. The anterior two-thirds, or oral part, of the dorsum faces upwards towards the hard palate, and the posterior one-third, or pharyngeal part, faces backwards towards the oropharynx. The stratified squamous epithelium is keratinized on the oral part and non-keratinized on the pharyngeal part. The tip is the most anterior and mobile part and merges into the inferior surface. The mucous membrane of the inferior surface is thin and smooth, similar to that of the floor of the mouth and cheek.

The oral **anterior two-thirds of the dorsum** of the tongue is covered by mucous membrane into which the underlying muscles are inserted. The surface is roughened by the presence of three types of **papillae**: filiform, fungiform and vallate. The *filiform papillae* are minute conical projections that give rise to the velvety appearance of the tongue. *Fungiform papillae* are visible as discrete pink pinheads, more numerous towards the edges of the tongue; each bears a few taste buds (there are none on filiform papillae). The *vallate papillae* are about a dozen in number and are arranged in the form of a V with the apex pointing backwards, just in front of an ill-defined shallow groove, the *sulcus terminalis*, which marks the junction of the oral and pharyngeal parts of the tongue. Each is a cylindrical projection surrounded by a circular sulcus and a raised outer wall (Fig. 6.33). There are many taste buds and serous glands in the sulcus that surrounds each vallate papilla. There are no other glands on the dorsum of the anterior two-thirds of the tongue. The vallate papillae are far back on the oral surface and so not in contact with the food being chewed, but food juices and saliva reach them and so flavours are transmitted to them.

There are scattered mucous and serous glands under the tip and sides. On the undersurface behind the tip there is a rather large mixed gland, the *anterior lingual gland*, on each side of the midline. From each gland small ducts open on the undersurface of the tongue. A retention cyst of this gland is the probable cause of the clinical condition known as a ranula.

The **posterior third of the dorsum** of the tongue slopes downwards from the sulcus terminalis as the anterior wall of the oropharynx. At the apex of the sulcus is a small depression, the *foramen caecum*, the remains of the upper end of the thyroglossal duct (see p. 28). There are no papillae behind the sulcus. The smooth mucous membrane has a nodular appearance from the presence of underlying masses of mucous and serous glands and aggregations of lymphoid follicles. The latter constitute the 'lingual tonsil', part of Waldeyer's ring (see p. 402). Between the tongue and epiglottis there is a midline flange of mucous membrane, the *median glossoepiglottic*

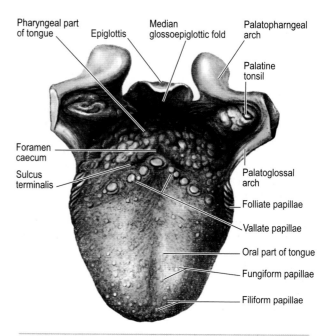

Fig. 6.33 Dorsum of the tongue.

fold, on each side of which is a depression, the *vallecula* (see p. 402), bounded laterally by a similar mucosal fold, the *lateral glossoepiglottic fold*, extending from the side of the epiglottis to the wall of the pharynx; as the latter fold is not attached to the tongue it would be better named pharyngoepiglottic.

When the tip of the tongue is raised to the roof of the mouth, the **inferior surface** of the tongue can be inspected. A small midline septum of mucous membrane (lingual frenulum) unites it to the floor of the mouth. Lateral to this the deep lingual vein can usually be seen through the mucosa (the lingual artery and nerve that are near it are not visible), and farther laterally still is another fold of mucosa, the fimbriated fold. *Foliate papillae* are a series of parallel folds of mucous membrane on the sides of the posterior part of the tongue (Fig. 6.33). They are the site of numerous taste buds.

The **palatoglossal arches** (anterior pillars of the fauces) are ridges of mucous membrane raised up by the palatoglossus muscles. They extend from the undersurface of the front of the soft palate to the sides of the tongue in line with the vallate papillae. The whole constitutes the **oropharyngeal isthmus**. In front of it is the mouth, behind it is the pharynx; and it is narrower than either. It is closed by depression of the palate and elevation of the dorsum of the tongue, and narrowed by contraction of the palatoglossus muscles.

Muscles

The muscles of the tongue are divided into intrinsic and extrinsic groups; the *intrinsic muscles* are wholly within the tongue and not attached to bone, while the *extrinsic muscles* have a bony attachment. There are four muscles in each group in each half of the tongue, with a midline fibrous *septum* dividing the organ into two symmetrical halves. The muscles of the intrinsic group are the *superior* and *inferior longitudinal, transverse* and *vertical*, and the extrinsic group comprises genioglossus (which is the largest of all the muscles and makes up the bulk of the tongue), hyoglossus, styloglossus and palatoglossus.

Genioglossus arises from the superior mental spine (genial tubercle) of the mandible (see Fig. 8.5B, p. 533), whence the fibres radiate backwards in a fan-shaped manner to be inserted into the mucous membrane of the tongue, with the lowest fibres passing down to the hyoid body.

Hyoglossus arises from the length of the greater horn of the hyoid bone and from the lateral part of its body. It extends upwards as a quadrilateral sheet, its upper border interdigitating at right angles with the fibres of styloglossus, and is attached to the side of the tongue. Superficial (lateral) to the muscle from above downwards lie the lingual nerve, submandibular duct, and the hypoglossal nerve with its accompanying veins, while passing deep to its posterior border from above downwards are the glossopharyngeal nerve, stylohyoid ligament and the lingual artery with its accompanying veins lying on the anterior fibres of the middle constrictor (Fig. 6.24).

Styloglossus arises from the front of the lower part of the styloid process and the upper part of the stylohyoid ligament. It passes forwards below the superior constrictor to be inserted into the side of the tongue, interdigitating with the upper fibres of hyoglossus.

Palatoglossus descends from the undersurface of the palatine aponeurosis to the side of the tongue, forming with its fellow of the opposite side the palatoglossal arch. It is described further with the soft palate (see p. 404).

Blood supply

The tongue is supplied by the **lingual artery** (see p. 355), which runs above the greater horn of the hyoid bone deep to hyoglossus and passes forwards to the tip. Beneath hyoglossus it gives off *dorsal lingual* branches into the posterior part. At the anterior border of hyoglossus it gives a branch to the sublingual gland and the floor of the mouth. There are small contributions from the tonsillar branch of the facial artery and from the ascending pharyngeal artery. The fibrous septum dividing the two halves of the tongue prevents any significant anastomosis of blood vessels across the midline.

Venous tributaries accompanying the lingual artery and its dorsal branches form the **lingual vein**. The venous return from the tip is by the *deep lingual vein*, visible on each side of the midline on the undersurface. It runs back superficial to hyoglossus and is joined at the anterior border of that muscle by the *sublingual vein* (from the sublingual gland) to form the *vena comitans of the hypoglossal nerve*. It continues backwards close to the nerve and has a variable ending, joining either the lingual, facial or internal jugular veins. The lingual vein usually joins the internal jugular near the greater horn of the hyoid bone.

Lymph drainage

A significant feature of the tongue's lymph drainage (Fig. 6.34), which is through the floor of the mouth or pharyngeal wall, is that lymph from one side, especially of the posterior part, may reach nodes of both sides of the neck (in contrast to the blood supply which remains unilateral). The tip may drain to submental nodes or directly to deep cervical nodes. Marginal lymphatics from the rest of the anterior part tend to drain to ipsilateral submandibular nodes and then, or sometimes directly, to deep cervical nodes. Central lymphatics from the anterior part descend between the genioglossi and drain to deep cervical nodes of either side. The posterior part drains directly and frequently bilaterally to deep cervical nodes. The deep cervical nodes usually involved are the jugulodigastric and jugulo-omohyoid nodes. All lymph from the tongue is believed to eventually drain through the jugulo-omohyoid node before reaching the thoracic duct or right lymphatic duct.

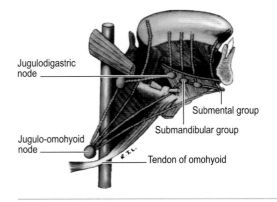

Fig. 6.34 Lymph drainage of the tongue. Of the deep cervical nodes, only the jugulodigastric and jugulo-omohyoid nodes are shown; other channels drain to other nodes of the group.

Nerve supply

All the muscles of the tongue, intrinsic and extrinsic, are supplied by the **hypoglossal nerve** (except palatoglossus, which, being essentially a palate muscle, is supplied by the pharyngeal plexus, see p. 404). The pathway of proprioceptive impulses from the tongue is probably via the lingual nerve.

The sensory supply of the mucous membrane of the oral part (anterior two-thirds), but not the region of the vallate papillae, is by the **lingual nerve**, whose trigeminal component mediates common sensibility (with cell bodies in the trigeminal ganglion) and whose **chorda tympani** component mediates taste (with cell bodies in the geniculate ganglion of the facial nerve). The parasympathetic secretomotor fibres to the anterior lingual gland run in the chorda tympani from the superior salivary nucleus, and relay in the submandibular ganglion.

The posterior one-third of the mucosa, together with the presulcal area that includes the vallate papillae, is mainly supplied by the **glossopharyngeal nerve**. This has fibres of both common sensibility and taste (with cell bodies in the glossopharyngeal ganglia in the jugular foramen). A small area of lingual mucosa forming the anterior wall of the vallecula is supplied by the nerve of the vallecular mucosa, the **internal laryngeal** (with cell bodies in the inferior vagal ganglion).

Movements

The intrinsic muscles alter the *shape* of the tongue, the extrinsic muscles stabilize the organ and by their contraction alter its *position*, as well as its shape. The tongue rests on the floor of the mouth (see p. 347) and this highly mobile shelf enhances the mobility of the tongue.

The position of the tongue is altered by the mylohyoid muscles, on which the tongue rests. The mobile floor of the mouth can be elongated or shortened, raised or lowered, thus still further altering the position of an already mobile organ.

In the first (voluntary) stage of swallowing contraction of the vertical intrinsic muscle makes a longitudinal groove on the dorsum; the heaped-up tip and edges are in contact with the hard palate and teeth. The liquid or moist bolus is thus imprisoned in the groove. Contraction of mylohyoid now raises the floor of the mouth, compressing the tongue against the hard palate. The vertical intrinsic fibres relax from before backwards obliterating the groove in the same sequence, forcing the bolus backwards.

In the unconscious, the tongue muscles relax and the organ may fall backwards to obstruct the pharyngeal part of the airway. Pulling the tongue forwards is an important element in restoring a patent airway in cardiopulmonary resuscitation.

Development

Tongue muscles are derived from *occipital myotomes* which migrate forwards carrying their nerve supply with them (hypoglossal nerve). The migration passes ventrally medial to the internal jugular vein and around the internal and external carotid arteries. The epithelium is derived from the lining of the floor of the pharynx (see p. 400), and comes from parts of the *first*, *third* and *fourth arches*. The mucosa of the anterior two-thirds is from the ectodermal lining of the midline tuberculum impar and the pair of lateral lingual swellings of the first arch (lingual and chorda tympani nerves, see Fig. 1.20, p. 26). The mucosa of the posterior third is from the endodermal lining of the midline hypobranchial eminence of the third arch (glossopharyngeal nerve), with a small contribution from the fourth arch (internal laryngeal nerve). Tissue of the second arch is not represented because third arch tissue overgrows it in a forward direction to meet that from the first arch. The thyroglossal duct grows downwards from the junction between the tuberculum impar and the hypobranchial eminence, the site being indicated by the foramen caecum.

The **sublingual gland** is almond-shaped and lies in between mylohyoid and the side of the tongue (genioglossus), under the mucous membrane of the floor of the mouth. Laterally it lies against the sublingual fossa of the mandible (see Fig. 8.5B, p. 533). Its upper surface raises the sublingual fold in the floor of the mouth. At the front the two glands almost meet each other. The gland is mucus-secreting and of its 15 or so ducts half open into the submandibular duct, the remainder separately on the sublingual fold.

It is supplied by the lingual artery and by branches of the submental artery which pierce mylohyoid muscle to reach it. The venous return is by corresponding veins. Postganglionic parasympathetic secretomotor fibres are supplied to the gland by the lingual nerve; they originate from the submandibular ganglion where preganglionic chorda tympani fibres synapse (see p. 351).

PART TWELVE

Pharynx and soft palate

Pharynx

The pharynx is a fibromuscular tube, attached above to the base of the skull and continuous below with the oesophagus. It is about 12 cm in length. Its anterior wall is largely deficient so that it has wide communication with the nose, mouth and larynx. On account of these communications it is descriptively divided into three parts: nasal, oral and laryngeal, i.e. nasopharynx, oropharynx and laryngopharynx.

Muscles and fascia

The muscular wall is surprisingly thin. It consists of three curved sheets of muscle, the superior, middle and inferior constrictors (supplemented by three smaller muscles: stylopharyngeus, palatopharyngeus and salpingopharyngeus). They overlap posteriorly, being telescoped into each other like three stacked cups. But the muscle does not extend up to the base of the skull; here the immobile wall of the nasopharynx consists of a rigid membrane, the **pharyngobasilar fascia**. This is a fibrous thickening of the submucosa that fills in the gap between the skull and the upper border of the superior constrictor, making a fourth but fibrous cup stacked inside the other three. The attachment of this fascia to the base of the skull (Fig. 6.35) can be traced from the *pharyngeal tubercle*, a midline thickening, in front of the foramen magnum, which also receives fibres from the constrictor muscles. The attachment then passes laterally, convex forwards

over longus capitis to the petrous part of the temporal bone just in front of the carotid canal. From here it passes forwards and medially below the cartilaginous part of the auditory tube, to the sharp posterior border of the medial pterygoid plate, along which it continues down to the hamulus. Suspended from the base of the skull, and sweeping around from one medial pterygoid plate to the other, the pharyngobasilar fascia holds the nasopharynx permanently open for breathing. As it descends inside the superior constrictor it diminishes in thickness and peters out below the level of the hard palate.

The quadrangular area at the apex of the petrous bone in front of the carotid canal lies within a lateral recess of the pharynx. The levator palati muscle arises here and is intrapharyngeal, covered medially by mucous membrane. The cartilaginous part of the auditory tube enters the nasopharynx above the pharyngobasilar fascia, which is firmly attached to it.

Superior constrictor

The superior constrictor fibres arise from the lower part of the posterior border of the medial pterygoid plate down to the tip of the hamulus, outside the pharyngobasilar fascia, and from the pterygomandibular raphe,

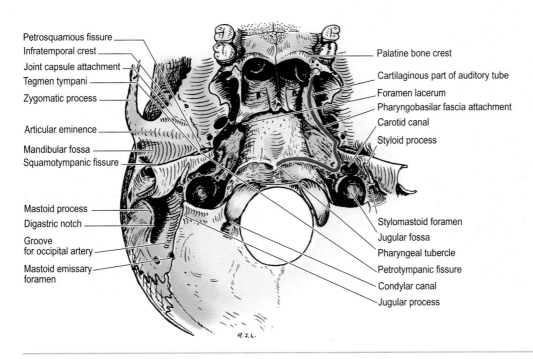

Petrosquamous fissure
Infratemporal crest
Joint capsule attachment
Tegmen tympani
Zygomatic process

Articular eminence

Mandibular fossa
Squamotympanic fissure

Mastoid process
Digastric notch
Groove for occipital artery
Mastoid emissary foramen

Palatine bone crest
Cartilaginous part of auditory tube
Foramen lacerum
Pharyngobasilar fascia attachment
Carotid canal
Styloid process

Stylomastoid foramen
Jugular fossa
Pharyngeal tubercle
Petrotympanic fissure
Condylar canal
Jugular process

R.J.L.

Fig. 6.35 External surface of the central and left part of the base of the skull.

which runs from the hamulus to the mandible just above the posterior end of the mylohyoid line. The superior constrictor passes backwards from the pterygomandibular raphe; buccinator passes forwards from it (Fig. 6.13).

From its origins the muscle sweeps around the pharynx, its fibres diverging mostly upwards to meet their opposite fellows in the midline *pharyngeal raphe* (Fig. 6.36) at the back. The upper end of this raphe forms a fibrous band which receives the uppermost constrictor fibres and is attached to the pharyngeal tubercle. The lowest fibres extend at the back as far down as the level of the vocal folds, lying within the middle constrictor.

There is a gap laterally between the superior and middle constrictors, through which stylopharyngeus passes down into the pharynx, and styloglossus and the glossopharyngeal and lingual nerves pass forwards to the tongue (Fig. 6.24).

Middle constrictor

The middle constrictor arises from the stylohyoid ligament, the lesser horn of the hyoid bone and the greater horn, deep to hyoglossus. Its fibres diverge upwards and downwards as they sweep backwards around the pharynx to end in the median raphe and enclose the superior constrictor; the lowest fibres arch down as far as the vocal folds, lying within the inferior constrictor.

The anterior gap between the middle and inferior constrictors is closed by the thyrohyoid membrane (see p. 407), which walls in the laryngeal part of the pharynx (Fig. 6.37). Passing through this gap by piercing the membrane are the internal laryngeal nerve and superior laryngeal vessels.

Inferior constrictor

This has two parts, named from their origins. The **thyropharyngeus** part arises from the oblique line of the thyroid cartilage and in continuity below this from a fibrous arch that spans the cricothyroid muscle (Fig. 6.37). It encloses the middle and superior constrictors as its fibres curve backwards and upwards around them to the midline raphe. The **cricopharyngeus**, rounded and thicker than the flat sheets of the other constrictors, extends

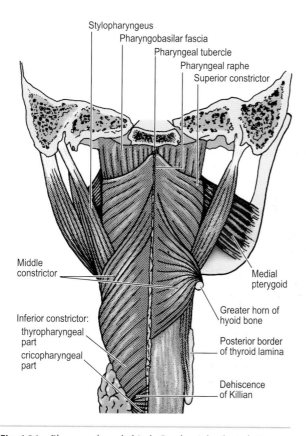

Stylopharyngeus
Pharyngobasilar fascia
Pharyngeal tubercle
Pharyngeal raphe
Superior constrictor
Middle constrictor
Medial pterygoid
Inferior constrictor:
thyropharyngeal part
cricopharyngeal part
Greater horn of hyoid bone
Posterior border of thyroid lamina
Dehiscence of Killian

Fig. 6.36   Pharynx, from behind. On the right the inferior constrictor has been removed to show the extent of the middle constrictor and the attachment of stylopharyngeus to the posterior border of the thyroid lamina.

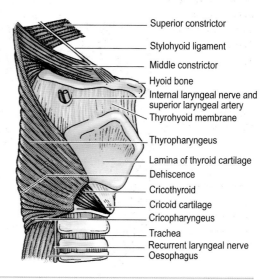

Superior constrictor
Stylohyoid ligament
Middle constrictor
Hyoid bone
Internal laryngeal nerve and superior laryngeal artery
Thyrohyoid membrane
Thyropharyngeus
Lamina of thyroid cartilage
Dehiscence
Cricothyroid
Cricoid cartilage
Cricopharyngeus
Trachea
Recurrent laryngeal nerve
Oesophagus

Fig. 6.37   Pharyngeal constrictors, from the right.

uninterruptedly from one side of the cricoid arch to the other around the pharynx. There is no raphe here. The muscle acts as a sphincter at the lower extent of the pharynx, and is continuous with the circular muscular coat of the oesophagus (Fig. 6.41). It is composed largely of fibres of the 'slow twitch' variety and is always closed, except for momentary relaxation during deglutition. It imparts some resistance to the passage of an endoscope (overcome by swallowing). The closure of the cricopharyngeus prevents air from being sucked into the upper oesophagus when intrathoracic pressure falls; air is sucked only into the permanently open trachea. Passing upwards deep to the lower border of the inferior constrictor are the recurrent laryngeal nerve and inferior laryngeal vessels.

The junction between the oblique fibres of thyropharyngeus and the horizontal fibres of cricopharyngeus near the midline is a potentially weak area at the back of the pharyngeal wall (Fig. 6.36), and through this area (*Killian's dehiscence*) a pouch of mucosa may become protruded (pharyngeal diverticulum) (Fig. 6.38).

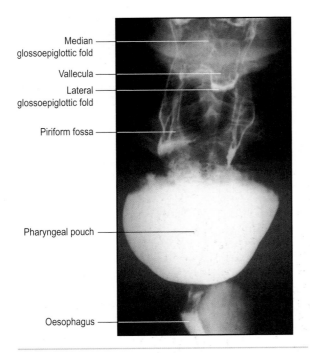

Median glossoepiglottic fold

Vallecula

Lateral glossoepiglottic fold

Piriform fossa

Pharyngeal pouch

Oesophagus

Fig. 6.38 Barium meal radiograph of a subject with a pharyngeal pouch. A residual film of barium sulphate has outlined the posterior surface of the tongue, the median and lateral glossoepiglottic folds and the piriform fossae.

Palatopharyngeus

Palatopharyngeus is described with the soft palate (see p. 404). As the muscle fibres pass down from the palate they lie internal to the superior constrictor (Fig. 6.41).

Salpingopharyngeus

Salpingopharyngeus is a very slender muscle that arises from the lower part of the cartilage of the auditory tube (see p. 434) and runs downwards (Fig. 6.41) to blend with palatopharyngeus.

Stylopharyngeus

Stylopharyngeus arises from the deep aspect of the styloid process high up. It slopes down across the internal carotid artery (Fig. 6.23), in front of which it crosses the lower border of the superior constrictor and passes down inside the middle constrictor, to be inserted with palatopharyngeus into the posterior border of the thyroid lamina (Fig. 6.36). The glossopharyngeal nerve curls round the posterior border of the muscle from medial to lateral, and supplies it.

Blood supply

Branches of many arteries supply the pharynx: ascending pharyngeal, ascending palatine and tonsillar (from facial), greater palatine and pharyngeal (from maxillary), lingual and the superior and inferior laryngeal arteries. Venous blood is largely collected into the pharyngeal venous plexus which like the nerve plexus (see below) is situated mainly at the back of the middle constrictor; it drains into the internal jugular vein and has connections with the pterygoid plexus.

Lymph drainage

Lymph passes to retropharyngeal lymph nodes and via these or directly to upper and lower deep cervical groups.

Nerve supply

The main motor nerve supply of the muscles of the pharynx is from the pharyngeal plexus. However, stylopharyngeus is supplied by the glossopharyngeal nerve and cricopharyngeus is also supplied by the recurrent and external laryngeal nerves. The cell bodies that supply all six muscles on each side are in the nucleus ambiguus.

The pharyngeal plexus lies on the posterolateral wall of the pharynx, mainly over the middle constrictor, and is formed by the union of pharyngeal branches from the vagus and glossopharyngeal nerves and the cervical sympathetic. The glossopharyngeal component is afferent; the pharyngeal fibres of the vagus carry motor fibres (derived from the cranial part of the accessory nerve). The sympathetic fibres are vasoconstrictor.

The mucosa of the nasopharynx is supplied by the pharyngeal branch of the maxillary nerve through the pterygopalatine ganglion. Most of the oropharynx receives its sensory supply from the glossopharyngeal nerve, but the internal laryngeal nerve supplies the valleculae and the lesser palatine nerves (maxillary) contribute to the supply of the tonsillar mucosa. The internal laryngeal nerve is sensory to the laryngopharynx.

Nasal part

The **nasopharynx** extends from the base of the skull to the upper surface of the soft palate, at the level of C1 vertebra. In front it communicates with the nose through the choanae. The space between the soft palate and the posterior pharyngeal wall through which the nasopharynx joins the oral part of the pharynx is the *oropharyngeal isthmus*. The soft palate becomes elevated during swallowing to meet the posterior wall, so closing the isthmus. The main features within the nasopharynx are the openings of the auditory tubes, the pharyngeal recesses and the pharyngeal tonsil (Fig. 6.39).

The **opening of the auditory tube** lies in the lateral wall and is triangular in appearance. The opening is guarded above, behind and in front by a prominent rounded ridge, the *tubal elevation*, formed by the trumpet-shaped medial end of the tubal cartilage as it underlies

the mucous membrane, which here contains lymphatic tissue, the *tubal tonsil*. The lower margin of the opening has a slight bulge due to the underlying levator palati muscle. The tubal elevation is in the shape of an inverted J, the long limb lying posteriorly and being continued downwards as the *salpingopharyngeal fold*, produced by the underlying salpingopharyngeus muscle.

The **pharyngeal recess** (fossa of Rosenmüller) is a narrow vertical gutter behind the opening of the auditory tube, resulting from the angular attachment of the pharyngobasilar fascia to the base of the skull in front of the carotid canal (Fig. 6.35). A catheter missing the tubal orifice and introduced into the recess may perforate the fascia and enter the internal carotid artery, which here lies against the wall of the pharynx.

In the mucous membrane high on the posterior wall is a collection of lymphoid nodules, prominent only in children and forming the **pharyngeal tonsil**. When enlarged the nodules are commonly known as the *adenoids*.

Oral part

The **oropharynx** extends from the lower surface of the soft palate to the upper border of the epiglottis (halfway down C3 vertebral body). The wall of the oropharynx is formed posteriorly by all three constrictors. It closes completely behind a swallowed bolus, but is otherwise open for breathing. Anteriorly in front of the gap between the soft palate and epiglottis there is a mobile wall, the posterior part of the tongue, above which the oropharynx communicates with the mouth. At the sides there are projecting ridges, the **palatopharyngeal** and

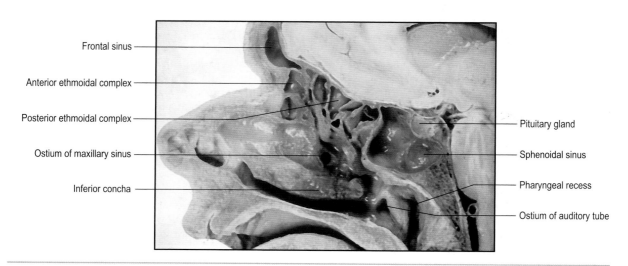

Frontal sinus

Anterior ethmoidal complex

Posterior ethmoidal complex

Ostium of maxillary sinus

Inferior concha

Pituitary gland

Sphenoidal sinus

Pharyngeal recess

Ostium of auditory tube

Fig. 6.39 Sagittal section of the head.

palatoglossal arches (*pillars of the fauces*), formed by the underlying corresponding muscles, with the palatine tonsils between them. The palatoglossal arches form the boundary between the pharynx and the mouth. The palatine and lingual tonsils and the valleculae are in the oropharynx.

The **palatine tonsil** (the pair commonly called simply 'the tonsils') is a large collection of lymphoid tissue which projects into the oropharynx from the *tonsillar fossa* between the palatopharyngeal fold behind and the palatoglossal fold in front (Fig. 6.33). The floor of the fossa (lateral wall) is the lower part of the superior constrictor. On its lateral aspect the glossopharyngeal nerve crosses the lower part of the bed, running obliquely downwards and forwards to reach the tongue by passing under the lower border of the constrictor.

The lymphoid tissue of the tonsil extends up to the soft palate and down to the dorsum of the tongue. The medial surface is covered by pharyngeal mucosa on which are the openings of several epithelial downgrowths, the *tonsillar crypts*. One large downgrowth near the upper pole is the *intratonsillar cleft*, which is the remains of the fetal second pharyngeal pouch (see p. 27). The lateral surface is covered by fibrous tissue which forms the tonsillar hemicapsule. (A peritonsillar abscess occurs outside the capsule.) The superior constrictor separates this surface from the facial artery and two of its branches, the ascending palatine and tonsillar. The internal carotid artery is about 2.5 cm posterolateral to the tonsil.

The palatine, lingual, pharyngeal and tubal tonsils collectively form an interrupted circle of lymphoid tissue (*Waldeyer's ring*) at the upper end of the respiratory and alimentary tracts.

Blood supply. The tonsillar branch of the facial artery forms the main arterial supply; it enters the tonsil by piercing the superior constrictor. There are smaller contributions from the lingual, ascending pharyngeal and ascending and greater palatine vessels.

The veins form a plexus round the capsule and pierce the superior constrictor to drain into the pharyngeal plexus. One large vein descends from the soft palate between the tonsillar hemicapsule and the superior constrictor before piercing the pharyngeal wall; this is the external palatine, or paratonsillar vein and, is the usual cause of haemorrhage after tonsillectomy.

Lymph drainage. Lymphatic channels pierce the superior constrictor to reach the deep cervical nodes, especially the jugulodigastric (or tonsillar) node below the angle of the mandible.

Nerve supply. The mucous membrane overlying the tonsil is supplied mainly by the tonsillar branch of the glossopharyngeal nerve, and to a small extent by the lesser palatine nerves. The glossopharyngeal nerve also supplies

the middle ear, through its tympanic branch, and tonsillitis may cause referred pain in the ear.

The **valleculae** lie between the epiglottis and the posterior surface of the tongue. They are shallow fossae separated by the median glossoepiglottic fold and limited inferolaterally by the lateral glossoepiglottic folds (Fig. 6.38). The nerve supply of the mucosa of the valleculae, including that of the part of the tongue that forms the anterior vallecular wall, is by the internal laryngeal nerve. A crumb that 'goes down the wrong way' is one that lodges in the vallecula and sets up a reflex bout of coughing (see p. 411) to dislodge it.

Laryngeal part

The **laryngopharynx** extends from the upper border of the epiglottis to the level of the cricoid cartilage (C6 vertebra) where it becomes continuous with the oesophagus. In the upper part of the anterior aspect is the opening into the larynx (aditus or *laryngeal inlet*) (see p. 408). The piriform recesses, broad above and narrow below, lie beside the aperture of the larynx. Below the inlet, the lower part of the pharynx (referred to clinically as the hypopharynx) possesses an anterior wall, comprising the arytenoids and the lamina of the cricoid cartilage (see p. 407) draped over with mucous membrane. The posterior wall of the laryngopharynx is formed by the three overlapping constrictors down to the level of the vocal folds (upper border of cricoid lamina). Below this (i.e. behind the cricoid lamina) there is only the inferior constrictor, the site of the dehiscence of Killian, and finally the cricopharyngeal sphincter.

At each side of the epiglottis the *lateral glossoepiglottic fold* separates the oropharynx from the laryngeal part. Below the fold is the **piriform recess** (piriform fossa) (Fig. 6.38). This mucosa-lined space is bounded medially by the quadrangular membrane of the larynx, (see p. 407), and laterally by the thyrohyoid membrane above and the lamina of the thyroid cartilage below (Fig. 6.40). A malignancy may grow in the space provided by the piriform fossa without producing symptoms, until the patient presents with metastatic cervical lymphadenopathy. The recesses are danger sites for perforation by an endoscope.

Soft palate

The soft palate hangs down from the back of the hard palate as a mobile flap that fuses at the sides with the lateral wall of the pharynx and which can be raised so that the posterior part of its superior surface makes contact with the posterior wall of the pharynx to close

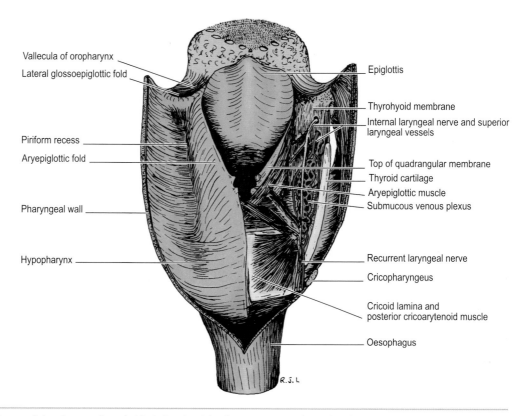

Fig. 6.40 Laryngeal part of the pharynx from behind. On the right the mucous membrane has been removed to show the anastomoses within the pharynx of the superior and inferior laryngeal vessels and of the internal and recurrent laryngeal nerves. There is no such overlap in the larynx; the vocal folds are a complete 'watershed'.

off the nasopharynx during swallowing. It consists of an **aponeurosis** that is acted upon by attached muscles to alter its shape and position, but much of its bulk is due to mucous and serous glands. There are five paired **muscles**: tensor palati, levator palati, palatoglossus (which also belongs to the tongue), palatopharyngeus (which also belongs to the pharynx) and the muscle of the uvula. The tensor and levator are properly called tensor veli palatini and levator veli palatini, but the older and simpler name is retained here.

Tensor palati

This muscle arises outside the palate from the scaphoid fossa at the upper end of the medial pterygoid plate, the lateral side of the cartilaginous part of the auditory tube, and the spine of the sphenoid (Figs 6.19 and 6.35). From this origin the triangular muscle passes down between the medial and lateral pterygoid plates converging to a tendon that turns medially around the pterygoid hamulus, above the fibrous arch in the origin of the buccinator (Fig. 6.13), and so gets inside the pharynx. As to whether the tendon now is attached to the palatine aponeurosis, or flattens to become the fibrous aponeurosis, is academic. The triangular aponeurosis is attached anteriorly to the inferior surface of the hard palate behind the crest of the palatine bone (Fig. 6.35). The posterolateral borders of the aponeurosis blend with the side wall of the pharynx in front, but hang free behind, forming the edge of the soft palate and meeting at the dependent uvula in the midline. The aponeurosis is not flat, but concave towards the mouth; when tensed by contraction of the tensor muscle it is flattened and therefore depressed somewhat. The increased rigidity, however, enables the levator palati to elevate the soft palate during swallowing. The main action of the tensor palati is to tense the palatine aponeurosis so that other muscles may elevate and depress it without altering its shape. When the tensor palati contracts (e.g. in swallowing and yawning) it pulls upon the cartilage of the auditory tube, opens the tube, and permits equalization of air pressure between the middle ear and nose. This action is impaired in children with cleft palate, who hence have a higher incidence of middle ear problems.

Levator palati

This muscle arises from the quadrate area on the inferior surface of the apex of the petrous bone anterior to the carotid canal and from the adjacent medial side of the cartilaginous part of the auditory tube, it forms a rounded belly that is inserted into the nasal surface of the palatine aponeurosis between the two heads of palatopharyngeus. The two levator muscles in passing down to the palate are directed forwards and medially, together forming a V-shaped sling. Their contraction pulls the palate upwards and backwards. Contraction of the levator also opens the cartilaginous tube and equalizes air pressure between the middle ear and the nose.

Palatoglossus

The muscle arises from the undersurface of the palatine aponeurosis and passes downwards to interdigitate with styloglossus. The muscle raises the palatoglossal fold of mucous membrane in front of the tonsil (the anterior pillar of the fauces), marking the junction between mouth and pharynx. Its action is sphincteric at the oropharyngeal isthmus; it raises the tongue and narrows the transverse diameter of the isthmus.

Palatopharyngeus

The muscle arises from two heads. The *anterior head* arises from the posterior border of the hard palate and the anterior part of the upper surface of the palatine aponeurosis (Fig. 6.42). The *posterior head* arises further back on the upper surface of the aponeurosis. The two heads arch downwards over the lateral edge of the aponeurosis, join, and form a muscle that passes downwards beneath the mucous membrane and submucosa of the lateral wall of the pharynx just behind the tonsil (Figs 6.41 and 6.42). The upper part of the muscle raises the palatopharyngeal fold of mucous membrane that constitutes the posterior pillar of the fauces; the lower part (blending with stylopharyngeus and salpingopharyngeus) is inserted chiefly into the posterior border of the thyroid lamina and its horns; the muscle ought rightly to be named palatolaryngeus. Some of the anterior fibres are inserted into the upper border of the thyroid lamina just in front of the superior horn. Some of the

posterior ones merge with the surrounding fibres of the inferior constrictor.

The muscle is an elevator of the larynx and pharynx. It arches the palate, making it more concave on its oral surface.

Palatopharyngeal sphincter

The uppermost fibres of palatopharyngeus, arising with the anterior head, run horizontally at the level of C1 vertebra, from the anterior part of the lateral edge of the aponeurosis on one side to that on the other side. These fibres form the palatopharyngeal sphincter (Fig. 6.42); when they contract they draw the posterior wall of the pharynx forwards as a ridge (*Passavant's ridge*), against which the upper surface of the elevated soft palate comes into contact during swallowing. The palatopharyngeus is hypertrophied in children with cleft palate.

The *musculus uvulae* consists of two strips of muscle on the upper surface of the aponeurosis on either side of the midline, running from the posterior nasal spine of the palatine bone to the mucosa of the uvula. They aid palatopharyngeal closure.

Blood supply

Lesser palatine branches of the maxillary artery, the ascending palatine branch of the facial artery, and palatine branches of the ascending pharyngeal artery supply the soft palate. The venous drainage passes through the pharyngeal wall into the pharyngeal venous plexus and the pterygoid plexus.

Lymph drainage

Lymphatics from the soft palate empty into retropharyngeal and upper deep cervical lymph nodes.

Nerve supply

All the muscles of the soft palate are supplied by the pharyngeal plexus except for tensor palati, which is supplied by a branch from the nerve to the medial pterygoid (from the mandibular branch of the trigeminal nerve). The plexus fibres to the palate are from the nucleus ambiguus via the cranial part of the accessory nerve and the pharyngeal branch of the vagus. Postganglionic secretomotor fibres to the palatal glands from the pterygopalatine ganglion run with the lesser palatine nerves. They are activated from the superior salivary nucleus in the pons by way of the nervus intermedius and the greater petrosal nerve (see p. 468); these nerves

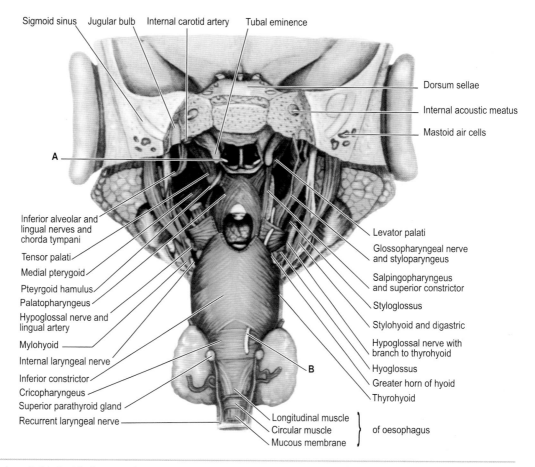

Sigmoid sinus   Jugular bulb   Internal carotid artery   Tubal eminence

Dorsum sellae

Internal acoustic meatus

Mastoid air cells

A

Inferior alveolar and
lingual nerves and
chorda tympani

Tensor palati

Medial pterygoid

Pteyrgoid hamulus

Palatopharyngeus

Hypoglossal nerve and
lingual artery

Mylohyoid

Internal laryngeal nerve

Inferior constrictor

Cricopharyngeus

Superior parathyroid gland

Recurrent laryngeal nerve

Levator palati

Glossopharyngeal nerve
and styloparyngeus

Salpingopharyngeus
and superior constrictor

Styloglossus

Stylohyoid and digastric

Hypoglossal nerve with
branch to thyrohyoid

Hyoglossus

Greater horn of hyoid

Thyrohyoid

B

Longitudinal muscle   }
Circular muscle   } of oesophagus
Mucous membrane   }

Fig. 6.41   Pharynx from behind with the nasopharynx opened to show the soft palate musculature: **A** is a probe entering the opening of the auditory tube; **B** is a probe passed down between middle and inferior constrictors, emerging through Killian's dehiscence. The diagram is based on a prosection in the Anatomy Museum of the Royal College of Surgeons of England.

also carry taste fibres (cell bodies in geniculate ganglion) from the few taste buds on the oral surface of the soft palate. Common sensation from the mucous membrane of the soft palate is transmitted by the lesser palatine nerves to the maxillary division of the trigeminal nerve, through the pterygopalatine ganglion without relay. On the oral surface there is slight overlap of glosso-pharyngeal sensory fibres from the lateral wall of the pharynx.

Elevation of the palate and contraction of pharyngeal muscles—the **gag reflex**—occur when the palate, tonsil, posterior part of the tongue or posterior pharyngeal wall are touched by an unfamiliar object, as when testing with a swab (but the passage of food over the same areas does not cause the reflex, due to conditioned familiarity).

The afferent side of the reflex is glossopharyngeal and the efferent is vagal.

Structure

The soft palate is covered with non-keratinized stratified squamous epithelium on its oral surface, and on the posterior part of its nasal surface up to where it comes into contact with Passavant's ridge. The anterior part of its nasal surface is covered with respiratory mucous membrane. In the submucosa on both surfaces are mucous glands, which are most plentiful around the uvula and on the oral aspect of the soft palate. On this surface there are also scattered taste buds and lymphoid follicles.

405

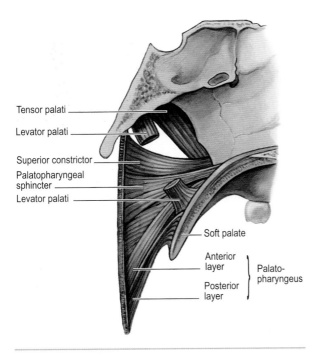

Tensor palati

Levator palati

Superior constrictor

Palatopharyngeal
sphincter

Levator palati

Soft palate

Anterior
layer

Posterior
layer

Palato-
pharyngeus

Fig. 6.42 Muscles of the left half of the soft palate, viewed from within the pharynx. Part of the levator palati muscle has been removed.

PART **THIRTEEN**

Larynx

The larynx is a respiratory organ, set in the respiratory tract between the pharynx and trachea. Although phonation is important in man, the main function of the larynx is to provide a protective sphincter for the air passages. The larynx lies below the hyoid bone in the midline of the neck at the level of C4–6 vertebrae.

Skeleton of the larynx

The framework of the larynx consists of cartilages, ligaments and membranes. There are three single cartilages (thyroid, cricoid and epiglottic) and three pairs of cartilages (arytenoid, corniculate and cuneiform). The ligaments and membranes are extrinsic (thyrohyoid membrane and cricotracheal, hyoepiglottic and thyroepiglottic ligaments) and intrinsic (quadrangular membrane and cricothyroid ligament). The vocal cords are the upper part of the cricothyroid ligament (cricovocal membrane).

Cartilages

The thyroid, cricoid and arytenoid cartilages are composed of hyaline cartilage and with age parts of them may calcify or ossify; the epiglottic, corniculate and cuneiform cartilages are elastic fibrocartilage.

The **thyroid cartilage** consists of two *laminae* whose anterior borders are fused at a median *angle*, or *laryngeal prominence*. A thyroid notch marks the upper end of the prominence. The posterior borders are free and projected upwards and downwards as the *superior and inferior horns* (Fig. 6.43). Each inferior horn articulates with the cricoid cartilage to form the cricothyroid joint. The outer surface of each lamina possesses an oblique ridge running downwards and forwards, and bounded above and below by a tubercle.

The **cricoid cartilage** is the foundation of the larynx; to this signet-ring structure (Fig. 6.44) the thyroid and

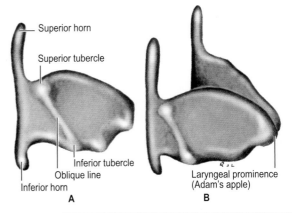

Superior horn

Superior tubercle

Inferior tubercle

Oblique line

Inferior horn

Laryngeal prominence
(Adam's apple)

A   **B**

Fig. 6.43 Thyroid cartilage: **A** from the right; **B** from the right and above and slightly in front.

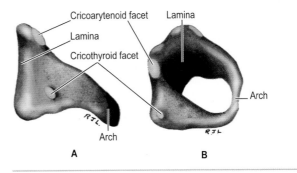

Cricoarytenoid facet   Lamina

Lamina

Cricothyroid facet

Arch

Arch

A   **B**

Fig. 6.44 Cricoid cartilage: **A** from the right; **B** from the right, above and in front.

arytenoid cartilages are articulated by synovial joints. It is the only complete cartilaginous ring in the whole of the air passages. The anterior part of the ring is the *arch*; posteriorly it is projected upwards as a quadrangular flat *lamina*. Near the junction of the arch and lamina is an articular facet for the inferior horn of the thyroid cartilage. The upper part of the lamina has sloping shoulders, which carry articular facets for the arytenoids. A vertical ridge in the midline of the lamina produces a shallow concavity on each side for the attachment of the posterior cricoarytenoid muscle; the ridge gives attachment to longitudinal muscle fibres of the oesophagus (see p. 216).

The **epiglottic cartilage** is a slightly curled, leaf-shaped structure, prolonged below into a slender process (the stalk of the leaf) attached in the midline to the back of the laryngeal prominence, below the thyroid notch. The epiglottic cartilage leans back from its attached stalk to overhang the vestibule of the larynx. Fibrous tissue attaching the front and sides of the epiglottis to the body and greater horns of the hyoid bone (hyoepiglottic ligaments) form the framework of the glossoepiglottic folds that bound the valleculae (see p. 402). The posterior surface below the apex is pitted by mucous glands. A bulge on the lower part of this surface is the tubercle of the epiglottis.

Each of the pair of **arytenoid cartilages** is a three-sided pyramid with anterolateral, medial and posterior surfaces. The inferior base has a forward projection, the vocal process, and a lateral projection, the muscular process. The base articulates with the sloping shoulder on the upper border of the cricoid lamina. A very small *corniculate cartilage* articulates with the apex of each arytenoid cartilage and a tiny *cuneiform cartilage* lies nearby in the aryepiglottic fold; they are unimportant.

Joints

The **cricothyroid joint**, between the inferior horn of the thyroid cartilage and the facet on the side of the arch of the cricoid, is synovial. Movement between the cricoid and thyroid occurs round an axis that passes transversely between the two joints, so that one cartilage can rock backwards and forwards on the other. The recurrent laryngeal nerve lies immediately behind this joint.

The **cricoarytenoid joint** is also synovial. The capsule here is lax, allowing both rotary and lateral gliding movements. When the arytenoids are pulled laterally and downwards they slide apart from one another along the sloping shoulders of the cricoid lamina. This gliding of the arytenoids opens the gap between the vocal folds (the rima of the glottis) in the shape of a V; rotation opens the glottis in the shape of a diamond. In man there

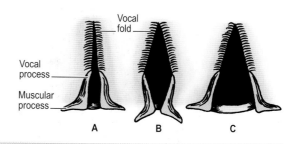

Fig. 6.45 Movements of the arytenoid cartilages. In **A**, the vocal folds are adducted. In **B**, rotation of the arytenoids, as in animals, produces a diamond-shaped opening. In **C**, lateral excursion of the arytenoids produces the human V-shaped opening.

is a greater range of gliding than of rotary movement, and the open human glottis resembles a V and not a diamond (Fig. 6.45).

Ligaments and membranes

Of the *extrinsic membranes*, the **thyrohyoid membrane** connects the whole length of the upper border of the thyroid laminae and the superior horns to the body and greater horns of the hyoid bone (Fig. 6.46). The thyrohyoid membrane passes up behind the body of the hyoid bone to be attached to its upper border; a bursa lies between the membrane and the back of the bone. It is here that remnants of the thyroglossal duct (see p. 28) may persist, necessitating resection of the central part of the bone to give adequate removal.

The thyrohyoid membrane forms the lateral wall of the piriform recess and is perforated by the internal laryngeal nerve and the superior laryngeal vessels. It is not part of the larynx, but anchors the skeleton of the larynx to the hyoid bone.

The epiglottis is attached to the hyoid bone and thyroid cartilage by the *hyoepiglottic* and *thyroepiglottic ligaments*. The former are described above; the latter is a strong band attaching the stalk of the cartilage to the angle between the thyroid laminae just below the thyroid notch.

The *cricotracheal membrane* connects the lower border of the cricoid cartilage to the first cartilaginous ring of the trachea.

Of the *intrinsic membranes*, the **quadrangular membrane** is a thin fibroelastic membrane that extends between the arytenoid cartilage and the epiglottis (Fig. 6.46). Its anterior border is attached to the side of the lower half of the epiglottis. Its posterior border, much shorter, is attached to the anterolateral surface of the arytenoid.

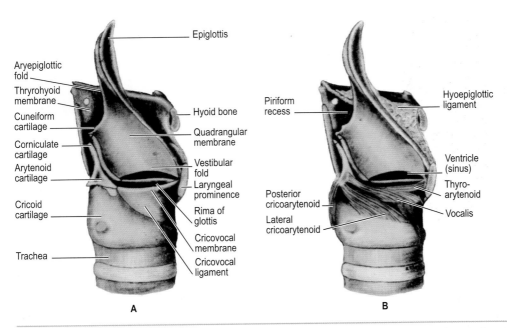

Fig. 6.46   Skeleton of the larynx: **A** interior, viewed from the right with the right quadrangular membrane and the right halves of the thyroid cartilage and hyoid bone removed; **B** similar view showing muscles attached to the right arytenoid cartilage.

Its lower border is free, constituting the **vestibular ligament** ('false vocal cord'). The mucous membrane covering its much longer upper border constitutes the **aryepiglottic fold.** The two aryepiglottic folds form the margins of the oval **inlet of the larynx.**

The other intrinsic ligament is the **cricothyroid ligament.** This is composed of mainly elastic tissue and has distinct anterior and lateral parts, continuous with each other. The anterior part is a thick band in the midline connecting the upper border of the cricoid to the lower border of the thyroid, the *anterior (median) cricothyroid ligament.* The paired, thinner *lateral cricothyroid ligaments* (also termed cricothyroid or **cricovocal membranes**) are attached below to the upper border of the cricoid, but as they ascend they converge and pass up deep to the lamina of the thyroid on each side (Fig. 6.46). Each lateral ligament has a free, thickened superior edge, attached in front to the back of the angle of the thyroid cartilage, midway between the notch and the lower border, and at the back to the vocal process of the arytenoid cartilage. This free edge constitutes the **vocal ligament** or vocal cord (hence the term cricovocal membrane). The free edge of the quadrangular membrane, the vestibular ligament, lies above the vocal ligament and there is a gap between the two ligaments. The quadrangular and cricovocal membranes are lined on their inner aspects by mucous membrane, and that part

of it which covers the vestibular and vocal ligaments forms the **vestibular** and **vocal folds** respectively.

Cavity of the larynx

The **inlet** (aditus) of the larynx, through which it communicates with the pharynx, faces backwards and upwards and is bounded in front by the upper edge of the epiglottis, at the sides and back by the aryepiglottic folds, and in the posterior midline by the transverse mucosal fold between the arytenoids (Figs 6.40 and 6.47). The space below the level of the inlet down as far as the vestibular folds is the **vestibule.** In the gap between the vestibular and vocal ligaments, the mucous membrane of the larynx bulges outwards, forming a deep horizontal groove, the **ventricle** or *laryngeal sinus* (Fig. 6.48). Opening from its anterior end is a small pouch of mucous membrane, the *laryngeal saccule,* which extends upwards between the vestibular fold and the thyroid lamina.

The gap between the vocal folds is the **rima of the glottis** (or simply 'the glottis'), the anteroposterior slit through which air passes (Fig. 6.45). The anterior 60% of the glottis (*intermembranous part*) is bounded on each side by the vocal fold itself. The posterior 40% (*intercartilaginous part*) lies between the vocal processes of the arytenoid cartilages and the medial margins of

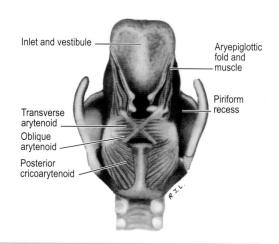

Inlet and vestibule

Aryepiglottic fold and muscle

Piriform recess

Transverse arytenoid

Oblique arytenoid

Posterior cricoarytenoid

Fig. 6.47 Larynx from behind after removal of the mucous membrane of the laryngopharynx.

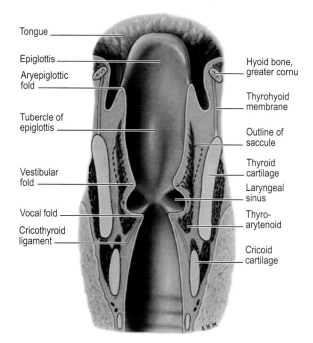

Tongue

Epiglottis

Aryepiglottic fold

Tubercle of epiglottis

Vestibular fold

Vocal fold

Cricothyroid ligament

Hyoid bone, greater cornu

Thyrohyoid membrane

Outline of saccule

Thyroid cartilage

Laryngeal sinus

Thyro-arytenoid

Cricoid cartilage

Fig. 6.48 Anterior half of the larynx and upper trachea which have been sectioned in the coronal plane.

their bases (covered of course by mucous membrane). In the resting state during quiet respiration, the glottis is triangular and about 8 mm wide at the back; the sagittal length is about 23 mm in the male and 17 mm in the female. On looking down into the larynx from above,

as with a laryngoscope, the vestibular folds appear as bulges of mucosa above and lateral to the vocal folds, which are lower and closer together and move with respiration and phonation.

Below the glottis the infraglottic part of the larynx extends down to the level of the lower border of the cricoid cartilage where it becomes continuous with the trachea.

Mucous membrane

As part of the respiratory tract, the larynx in general is lined by pseudostratified columnar ciliated epithelium. The anterior surface of the epiglottis (not in the larynx) faces the tongue. Its mucosa is covered by stratified squamous epithelium, which 'climbs over' from the front of the epiglottis on to the aryepiglottic folds and the upper part of the posterior epiglottic surface, before being replaced by the ciliated variety. However, over the vocal folds the epithelium is always stratified squamous. The folds are a whitish colour since blood vessels do not show through here, due to the firm attachment of the mucosa to the vocal ligaments. The saccules contain many mucous glands whose secretion flows down to lubricate the vocal folds, where mucous glands are absent. Taste buds are present on the posterior epiglottic surface and the aryepiglottic folds.

The *lamina propria* is loose in all parts except over the vocal folds where it is very firmly attached. It therefore allows great swelling except at the glottis; in '*oedema of the glottis*' the swelling accumulates above the rima, but may still cause dangerous obstruction to the airflow.

Muscles

The muscles of the larynx alter the size and shape of the inlet, or affect the vocal ligaments causing their movements or changing their tension. The muscles that act on the inlet are the aryepiglottic and oblique arytenoid muscles, assisted by the transverse arytenoid and thyro-epiglottic muscles. Those that affect the vocal ligaments are the posterior and lateral cricoarytenoids, oblique and transverse arytenoids, thyroarytenoids and vocalis, and the cricothyroids.

The **transverse arytenoid** is the only unpaired intrinsic muscle. It is attached to the posterior surfaces of the arytenoid cartilages (Fig. 6.47). It draws the arytenoids (and their vocal processes) nearer to each other and adducts the vocal folds, helping to close the glottis. The **oblique arytenoids** pass from the back of the muscular process of one arytenoid to the apex of the opposite one, crossing each other on the posterior surface of the transverse arytenoid, and have the same action. Some fibres

409

continue from the arytenoid apex into the aryepiglottic fold and reach the edge of the epiglottis, so forming the **aryepiglottic muscle** (Fig. 6.40); they approximate the aryepiglottic folds and close the laryngeal inlet.

The **posterior cricoarytenoid** arises from the concavity on the back of the lamina of the cricoid whence its fibres converge on the back of the muscular process of the ipsilateral arytenoids (Fig. 6.47). Its upper fibres are almost horizontal, its lower lateral fibres almost vertical. Their combined action is to move the arytenoid laterally and rotate its vocal process outwards. It is the most important muscle of the larynx as it is the only muscle that abducts the vocal folds and opens the glottis.

The **lateral cricoarytenoid** arises from the upper border of the cricoid arch and passes upwards and backwards to be attached to the front of the muscular process of the arytenoid (Fig. 6.46B). By drawing the muscular process forwards it rotates the vocal process inwards and closes the glottis.

The **thyroarytenoid** muscle extends backwards and laterally from the angle of the thyroid to the antero-lateral surface of the arytenoid and the lateral surface of its vocal process (Fig. 6.46B). It shortens and relaxes the vocal ligament, thereby altering the pitch of the voice. A part of this muscle runs parallel and lateral to the vocal ligament, and some of its fibres arise from the ligament rather than the thyroid; these form the **vocalis** muscle and act on the posterior part of the vocal ligament.

Many thyroarytenoid fibres ascend up to the aryepiglottic fold and some even reach the side of the epiglottis. They constitute the **thyroepiglottic muscle** and they open the laryngeal inlet by abducting the aryepiglottic fold. Some of these fibres pass lateral to the saccule, which they compress.

The **cricothyroid** muscle is a fan-shaped muscle on the outer surface of the larynx; it arises from the lateral aspect of the cricoid arch and is attached to the inferior horn and adjacent lower border of the thyroid lamina (Fig. 6.49). Its contraction makes the thyroid tilt slightly downwards and forwards, thereby lengthening and tensing the vocal ligament.

Swallowing. Protection of the inlet during swallowing is provided by the sphincteric action of the aryepiglottic muscles. A second sphincter is provided by closure of the glottis, but swallowed material very rarely enters the vestibule. Elevation of the larynx beneath the posteriorly bulging tongue displaces the epiglottis backwards, assisting closure of the larynx. A large passing bolus may fold the epiglottis over the closed inlet, but the epiglottis is not essential for the protection of the airway. Indeed the epiglottis often stays upright during swallowing, food passing beside it on either side into the piriform fossa (the lateral food channel; see Fig. 6.38).

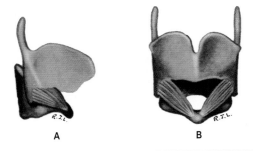

Fig. 6.49 Cricothyroid muscle: **A** from the right; **B** from the front.

Phonation. Phonation or voice production involves the making of sounds that can be varied in pitch, intensity and quality (timbre). The stream of air emitted during phonation emerges as a series of discrete jets, as from a siren. This is not only a more effective means of sound production, but is very economical of expired air. At rest the vocal folds are separated. During phonation they are held together. The apposed vocal folds are blown apart by the pressure of the air below them, and elastic recoil returns them to their original position; the rapid repetition of these movements results in vibration of the folds, so giving rise to sound waves with a certain *pitch*. The frequency of emission of the jets depends on the length and tension of the folds, and it is these features that are adjusted by the intrinsic muscles to vary the pitch. The *intensity* of the sound varies with the pressure of the air forced through the glottis. The *quality* or timbre of the voice depends on the resonating chambers above the glottis; these include the vestibule of the larynx, pharynx, mouth, nose and paranasal sinuses, and their overall shape and volume can be altered by the soft palate, tongue and other muscles. Depression of the larynx (see p. 348) increases the volume of the resonating chambers. *Articulation* depends on breaking up the sound into recognizable consonants and vowels by the use of tongue, teeth and lips.

In *whispering* the vocal folds are separated, and vibrations are imparted to a constant stream of expired air. This is inefficient as a means of sound production, and is very wasteful of air.

Various muscular efforts such as heavy lifting, coughing and abdominal straining are accompanied by closure of the glottis, and also by some medial movement of the vestibular folds and compression of the laryngeal ventricle.

A **cough** or sneeze is an explosion of compressed air. The vocal folds are powerfully adducted, a strong expiratory contraction is made to build up the intrathoracic pressure (see p. 193), the folds are then suddenly abducted and the blast of compressed air explodes through the larynx (its expulsive force increased by the simultaneous 'choke-barrel' narrowing of the trachea). In the **cough reflex**, afferents from the mucous membrane supplied by the glossopharyngeal and vagus nerves pass to the nucleus of the tractus solitarius (see p. 499). There are widespread connections in the brainstem and spinal cord for the efferent side of the reflex, which involves muscles of the larynx, pharynx, palate, tongue, diaphragm and other thoracic and abdominal muscles.

Abdominal straining is made more effective by adduction of the vocal folds. The diaphragm is weaker than the muscles of the anterior abdominal wall. To prevent loss of intra-abdominal pressure by upward displacement of the diaphragm the folds are closed after a deep breath and the diaphragm is held down by a cushion of compressed air. This manoeuvre is used for evacuation of pelvic effluents and also for the straining of heavy lifting. Escape of a jet of compressed air causes the characteristic grunt.

Blood supply

Above the vocal folds blood is brought to the larynx by the superior laryngeal branch of the superior thyroid artery. This enters the piriform recess below the internal laryngeal nerve by piercing the thyrohyoid membrane (Fig. 6.40). The superior laryngeal veins accompany the artery and empty into the superior thyroid veins.

The lower half of the larynx is supplied from the inferior laryngeal branch of the inferior thyroid artery; it accompanies the recurrent laryngeal nerve beneath the inferior constrictor of the pharynx. Venous return is by the inferior laryngeal veins to the inferior thyroid veins.

Lymph drainage

From the supra- and infraglottic parts of the larynx, lymphatics accompany the superior or inferior thyroid vessels and drain to the upper or lower groups of deep cervical nodes respectively. A few infraglottic lymphatics pass through the cricothyroid membrane and drain initially to prelaryngeal and to pretracheal nodes.

Nerve supply

All the *muscles* of the larynx are supplied by the **recurrent laryngeal nerve** except cricothyroid which is innervated by the **external laryngeal nerve**. All the motor fibres in both nerves are from cell bodies in the nucleus ambiguus derived mainly via the cranial part of the accessory nerve.

The recurrent laryngeal nerve enters the pharynx by passing upwards under the lower border of the inferior constrictor behind the cricothyroid joint. By this stage it has often divided into an anterior (motor) and a posterior (sensory) branch, at the level of the upper border of the isthmus of the thyroid gland. The nerve reaches the lower part of the piriform recess and then penetrates the laryngeal wall.

With complete recurrent laryngeal nerve paralysis the vocal fold takes up a variable position. Respiratory problems are rare but there may be stridor (noisy respiration) if the airflow is substantially increased for any reason. The voice is initially hoarse but with compensatory movement of the other vocal fold disability is reduced. With acute bilateral complete palsies there is significant inspiratory stridor and an immediate tracheostomy may be needed. The position of the vocal folds following partial lesions of the recurrent laryngeal nerves is contentious. The traditional view, that the only abductor muscle (posterior cricoarytenoid) is more vulnerable, is disputed and the vocal folds may assume a paramedian or intermediate (half abducted) position with differing effects on phonation and respiration.

Paralysis of the external laryngeal nerve affecting cricothyroid may pass unnoticed, or perhaps cause some hoarseness of the voice which appears to recover (due to hypertrophy of the opposite cricothyroid) but with a residual inability to produce higher frequencies, as in the higher notes in singing. Examination reveals that the vocal fold on the damaged side is slightly bowed and at a lower level than the normal, due to loss of the tension normally provided by cricothyroid.

The *mucous membrane* of the larynx above the level of the vocal folds is supplied by the **internal laryngeal nerve**; that of the folds and the larynx below them is supplied by the **recurrent laryngeal nerve**.

The sympathetic supply (vasoconstrictor) comes in with the superior and inferior laryngeal arteries from the middle and inferior cervical sympathetic ganglia.

Development

The larynx develops from the tracheobronchial groove at the caudal end of the floor of the primitive pharynx, with the laryngeal cartilages being derived from the fourth and sixth arches (see p. 27).

Laryngotomy

In very acute airway obstruction at the level of the glottis or above, when an endotracheal tube cannot be successfully introduced through the oral or nasal cavities, an emergency laryngotomy is preferred to tracheostomy (see p. 353). The laryngeal prominence and cricoid cartilage are palpated and entry is made through the cricothyroid ligament between the cricoid and the lower border of the thyroid cartilage. There are no large midline vessels here; an anastomosis between the small cricothyroid branches of the superior thyroid arteries, high up on the cricothyroid ligament, does not usually cause problems. The proximity of the vocal cords, at the level of the middle of the thyroid angle, must be borne in mind both during the procedure and thereafter; an airway introduced through a laryngotomy is usually not maintained for more than 48 hours, lest it leads to subglottic stenosis. This site is also used for the insertion of a minitracheal tube (for suction rather than as an airway).

PART **FOURTEEN**

Orbit and eye

The **eye** (eyeball) is the organ of vision and the principal component of the visual apparatus. This is lodged in the orbit, together with the extraocular muscles which move the eye, nerves, vessels, the lacrimal gland, fascia and fat.

Orbit

The orbit is a bony cavity shaped like a four-sided pyramid lying on its side, with the apex at the back and the base forming the orbital margin on the front of the facial skeleton (Fig. 6.50). The *orbital fascia* is the periosteum of the orbit which, at the back, becomes continuous with the dura mater and the sheath of the optic nerve, which enters the orbit through the optic canal at the apex.

The relations of the orbit are important. Above is the anterior cranial fossa, with the meninges and the frontal lobe of the cerebral hemisphere. Medially are the nasal cavity, ethmoid sinuses and the sphenoid sinus. Below lies the maxillary sinus. Posterolaterally are the infratemporal fossa and the middle cranial fossa.

The **roof** of the orbit is the orbital part of the frontal bone, with the lesser wing of the sphenoid at the most posterior part. The frontal sinus frequently extends into its anteromedial part.

The **medial wall**, 5 cm long, extends in front from the anterior lacrimal crest on the frontal process of the maxilla, backwards across the lacrimal bone and the paper-thin orbital plate of the ethmoid, to the body of the sphenoid. The posterior lacrimal crest is a vertical ridge on the lacrimal bone. Between the two crests is the *fossa for the lacrimal sac*, which leads down into the *nasolacrimal canal*. At the junction of medial wall and roof lie the *anterior* and *posterior ethmoidal foramina*, between the ethmoid and frontal bones; the anterior foramen is about 24 mm behind the anterior lacrimal crest, the posterior foramen about 12 mm behind this and the optic nerve emerges through the optic canal about 6 mm further back. A knowledge of these mean measurements is of particular value during endoscopic surgical procedures on the ethmoid sinuses. The medial walls lie anteroposterior, parallel with each other. The very thin bone of the orbital plate separates the orbits from the ethmoidal air cells.

The **lateral wall**, 5 cm long, is composed of the zygomatic bone (the thickest and strongest part of the orbit walls) and the greater wing of the sphenoid. Posteriorly there is a gap, the *superior orbital fissure*, between lateral wall and roof (greater and lesser wings of the sphenoid), leading into the middle cranial fossa (Fig. 6.50). Another gap, the *inferior orbital fissure*, diverges from the medial

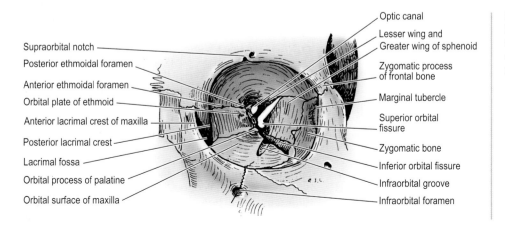

Supraorbital notch
Posterior ethmoidal foramen
Anterior ethmoidal foramen
Orbital plate of ethmoid
Anterior lacrimal crest of maxilla
Posterior lacrimal crest
Lacrimal fossa
Orbital process of palatine
Orbital surface of maxilla

Optic canal
Lesser wing and Greater wing of sphenoid
Zygomatic process of frontal bone
Marginal tubercle
Superior orbital fissure
Zygomatic bone
Inferior orbital fissure
Infraorbital groove
Infraorbital foramen

Fig. 6.50 Bones of the left orbit, viewed along the orbital axis which is at 25° to the sagittal plane.

end of this fissure between lateral wall and floor (greater wing and maxilla); it leads into the pterygopalatine and infratemporal fossae. The lateral wall slopes at 45° to the sagittal plane; the two lateral walls are at right angles to each other, and, if prolonged backwards, would meet at a right angle in the pituitary fossa.

The **floor**, formed mainly by the orbital surface of the maxilla (grooved and canalized by the infraorbital nerve), is completed laterally by the zygomatic bone and posteriorly by the tiny orbital process of the palatine bone. Blunt force applied to the face may cause a 'blow-out' fracture of the thin bone of the orbital floor or medial wall. Fracture of the floor may lead to herniation of orbital fat into the maxillary sinus, entrapment of an extraocular muscle (causing diplopia) or injury to the infraorbital nerve.

The **orbital margin** has four curved sides. The supraorbital margin (frontal bone) is notched or canalized a third of the way from its medial end for the passage of the supraorbital nerve and artery. The lateral margin is formed by corresponding processes of the frontal and zygomatic bones, which meet at a palpable suture line. The infraorbital margin is formed by the zygomatic bone and maxilla. The infraorbital foramen lies about 1 cm below the middle of this margin. The medial margin of the orbit is formed by the anterior lacrimal crest (maxilla) and the frontal bone.

Eyelids

The eyelids protect the eye from injury and assist in the distribution of tears over the anterior surface of the eyeball. They are covered in front with loose skin and behind with adherent conjunctiva. Their fibrous framework is the orbital septum, thickened at the margins of the lids to form the tarsal plates. The orbicularis oculi muscle lies in front of the septum. The eyelids meet at the medial and lateral angles (or canthi). The lateral canthus is in direct contact with the eyeball. The medial canthus is separated by a small triangular space, the lacus lacrimalis, in the centre of which is a small pink elevation, the caruncle. A semilunar conjunctival fold lies on the lateral side of the caruncle.

The **orbital septum** is attached to the margins of the orbit (Fig. 6.51). It has a wide 'buttonhole' in it: the palpebral fissure between the lids. It is greatly thickened above and below the buttonhole to form the crescent-shaped **superior** and **inferior tarsal plates**. The plates are formed of dense fibrous tissue, not cartilage as might be imagined from their stiffness. From the medial end of the buttonhole a thick **medial palpebral ligament** anchors the tarsal plates to the anterior lacrimal crest. The corresponding, much thinner, **lateral palpebral ligament**

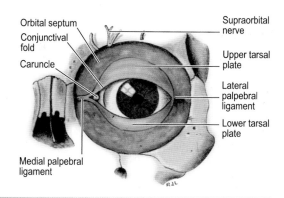

Fig. 6.51   Left orbital septum.

is attached to the marginal tubercle (of Whitnall) on the zygomatic bone just inside the orbital margin (Fig. 6.50). The levator palpebrae superioris is attached to the superior tarsal plate (see p. 415). The **tarsal** (**Meibomian**) **glands** are modified sebaceous glands embedded within the substance of the tarsal plates. Their ducts discharge an oily secretion at the eyelid margin; this delays evaporation of tears and discourages spilling of excess tears.

The thin skin of the eyelids is adherent to the margins of the palpebral fissure where it becomes continuous with the conjunctiva. The eyelashes are located here; they do not possess arrector pili muscles. Sebaceous glands open into each hair follicle. Ciliary glands (modified sweat glands) between the follicles open on to the eyelid margin. A hordeolum, or stye, is an infection of these glands.

Movements. The lower lid possesses very little mobility, the upper lid a great deal. The lids are closed gently by the palpebral fibres and forcibly when the orbital fibres of the orbicularis oculi join in (see p. 363). The lids are opened in the ordinary way by levator palpebrae superioris (see p. 415). The levators hold the lids open while the orbital fibres of orbicularis are contracting to lower the eyebrows as a pair of sun visors. The sun visors can be brought together by corrugator supercilii, causing (unwanted) vertical wrinkles between them. This small muscle arises medially from the frontal bone and passes laterally through orbicularis to skin above the middle of the supraorbital margin.

The **conjunctiva** is a transparent membrane attached to the sclera at the margins of the cornea, with which it blends. It is loosely attached elsewhere over the anterior part of the sclera and thence reflected to the inner surfaces of the eyelids. It is firmly attached to the tarsal plates and blends with the skin at the margins of the lids. The subtarsal sulcus is a shallow groove on the back of the lids, about 2 mm from the margin, where foreign bodies tend to lodge. The conjunctival epithelium is stratified columnar, except near the eyelid margin and close to the corneoscleral junction, where it changes to non-keratinized stratified squamous. Mucus-secreting goblet cells are scattered in the conjunctival epithelium and small accessory lacrimal glands are scattered in the subconjunctival connective tissue.

The **blood supply** of the eyelids is from the medial palpebral branches of the ophthalmic artery and the lateral palpebral branches of the lacrimal artery (branch of ophthalmic), which form a pair of arcades in each lid. The palpebral (eyelid) conjunctiva is very vascular (hence the pink colour); the bulbar (ocular) is only slightly vascular and is transparent. The venous drainage of the lids is to ophthalmic and angular veins. Lymphatic drainage from the lateral two-thirds of the lids (and lacrimal gland) is to preauricular nodes, and from the medial third to submandibular nodes.

The skin of the upper lid receives **nerve supply** from the lacrimal, supraorbital, supratrochlear and infratrochlear nerves, and that of the lower lid from the infraorbital nerve. The same nerves supply the corresponding palpebral and bulbar conjunctiva. The cornea has a separate supply from the long and short ciliary nerves (see p. 418).

Lacrimal apparatus

The production of tears and the removal of excess tears is the function of the lacrimal apparatus, which consists of the lacrimal gland, lacrimal canaliculi, lacrimal sac and the nasolacrimal duct.

Lacrimal gland

This is a serous gland with a large orbital and a small palpebral part. The orbital part lies in the lacrimal fossa on the lateral part of the roof of the orbit, above the lateral part of the aponeurotic tendon of levator palpebrae superioris. The gland curls round the lateral margin of the tendon and the palpebral part is visible through the superior fornix of the conjunctiva. The gland drains by a dozen ducts that run from the palpebral part into the lateral extent of the superior fornix. Closure of the eyelids begins at the lateral side of the upper lid and moves medially, so spreading tears across the eye. Under normal conditions the lacrimal gland secretes just enough tears to replace those lost by evaporation. Secretomotor fibres from the superior salivary nucleus travel in the greater petrosal nerve and relay in the pterygopalatine ganglion. The postganglionic fibres run with the zygomatic branch of the maxillary nerve, and reach the gland via its anastomotic branch with the lacrimal nerve.

At the medial end of each lid margin is a low elevation, the *lacrimal papilla*, surmounted by a minute *lacrimal punctum*. This opens into a *lacrimal canaliculus*, a tiny canal which conveys excessive tears to the lacrimal sac (Fig. 6.52).

The **lacrimal sac** lies in the lacrimal groove formed by the maxilla and lacrimal bone, crossed in front by the medial palpebral ligament, and some of the palpebral fibres of orbicularis oculi are inserted into the walls of the sac. When the palpebral and lacrimal parts of orbicularis oculi contract, the lids are closed and the puncta turned inwards to dip into the lacus lacrimalis. Simultaneously the sac is drawn widely open, so that tears are sucked in through the canaliculi.

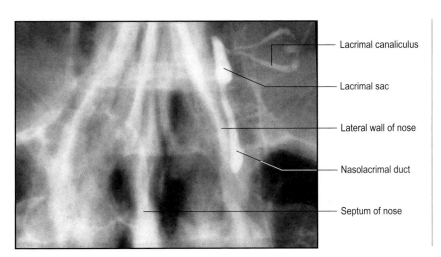

Fig. 6.52 Magnified view of a left dacrocystogram (lacrimal canaliculogram).

Lacrimal canaliculus

Lacrimal sac

Lateral wall of nose

Nasolacrimal duct

Septum of nose

The **nasolacrimal duct**, 2 cm long, slopes downwards, backwards and laterally, in conformity with the pear-shaped nasal cavity, to open high up in the anterior part of the inferior meatus 2 cm behind the nostril. The mucous membrane is raised into several variable folds which act as valves to prevent air being blown up the duct into the lacrimal sac. The duct and sac are lined by ciliated columnar epithelium.

Muscles of the orbit

The eyeball is moved by extrinsic or **extraocular muscles**: four rectus (superior and inferior, medial and lateral) and two oblique (superior and inferior). The orbit also contains the levator palpebrae superioris for moving the upper lid.

The two eyes face forwards and the long axes of the eyes lie in the sagittal plane, parallel with each other and with the medial walls of the orbits, but the lateral walls slope backwards and medially, making a right angle with each other. The optic nerve and ocular muscles come from the apex of the orbit, at the back of the medial wall, and pass forwards and laterally to their ocular attachments. The actions of the superior and inferior recti are therefore not 'straight', despite their names. Hence the need for two oblique muscles, to act in concert with these two recti and produce direct upward and downward movements of the eyes.

The superior orbital fissure is retort-shaped, with the broad end medially (Fig. 6.50). A *common tendinous ring* surrounds the 'bulb of the retort' and the optic canal (Fig. 6.53). It is attached to a small bony projection on the inferior margin of the fissure, and is adherent to the dural sheath of the optic nerve. From the ring the four recti arise; from the bone above the ring the levator palpebrae superioris and the superior oblique take origin. As these muscles pass forwards from the apex of the orbit they broaden out, to form a cone of muscles around the eye. Many nerves pass through the superior orbital fissure (Fig. 6.29). Three pass through the lateral part, outside the fibrous ring, and they remain outside the cone of muscles. They are the lacrimal, frontal and trochlear nerves. The rest of the lateral part of the fissure is closed by the fibrous layer of the dura mater of the middle cranial fossa. The nerves that pass through the tendinous ring and enter the cone of muscles are the oculomotor, abducens and nasociliary. Only the posterior and anterior ethmoidal and infratrochlear branches of the nasociliary nerve come out of the cone.

Levator palpebrae superioris arises from the under-surface of the lesser wing of the sphenoid at the apex of the orbit. It is a flat muscle that broadens as it passes forwards (Fig. 6.54). The thick frontal nerve lies on its

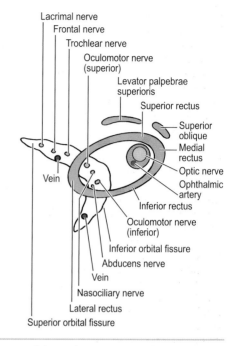

Fig. 6.53 Diagram of the tendinous ring muscle attachments, and of structures passing through the superior orbital fissure and optic canal.

upper surface, dividing towards the front of the orbit into its supraorbital and supratrochlear branches. At the anterior end the muscle forms an aponeurotic tendon that is widened on each side up to a crescentic margin. This broad tendon penetrates the orbital septum and is inserted into the front of the superior tarsal plate (Fig. 6.55). Some fibres are attached to the skin of the upper lid. A thin sheet of smooth muscle lies beneath the main tendon and is inserted into the upper margin of the tarsal plate.

The superior division of the oculomotor nerve supplies the muscle. The branch either pierces the superior rectus or passes on its medial side to enter the lower surface of the levator. The nerve also carries postganglionic sympathetic fibres (from the superior cervical ganglion, via the internal carotid plexus) for the smooth muscle part.

The muscle opens the eye by elevating the upper lid. Complete oculomotor palsy causes complete ptosis (drooping of the upper lid); division of the cervical sympathetic chain causes partial ptosis.

The **superior, medial, inferior** and **lateral rectus** muscles arise from the common tendinous ring. The superior and medial recti also have origin from the dural sheath of the optic nerve. The superior, inferior and lateral muscles pass forwards and laterally, the medial directly

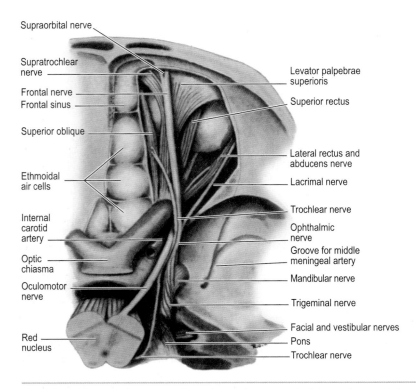

- Supraorbital nerve
- Supratrochlear nerve
- Frontal nerve
- Frontal sinus
- Superior oblique
- Ethmoidal air cells
- Internal carotid artery
- Optic chiasma
- Oculomotor nerve
- Red nucleus
- Levator palpebrae superioris
- Superior rectus
- Lateral rectus and abducens nerve
- Lacrimal nerve
- Trochlear nerve
- Ophthalmic nerve
- Groove for middle meningeal artery
- Mandibular nerve
- Trigeminal nerve
- Facial and vestibular nerves
- Pons
- Trochlear nerve

Fig. 6.54   Right orbit. Dissection from above after removal of the roof (part of the anterior cranial fossa).

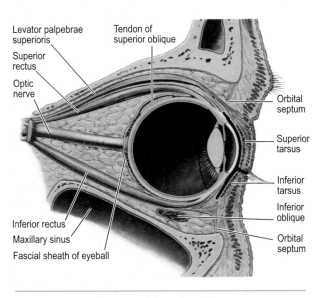

- Levator palpebrae superioris
- Superior rectus
- Optic nerve
- Tendon of superior oblique
- Orbital septum
- Superior tarsus
- Inferior tarsus
- Inferior oblique
- Orbital septum
- Inferior rectus
- Maxillary sinus
- Fascial sheath of eyeball

Fig. 6.55   Sagittal section of the right orbit.

forwards. They all pierce the fascial sheath of the eyeball and are inserted into the sclera anterior to the coronal equator of the eye.

The **superior oblique** arises from the body of the sphenoid, passes forward above the medial rectus (Fig. 6.54) and gives way to a slender tendon (Fig. 6.104), which passes through the trochlea (where it is lubricated by a synovial sheath). It then turns backwards and laterally to pierce the fascial sheath and pass under the superior rectus to be inserted into the posterosuperior lateral quadrant of the sclera (i.e. behind the coronal equator of the eye). The **trochlea** (pulley) is a loop of fibrocartilage attached to the trochlear fossa of the frontal bone just behind the orbital margin.

The **inferior oblique** arises from the maxilla on the floor of the orbit, near the anterior margin. The muscle passes obliquely backwards and laterally below inferior rectus (Fig. 6.56) and then curves upwards deep to lateral rectus to be attached to the posteroinferior lateral quadrant of the sclera (i.e. behind the coronal equator of the eye).

A mock 'chemical formula' is an aid to memorizing the nerve supplies of the eye muscles: LR_6SO_4. This signifies that the *Lateral Rectus* is supplied by the *sixth* (abducens) nerve, the *Superior Oblique* by the *fourth* (trochlear) nerve. All the other muscles (superior, medial and inferior rectus and inferior oblique) are supplied by the *third* (oculomotor) nerve. The nerves all enter the ocular surfaces of the respective muscles, except the trochlear which enters the superior surface of superior oblique. Because of the decussation of fibres in the mid-brain (see p. 496), the trochlear nerve nucleus of one side supplies the superior oblique of the eye of the opposite side.

The actions of the muscles that move the eyes are considered below.

Fascial sheath of the eye

A thin fascial sheath of the eye (fascia bulbi or Tenon's capsule) closely surrounds the eyeball and separates it from orbital fat. Anteriorly the sheath is attached to the sclera just behind the corneoscleral junction. Posteriorly the sheath is pierced by ciliary vessels and nerves, and fuses with the sclera and the dura around the optic nerve at its attachment to the eye. The sheath is pierced by the tendons of the four recti and two obliques and is reflected as a sleeve proximally (i.e. away from the eye) around each tendon. Triangular expansions from the sleeves of the medial and lateral recti form the **medial** and **lateral check ligaments**, which are attached respectively to the lacrimal and zygomatic bones. The sleeve of the inferior rectus is thickened on its underside and blends with the sleeve of the inferior oblique as well as with the check ligaments, forming a hammock-like support for the eye, the **suspensory ligament** (of Lockwood). If the suspensory ligament remains intact when the floor of the orbit is fractured, or the maxilla removed surgically, the eye does not sag. Double vision (diplopia) following a blow-out fracture of the orbital floor is usually due to entrapment of the inferior rectus.

Nerves of the orbit

The **optic nerve** enters the orbit through the optic canal, accompanied by the ophthalmic artery below and lateral to the nerve. The nerve is really an extension of the white matter of the brain; it is covered by pia, arachnoid and dura mater as far as the back of the eye. Its length in the orbit is 25 mm. It curves laterally and downwards as it passes forwards to meet the sclera 3 mm medial to the posterior pole. The central artery and vein of the retina pierce the nerve about halfway along its course to the eye. After passing within the fibrous ring, the optic nerve is usually crossed above from lateral to medial by

the ophthalmic artery, with the nasociliary nerve and the superior ophthalmic vein behind the artery. The ciliary ganglion (see below) lies on the lateral side of the optic nerve one-third of the way from optic canal to eye, and the anterior part of the nerve is closely surrounded by the short ciliary nerves and vessels.

The continuation of the subarachnoid space around the optic nerve accounts for the appearance of papilloedema in increased intracranial pressure.

The **infraorbital nerve** enters the orbit through the inferior orbital fissure accompanied by the zygomatic nerve and infraorbital artery. The infraorbital nerve and artery occupy the groove in the posterior part of the orbital floor. Both enter the infraorbital canal and proceed to the face, also supplying the maxillary sinus and some upper teeth (see p. 390).

The **zygomatic nerve** passes along the lateral wall and divides into its *zygomaticotemporal* and *zygomaticofacial* branches. The former gives a *communicating branch* to the lacrimal nerve, so providing the secretomotor fibres for the lacrimal gland, and traverses a canal in the zygomatic bone to enter the infratemporal fossa; the latter traverses a separate canal to emerge on the face.

The lacrimal, frontal and trochlear nerves enter the orbit through the superior orbital fissure, outside the tendinous ring (Figs 6.53 and 6.54).

The **lacrimal nerve**, the smallest of the three main branches of the ophthalmic, runs forward on the lateral wall of the orbit along the upper border of the lateral rectus muscle. It picks up a secretomotor branch from the zygomaticotemporal nerve which it gives off to the lacrimal gland. It pierces the orbital septum to supply both surfaces of the conjunctiva in the upper fornix and the skin of the outer part of the upper lid.

The **frontal nerve** is a large main branch of the ophthalmic nerve which runs straight forward above the levator muscle in contact with the periosteum of the orbital roof. It divides into the small supratrochlear and (laterally) the large supraorbital nerves which pass to the forehead.

The **trochlear nerve** (fourth cranial), lying medial to the frontal nerve, passes forward and sinks into the superior oblique muscle (Fig. 6.54).

The **oculomotor nerve** enters the tendinous ring in two divisions, superior and inferior, with the nasociliary nerve between them and the abducent nerve below all three (Figs 6.53 and 6.29).

The *superior division* of the oculomotor nerve (third cranial) runs forwards above the optic nerve and supplies the overlying superior rectus and levator palpebrae muscles. It carries sympathetic fibres from the internal carotid cavernous plexus to the smooth muscle part of the levator.

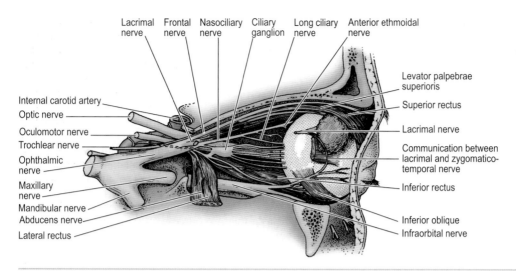

Fig. 6.56 Nerves of the right orbit and the ciliary ganglion: lateral aspect.

The *inferior division* of the oculomotor nerve is larger; it gives off the nerve to the inferior rectus and the nerve to the medial rectus, which passes below the optic nerve to reach that muscle. The rest of the inferior division continues as the nerve to the inferior oblique; it gives off the parasympathetic root to the ciliary ganglion (Fig. 6.56).

The **abducens nerve** (sixth cranial) simply passes forward, diverging away from the optic nerve, and enters the lateral rectus muscle (Fig. 6.29).

The **nasociliary nerve**, the third branch of the ophthalmic, runs forward and then crosses from lateral to medial above the optic nerve (Fig. 6.56) and behind the ophthalmic artery to approach the medial wall of the orbit. Here it becomes the **anterior ethmoidal** by entering the anterior ethmoidal foramen (Fig. 6.104), under the frontal bone and above the ethmoidal labyrinth; it then runs forward in a groove on the cribriform plate and enters the nose through a slit at the side of the crista galli. Before entering the foramen, the nasociliary gives off the **infratrochlear nerve** which passes forward on the medial wall of the orbit just below the trochlea, supplies the lacrimal sac and conjunctiva, and continues above the medial palpebral ligament to skin of the upper lid and bridge of the nose.

The nasociliary nerve gives off the **posterior ethmoidal nerve**, which leaves the orbit through the posterior ethmoidal foramen to supply the posterior ethmoidal and sphenoidal air sinuses.

The nasociliary nerve also gives off a sensory branch to the ciliary ganglion, and a pair of **long ciliary nerves** which pierce the sclera medial to the short ciliary nerves. The long ciliary nerves supply the ciliary body, iris and cornea, and carry postganglionic sympathetic fibres from the superior cervical ganglion (derived from the internal carotid plexus) for the dilator pupillae.

The **ciliary ganglion** is a minute body (2 mm diameter) lying on the lateral side of the optic nerve (Fig. 6.56), between the nerve and the lateral rectus. Three roots enter its posterior end (see Fig. 1.16, p. 23). The *sensory root* is a branch of the nasociliary nerve and passes through the ganglion without relay to supply the eye, but not the conjunctiva. The *sympathetic root* is a branch from the internal carotid plexus, which enters through the fibrous ring and passes through the ganglion without relay, carrying vasoconstrictor fibres to the vessels of the eye. The *parasympathetic root* is from the nerve to the inferior oblique, the cell bodies being in the Edinger–Westphal nucleus (see p. 496); the fibres relay in the ganglion and supply the ciliary body (for accommodation) and the sphincter pupillae. The branches of the ganglion are the 8–10 **short ciliary nerves**, which contain fibres from all three roots of the ganglion. The nerves pierce the back of the sclera around the attachment of the optic nerve.

Vessels of the orbit

The **ophthalmic artery** is a branch of the internal carotid given off as the vessel emerges from the roof of the cavernous sinus. It passes through the optic canal, inferolateral to the optic nerve and within its dural sheath. In the orbit it pierces the dura and spirals around the lateral side of the optic nerve to pass forwards above the nerve, anterior to the nasociliary nerve. Its many branches accompany all the branches of the nasociliary, the frontal and the lacrimal nerves. Thus it supplies the ethmoidal air cells, nasal cavity, external nose, eyelids and forehead, in all of which places its branches anastomose with branches of the external carotid, establishing connections between internal and external carotid systems.

Within the orbit the ophthalmic artery supplies all the extraocular muscles, the lacrimal gland and the eye. This last is by two sets of vessels. The *central artery* supplies the optic nerve and retina, while the *posterior ciliary arteries* pierce the sclera to enter the choroid coat of the eye. Choroidal capillaries supply the outer layers of the retinae, but there is no anastomosis between the two sets of vessels; the central artery is an end artery. *Anterior ciliary arteries*, from the *muscular branches* to the recti, pierce the anterior part of the eye.

Two ophthalmic veins drain the orbit and receive tributaries that correspond in the main with the branches of the ophthalmic artery. The **superior ophthalmic vein** commences above the medial palpebral ligament and passes back above the optic nerve to drain into the cavernous sinus through the superior orbital fissure. It communicates at its commencement with the angular vein. The **inferior ophthalmic vein** commences at the front of the orbital floor and runs back to drain through the inferior orbital fissure into the pterygoid plexus and either directly into the cavernous sinus through the superior orbital fissure or by joining the superior ophthalmic vein.

There are no lymphatics in the eyeball. The lymphatics of the eyelids drain with those of the face.

Movement of the eyes

Normal binocular vision depends on the properly coordinated activity of the 12 muscles that move the two eyes. Three of the rectus muscles—medial, superior and inferior—are concerned with turning the eye in, and the lateral rectus and the two obliques turn it out.

The actions of the *medial* and *lateral recti* are simple. Each lies in a horizontal plane and turns the eye *in* or *out* respectively. There are no secondary movements.

The actions of the superior and inferior recti and obliques are more complex. Each is inserted in front of the coronal equator, and the line of pull passes medial to the axis of rotation of the eye. Thus the *superior rectus* turns the eye *up and in*, and in the *inferior oblique* turns it *up and out*; combined they produce a *vertical upward* movement, for their medial and lateral components cancel each other out. Similarly the *inferior rectus*

turns the eye *down and in*, the *superior oblique down and out*; combined they turn it *vertically down*. Pure up and down movement is thus produced by one rectus acting with its oppositely named oblique (superior rectus and inferior oblique, inferior rectus and superior oblique).

On account of the concurrent action of the superior and inferior recti, the *elevating* action of the *inferior* oblique and the *depressing* action of the *superior* oblique only become independently demonstrable when the eye is turned in; the more the eye is turned out, the less is their contribution to the up or down movement. Hence the function of the trochlear nerve (action of superior oblique) is tested by asking the subject to look downwards and inwards at the tip of the nose. Similarly the elevating and depressing actions of the superior and inferior recti are best demonstrated when the eye is turned out.

The obliquity of pull of the superior and inferior recti and obliques produces a certain amount of *torsion* or wheel rotation of the eye around an anteroposterior axis. Thus, as viewed by an observer from the front, 12 o'clock on the right cornea rotates to 1 o'clock (*intorsion*) by the action of superior rectus and oblique, or to 11 o'clock (*extorsion*) by the action of inferior rectus and oblique.

Control of conjugate gaze

Moving the eyes from side to side implies turning one eye in and the other out; this is *conjugate horizontal gaze* and, if looking to the left for example, depends essentially on the coordinated activity of the left lateral rectus and right medial rectus. The neural pathways (Fig. 6.57) involve fibres from the visual cortex to the frontal eye field in the middle frontal gyrus, from which fibres pass to a region of the reticular formation of the opposite side adjacent to the abducens nucleus in the pons, the pontine paramedian reticular formation. From here some fibres pass to the abducens nucleus of the same side, so activating the lateral rectus of that eye; other fibres cross the midline to join the medial longitudinal fasciculus and run to the part of the oculomotor nucleus that controls the medial rectus of the other eye.

Similar pathways for control of *conjugate vertical gaze* involve the oculomotor and trochlear nuclei and a rostral interstitial nucleus of the medial longitudinal fasciculus in the midbrain.

Ocular nerve paralyses

Each complete nerve lesion produces a characteristic pattern of strabismus (squint) and diplopia (Fig. 6.58). The simplest nerve lesion is that of the sixth nerve

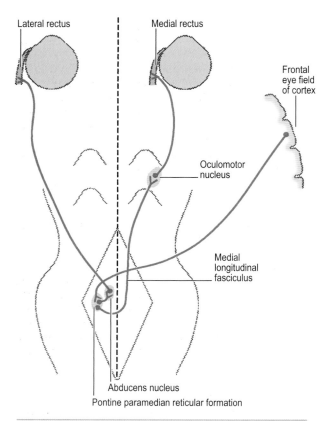

Lateral rectus | Medial rectus

Frontal eye field of cortex

Oculomotor nucleus

Medial longitudinal fasciculus

Abducens nucleus

Pontine paramedian reticular formation

Fig. 6.57 Pathway for conjugate gaze. The para-abducent nucleus (pontine paramedian reticular formation) projects to the abducens nucleus of the same side and the oculomotor nucleus of the opposite side.

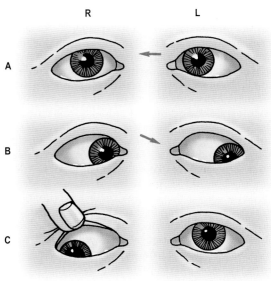

R   L

A

B

C

Fig. 6.58 Position of the right eye in right ocular nerve paralyses, when attempting to look in the direction of the arrow in **A** and **B**, and looking forward in **C**. **A** Abducens nerve; **B** trochlear nerve; **C** oculomotor nerve.

(abducens). The eye cannot look outwards due to paralysis of the lateral rectus (Fig. 6.58A) and, when trying to look straight ahead, it is turned in by the un-opposed action of the medial, superior and inferior recti (oculomotor nerve).

With a fourth nerve paralysis (trochlear), the eye cannot look downwards as far as it should when the eye is turned in (Fig. 6.58B) because of the superior oblique paralysis, so that the patient complains of diplopia when reading or difficulty going down stairs. There is also some degree of extorsion, because the superior oblique which normally produces intorsion is not available to counteract the extorting effect of the inferior oblique. To compensate for the extorsion, the patient characteristically tilts the head towards the opposite shoulder, in order to bring (for example in a right fourth nerve palsy) the 11 o'clock position on the cornea up to 12 o'clock; at the same time the good eye (the left in this example) uses its intact control mechanisms to produce intorsion.

With a third nerve lesion (oculomotor), the most obvious feature is ptosis of the upper lid due to paralysis of the levator. When the lid is manually lifted up, the eye is seen to be looking down and out (Fig. 6.58C) due to the unopposed actions of the lateral rectus (sixth nerve) and superior oblique (fourth nerve). The eye cannot be turned up, in or further down due to paralysis of the superior, medial and inferior recti, but on looking outwards the diplopia will disappear because the lateral rectus (sixth nerve) is acting normally. The pupil is dilated and does not react to light or on accommodation, due to interruption of the parasympathetic fibres that run in the oculomotor nerve (see p. 423) though the consensual reflex in the opposite eye is preserved.

Structure of the eye

The eye contains the light-sensitive retina and, like a camera, it is provided with a lens system for focusing images (the cornea, lens and refractive media) and with means of controlling the amount of light admitted (the iris diaphragm). Like a camera, its inside is black to prevent internal reflections. The relatively large area behind the lens is occupied by the vitreous body. In front of the lens is the small area filled by aqueous humour and incompletely divided into anterior and posterior chambers by the iris. The space bounded by the inner margin of the iris is the pupil.

The wall of the eye, enclosing the refractive media, is made up of three coats. The outer coat is *fibrous* and consists of the sclera and cornea; a *vascular* coat (the choroid, ciliary body and iris) intervenes between this and the innermost *nervous* coat (the retina). The sclera can be regarded as a cup-like expansion of the dural sheath of the optic nerve. The choroid, similarly, is an expansion of the arachnoid and pia, the retina being an expansion of the brain substance of the optic nerve.

Fibrous coat

The **sclera** is the posterior five-sixths of the outer coat of the eyeball. The sclera is opaque (the 'white' of the eye) and consists of dense collagen fibres, interspersed with elastic fibres. It is thinnest at the equator and where it is pierced by the recti. It is thickest at the back but weakest at the entrance of the optic nerve, whose perforating fibres give it a sieve-like appearance, the **lamina cribrosa.**

If a sustained increase of intraocular pressure occurs (chronic glaucoma) the lamina cribrosa yields and bulges posteriorly ('cupping' of the disc).

The sheath of dura mater around the optic nerve blends with the sclera. The sclera receives the insertions of the ocular muscles. It is pierced by the ciliary nerves and arteries around the entrance of the optic nerve, and by the venae vorticosae (the choroid veins) just behind the coronal equator. The anterior ciliary arteries (from muscular branches to the recti) perforate the sclera near the corneoscleral junction.

The fascial sheath of the eye and the bulbar conjunctiva are connected to the sclera by loose connective tissue, which is vascular under the conjunctiva; engorgement of these vessels produces a circumcorneal injection indicative of inflammation within the eye. The rest of the sclera is almost avascular.

Just behind the corneoscleral junction, within the sclera is a circularly running canal, the *sinus venosus sclerae (canal of Schlemm)* (Fig. 6.59). Posterior to the canal is a triangular projection, the *scleral spur*, pointing forwards and inwards, to which the ciliary muscle is attached. The canal is lined with endothelium. Aqueous humour from the anterior chamber filters into the canal

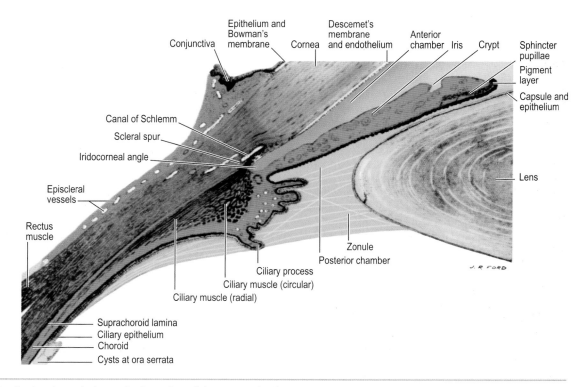

Fig. 6.59   Section through the eye in the region of the corneoscleral junction.

through trabecular tissue on its anterior wall. The canal is connected with anterior scleral veins, into which it drains.

Anteriorly the **cornea** is continuous with the sclera (Fig. 6.59), with the difference that its laminae of fibrous tissue are transparent instead of opaque white. It bulges forward from the sclera at the *corneoscleral junction* or *limbus*, being the segment of a smaller sphere. It occupies the anterior one-sixth of the eye and is completely avascular. At the limbus the conjunctival epithelium becomes continuous with the *corneal epithelium*, which is a very regular stratified squamous type of about five layers of cells. It is separated from the corneal stroma by the *anterior limiting layer* (Bowman's membrane), a homogeneous layer with scattered collagen fibrils and much ground substance.

The *corneal stroma* or substantia propria consists of over 200 lamellae of collagen fibrils, with scattered fibroblasts. The transparency is due to the precise lattice arrangement of its lamellae embedded in a ground substance. The normal lack of vascularity (and of lymph vessels) accounts for the success of corneal grafts, which are thus not invaded by T lymphocytes. The inner surface of the stroma lies against the *posterior limiting layer* (Descemet's membrane), which is the basement membrane of the innermost single layer of *corneal endothelium*.

The cornea is supplied by the short (mainly) and long ciliary nerves. The corneal reflex is elicited clinically by the gentlest touching of the cornea (not the conjunctiva) with a wisp of cotton wool; both eyes should shut. The pathway is via the trigeminal ganglion to the main sensory nucleus, whence impulses pass by way of the reticular formation to reach both facial nerve nuclei and so stimulate both orbicularis oculi to close the lids on both sides.

Vascular coat

The intermediate coat of the eye, frequently known as the **uveal tract**, consists of a continuum of vascular tissue which is made up of the choroid, the ciliary body and iris.

The **choroid** is a thin, pigmented layer lining the inner surface of the sclera, with the delicate connective tissue of the suprachoroid lamina intervening. Anteriorly it merges into the ciliary body (Fig. 6.59). Posteriorly it is perforated by the optic nerve, to which it is firmly attached. Its inner surface is firmly attached to the pigment layer of the retina, and the choroid capillaries provide nutrition for the rods and cones of the retina. The veins collect into four or five large *venae vorticosae*, which pass through the sclera just behind the equator.

The **ciliary body** is continuous with the choroid behind, and the iris in front. It lies as a flat ring applied to the inner surface of the sclera. Being thicker in front and thinner behind, the ciliary body appears triangular in section. The two long sides of the triangle are in contact with the sclera externally and the vitreous body internally. The periphery of the iris is attached halfway along the short anterior base of the triangle. The scleral surface of the ciliary body contains the ciliary muscle. The vitreous surface of the ciliary body is lined by two layers of epithelium. The outer layer is pigmented and the inner layer non-pigmented; they respectively represent the pigmented layer and the nervous part of the retina. This surface appears smooth where it is continuous with the choroid at the ora serrata, but further forward this surface is projected into 70–80 small *ciliary processes* which lie in reciprocal grooves on the anterior surface of the vitreous body.

The **ciliary muscle** consists of smooth muscle; its function is to focus the lens for near vision. Its outermost fibres are longitudinal and pass back into the stroma of the choroid; the innermost are circular and run circumferentially near the periphery of the lens. Between the two are radial fibres which radiate in from the scleral spur. Contraction of the ciliary muscle relaxes the suspensory ligament, allowing the lens to bulge and focus near objects on the retina. The muscle is supplied from the Edinger–Westphal part of the oculomotor nucleus in the midbrain, by fibres which relay in the ciliary ganglion and enter the eye in the short ciliary nerves.

The **iris** is attached at its periphery to the middle of the anterior surface of the ciliary body; peripheral to this attachment the ciliary body itself and a narrow rim of sclera form the iridocorneal angle of the anterior chamber (Fig. 6.59). From its peripheral attachment the iris is pushed slightly forwards, in the form of a very low cone, by contact with the anterior convexity of the lens. The iris is perforated centrally by the pupil, the varying size of which controls the amount of light entering the eye.

The main bulk of the iris is made up of vascular connective tissue in which melanocytes are present. Behind the stroma are two epithelial layers. The cells of the anterior layer contain few melanin granules, while those of the posterior layer are packed with melanin granules. The colour of the iris is determined by the amount of pigment in the iris. When pigment is lacking, as at birth, the iris is blue. As the amount of pigment cells increase the iris colour becomes darker. The colour of the pigment, too, varies in different individuals.

The **sphincter pupillae** is a circular band of smooth muscle lying in the stroma of the iris at the margin of the pupil. It is supplied, like the ciliary muscle, from the Edinger–Westphal part of the oculomotor nucleus. The dilator pupillae is a thin sheet of radial fibres of smooth muscle at the back of the stroma of the iris, extending from the ciliary body to the sphincter pupillae. It is supplied by the cervical sympathetic. The preganglionic cells lie in T1 segment of the spinal cord. The stroma of the iris and the sphincter and dilator muscles are derived from the neural crest (see p. 25).

Control of the pupil and reflexes

The size of the pupil depends on the interplay between the sphincter innervated by parasympathetic fibres and the dilator which receives a sympathetic supply. When a light is shone into one eye, the pupil of that eye constricts; this is the **direct pupillary light reflex**. The pupil of the other eye also constricts; this is the *indirect* or **consensual light reflex**. The neural pathway is as follows (Fig. 6.60). Some fibres of the optic tract bypass the lateral geniculate body by running in the superior brachium to reach the midbrain at the level of the superior colliculus and enter the pretectal nucleus. From there the cell bodies send their axons to the Edinger–Westphal nucleus, from which fibres reach the ciliary ganglion via the oculomotor nerve and its branch to the inferior oblique. The short ciliary nerves from the ganglion supply the sphincter pupillae. Because the pretectal nucleus sends fibres to the Edinger–Westphal nucleus of both sides, both pupils will constrict. The partial crossing

of the fibres of one optic nerve in the optic chiasma also ensures that both pretectal nuclei are stimulated.

Pathological studies indicate that in the main oculomotor nerve trunk the pupillary fibres lie on the surface of the nerve and have a blood supply from vessels of the nerve sheath, not from those of the nerve trunk. Thus these fibres may be affected by pressure (e.g. from an aneurysm of the posterior communicating artery) but not by infarction of the nerve trunk (as in diabetes).

The eye automatically focuses and converges for near vision, and this change in lens curvature is accompanied by pupillary constriction to sharpen the focus. These three components—accommodation, convergence and pupillary constriction—constitute the **accommodation–convergence reflex**, or *near reflex*. The changes accompany conscious vision: they involve cortical as well as subcortical pathways. From the visual cortex an association bundle reaches the frontal eye field of the middle frontal gyrus. Cell bodies in this cortex send their efferent fibres via the anterior limb of the internal capsule to the oculomotor nucleus including the Edinger–Westphal part, which by ciliary ganglion relay activates the ciliary muscle and the sphincter pupillae. Contraction of the ciliary muscle releases tension on the suspensory ligament of the lens, so allowing the lens by its own elasticity to thicken and focus for near vision. Accompanying the accommodation changes, the medial rectus muscle of each eye contracts to provide the necessary convergence for near vision.

The sympathetic path to the pupil is very long (Fig. 6.61). From cells in the hypothalamus (whose cortical control is uncertain), fibres run down through the brainstem and spinal cord to lateral horn cells in T1 segment of the cord. Preganglionic fibres enter the sympathetic trunk via the white ramus communicans of T1 nerve and pass up to the superior cervical ganglion. From there postganglionic fibres accompany the internal carotid artery into the skull and cavernous sinus, leaving the artery to join the ophthalmic nerve and become distributed to the eye by the nasociliary and then the long ciliary branches.

Damage to any of the above fibres can interrupt this pathway. Thus such conditions as vascular or degenerative lesions of the brainstem or spinal cord, pressure on the T1 nerve root by a cervical rib, involvement of the sympathetic trunk by carcinoma of the lung, thyroid or oesophagus, or metastatic lymph nodes, may give rise to **Horner's syndrome**. The characteristic features include *slight constriction of the pupil* (due to unopposed parasympathetic activity and really a failure of dilatation) but which still reacts to light and accommodation, *partial ptosis* (due to paralysis of the smooth muscle part of levator palpebrae) and *reduction of sweating* on the

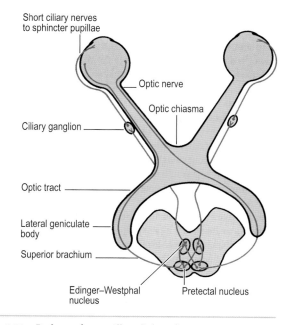

Fig. 6.60 Pathway for pupillary light reflexes.

Short ciliary nerves to sphincter pupillae

Optic nerve

Optic chiasma

Ciliary ganglion

Optic tract

Lateral geniculate body

Superior brachium

Edinger–Westphal nucleus

Pretectal nucleus

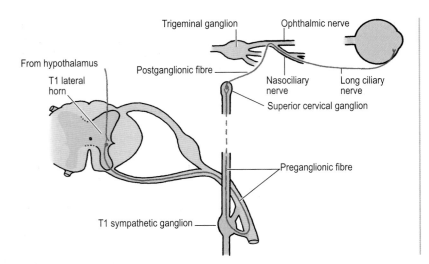

Fig. 6.61   Sympathetic pathway to the pupil.

forehead or a larger area of the head (unless the lesion is above the superior cervical ganglion, when there is no loss of sweating).

Nervous coat

The **retina** is the delicate innermost membrane of the eye. Its outer surface is attached to the choroid, and its inner surface is in contact with the vitreous body. The light-sensitive area ends abruptly, halfway between equator and corneoscleral junction, at a dentate line, the **ora serrata**. Forward of this a thin insensitive layer passes on in continuity as the epithelial layers of the ciliary body and iris. At the entrance of the optic nerve is a circular pale area, 1.5 mm in diameter; this is the **optic disc**. It overlies the lamina cribrosa of the sclera. The optic disc is excavated to a variable degree, producing the physiological cup. There are no rods or cones in the optic disc, hence it is insensitive to light: the '*blind spot*'. The disc and whole surrounding area of the back of the eye as seen with the ophthalmoscope constitute the *fundus* of the eye.

At the posterior pole of the eye (3 mm lateral to the optic disc) is a shallow depression; it is completely free of blood vessels and is yellowish, hence called the **macula lutea**. In the centre of the macula is a shallow pit, the **fovea centralis**, of comparable size to the disc. This is the thinnest part of the retina. There are no blood vessels and no rods here, but there is a high concentration of cones. It is the area of the most acute vision.

The outer layer of the retina consists of a single layer of pigmented epithelial cells firmly attached to the choroid. Next to this layer lie the light receptors (the rods and cones), forming a layer less firmly attached to the pigment cells, so that in detachment of the retina the pigment cells remain in position while the rods and cones, with the other layers of the retina, become displaced inwards from them.

The physiological arrangement of the nervous elements is very similar to that in any other sensory pathway (e.g. in the spinal cord). From the sense receptor, the first neuron has its cell body peripherally placed (in the retina this is the bipolar cell). It leads by synapse to the second neuron (in the retina this is the ganglion cell) whose axon passes to the thalamus (in this case the lateral geniculate body) whence, after relay, the third neuron leads through the retrolentiform part of the internal capsule to the visual cortex (see Fig. 7.9, p. 483).

The light receptors are of two kinds, rods and cones. Only the **rods** contain the photoreceptor protein rhodopsin, or visual purple. (Cones contain related photosensitive pigments with different absorption properties.) Rods do not register colour, but are sensitive to dim light (*scotopic vision*). The periphery of the retina contains rods only. Several rods by their bipolar cells share one ganglion cell (from which one axon passes to the lateral geniculate body). They are of low threshold; together they 'whisper up the line' to the thalamus and cortex. The **cones** have a higher threshold (*photopic vision*) and they register colour. Cones alone occupy the fovea centralis. Beyond this they share equally with the rods, but they fall short of the periphery of the retina. Each cone is connected to a separate ganglion cell; alone it 'shouts up the line' to the thalamus and cortex.

Customarily 10 retinal layers are distinguished from outside inwards; they are as follows:

1. Pigment epithelium
2. Rods and cones (processes)
3. External limiting lamina
4. Outer nuclear layer (rod and cone cell bodies with their nuclei)
5. Outer plexiform layer
6. Inner nuclear layer (bipolar cells)
7. Inner plexiform layer
8. Ganglion cell layer
9. Nerve fibre layer (axons of ganglion cells which pass into the optic nerve at the disc)
10. Inner limiting lamina.

The central artery of the retina passes through the lamina cribrosa within the optic nerve and in the optic disc divides into an upper and lower branch. Each gives off nasal and temporal branches. The upper and lower temporal branches curve up and down respectively to clear the macula lutea. The branches of the central artery are end arteries. They supply the neurons (bipolar and ganglion cells) of the retina. The light receptors (rods and cones and their nuclei in the outer nuclear layer) are supplied by diffusion from the capillaries of the choroid. The retinal veins run with the branches of the central artery. The central vein leaves via the optic disc and emerges from the optic nerve and its coverings to join the superior ophthalmic vein.

Development. The retina is developed from a hollow outgrowth, the *optic vesicle*, which protrudes from the cerebral vesicle. The optic vesicle becomes invaginated to form the *optic cup*, consisting of two layers of cells.

The outer layer differentiates to form the pigment cell layer. The inner layer forms the remaining layers of the retina with the rods and cones outermost (next to the pigment cells). The ganglion cells and their axons are innermost; light has therefore to pass through them to activate the receptors.

Refracting media

Most of the refraction of light takes place at the junction of air and corneal epithelium. Beyond the cornea light passes through the aqueous humour, the lens and vitreous body to reach the retina.

The **aqueous humour** is a clear fluid that lies between the back of the cornea and the front of the lens. The space is divided by the iris into anterior and posterior chambers, which communicate with each other through the pupil (Fig. 6.62). The anterior chamber is 3 mm deep centrally. Aqueous humour is produced by the ciliary processes by diffusion from the capillaries and transported by the ciliary epithelium into the posterior chamber, it passes through the pupil into the anterior chamber. At the margin of the anterior chamber is the iridocorneal angle (see p. 422) and here aqueous humour filters through trabecular tissue into the canal of Schlemm (see p. 421). Obliteration of the angle therefore prevents absorption of aqueous humour, with consequent rise of intraocular tension, leading to the condition of glaucoma. Aqueous humour is an avenue for nutrients and metabolic exchange for the avascular cornea and lens.

The posterior chamber is bounded in front by the iris and behind by the lens and its suspensory ligament. It is triangular in cross-section (pupil and lens in contact with

Fig. 6.62 Horizontal section of the right eyeball: superior aspect.

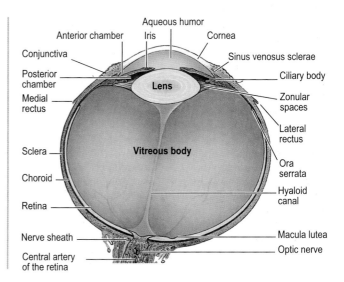

each other forming the apex of the triangle). The base of this triangle is formed by the ciliary processes. Aqueous humour lies between the fibres of the suspensory ligament as far back as the anterior surface of the vitreous.

The **lens** is a transparent biconvex body enclosed in a transparent elastic capsule. It is 10 mm in diameter and 4 mm thick. Its posterior surface, resting on the vitreous, is more highly convex than the anterior. The latter surface is in contact with the pupillary margin of the iris. The *lens capsule* is an elastic membrane that envelops the whole lens. The *capsular epithelium* lies anteriorly, deep to the capsule. Centrally it is a single layer of cubical cells, but more peripherally the cells elongate to produce *fibres* which, by their accumulation, make up the lens substance.

The **suspensory ligament** of the lens, or *zonule*, is a series of delicate fibrils attached to the ciliary processes and, through the furrows between them, further back on the ciliary body. The fibres pass centrally to attach themselves to the lens, mostly in front of, but a few behind, the circumference. In the rest position they hold the lens flattened under tension; when relaxed by contraction of the ciliary muscle, elasticity of the lens causes its anterior surface to bulge, so thickening it (as in accommodation, see p. 423).

The **vitreous body** is a colourless, jelly-like mass which occupies the posterior four-fifths of the eyeball. It comprises about 99% water and a sparse cellular and fibrous content. It is indented in front by the posterior convexity of the lens and, beyond this, has radial furrows reciprocal with the ciliary processes. It is traversed from the front towards the optic disc by the tiny hyaloid canal, the site of the embryonic hyaloid artery. The vitreous body is attached to the optic disc and just in front of the ora serrata; elsewhere it lies free, in contact with the retina.

PART **FIFTEEN**

Lymph drainage of head and neck

All the lymph drainage from the head and neck goes to the deep cervical nodes. They receive afferents from other lymph node groups in the head and neck as well as directly from organs in these regions. Efferents from the **deep cervical nodes** form the *jugular trunk* which on the left drains into the *thoracic duct* and on the right into the *right lymphatic duct*. The thoracic duct and the right lymphatic duct usually empty into the junction of the subclavian and internal jugular veins on their respective sides; otherwise they open into either of these veins.

There is a horizontal, encircling band of lymph node groups at the craniocervical junction. Nodes in all these groups are clinically palpable when enlarged. *Submental nodes* lie across the midline, below the chin in the submental triangle (see p. 357). The other lymph node groups in the horizontal band are bilaterally represented. *Submandibular nodes* lie in the digastric triangle in relation to the submandibular salivary gland (see p. 349). *Preauricular nodes* are found both superficial and deep to the fascial capsule of the parotid, as well as within the gland (see p. 372). A small *mandibular node* is frequently present where the facial vessels cross the lower border of the mandible, and a small *buccal node* may lie on the lateral surface of the buccinator. One or two *mastoid* (postauricular) *nodes* lie on the mastoid process and two or three *occipital nodes* are present at the apex of the posterior triangle of the neck (see p. 345). The organs and areas that drain to all these nodes are mentioned in connection with the descriptions of the relevant regions.

A few *superficial cervical nodes* lie along the external jugular vein, on the superficial surface of the sterno-cleidomastoid, and drain the lobule of the auricle, floor of the external acoustic meatus and skin over the lower parotid region, as well as the lateral cervical skin. Anterior cervical skin drains to a few superficially located *anterior cervical nodes* along the anterior jugular veins; one such node frequently lies in the suprasternal space.

Deep to the investing fascia at the front of the neck are *infrahyoid nodes* lying on the thyrohyoid membrane, *prelaryngeal nodes* on the cricothyroid membrane and *pretracheal nodes* on the tracheal rings. They drain the anterior cervical nodes and receive lymph from the larynx, trachea and thyroid gland. *Paratracheal nodes* on either side of the trachea and oesophagus receive lymph from pretracheal nodes and directly from the trachea and oesophagus. *Retropharyngeal nodes* lie posterior to the pharynx and anterior to the prevertebral fascia. They drain the pharynx, soft palate, posterior parts of hard palate and nose, and the cervical vertebrae. When enlarged, these nodes can cause difficulty in swallowing (dysphagia) due to pressure on the pharynx.

Many of the deep cervical nodes are closely related to the internal jugular vein, some within the carotid sheath, some on the surface of the sheath. They are descriptively divided into upper and lower groups (*superior* and *inferior deep cervical nodes*) and are mainly under cover of the sternocleidomastoid. Some nodes of the lower group extend into the lower part of the posterior triangle and are related to the brachial plexus and subclavian vessels; these are also termed supraclavicular nodes. One or two nodes lie in contact with the accessory nerve at a higher level in the posterior triangle. One or two

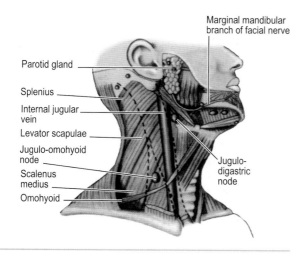

Fig. 6.63 Jugulodigastric and jugulo-omohyoid nodes of the deep cervical chain. Sternocleidomastoid is indicated in dotted outline.

nodes of the upper group of deep cervical nodes, the *jugulodigastric nodes*, lie behind the posterior belly of the digastric in front of the internal jugular vein (Fig. 6.63). When enlarged, as a result for instance of pathology in the palatine tonsil, these are easily palpable behind and below the angle of the mandible. The *jugulo-omohyoid node* is a lower group node that lies above the intermediate tendon of omohyoid posterior to the internal jugular vein. All the lymph drainage from the tongue is believed to reach this node on the two sides of the neck before entering the jugular trunks. The node lies deep to sternocleidomastoid and needs to be considerably enlarged to be clinically palpable.

Surgical approach

Surgeons treating malignant lymph nodes in the neck tend to classify them by levels. Level I nodes are in the submental and submandibular triangles. Level II–IV nodes are deep cervical nodes, Level II being from the base of the skull to the carotid bifurcation (hyoid bone), Level III from there to the intermediate tendon of omohyoid (cricoid cartilage), and Level IV from there down to the clavicle and including the supraclavicular nodes. Level V nodes are in the posterior triangle of the neck, related to the accessory nerve. Level VI nodes are nodes surrounding the midline visceral structures and include the pretracheal and paratracheal nodes. Level VII nodes are in the superior mediastinum. Classical radical neck dissection removed Level I–V nodes with the sternocleidomastoid muscle, internal jugular vein and accessory nerve. Modified radical neck dissection (also called functional neck dissection) preserves some or all of these latter three structures. Selective neck dissection removes some but not all Level I–V nodes.

PART SIXTEEN

Temporomandibular joint

The temporomandibular joint is a synovial joint between the head (condyle) of the mandible and the mandibular fossa on the undersurface of the squamous part of the temporal bone. The mandible is a single bone with a horizontal horseshoe-shaped body, which is continuous at its posterior ends with a pair of vertical rami, each ramus being surmounted by a head or condyle. The cranium, with which the mandible articulates, is also mechanically a single component, with a mandibular fossa on each side. This complex is in effect one functioning joint, as movement cannot take place at one temporomandibular joint without a concomitant movement occurring at the joint on the opposite side. The temporomandibular joints are thus the bilateral components of a craniomandibular articulation.

The joint is separated into upper and lower cavities by a fibrocartilaginous disc within it. Both bone surfaces are covered with a layer of fibrocartilage identical with that of the disc. Though termed fibrocartilage, the articular cartilage and disc consist mainly of collagen fibres with few cartilage cells. There is no hyaline cartilage in this joint, so it is an atypical synovial joint.

The **capsule** is attached high up on the neck of the mandible anteriorly, near the articular margin of the head, but lower down the neck posteriorly. Above, it is attached anteriorly just in front of the articular eminence of the temporal bone (Fig. 6.35), posteriorly to the squamotympanic fissure, and medially and laterally to the margins of the mandibular fossa. It is lax above the disc, but taut below. The synovial membrane lines the inside of the capsule and the intracapsular posterior aspect of the neck of the mandible.

The articular **disc** is attached around its periphery to the inside of the capsule and to the medial and lateral poles of the head of the mandible. Its upper surface is anteroposteriorly concavoconvex in the sagittal plane to fit the articular eminence and fossa; the inferior surface is concave in adaptation to the condyle (Fig. 6.64). Anteriorly the disc is continuous through its capsular attachment with the tendon of lateral pterygoid. Posteriorly the disc divides into two laminae. The upper fibroelastic lamina is attached to the margin of the mandibular fossa; the lower non-elastic fibrous lamina is attached to

427

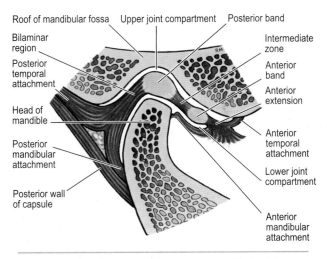

Roof of mandibular fossa   Upper joint compartment   Posterior band

Bilaminar region

Posterior temporal attachment

Head of mandible

Posterior mandibular attachment

Posterior wall of capsule

Intermediate zone

Anterior band

Anterior extension

Anterior temporal attachment

Lower joint compartment

Anterior mandibular attachment

Fig. 6.64   Sagittal section of the temporomandibular joint.

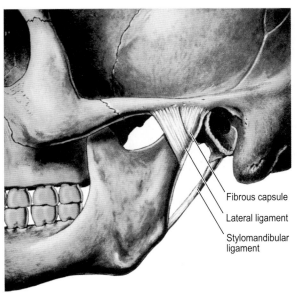

Fibrous capsule

Lateral ligament

Stylomandibular ligament

Fig. 6.65   Capsule and ligaments of the left temporomandibular joint: lateral aspect.

the neck of the mandible. Between the two laminae is a pad of loosely textured tissue containing many blood vessels and sensory nerve endings. The disc has two transverse thickened bands, the posterior being thickest; between these bands it is thinnest and relatively avascular.

The **lateral temporomandibular ligament** is a stout band of fibrous tissue passing obliquely down and back from the articular tubercle of the zygomatic arch (see p. 527) to the lateral surface and posterior border of the neck of the mandible (Fig. 6.65). On its deep aspect a narrow band runs transversely from the articular tubercle to the lateral pole of the mandibular head.

The **sphenomandibular ligament**, running between the spine of the sphenoid and the lingula of the mandible (Fig. 6.66), is an accessory ligament of the joint.

The nerve supply of the joint is from the auriculo-temporal nerve and the nerve to masseter.

Stability

The joint is much more stable with the teeth in occlusion than when the jaw is open.

In **occlusion** the teeth themselves stabilize the mandible on the maxilla and no strain is thrown on the joint when an upward blow is received on the mandible. In the occluded position apart from the stabilizing effect of the teeth, forward movement of the condyle is discouraged by the prominence of the articular eminence and by contraction of the posterior fibres of temporalis, while backward movement is prevented by the fibres of the lateral ligament and by contraction of the lateral pterygoid.

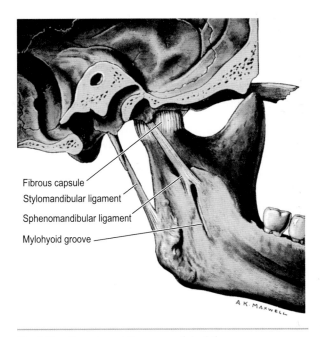

Fibrous capsule

Stylomandibular ligament

Sphenomandibular ligament

Mylohyoid groove

Fig. 6.66   Capsule and ligaments of the left temporomandibular joint: medial aspect.

In the **open position** the joint is less stable as the condyle lies forward on the slope of the articular eminence. Forward dislocation is the most common form of displacement. Forward dislocation is normally opposed by the articular eminence, by the tension of the lateral ligament and by contraction of the masseter, temporalis and medial pterygoid muscles. But when the condyle is dislocated forwards, reduction is prevented by spasm of these same muscles, which hold the dislocated jaw open with the condyle in front of the eminence. The spasm must be overcome (with or without an anaesthetic) by the operator's thumbs pressing downwards on the molar teeth or alveoli, before the condyle can be guided back into the fossa. Anterior dislocation readily occurs in the edentulous. In addition to the loss of stability resulting from the lack of proper occlusion in the elderly, increased postural elevation of the edentulous mandibular body lowers the mandibular head and neck and elongates the lateral ligament.

Movements

There are three sets of mandibular movements at the temporomandibular joint. These are depression and elevation (opening and closing the jaws), side-to-side (grinding) movements, protraction and retraction (pro-trusion and retrusion). The group of muscles commonly classified as the muscles of mastication—temporalis, masseter and medial and lateral pterygoids—play major roles in these movements; others taking part can be called accessory muscles of mastication (Fig. 6.67).

When the mouth is opened, the mandibular head rotates around a horizontal axis in a hinge-like movement that occurs in the lower compartment of the temporo-mandibular joint, between the head and the inferior aspect of the disc, while a gliding movement occurs in the upper compartment between the disc and the mandibular fossa of the temporal bone. In this sequence of events, the mandible is depressed by the digastric, mylohyoid and geniohyoid muscles, while the infrahyoid muscles act to stabilize the hyoid bone. Forward movement of the mandibular head on to the articular eminence of the temporal bone is effected by the lateral pterygoid muscle, principally its inferior head.

Elevation of the mandible (closing the jaw) is produced by the masseters, medial pterygoids and temporalis muscles.

Side-to-side movements are the result of medial and lateral pterygoid activity on one side, alternating with similar activity on the other side. Simultaneous contraction of lateral and medial pterygoid muscles of one side rotates the mandible in the horizontal plane around

Fig. 6.67 Muscles producing movements of the temporomandibular joint. The direction of their actions is indicated by the arrows.

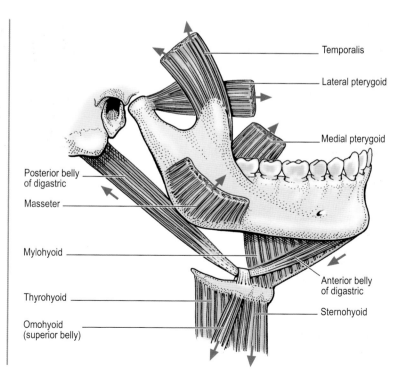

Temporalis

Lateral pterygoid

Medial pterygoid

Posterior belly of digastric

Masseter

Mylohyoid

Thyrohyoid

Omohyoid (superior belly)

Anterior belly of digastric

Sternohyoid

a vertical axis passing a little behind the mandibular head on the opposite side, which moves slightly laterally, while the head on the side of the contracting muscles is drawn forwards on to the articular eminence.

During protraction (as when jutting the chin forwards), all four pterygoid muscles contract, such that the head and disc are drawn forwards, without depression or elevation of the mandibular body. The normal position is restored by passive recoil of stretched joint structures, aided by contraction of the posterior fibres of temporalis and the deep fibres of masseter.

PART SEVENTEEN

Ear

The ear, which houses the peripheral parts of the auditory and vestibular apparatus, is descriptively divided into the external, middle and internal ear. The external ear consists of the auricle or pinna and the external acoustic meatus, at the medial end of which lies the tympanic membrane, separating the external ear from the middle ear. The middle ear or tympanic cavity (tympanum) is a small space in the temporal bone containing the auditory ossicles (malleus, incus and stapes) and air that communicates with the nasopharynx by the auditory tube. By its medial wall the middle ear adjoins the inner ear, which is composed of the osseous labyrinth, another space within the temporal bone, inside which is the membranous labyrinth containing the auditory and vestibular nerve receptors.

External ear

The **auricle** or pinna has a skeleton of resilient yellow elastic cartilage which is thrown into folds. The folds give the auricle its characteristic shape. The cartilage is covered on both surfaces with adherent hairy skin; it does not extend into the lobule of the ear. The lobule is a tag of skin containing soft fibrofatty tissue; it is easily pierced for earrings. The cartilage of the auricle is prolonged inwards in tubular fashion as the cartilaginous part of the external acoustic meatus, whose attachment to bone stabilizes the auricle in position. Small anterior, superior and posterior auricular muscles attach the auricle to the scalp and skull, and all are supplied by the facial nerve.

The **external acoustic meatus** is a sinuous tube nearly 3 cm in length; it is straightened for introduction of an otoscope by pulling the auricle upwards and backwards. Due to the obliquity of the tympanic membrane at the deep end of the meatus, separating it from the tympanic cavity, its anteroinferior wall is longest and its postero-superior wall shortest (Fig. 6.68). Its outer third is cartilage, its inner two-thirds bone; in both zones the skin is firmly adherent.

The bony part is formed by the tympanic part of the temporal bone, C-shaped in cross-section, the gap in the C being applied to the under surface of the squamous and petrous parts. The cartilaginous portion is likewise C-shaped; the gap is filled with fibrous tissue. Hairs and sebaceous glands abound in the cartilaginous part. Here also are the *ceruminous glands*, long coiled tubules like modified sweat glands, which secrete a yellowish-brown

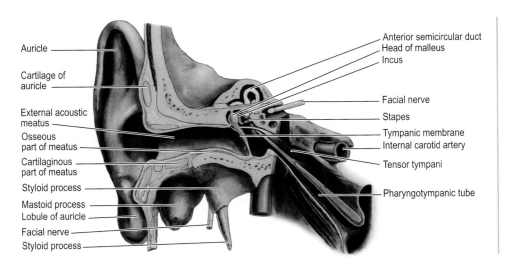

Auricle

Cartilage of auricle

External acoustic meatus

Osseous part of meatus

Cartilaginous part of meatus

Styloid process

Mastoid process

Lobule of auricle

Facial nerve

Styloid process

Anterior semicircular duct
Head of malleus
Incus

Facial nerve

Stapes

Tympanic membrane
Internal carotid artery

Tensor tympani

Pharyngotympanic tube

Fig. 6.68 Oblique section through the right external ear, middle ear and pharyngotympanic tube: anterior aspect.

wax. The meatus is narrowest at the isthmus, a few millimetres from the membrane.

The auricle and external meatus are mainly supplied by the posterior auricular and superficial temporal arteries, with the deeper part of the meatus receiving the deep auricular artery (from the maxillary) which enters the meatus through the squamotympanic fissure. There are corresponding veins.

Lymphatic drainage is to occipital, preauricular and superficial cervical nodes.

The main cutaneous nerves are the great auricular and auriculotemporal nerves, with a small contribution from the vagus. The great auricular supplies the whole of the cranial surface of the auricle (C2, with a little overlap from the lesser occipital at the top) and the lower part of the lateral surface. The auriculotemporal supplies the upper part of the lateral surface and most of the meatal skin. The auricular branch of the vagus (Arnold's nerve) supplies small areas of skin on the cranial auricular surface, posterior wall and floor of the meatus and adjoining part of the tympanic membrane. The facial nerve may also contribute via a communication with the vagus.

Middle ear

The middle ear is an air space in the temporal bone (Fig. 6.68). It contains the three auditory ossicles whose purpose is to transmit sound vibrations from the tympanic membrane in its lateral wall to the inner ear via its medial wall. The cavity of the middle ear, the tympanic cavity or tympanum, is really the intermediate portion of a blind diverticulum from the respiratory mucous membrane of the nasopharynx. From front to back the diverticulum consists of the *auditory tube*, the *tympanic cavity*, and the *mastoid antrum and air cells*.

Tympanic cavity

The tympanic cavity, about 15 mm in anteroposterior and vertical diameters, is the shape of a biconcave lens. Its *lateral wall* is largely occupied by the tympanic membrane, which extends upwards for 10 mm from the floor and bulges inwards to within a couple of millimetres of the medial wall. Above the membrane the temporal bone is hollowed out into the *epitympanic recess*.

The **tympanic membrane** is a thin fibrous structure covered externally with a thin layer of stratified squamous epithelium and internally with low columnar epithelium. The framework consists of collagen fibres. The membrane is circular, 1 cm in diameter, and lies obliquely at 55° with the external acoustic meatus, facing downwards, forwards and laterally (Fig. 6.68). It is concave towards the meatus. At the depth of the concavity is a small depression, the *umbo*. When the drum is illuminated for inspection, the concavity of the membrane produces a 'cone of light' radiating from the umbo over the antero-inferior quadrant. The handle of the malleus is firmly attached to the inner surface of the membrane. From the lateral process of the malleus two thickened fibrous folds (mallear folds) diverge up to the margins of the tympanic bone; between them the small upper segment of the membrane is lax (pars flaccida, Shrapnell's membrane). This part and the handle of the malleus are crossed internally by the chorda tympani. The rest of the membrane, the main part, is the pars tensa. It is held tense by the inward pull of the tensor tympani muscle. Its tension is affected by difference of pressure in the tympanic cavity and external meatus in cases of auditory tube obstruction. The tympanic membrane is thickened at its circumference and slotted into a groove in the tympanic plate.

The tympanic membrane is supplied by the deep auricular artery (maxillary) on the meatal side, and on the mucosal side the stylomastoid artery (posterior auricular) forms a circular anastomosis with the anterior tympanic branch of the maxillary round the margin of the membrane.

On the meatal surface the tympanic membrane is supplied by the auriculotemporal nerve, supplemented by the vagus. The tympanic branch of the glossopharyngeal nerve, via the tympanic plexus, supplies the mucosal surface.

The *medial wall* of the tympanic cavity (which is also the lateral wall of the internal ear) has as its most prominent feature the *promontory* (Fig. 6.69), due to the first turn of the cochlea and indented with fine grooves by the tympanic plexus. Above it is a horizontal ridge for the *canal for the facial nerve*, and immediately above that is the (horizontal) bulge due to the *lateral semicircular canal*. Above and behind the promontory is the *oval window* (fenestra vestibuli), closed in life by the foot-piece of the stapes. *Below and behind* the promontory is the *round window* (fenestra cochleae), closed in life by the fibrous secondary tympanic membrane.

The **roof** of the tympanum is the *tegmen tympani*, a laminar projection of petrous bone that roofs in also the canal for the tensor tympani and the tympanic antrum. Above it the temporal lobe lies in the middle cranial fossa (Fig. 6.69).

The **floor** is a thin plate of bone above the jugular fossa. At the anterior end is the internal opening of the tympanic canaliculus, where the tympanic branch of the glossopharyngeal nerve enters, from the jugular fossa, the external opening of the canaliculus being on the ridge of bone between the fossa and the carotid canal (Fig. 6.19).

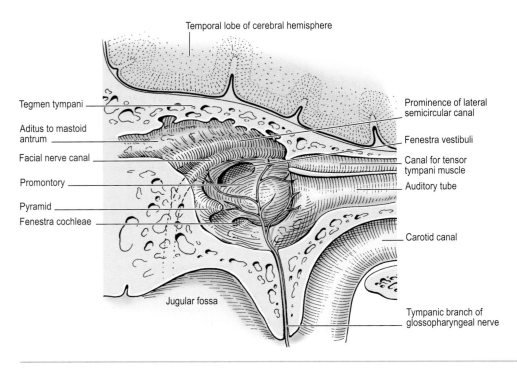

Fig. 6.69   Medial wall of the right middle ear.

The **anterior wall** is shortened by approximation of roof and floor. It is perforated by the openings of two canals: the lower and larger of these is the bony part of the *auditory tube*, the upper and smaller is the *canal for the tensor tympani* muscle (Fig. 6.68). The lower part of this wall forms the posterior wall of the carotid canal and is perforated by tympanic branches of the internal carotid artery and sympathetic fibres from the internal carotid plexus.

The **posterior wall** is deficient above, where there is an aperture, the *aditus*, which leads back into the tympanic antrum. The ridge for the canal for the facial nerve and the bulge due to the lateral semicircular canal continue backwards along the medial wall of the aditus. Below the aditus a hollow cone, the *pyramid*, projects into the tympanic cavity (Fig. 6.69); its apex is perforated by the tendon of stapedius. Close to the posterior margin of the tympanic membrane is the tiny posterior canaliculus for the chorda tympani.

The **auditory ossicles** form by synovial joints a bony chain for transmission of vibrations from the tympanic membrane to the internal ear. The malleus and incus are developed from the proximal end of the first arch cartilage (see Fig. 1.21, p. 27), the stapes comes from the second arch cartilage (see Fig. 1.22, p. 27).

The **malleus** is shaped like a round-headed club. There is a constriction, the neck, between head and handle. The convex *head* lies in the epitympanic recess (Fig. 6.68). Its posterior surface has an articular facet for the incus. The narrow *neck* lies against the pars flaccida of the tympanic membrane. The chorda tympani crosses medial to the neck. The *handle* projects somewhat backwards down to the umbo; its upper end has a projection, the *lateral process*. The two form a lateral concavity moulded to the medial convexity of the tympanic membrane; the periosteum of lateral process and handle is firmly fixed to the fibrous layer of the membrane. The mallear folds are attached to the apex of the lateral process. The tiny *anterior process* is directed forwards from just below the neck; it is embedded in the fibres of the anterior ligament, which passes through the petrotympanic fissure to the spine of the sphenoid; like the sphenomandibular ligament it is derived from the perichondrium of the first arch cartilage.

The **incus** has a relatively large body and two slender processes or limbs. The *body* is rounded and laterally compressed. It lies in the epitympanic recess and articulates anteriorly with the head of the malleus (Fig. 6.65). The *short limb* projects backwards to lie in a shallow fossa in the posterior wall just below the aditus. The *long limb* projects down into the cavity of the middle ear, just behind and parallel with the handle of the malleus. Its tip hooks medially and is bulbous—the lentiform nodule—for articulation with the stapes.

The **stapes** has a small *head* showing a concave facet for articulation with the lentiform nodule. A narrower *neck* diverges into slender anterior and posterior *limbs*, which are attached to the *base* (or footpiece) like a rider's stirrup. This is attached to the oval window by an annular ligament.

The **tensor tympani** arises from and occupies the canal above the bony part of the auditory tube. The slender muscle ends in a round tendon which passes across the cavity of the middle ear and is inserted into the handle of the malleus. Its nerve supply is from the mandibular nerve via its branch to the medial pterygoid (see p. 378). Contraction of the muscle draws the handle of the malleus inwards, making the drum more highly concave and therefore more tense.

The **stapedius** arises from the interior of the hollow pyramid. Its tendon emerges from the apex of the pyramid and is inserted into the back of the neck of the stapes. The muscle is supplied from the facial nerve by a branch given off in the facial (stylomastoid) canal. Its action is to retract the neck of the stapes, thus tilting the footpiece in the oval window. Paralysis of the stapedius causes an abnormally increased power of hearing (hyperacusis).

Mastoid antrum and air cells

The **mastoid (tympanic) antrum** lies behind the epitympanic recess in the petrous part of the temporal bone. It is connected to the recess by the *aditus*. Its size is very variable; it may be up to 1 cm in diameter. When large it is covered by a thin layer of bone, when small by a thick layer. Its lateral wall corresponds to the supra-meatal triangle at the posterosuperior margin of the external acoustic meatus (see p. 529) and the antrum lies about 15 mm deep to the surface of the bone here. It is roofed by the tegmen tympani.

The mastoid antrum is present at birth and is then almost adult size. During the first year **mastoid air cells**, lined with adherent mucoperiosteum, burrow out from the mastoid antrum into the thin plate of bone at the bottom of the groove for the sigmoid sinus. Later they pneumatize the mastoid process for a variable distance, even to the tip. They may be separated from the sigmoid sinus and posterior cranial fossa by extremely thin bone.

The thin **mucous membrane** of the middle ear, continuous with that of the auditory tube and mastoid antrum, adheres to all the structures enumerated above: the walls; ossicles; ligaments; and muscles. The lining epithelium is columnar and ciliated, but squamous and non-ciliated in the antrum and air cells.

The anterior tympanic from the maxillary, the stylomastoid from the posterior auricular (or occipital), and tympanic branches from the internal carotid, middle meningeal and ascending pharyngeal arteries supply the middle ear. Venous drainage is to the pterygoid plexus and superior petrosal sinus. Thrombophlebitis from suppuration in the middle ear may lead to meningitis, and by retrograde venous spread to a cerebral abscess in the temporal lobe. Veins from the mastoid antrum communicate via the mastoid emissary vein with the posterior auricular vein and the sigmoid sinus. Spreading infection from the mastoid antrum and air cells can lead to sigmoid sinus thrombosis, meningitis and a cerebellar abscess.

Lymphatic drainage from the middle ear is to preauricular, retropharyngeal and upper deep cervical nodes.

The mucous membrane of the middle ear is supplied by branches of the **tympanic plexus**. This is mainly formed by the tympanic branch of the glossopharyngeal nerve (Jacobson's nerve), which forms a fine plexiform network on the promontory (Fig. 6.69). It is joined by sympathetic fibres from the internal carotid plexus which enter the tympanic cavity through the wall of the carotid canal.

Since the middle ear and the external ear are supplied by branches of the trigeminal, glossopharyngeal and vagus nerves, pain in the ear (otalgia) may be referred from other areas supplied by these nerves, especially the pharynx, larynx, posterior part of tongue and teeth.

The plexus gives off the **lesser petrosal nerve**. This contains preganglionic parasympathetic fibres from the inferior salivary nucleus, destined to supply the parotid gland via the otic ganglion. The fibres enter the plexus with the glossopharyngeal tympanic branch. The nerve leaves the middle ear through a canaliculus in the anterior wall above the auditory tube and emerges in the middle cranial fossa through a small hiatus lateral to that for the greater petrosal nerve (see Fig. 8.4, p. 529); it then passes through the foramen ovale to reach the otic ganglion (Figs 6.21 and 6.27).

Facial nerve and the ear

The **facial nerve** itself is not within the middle ear cavity but passes through the petrous bone from the internal acoustic meatus to the stylomastoid foramen in three directions, laterally, posteriorly and downwards, in that order. First the main trunk of the nerve runs laterally from the internal acoustic meatus with the nervus intermedius, which contains the parasympathetic fibres for the pterygopalatine and submandibular ganglia (see

Fig. 1.16, p. 23), and also taste fibres from the anterior part of the tongue and the soft palate. The two parts of the facial nerve here lie above the vestibule, with the cochlea in front and the semicircular canals behind. The nervus intermedius now joins the main nerve at the geniculate ganglion. The greater petrosal nerve passes forwards from the ganglion through a canal in the petrous bone and emerges from a hiatus into the middle cranial fossa (Fig. 6.101), which it leaves through the foramen lacerum to become part of the nerve of the pterygoid canal (see p. 384).

The facial nerve now passes backwards from the ganglion in the canal which raises the ridge on the medial wall of the tympanic cavity above the promontory and below the prominence of the lateral semicircular canal (Fig. 6.69). Finally the nerve passes downwards medial to the aditus to the antrum and emerges from the stylomastoid foramen. The nerve to stapedius and the chorda tympani leave this part of the nerve in the middle ear.

The **chorda tympani** is a mixed visceral nerve, containing taste fibres from the tongue (cell bodies in the geniculate ganglion) and secretomotor fibres for the salivary glands of the floor of the mouth (cell bodies in the superior salivary nucleus in the pons). At about 6 mm above the stylomastoid foramen the chorda tympani leaves the facial nerve in the facial canal and pierces the posterior wall of the tympanic cavity (Fig. 6.27). It runs forward over the pars flaccida of the tympanic membrane and the neck of the malleus, lying just beneath the mucous membrane (Fig. 6.21). It passes out of the front of the middle ear and emerges from the medial end of the petrotympanic fissure (Fig. 6.35), grooves the medial side of the spine of the sphenoid, and joins the lingual nerve 2 cm below the base of the skull.

Auditory tube

The auditory tube (pharyngotympanic tube, Eustachian tube) connects the nasopharynx with the middle ear. Over 3 cm long, it slopes from the middle ear forwards and medially at 45° and downwards at 30°. Like the external acoustic meatus it has bony and cartilaginous parts, but the proportions are reversed.

The **bony part**, over 1 cm long, tapers down from the anterior wall of the middle ear to its orifice. This is the narrowest part of the tube, the *isthmus*; it lies posteromedial to the spine of the sphenoid and lateral to the carotid canal. The bony part perforates the petrous part of the temporal bone and is lined with adherent mucoperiosteum. It is surfaced by ciliated columnar epithelium and, as in the middle ear, has no glands.

The **cartilaginous part**, over 2 cm long, joins the bony orifice at the isthmus and is lodged in the groove between the greater wing of the sphenoid and the apex of the petrous part of the temporal bone (Fig. 6.35). It is made of elastic cartilage, which in transverse section resembles an inverted J (long limb medial) open inferolaterally where it is closed by fibrous tissue. It enlarges from the isthmus like a trumpet, with its open end expanded, particularly the long posterior limb which forms the *tubal elevation* in the lateral wall of the nasopharynx (Fig. 6.39). The mucosa is lined by ciliated columnar cells and has mucous glands. The cilia beat towards the nasopharynx, thus protecting the middle ear from airborne particles, including bacteria.

The **ostium** (opening) of the tube is attached to the back of the medial pterygoid plate just below the skull base. The tubal elevation is made more prominent, especially in the young, by lymphoid follicles in the mucous membrane (tubal tonsil). The posterior limb is elongated by the vertical salpingopharyngeal fold, draped over salpingopharyngeus.

The pharyngobasilar fascia is attached to the lower part of the tube; lateral to this the tensor palati arises outside the pharynx, and medial to this the levator palati arises inside the pharynx. Both are attached in part to the tube and contract during swallowing which opens the tube and allows equalization of air pressure on the two sides of the tympanic membrane. Air is slowly lost from the middle ear and mastoid cavities by absorption into the capillaries thereof.

The blood supply of the tube is from the ascending pharyngeal and middle meningeal arteries. Its veins drain into the pharyngeal plexus. The lymphatic drainage is to retropharyngeal lymph nodes. The nerve supply is by the pharyngeal branch of the pterygopalatine ganglion (maxillary nerve) and the tympanic plexus (glossopharyngeal nerve).

Internal ear

The internal ear is buried in the petrous part of the temporal bone and is practically full adult size at birth. It consists of a complex series of connected cavities, the *osseous labyrinth*, within which lies a correspondingly complex fluid-filled sac, the *membranous labyrinth*. The fluid it contains is *endolymph* and, because the membranous labyrinth is smaller than the osseous, its walls are not all pressed tightly against the bone but are mostly separated from it by another fluid, *perilymph*. The endolymph and perilymph do not communicate with one another.

The parts of the osseous labyrinth, in order from front to back, are the *cochlear canal* (or *cochlea*), the *vestibule*, and the *semicircular canals* (Figs 6.70 and 6.71; these illustrations depict casts of the bony cavity).

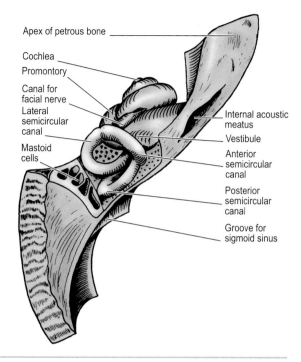

Apex of petrous bone

Cochlea
Promontory
Canal for
facial nerve
Lateral
semicircular
canal
Mastoid
cells

Internal acoustic
meatus
Vestibule
Anterior
semicircular
canal
Posterior
semicircular
canal
Groove for
sigmoid sinus

Fig. 6.70 Left osseous labyrinth in the temporal bone, from above and behind. The cochlea is at the front, the vestibule in the middle and the semicircular canals at the back.

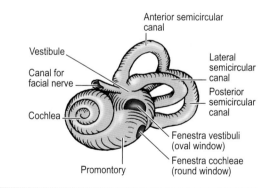

Anterior semicircular
canal
Vestibule
Canal for
facial nerve
Cochlea
Lateral
semicircular
canal
Posterior
semicircular
canal
Fenestra vestibuli
(oval window)
Fenestra cochleae
(round window)
Promontory

Fig. 6.71 Left osseous labyrinth, from the lateral side.

The parts of the membranous labyrinth (Fig. 6.72) are the *cochlear duct* (within the cochlear canal and concerned with hearing), the *utricle* and *saccule* (within the vestibule and concerned with static balance), and the *semicircular ducts* (within the semicircular canals and concerned with kinetic balance).

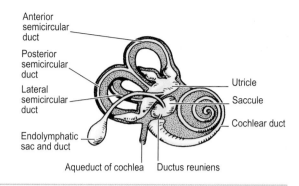

Anterior
semicircular
duct
Posterior
semicircular
duct
Lateral
semicircular
duct
Endolymphatic
sac and duct
Aqueduct of cochlea   Ductus reuniens
Utricle
Saccule
Cochlear duct

Fig. 6.72 Left membranous labyrinth, from the medial side. The stippled part represents the osseous labyrinth.

Osseous labyrinth

The cavity of the osseous labyrinth is lined by endosteum and opens into the medial wall of the middle ear through the oval window (closed in life by the footpiece of the stapes) and the round window (closed in life by the secondary tympanic membrane) (Figs 6.71 and 6.69). It also opens into the posterior cranial fossa through the aqueduct of the vestibule (Fig. 6.105), closed in life by the endolymphatic duct, and through the aqueduct of the cochlea (Fig. 6.72) through which perilymph is believed to drain into the cerebrospinal fluid. The source of perilymph is uncertain; it may be derived from cerebrospinal fluid or as an ultrafiltrate from perilymphatic blood capillaries.

The **cochlea** is a conical snail-shaped cavity in the petrous bone. It consists of two and three-quarter spiral turns of a tapering canal. The bony canal is of greatest calibre at the basal turn; this part projects laterally, producing the promontory on the medial wall of the middle ear (Fig. 6.69).

The axial bony stem around which the canal spirals is the *modiolus*. The base of the modiolus lies at the fundus of the internal acoustic meatus and its apex lies across the long axis of the petrous bone, pointing towards the middle ear. The apex of the modiolus is overlaid by the blind extremity of the apical turn of the cochlea.

From the modiolus a spiral shelf of bone projects into the canal, like a thread projecting from a screw. This is the *spiral lamina*. Its projection is widest in the basal and narrowest in the apical turn. The membranous cochlear duct (Figs 6.72 and 6.73) is attached to the spiral lamina and to the outer bony wall of the canal.

The bony canal of the cochlea is thus partitioned by the spiral lamina and the membranous cochlear duct, which contains endolymph. The canal on the apical

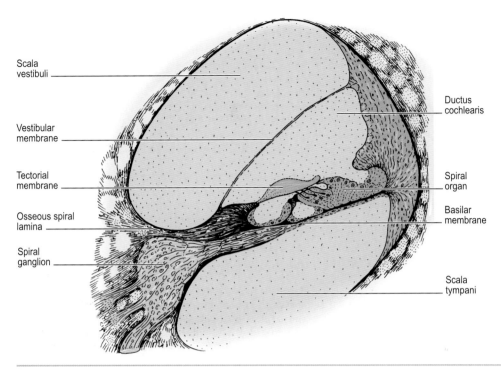

Scala vestibuli

Vestibular membrane

Tectorial membrane

Osseous spiral lamina

Spiral ganglion

Ductus cochlearis

Spiral organ

Basilar membrane

Scala tympani

Fig. 6.73   Transverse section through a single turn of the cochlea.

side of the partition is the *scala vestibuli*, that on the basal side the *scala tympani* (Fig. 6.73); they contain perilymph. They communicate with each other around the blind apical extremity of the cochlear duct.

The basal turn of the cochlea sees the termination of the spiral lamina. Here the scala tympani is sealed off into a blind end. There are two holes in this cul-de-sac. One leads laterally into the middle ear—the round window—which is closed in life by the secondary tympanic membrane. The other is the beginning of a canal, the *aqueduct of the cochlea* (perilymphatic duct), which leads down through the substance of the petrous bone and opens into the *cochlear canaliculus*, below the internal acoustic meatus, in the anterior compartment of the jugular foramen. The aqueduct of the cochlea is patent in life. The arachnoid mater is attached to the margin of its opening, so that perilymph draining down the aqueduct is received into the cerebrospinal fluid in the subarachnoid space.

The modiolus is perforated spirally at its base in the internal acoustic meatus by the branches of the cochlear nerve (Fig. 6.108). These run into the modiolus and fan out spirally towards the base of the spiral lamina, where the *spiral ganglion* containing their bipolar cell bodies

lies in the spiral canal of the modiolus (Fig. 6.73). This is the counterpart of the posterior root ganglion of a spinal nerve (i.e. it contains the cell bodies of the first neuron of a sensory pathway). The spiral ganglion (cochlear nerve) connects the sound receptors in the spiral organ (see below) with the cochlear nuclei in the brainstem.

The **vestibule** is a hollow in the petrous bone which contains the membranous saccule and utricle (Figs 6.70 and 6.72). The scala vestibuli of the cochlea opens into the front of the vestibule and the five orifices of the semicircular canals open posteriorly.

The medial wall abuts on the internal acoustic meatus and is perforated by minute foramina for the branches of the vestibular nerve to the saccule, utricle and semicircular canals.

The lateral wall of the vestibule abuts on the middle ear behind the promontory. Here is the opening of the oval window (Fig. 6.71), closed in life by the foot-piece of the stapes and its annular ligament.

The **semicircular canals** lie in three planes at right angles to each other (Fig. 6.71). Each is about two-thirds of a circle; in length along the curve they measure about 20 mm. Their calibre is 1 mm except at one end, where each is dilated as the ampulla to a calibre of 2 mm.

The *anterior (superior) semicircular canal* is placed in a vertical plane across the long axis of the petrous bone, convexity upwards, ampulla laterally (Fig. 6.70). Its convexity produces the arcuate eminence on the upper surface of the petrous bone in the middle cranial fossa (see p. 465). It lies highest of the three canals.

The *posterior semicircular canal* is placed in a vertical plane in the long axis of the petrous bone, convexity backwards, ampulla below. The ampulla is innervated separately by a branch of the vestibular nerve which pierces the foramen singulare in the internal acoustic meatus (Fig. 6.108).

The *lateral semicircular canal* is placed 30° off the horizontal plane, convexity backwards and laterally, ampulla anteriorly. The ampulla bulges the medial wall of the aditus and epitympanic recess above the facial canal. The lateral semicircular canal lies horizontal if the head nods 30° forwards. The canal opens by each end separately into the back of the vestibule. The anterior and posterior canals open separately at their ampullated ends, but their non-ampullated ends fuse into a common canal. Thus only five openings connect the three canals with the cavity of the vestibule.

The anterior and posterior canals, lying across and along the axis of the petrous bone, are each at 45° with the sagittal plane. Thus the posterior canal of one side lies parallel with the anterior canal of the opposite side.

Membranous labyrinth

The membranous labyrinth is a reduced replica of the hollow bony labyrinth (Fig. 6.72). It consists of one continuous closed cavity containing endolymph. The membranous covering consists of three layers. The outer fibrous layer is vascular and in places adherent to the endosteum of the bony labyrinth forming the stria vascularis which produces endolymph. The intermediate layer is homogeneous like a basal lamina and the inner epithelial layer is elaborated in three places into receptors of sound, static balance and kinetic balance, supplied by the cochlear (hearing) and vestibular (balance) divisions of the eighth nerve.

The **cochlear duct** is the spiral anterior part of the membranous labyrinth which contains the sound receptors. It is attached to the apical surface of the spiral lamina and to the outer bony walls of the cochlea. It commences at a blind extremity at the apex of the cochlea and after two and three-quarter spiral turns ends in a bulbous extremity in the basal turn of the cochlea. The minute ductus reuniens connects this extremity with the saccule (Fig. 6.72).

Two membranes enclose the duct of the cochlea. It is triangular in cross-section (Fig. 6.73). One side of the triangle is formed by the *basilar membrane* which extends in the line of the spiral lamina to the outer bony wall of the cochlea. Throughout its length it supports the spiral organ.

Another side is formed by the delicate *vestibular (Reissner's) membrane* which passes obliquely across the cochlea on the apical side of the basilar membrane. Connecting the two membranes, and completing the triangle, is the endosteum of the outer wall of the cochlea, which is thickened here to form the spiral ligament.

In the *spiral organ* (of Corti) the sensory hair cells, the receptors for hearing, are lodged on supporting cells. The 'hairs' are modified microvilli (stereocilia) and are overlaid by the tectorial membrane, a sheet of keratin-like protein that projects from beneath the inner attachment of the vestibular membrane (Fig. 6.73). The hair cells are supplied by the dendrites of the *spiral ganglion*.

The mechanism of the organ of Corti is not fully understood. It is probable that sound vibrations are communicated from the perilymph to the endolymph through the delicate vestibular membrane and cause appropriate fibres in the basilar membrane to bulge. The overlying hair cells are thus stimulated.

The **saccule** is a fibrous sac that lies in the lower front part of the vestibule, connected to the basal part of the cochlear duct by the very small ductus reuniens. The **utricle** is a similiar sac in the upper and back part of the vestibule and receives the five openings of the three semicircular ducts (Fig. 6.72). The two sacs lie with their adjacent walls in contact; a small duct leads from each and they unite in a Y-shaped manner to form the *endolymphatic duct*. This lies in the aqueduct of the vestibule and projects as a blind diverticulum, the *endolymphatic sac*, beneath the dura mater of the posterior cranial fossa. Endolymph is absorbed by the epithelium of the sac.

The medial wall of the saccule and the floor of the utricle are thickened to form the *maculae*, the areas that contain the sensory receptors for static balance. As in the cochlear duct, they are called hair cells (with stereocilia), and are here overlaid by the gelatinous otolithic (stato-conial) membrane which contains particles of calcium carbonate (otoliths or statoconia).

The **semicircular ducts** are only a quarter the calibre of the bony canals except at the ampullae, which they almost fill. Each membranous duct is adherent by its convexity to the wall of the bony canal in which it lies. The ducts open into five orifices in the back of the utricle inside the elliptical recess.

A transverse crest on the medial surface of each ampulla forms the *crista*, containing the sensory receptors (hair cells) for kinetic balance, here overlaid by the gelatinous cupula.

The hair cells of the maculae of the utricle and saccule, and the cristae of the semicircular ducts, are stimulated by movements of the otolithic membranes or cupulae respectively in response to head movements, e.g. changes in position, speed of change, etc. They are supplied by the vestibular nerve.

Blood supply of the labyrinth

The *labyrinthine artery* (from the basilar or its anterior inferior cerebellar branch) divides in the internal acoustic meatus into branches which accompany the cochlear and vestibular nerves to the labyrinth. Branches of the stylomastoid artery assist. The veins unite to form a labyrinthine vein which leaves the internal acoustic meatus and joins the inferior petrosal sinus. Various irregular veins penetrate the petrous bone independently to open into the superior petrosal sinus. A small vein lies in each aqueduct; that in the aqueduct of the cochlea joins the inferior petrosal sinus, that in the aqueduct of the vestibule joins the superior petrosal sinus.

Distribution of the eighth nerve

The **cochlear nerve** enters the front of the inferior part of the fundus of the internal aconstic meatus in spiral fashion to reach the organ of hearing (Fig. 6.108). The *lower division* of the **vestibular nerve** supplies the macula of the saccule and, through the foramen singulare, the ampulla of the posterior semicircular duct. The *upper division* of the vestibular nerve supplies the macula of the utricle and the ampullae of the anterior and lateral semicircular ducts. The cell bodies of the cochlear fibres lie in the spiral ganglion in the base of the spiral lamina. The cell bodies of the vestibular fibres lie in the vestibular ganglion in the depths of the internal acoustic meatus.

PART EIGHTEEN

Vertebral column

The **vertebral column** (spine) forms the central axis of the skeleton. It supports the skull and gives attachment, by way of the ribs, to the thoracic cage and, by way of this cage, to the pectoral girdle and upper limb. By the pelvic girdle it is strongly united to the lower limbs, which serve the double function of support and propulsion. The great strength of the column comes from the size and architecture of the bony elements, the vertebrae, and the ruggedness of the ligaments and muscles that hold them together. This great strength is combined with great flexibility; the column is flexible because it has so many joints so close together. Finally, the vertebral column contains in its cavity the spinal cord, to which it gives protection.

The vertebral column is made up of five parts with individual vertebrae peculiar to each: cervical, thoracic, lumbar, sacral and coccygeal.

In the fetus in utero the column lies flexed in its whole extent, like the letter C. This anterior flexion or concavity is the *primary curvature* of the column, and it is retained throughout life in the thoracic, sacral and coccygeal parts. After birth secondary extension of the column produces the *secondary curvatures* with an anterior convexity (i.e. lordosis) in the cervical and lumbar regions, the former associated with muscular support of the head and the latter with that of the trunk (see p. 37).

As the secondary curvatures develop in the neck and lumbar regions the vertebral column is opened out from its original C shape, and elongated into a vertical column characterized by gentle sinuous bends. These bends give a certain resilience to the column, but the actual shock-absorbing factors in the spinal column are the intervertebral discs.

General features of vertebrae

The general features of vertebrae are best exemplified by a thoracic vertebra. It consists of a ventral *body* and a dorsal vertebral or neural *arch*; they enclose between them the *vertebral foramen* (vertebral *canal* is the collective name given to the whole series of foramina when the vertebrae are strung together as a column). From the neural arch three processes diverge; in the posterior midline, the spinous process or *spine*, and on either side the *transverse processes*. That part of the neural arch between spinous process and transverse process is the *lamina*, that between transverse process and body is called the *pedicle*. The vertical height of the pedicle is less than that of the body, to allow room for passage of the spinal nerve through the *intervertebral foramen* between the pedicles of adjacent vertebrae (Fig. 6.76). At the junction of lamina and pedicle (i.e. at the root of the transverse process) are *articular processes, superior and inferior*, which have hyaline cartilage facets for the synovial joints between the neural arches. The direction of the facets determines the nature of the movement possible between adjacent vertebrae.

Each cervical vertebra has a foramen in the transverse process (*foramen transversarium* or *vertebrarterial foramen*) and it has no costal facets. Each thoracic vertebra has costal facets on the side of the body. Each lumbar vertebra has neither a foramen in the transverse process nor costal facets. These two features, foramen in the transverse process and presence or absence of costal facets, serve to distinguish cervical, thoracic and lumbar vertebrae.

During its development a vertebra ossifies in three parts, the *centrum* and the right and left halves of the *neural arch*. In the thoracic region *costal elements* develop separately as the ribs, which articulate with the vertebrae. The centrum is not the same thing as the anatomical body of a vertebra. Part of the neural arch is incorporated into the body of the vertebra, and the *neurocentral junction* lies anterior to the *costal facets* on the body of a thoracic vertebra; hence these facets lie on the neural arch, and not on the centrum.

Costal elements develop in association with all vertebrae. But, except in the thoracic region, the costal elements are vestigial and fuse with the neural arches to become incorporated into the vertebrae. The foramen in the transverse process of a cervical vertebra is produced by this fusion (Fig. 6.74). The costal element consists

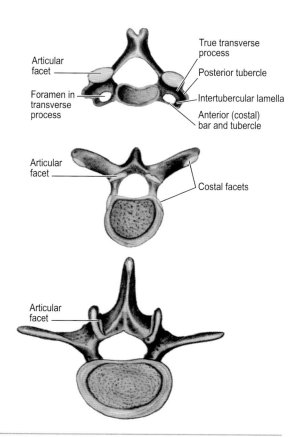

Fig. 6.74 Essential characteristics of cervical, thoracic and lumbar vertebrae (as viewed from above).

Labels in figure:
Articular facet
Foramen in transverse process
True transverse process
Posterior tubercle
Intertubercular lamella
Anterior (costal) bar and tubercle
Articular facet
Costal facets
Articular facet

of the anterior bar and tubercle, the intertubercular lamella and the posterior tubercle.

A *cervical rib* is due to the elongation of the costal element of C7 vertebra. It presents as either bony elements or fibrous tissue bands, passing down from C7 vertebra to the first rib (Fig. 6.75). The subclavian artery and lowest root (T1) of the brachial plexus become displaced upwards over such a rib or band, and pressure upon the neurovascular structures from below may cause severe symptoms. The pressure produced by a thin fibrous band may do more harm than that due to a smooth bony rib. The presence of a fibrous band may be inferred if the anterior tubercle of C7 vertebra is enlarged. The patient whose radiograph is shown in Figure 6.75 had symptoms on the right side which were due to a fibrous band, and the well-ossified cervical rib on the left side produced no symptoms. When a cervical rib is well developed the brachial plexus is more likely to be prefixed (i.e. its roots are C4–8), thus preserving the normal nerve to rib relationship.

The so-called transverse processes of the lumbar vertebrae are in reality costal elements. The true transverse process is contracted into a small mass of bone which is grooved by the medial branch of the posterior ramus of the spinal nerve. Above the groove lies the small mamillary process (on the superior articular facet) and below the groove is found the tiny accessory tubercle (Figs 6.94 and 6.96).

The five sacral vertebrae are fused into a single bone and so, too, are the five costal elements. The latter produce the lateral mass of the sacrum, lying lateral to the transverse tubercles on the back of the sacrum and extending between the anterior sacral foramina on the front of the bone. The auricular surface for the sacroiliac joint lies wholly on the lateral mass.

Vertebral joints

Adjacent vertebrae are held together by strong ligaments and small joints. The vertebrae articulate between their bodies and between their neural arches. These joints are very different from each other, and they allow a greater range of movement between the neural arches than between the bodies.

Joints between the bodies

The bodies of adjacent vertebrae are held together by the strong intervertebral disc, and by the anterior and posterior longitudinal ligaments.

An **intervertebral disc** is a secondary cartilaginous joint, or symphysis. The upper and lower surfaces of each vertebral body are covered completely by a thin

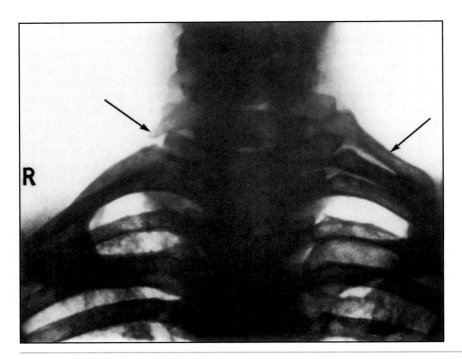

Fig. 6.75   Radiograph of a left cervical rib. On the right the anterior tubercle of C7 vertebra is greatly enlarged; a fibrous band passed from this tubercle to the first rib.

plate of hyaline cartilage. These plates are united by a peripheral ring, the **annulus fibrosus**, which has a narrow outer collagenous zone and a wider inner fibrocartilaginous zone. It consists of concentric laminae, the fibres of which lie at 25–45° with the horizontal plane. Alternate layers of the annulus contain fibres lying at right angles to each other. By this means the annulus is able to withstand strain in any direction. Inside the annulus is a bubble of semiliquid gelatinous substance, the **nucleus pulposus**, derived from the embryonic notochord. (The notochord extended originally as far cranially as the sella turcica, but it disappears except in the nucleus pulposus of each intervertebral disc and in the apical ligament of the atlas.) The nucleus pulposus in the embryo lies at the centre of the disc. Subsequent growth of the vertebral bodies and discs occurs in a ventral and lateral direction (the spinal cord prevents a corresponding growth dorsally). Thus in the adult and especially in the lumbar region the nucleus pulposus lies nearest to the back of the disc (Fig. 6.76) and if it herniates through the annulus it will be most likely to do so posteriorly and press on the roots of a spinal nerve near the intervertebral foramen, or on the spinal cord itself.

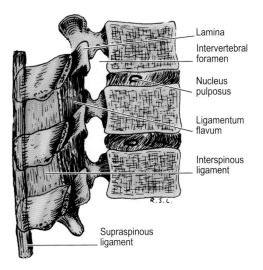

Lamina
Intervertebral foramen
Nucleus pulposus
Ligamentum flavum
Interspinous ligament
Supraspinous ligament

Fig. 6.76   Bisected vertebral column (lumbar region). The left half is seen from the right, so showing the inside of the vertebral canal, intervertebral discs in section, and the boundaries of two intervertebral foramina.

The nucleus pulposus accounts for 15% of the whole disc. It contains about 90% water at birth, and this diminishes to about 70% in old age. The water content keeps the nucleus under constant pressure since its mucoprotein (proteoglycan) component has the property of imbibing and retaining water. Imbibition of water by the nucleus accounts for the overnight increase in height of a young adult by 1 cm; when upright during the day, water is squeezed out. In old age there is little height change between night and morning; imbibition pressure becomes less and the nucleus more fibrous. In astronauts, who have been relieved of gravity, there may be a height increase of several centimetres.

The relationship of nerve roots to intervertebral discs is of great importance, and is best understood by considering the lowest disc—the fifth lumbar or lumbosacral disc—which is the one most frequently herniated or prolapsed ('slipped disc'), with its nucleus pulposus being extruded posterolaterally. At the level of this fifth lumbar disc, the fifth lumbar nerve roots within their dural sheath have already emerged from the intervertebral foramen, hugging the pedicle of L5 vertebra and so not lying low enough to come in contact with the fifth lumbar disc. The roots that lie behind the posterolateral part of this disc are those of the first sacral nerve, and these are the ones liable to be irritated by a prolapse. Thus the general rule throughout the vertebral column is that when a disc herniates (usually posterolaterally rather than in the midline) it may irritate the nerve roots numbered one below the disc: S1 nerve by L5 disc; L5 nerve by L4 disc; and C8 nerve by C6 disc (there are 8 cervical nerve roots and 7 cervical vertebrae). These are the commonest clinical examples.

The posterolateral lip, or uncus, on the upper surface of cervical vertebrae 3 to 7 (see p. 450) may appear to form a joint with the side of the vertebra above because a small cavity may develop in this region (the so-called neurocentral, uncovertebral or *Luschka's joint*). It is disputed as to whether these are synovial joints, or are due to degenerative changes in the adjacent disc.

The **anterior longitudinal ligament** extends from the basiocciput of the skull and the anterior tubercle of the atlas to the front of the upper part of the sacrum. It is firmly united to the periosteum of the vertebral bodies, but is less so over the intervertebral discs. It is a flat band, broadening gradually as it passes downwards.

The **posterior longitudinal ligament** extends from the back of the body of the axis to the anterior wall of the upper sacral canal. It narrows gradually as it passes downwards. It has serrated margins, being broadest over the discs to which it is firmly attached, and narrow over the vertebral bodies to which it is more loosely attached in order to give free exit to the basivertebral veins emerging from the backs of the bodies (Fig. 6.10). At the top the ligament is continued above the body of the axis as the tectorial membrane (see p. 443).

Joints between the arches

The pedicles of adjacent vertebrae are not attached to one another, so leaving a space—the intervertebral foramen—for the emergence of the spinal nerve. All other parts of the neural arch and its processes are joined to their adjacent companions: the articular processes by synovial joints, and the remainder by ligaments, of which the most important are the ligamenta flava and the supraspinous ligament.

The joints between the articular facets of the superior articular processes of one vertebra and the articular facets of the inferior articular processes of the vertebra above are termed the *zygapophyseal joints* (or simply known as **facet joints**). They are synovial with a simple capsule which blends medially with a ligamentum flavum. The articular surfaces allow gliding of one on the other; the direction of the surfaces determines the direction of the possible movements between adjacent vertebrae. The joints have a nerve supply from the nerve of their own segmental level and from the nerve of the segment above. One nerve thus supplies two joints; this may be important when considering nerve root pain which can be referred from facet joints. Although most of the weight transmission by the vertebral column takes place via the vertebral bodies and intervening discs, a small amount does occur through these joints.

The paired **ligamenta flava** are yellowish from their high content of elastic fibres. They join the contiguous borders of adjacent laminae (Fig. 6.76). They are attached above to the front of the upper lamina and below to the back of the lower lamina. Thus adjacent laminae and ligamenta flava overlap each other slightly like the tiles of a roof. The ligamenta extend from the facet joints to the midline where they partially fuse; small veins connecting the internal and external vertebral venous plexuses may pass between a pair of ligamenta. They are stretched by flexion of the spine; in leaning forward their increasing elongation becomes an increasing antigravity support.

The **supraspinous ligaments** join the tips of adjacent spinous processes (Fig. 6.76). They are strong bands of white fibrous tissue and are lax in the extended spine. They are drawn taut by full flexion, and then support the spine (no action currents can be obtained from the erector spinae muscles when the spine is fully flexed, as in touching the toes). They are indistinct below the L4 spine where the lumbar fascia is thick. In the neck they are replaced by the ligamentum nuchae (see p. 447).

The **interspinous ligaments** are relatively weak sheets of fibrous tissue uniting spinous processes along their adjacent borders (Fig. 6.76). They are well developed only in the lumbar region. They fuse with the supraspinous ligaments.

The **intertransverse ligaments** are similar weak sheets of fibrous tissue joining the transverse processes along their adjacent borders.

Vertebral column

In the normal erect posture the vertebral column supports the head and trunk on the pelvis. (The pelvis is supported by the lower limbs in standing and by its own ischial tuberosities in sitting.) This support is maintained by the bodies of the vertebrae and the intervertebral discs, which thus become progressively larger from above downwards. The curvatures of the spine are produced partly by the wedge-shape of the vertebral bodies, but mostly by the wedge-shape of the intervertebral discs. This is particularly noticeable in the lower part of the spine; L5 vertebra is usually wedge-shaped and the disc between it and the sacrum is very thick anteriorly.

The **vertebral canal** (see p. 438) becomes progressively smaller from above downwards. It is closed anteriorly by the vertebral bodies, the intervertebral discs and the posterior longitudinal ligament and posteriorly by the laminae and the ligamenta flava. Laterally it is occupied by the pedicles, which are narrower than the height of the vertebral bodies. Thus a series of **intervertebral foramina** is produced between adjacent pedicles which form the upper and lower boundaries of each foramen. In the thoracic and lumbar regions each intervertebral foramen is bounded in front by the lower part of a body of a vertebra (mainly in the thoracic region; Fig. 6.92) and the adjacent intervertebral disc (mainly in the lumbar region; Fig. 6.93), and behind by the facet joint and its capsule. In the cervical region, because the pedicle arises from a little lower down the back of the body, a small part of the vertebral body below the disc is also included in this anterior boundary (Fig. 6.88). The intervertebral foramina lodge the spinal nerves and posterior root ganglia and give passage to the spinal arteries and veins.

Movements of the vertebral column

In general the movements of the spine are simple enough. Flexion and extension, and lateral flexion (abduction) are possible in cervical, thoracic and lumbar regions, though in varying degree in the three parts. Rotation occurs mainly in the thoracic region. Movements of the head occur at the specialized atlanto-occipital and atlantoaxial joints.

Lumbar region

The articular facets lie in an anteroposterior plane; they lock, and greatly limit rotation of the bodies on each other. Flexion and extension are free, and a good deal of lateral flexion is possible.

Thoracic region

The synovial joints between T12 and L1 are lumbar in type (Fig. 6.93); elsewhere the direction of the articular facets on the neural arches is quite different. On any one neural arch the upper facets face backwards and laterally (Fig. 6.74); they lie on the circumference of a circle whose centre lies in the vertebral body. The lower facets are reciprocal. Thus rotation of the bodies on each other is possible, though restricted by the splinting effect of the ribs. As in the lumbar region, flexion and extension occur, as well as 'lateral flexion'. The thoracic spine is thus the most versatile region of all, but the range of movements is limited by the ribs.

Cervical region

The atlanto-occipital and atlantoaxial joints are specialized for head nodding and head rotation. They are considered below.

The upper articular facets of the other joints face backwards and upwards; the lower facets face, reciprocally, forwards and downwards. While flexion and extension are free, pure rotation is impossible. Lateral flexion is not a simple movement. The neural arch of the abducted vertebra slides downwards (and therefore backwards) on the concave side and upwards (and therefore forwards) on the convex side, thus inevitably producing slight concomitant rotation.

Special vertebrae and joints

The **atlas** (Fig. 6.77) lacks a centrum (see p. 439). The vertebral arch has become modified to form a thick *lateral mass* on each side, joined at the front by a short *anterior arch* and with a longer *posterior arch* at the back. The articular facets on the upper and lower surfaces of the lateral mass differ markedly. The upper surface is kidney-shaped and concave for articulation with the occipital condyle, while the lower is round or oval and nearly flat for the lateral atlantoaxial joint. The articular facets are in line with the uncovertebral joints (see p. 441) of the other cervical vertebrae, not with the articular facets on the neural arches. Thus the C1 and C2 nerves send their anterior rami behind, and not in front of, the joints.

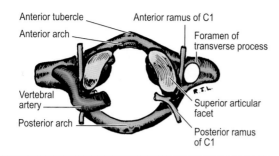

Fig. 6.77 Superior surface of the atlas. C1 nerve divides into anterior and posterior rami just behind the atlanto-occipital joint (right side), where it lies in the groove beneath the vertebral artery (left side).

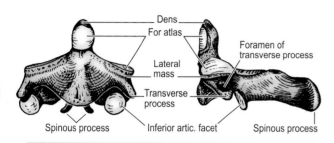

Fig. 6.78 Anterior and lateral views of the axis.

The **axis** is characterized by the dens and a large spinous process (Fig. 6.78). The *dens (odontoid process)* has an articular facet at the front for the joint with the anterior arch of the atlas. It bears no weight. The weight of the skull is transmitted through the lateral mass of the atlas to the superior articular process of the axis which lies immediately lateral to the dens. The lower articulations of the axis are as for the ordinary cervical vertebrae: body to body with intervening disc and the two uncovertebral joints, and the ordinary articular facets on the neural arch. From the axis downwards the weight of the skull is supported by the vertebral bodies. The *bifid spinous process* is very large, due to the attachments of muscles of the suboccipital triangle above (Fig. 6.84).

The atlanto-occipital and the atlantoaxial joints are adapted to provide freedom of head movement, the former for nodding and lateral flexion, the latter for rotation.

The **atlanto-occipital joint** is a synovial joint between the convex occipital condyle and the concave facet on the lateral mass of the atlas. Both surfaces are covered with hyaline cartilage. The synovial cavity of the joint is

contained in a lax but strong capsule, which is attached to the articular margins of both bones and is innervated by C1 nerve.

The **anterior** and **posterior atlanto-occipital membranes** are attached to the upper borders of the respective arches of the atlas and to the outer margins of the foramen magnum (Fig. 6.84). The posterior membrane is deficient at each lateral extremity to allow passage for the vertebral artery and C1 nerve; the lateral margin of the membrane sometimes ossifies, converting the groove for the vertebral artery into a foramen. The membranes are innervated by C1 nerve.

The curved surfaces of the joint are well adapted for head flexion and extension, and allow also for a considerable amount of lateral flexion of the skull on the atlas. In the ordinary erect position the centre of gravity of the skull lies in front of the joint and the head is maintained in position by the tonus of the extensor muscles, notably semispinalis capitis. It is flexed by relaxation of the extensors (i.e. by gravity) and, actively, by longus capitis and the two sternocleidomastoids acting together. The effect of gravity is considerable on account of the weight of the head and, of course, varies with position. Lateral flexion is produced by unilateral contraction of such muscles as sternocleidomastoid, trapezius and splenius capitis. No rotation is possible at the atlanto-occipital joints.

The **median atlantoaxial joint** is where the dens articulates with the back of the anterior arch of the atlas (Fig. 6.79). The smooth facets seen on the dry bones are covered with hyaline cartilage in life, with a capsule attached to their margins to make this a small synovial joint. The dens is held in position by the transverse ligament; between the two is a relatively large bursa.

On each side there is a **lateral atlantoaxial joint** (also synovial) between the inferior articular facet of the atlas and the superior articular facet of the axis (Fig. 6.81). The joint surfaces are nearly circular and flat with hyaline cartilage lining, and there is a lax capsule supplied by C2 nerve.

Accessory ligaments connect the axis to the occiput, bypassing the atlas: the tectorial membrane, cruciform ligament, apical ligament and the paired alar ligaments.

The **tectorial membrane** extends upwards in continuity with the posterior longitudinal ligament. It is attached to the back of the body of the axis and diverges upwards to become attached to the margin of the anterior half of the foramen magnum. It lies in front of the spinal dura mater, which is firmly attached to it (Fig. 6.79).

The **transverse ligament** is a broad strong band that runs across (and grooves) the back of the dens from its attachment on each side to a tubercle in the 'hilum' of the kidney-shaped upper articular facet of the atlas. A

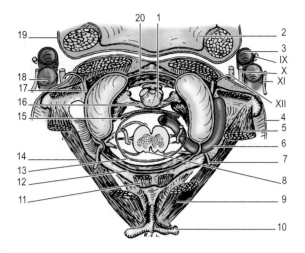

weaker longitudinal band runs from the back of the body of the axis to the basiocciput and together with the transverse ligament constitutes a *cruciform ligament* (Fig. 6.80). This lies in contact with the front of the tectorial membrane. They hold the dens in position; rupture of the ligament and membrane allows the dens to dislocate backwards with fatal pressure on the medulla.

The weak **apical ligament** joins the apex of the dens to the anterior margin of the foramen magnum, and is a fibrous remnant of the notochord (see p. 25).

The **alar ligaments** lie obliquely one on either side of the apical ligament. From the sides of the dens they diverge upwards to the margins of the foramen magnum. They are very strong and limit rotation of the head.

Movements at the atlantoaxial joints are simply those of rotation about a vertical axis passing through the dens. The atlas rotates by its anterior arch and transverse limb of the cruciform ligament gliding around the dens and by the lower flat facets on its lateral mass gliding on the superior facets of the axis. The head rotates with the atlas; the curved surfaces of the atlanto-occipital joints do not allow independent rotation of occiput on atlas.

The muscles chiefly responsible for rotation are sternocleidomastoid, splenius capitis and the inferior oblique.

The atlantoaxial region of the cervical spine can be visualized in transoral anteroposterior radiographs (Fig. 6.81). The transoral route is also utilized in surgical approaches to this region, with upward retraction of the soft palate and division of the posterior wall of the pharynx.

Fig. 6.79 Atlas and related structures. **1.** Dens of axis with apical and alar ligaments. **2.** Mucosa of nasopharynx over levator palati. **3.** Internal carotid artery and last four cranial nerves (Roman figures). **4.** Prevertebral fascia. **5.** Obliquus capitis superior. **6.** Vertebral artery. **7.** Posterior ramus of C1. **8.** Medulla/spinal cord junction (denticulate ligament, accessory nerve and roots of C1 not labelled). **9.** Rectus capitis posterior major. **10.** Spinous process of axis. **11.** Rectus capitis posterior minor, from posterior arch of atlas. **12.** Posterior atlanto-occipital membrane. **13.** Spinal dura and arachnoid. **14.** Obliquus capitis inferior. **15.** Tectorial membrane. **16.** Transverse band of cruciform ligament. **17.** Anterior ramus of C1 giving branch to hypoglossal nerve and ending in longus capitis. **18.** Internal jugular vein. **19.** Pharyngobasilar fascia. **20.** Anterior atlanto-occipital membrane.

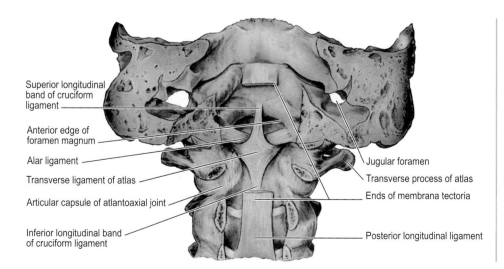

Superior longitudinal band of cruciform ligament

Anterior edge of foramen magnum

Alar ligament

Transverse ligament of atlas

Articular capsule of atlantoaxial joint

Inferior longitudinal band of cruciform ligament

Jugular foramen

Transverse process of atlas

Ends of membrana tectoria

Posterior longitudinal ligament

Fig. 6.80 Ligaments of the atlanto-occipital and atlantoaxial joints. The posterior part of the occipital bone and the laminae of the upper cervical vertebrae have been removed.

Fig. 6.81 Transoral anteroposterior radiograph.

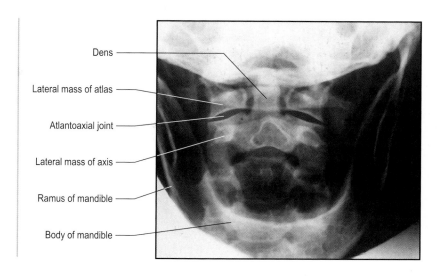

Dens

Lateral mass of atlas

Atlantoaxial joint

Lateral mass of axis

Ramus of mandible

Body of mandible

Blood supply of the vertebrae

The vertebrae are supplied segmentally by the vertebral, ascending and deep cervical, posterior intercostal, lumbar and lateral sacral arteries, which give multiple small branches to the vertebral bodies.

The richly supplied red marrow of the vertebral body drains through its posterior surface by a pair of large *basivertebral veins* into the **internal vertebral venous plexus**, which lies inside the vertebral canal, outside the dura (Fig. 6.110). It drains into the *external vertebral venous plexus*. This intramuscular plexus, which also receives blood from the neural arch, drains into the regional segmental veins (vertebral, posterior intercostal, lumbar and lateral sacral veins), which in turn drain into brachiocephalic veins, superior vena cava, inferior vena cava and internal iliac veins. Venous communication is thus established in the pelvis with veins draining the pelvic viscera, in the abdomen with the renal veins, in the thorax with the azygos venous system (and thereby with the venous drainage of the breast and bronchus), and in the neck with the inferior thyroid veins. In this way, by reflux blood flow through these largely valveless veins, malignant disease may spread from prostate, kidney, breast, bronchus and thyroid gland to the bodies of the vertebrae.

Extensor muscles of the spine

Running along the whole length of the vertebral column from skull to sacrum is a posterior mass of mainly longitudinal **extensor muscles**, derived from the outer of the three layers of the body wall and supplied segmentally by *posterior rami* of spinal nerves. They form a bulge on either side of the midline of the back, often best seen in the lumbar region. In the neck the posteriormost layer is the splenius muscle. Elsewhere the muscles are covered posteriorly by the thoracolumbar fascia.

The deepest muscles are the small interspinales and intertransversales. The remainder form intermediate and superficial masses collectively called transversospinalis and erector spinae, each of which is composed of three groups. Transversospinalis includes the rotatores, multifidus and semispinalis, while erector spinae comprises iliocostalis, longissimus and spinalis.

Deep layer

The *interspinales* join adjacent borders of spinous processes, alongside the interspinous ligaments. The *intertransversales* join adjacent transverse processes; they are best developed in the upper part of the vertebral column.

Transversospinalis (intermediate layer)

As a group these muscles run from transverse processes to spines, hence the name. The rotatores are small, but multifidus and semispinalis form larger muscle masses.

The *rotatores* are confined to the thoracic spine, the only region where pure rotation occurs. Each extends from the base of a transverse process to the root of the spinous process of the vertebra above (Fig. 6.82).

Multifidus fibres slope upwards from the back of the sacrum, mamillary processes of lumbar vertebrae,

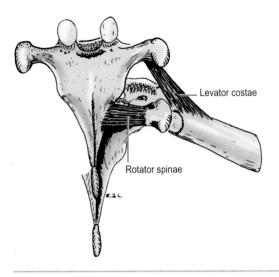

Fig. 6.82   Rotator spinae and levator costae muscles.

transverse processes of thoracic vertebrae and articular processes of cervical vertebrae to the spinous processes of vertebrae two or three above their level of origin. They commence at the upper part of the sacrum and extend to the upper part of the neck.

Semispinalis lies on the surface of multifidus. Its fibres arise from the transverse processes and slope steeply upwards to the spinous processes. It extends from the lower thoracic region to the skull. **Semispinalis thoracis** extends from the transverse processes of the lower thoracic vertebrae and each part is inserted into the spinous process six or more vertebrae higher. **Semispinalis cervicis** arises in continuity at a higher level; the uppermost part of the muscle is inserted into the concavity of the bifid spinous process of the axis.

Semispinalis capitis is the most powerful part of this layer. It arises from the transverse processes of the upper six thoracic and the articular processes of the lower four cervical vertebrae and is inserted into the occipital bone near the midline, between the superior and inferior nuchal lines (see p. 528). It lies beneath splenius and trapezius and is the chief extensor of the head. It contains a large plexus of veins within and around it.

Erector spinae (superficial layer)

This forms the most powerful muscle group. It commences below, deep to the lumbar fascia, on the back of the sacrum and the inner side of the iliac crest. The thick mass of fibres passes upwards and slightly outwards dividing as it does so into two main bundles, iliocostalis

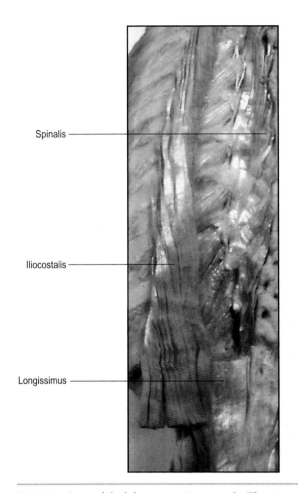

Fig. 6.83   Parts of the left erector spinae muscle. The most lateral mass is iliocostalis. Most of longissimus (whose lower part is seen adjacent to iliocostalis) has been removed to show various parts of spinalis. Prosection in the Anatomy Museum of the Royal College of Surgeons of England.

laterally and longissimus medially (Fig. 6.83). The **iliocostalis** fibres are inserted by shining tendons into the angles of the lower six ribs. From these attachments new muscle bundles arise and each runs up to be attached to the angle of the sixth rib above. From there further fibres run up to reach the transverse processes of the lower four cervical vertebrae. Iliocostalis forms the most lateral part of erector spinae.

The more medial longissimus bundle arising from the sacrum and iliac crest passes up to be inserted into the gutter between transverse processes and ribs; this is **longissimus thoracis**. At its insertion it is replaced by new fibres on the medial side that pass up to the transverse processes of the lower cervical vertebrae; this is **longissimus cervicis**. From these insertions new bundles arise and pass upwards as **longissimus capitis**; this muscle is inserted into the mastoid process deep to splenius capitis.

The most medial part of erector spinae is the **spinalis** part. Its fibres run alongside the spinous processes and are small and often indefinite.

Splenius

In the neck, the underlying extensor muscles are bound down by splenius, a flat sheet arising from upper thoracic spinous processes and the supraspinous ligament, and from the ligamentum nuchae. The fibres slope upwards and laterally, deep to trapezius and sternocleidomastoid (Fig. 6.4), and are inserted (as *splenius capitis*) into the mastoid process and the lateral third of the superior nuchal line, and (as *splenius cervicis*) into the transverse processes of the upper three or four cervical vertebrae (deep to levator scapulae). The whole muscle is like a bandage that holds down the deeper extensor muscles at the back of the neck. It, like the muscles deep to it, is supplied by posterior rami.

Back of the neck

The back of the neck consists of muscles connecting the skull to the spine and pectoral girdle. In the midline the **ligamentum nuchae** separates the muscles of the two sides. This is a triangular septum of fibroelastic tissue attached to the external occipital crest, the bifid spines of the cervical vertebrae, the tubercle of the spine of C7 vertebra and the investing layer of deep cervical fascia which encloses the trapezius muscles.

Beneath the trapezius and sternocleidomastoid lies the splenius, and beneath the splenius lie longissimus capitis and semispinalis capitis. When all these are removed the deeper structures of the back of the neck are seen to be divided into upper and lower portions by the prominent backward projection of the massive spinous process of the axis (C2 vertebra). Below this level semispinalis cervicis is seen converging almost vertically upwards to the internal surfaces of the bifid axial spine. Above the spine lie the right and left suboccipital triangles.

Suboccipital triangle

The suboccipital triangle is bounded by rectus capitis posterior major and the superior and inferior oblique muscles (Fig. 6.84). Its floor contains the posterior arch of the atlas and the posterior atlanto-occipital membrane. Across the floor runs the vertebral artery, and

through the floor emerges the suboccipital (C1) nerve. Across the roof run the greater occipital (C2) nerve and the occipital artery.

Rectus capitis posterior major arises from the outer surface of the bifid spinous process of C2 vertebra and extends obliquely upwards and outwards to be attached to the lateral part of the area below the inferior nuchal line. Its action is to extend the head and rotate it (with the atlas) back towards its own side.

The **inferior oblique (obliquus capitis inferior)** is attached between the outer surface of the bifid spine of the axis (below rectus capitis posterior major) and the back of the transverse process of the atlas. Its action is to rotate the atlas (and the skull with it) back towards its own side.

The **superior oblique (obliquus capitis superior)** extends from the upper surface of the transverse process of the atlas to the lateral part of the occipital bone between superior and inferior nuchal lines. It is a lateral flexor of the skull.

Rectus capitis posterior minor is the only muscle attached to the posterior arch of the atlas, from where it passes vertically upwards to be inserted into the medial part of the area below the inferior nuchal line. It weakly extends the head.

All four muscles are supplied by the posterior ramus of C1.

The second part of the **vertebral artery** ascends through the foramina in the transverse processes of the upper six cervical vertebrae, anterior to the emerging spinal nerves. It gives a *spinal branch* into each intervertebral foramen. Its course from C6 to C2 vertebra is vertical. Between the foramina in the transverse processes of the axis and atlas it passes laterally with a pronounced posterior convexity and then loops upwards beside the atlantoaxial joint (Figs 6.84, 6.85, 6.86 and 6.109). This must be to allow for taking up slack during rotation of the atlas on the axis.

On emerging from the foramen in the transverse process of the atlas, the third part of the vertebral artery curves backwards and medially behind the lateral mass of the atlas. Here it lies in the floor of the suboccipital triangle before piercing the lateral angle of the posterior atlanto-occipital membrane. It deeply grooves the posterior arch of the atlas before entering the skull through the foramen magnum.

The **vertebral veins** exist only in the neck, not inside the skull which the vertebral arteries enter. Blood from the veins in and around semispinalis capitis and from the muscles of the suboccipital triangle is collected in a plexus of veins that surrounds the second and third parts of the vertebral artery. The thin walls of these veins are adherent to the periosteum of the posterior arch of the

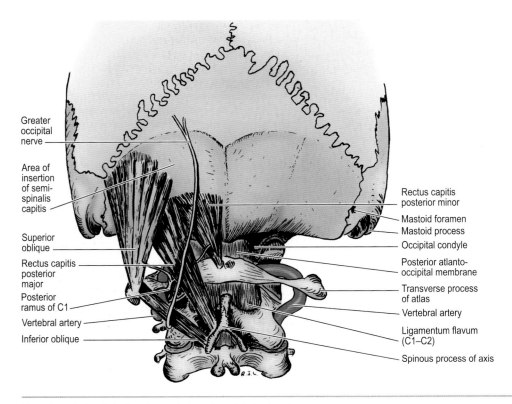

Greater
occipital
nerve

Area of
insertion
of semi-
spinalis
capitis

Superior
oblique

Rectus capitis
posterior
major

Posterior
ramus of C1

Vertebral artery

Inferior oblique

Rectus capitis
posterior minor

Mastoid foramen
Mastoid process

Occipital condyle

Posterior atlanto-
occipital membrane

Transverse process
of atlas

Vertebral artery

Ligamentum flavum
(C1–C2)

Spinous process of axis

Fig. 6.84   Suboccipital region and the suboccipital triangle.

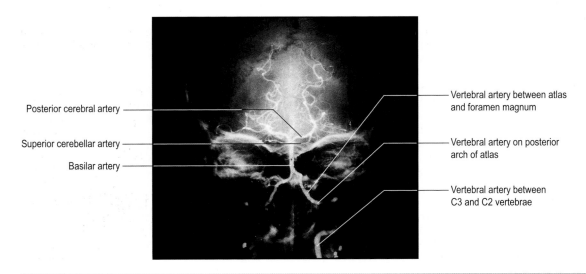

Posterior cerebral artery

Superior cerebellar artery

Basilar artery

Vertebral artery between atlas
and foramen magnum

Vertebral artery on posterior
arch of atlas

Vertebral artery between
C3 and C2 vertebrae

Fig. 6.85   Vertebral arteriogram: anteroposterior view.

Fig. 6.86 Vertebral arteriogram: lateral view.

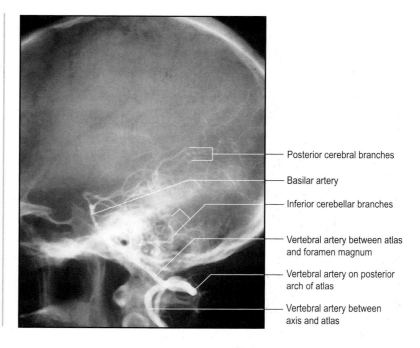

— Posterior cerebral branches

— Basilar artery

— Inferior cerebellar branches

— Vertebral artery between atlas and foramen magnum

— Vertebral artery on posterior arch of atlas

— Vertebral artery between axis and atlas

atlas and the foramina in the transverse processes. From this plexus two vertebral veins usually emerge, one from the sixth with the vertebral artery and one alone through the foramen in the transverse process of C7 vertebra, and join the brachiocephalic vein at the root of the neck (Fig. 6.9B).

In the groove between artery and bone on the posterior arch of the atlas lies the posterior ramus of the **suboccipital** (C1) **nerve**, as it passes backwards to supply the two recti, the two obliques and the upper fibres of semispinalis capitis. The anterior ramus winds round the lateral side of the lateral mass of the atlas between it and the vertebral artery, and passes forwards between rectus capitis lateralis and anterior to join the cervical plexus (Fig. 6.8). Neither branch reaches the skin.

The **greater occipital nerve** is the posterior ramus of C2 and emerges below the posterior arch of the atlas. It curls around the lower border of the inferior oblique muscle and passes upwards across the roof of the suboccipital triangle. It pierces semispinalis capitis (first supplying it) and extends up to supply the skin of the scalp up to the vertex.

The **occipital artery** is a large vessel that passes back along the occipitomastoid suture of the skull deep to digastric and longissimus capitis. It runs across the upper part of the roof of the suboccipital triangle and passes to the scalp. The companion veins form a rich plexus around and within semispinalis.

PART NINETEEN

Osteology of vertebrae

Cervical vertebrae

A typical cervical vertebra

The broad kidney-shaped *body* is the same size as, or smaller than, the vertebral foramen (Fig. 6.87). On each

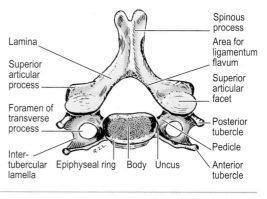

Lamina

Superior articular process

Foramen of transverse process

Inter-tubercular lamella

Spinous process

Area for ligamentum flavum

Superior articular facet

Posterior tubercle

Pedicle

Anterior tubercle

Epiphyseal ring   Body   Uncus

Fig. 6.87 C6 vertebra from above.

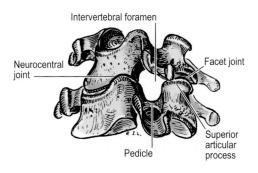

Fig. 6.88 C3 and C4 vertebrae articulated to show the boundaries of the intervertebral foramen.

side it is projected up into a posterolateral lip or *uncus*, and its lower margin laterally is bevelled reciprocal with this. The anterior surface of the body is concave from above down. Basivertebral veins emerge from the posterior surface.

The *pedicle* is attached below the upturned lip on the body. Thus an intervertebral foramen in the neck is bounded in front by both vertebral bodies and the uncovertebral joint and disc between them (Fig. 6.88). Attached to the pedicle and body is the lateral projection of the transverse process, perforated by its foramen. The proximal part of the posterior bar of bone that projects from the pedicle behind the foramen is the true transverse element; it ends in the *posterior tubercle*, which is part of the costal element, as is the bar of bone that projects from the body in front of the foramen ends and in the *anterior tubercle*. The anterior tubercles enlarge progressively from C3 to C6. The large C6 anterior tubercle is the *carotid tubercle* (of Chassaignac) because the common carotid artery can be compressed against it. The anterior and posterior tubercles are joined by the *intertubercular lamella*, on the concave upper surface of which lies the anterior ramus of the cervical nerve of the same number (Fig. 6.87). The vertebral artery, with its accompanying sympathetic nerve fibres, and the vertebral venous plexus lie in the foramen of the transverse process, and the posterior root ganglion of the nerve of the same number lies behind it (Fig. 6.109).

The *laminae* enclose a relatively large vertebral foramen, somewhat triangular in cross-section. At the junction of pedicle and lamina there are *superior* and *inferior articular processes*. The upper facets face obliquely up and back; the lower facets face down and forward.

The *spinous process* is usually bifid.

Atypical cervical vertebrae

The **seventh cervical vertebra** is often called the *vertebra prominens* because of its prominent spine. The vertebra is atypical in that its long spine is not bifid but ends in a rounded tubercle, and the foramen in the transverse process does not transmit the vertebral artery. The foramen is small, and contains the posterior vein when the vertebral vein is doubled. The anterior tubercle is very small; the suprapleural membrane is attached to it.

Some of the essential features of the **atlas** are described on page 442. Its distinctive feature is the lack of a body. The short *anterior arch* is projected into a *tubercle* in front (Fig. 6.89), for attachment of the anterior longitudinal ligament and longus colli. The longer *posterior arch* is grooved by the vertebral artery. The *lateral mass* carries the weight-bearing articular facets. The lateral mass is projected into the *transverse process*, which is perforated by the foramen. There are no anterior and posterior tubercles; but the blunt end of the transverse process represents a posterior tubercle and has corresponding muscle attachments: scalenus medius and levator scapulae. The atlas is the widest cervical vertebra, and the tip of its transverse process can be palpated with deep pressure behind the mandibular ramus, 1 cm below and in front of the apex of the mastoid process. The internal jugular vein, crossed by the accessory nerve, lies in front of the transverse process.

Some of the essential features of the **axis** are described on page 443. The *dens* (*odontoid process*) is characteristic, projecting up from the body between a pair of massive weight-bearing *lateral masses* (Fig. 6.78). The weight is communicated from these shoulders through the body to the body of C3 vertebra.

The *transverse process* has no anterior and posterior tubercles but ends in a rounded tip, which corresponds

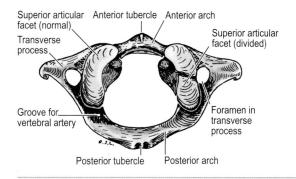

Fig. 6.89 Atlas, from above. The epiphyseal junction between the ossification centre of the anterior arch and that of the right lateral mass has not fused completely.

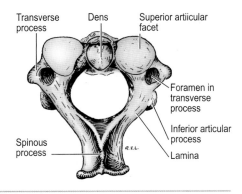

Fig. 6.90 Axis, from above.

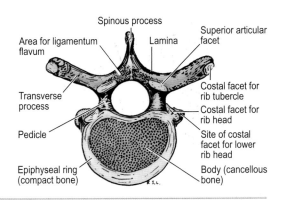

Fig. 6.91 Typical thoracic vertebra, from above.

with the posterior tubercles of lower cervical vertebrae with equivalent muscle attachments. The *foramen* in the transverse process is not vertical as in the other vertebrae, but is directed upwards and outwards (Fig. 6.90) to communicate a lateral bend to the vertebral artery to enable it to ascend to the transverse process of the wider atlas (Fig. 6.84). An inferior articular process extends down from the junction of pedicle and lamina; its articular facet faces downwards and forwards as in typical cervical vertebrae (Fig. 6.78). The *laminae* are thick and rounded and project posteriorly into a massive *spinous process* (Fig. 6.90), the lower surface of which is grooved and ends in a wide bifurcation; the tip of the spinous process thus resembles an inverted U (Fig. 6.84).

Thoracic vertebrae

A typical thoracic vertebra

The distinctive feature of a thoracic vertebra is the presence of costal facets (Fig. 6.91). On each side of the body of a typical thoracic vertebra there are a pair of semicircular demifacets (Fig. 6.92). The upper and larger of these is on the body at its junction with the upper border of the pedicle. The smaller lower facet is at the lower border of the body.

The *body* is concave from above down around its circumference. The posterior surface of the body is concave from side to side, making the body heart-shaped and the vertebral foramen almost circular in outline (Fig. 6.91). Two large foramina open centrally on the back of the body for the basivertebral veins. The upper and lower surfaces of the body have a heart-shaped ring of compact bone at their margins. This is the fused epiphyseal ring of the body, and it encloses a large central area in which cancellous bone reaches the surface.

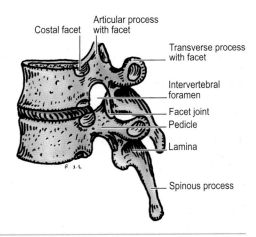

Fig. 6.92 Two articulated midthoracic vertebrae from the left. The intervertebral foramen is bounded in front by half of the body of the upper vertebra and the intervertebral disc, at the back by the facet joint, and above and below by pedicles.

The *pedicle* projects back from the upper half of the body. Its upper border is level with the upper surface of the body. The upper border of the pedicle curves up in a slight concavity to *a superior articular process*. The lower border curves markedly down to the *inferior articular process*, so making the upper boundary of the intervertebral foramen. This accommodates the thoracic nerve of the same number as the vertebra. The flat *laminae* slope downwards and backwards from the pedicles to unite in the midline and complete the neural arch. The superior articular process projects up from the junction of pedicle and lamina. It carries an oval articular facet facing backwards and slightly laterally; so the two articular surfaces lie on the arc of a wide circle, permitting rotation of adjacent bodies. The inferior articular facets are reciprocal, facing forwards and somewhat medially.

The *spinous processes* of successive thoracic vertebrae slope downwards with gradually increasing declivity as far as T7, below which they progressively level out to become almost horizontal at T12. Thus the tips of the upper four spines lie opposite the bodies of vertebrae one lower in the series, the next four spines (those of T5–8) opposite the upper margin of two vertebral bodies lower, and the lowest spines opposite one lower or their own vertebral bodies.

The *transverse process* projects backwards as well as laterally from the junction of pedicle and lamina. Its anterior surface expands towards the tip, to carry the characteristic costal facet. The upper six costal facets are concave, the lower ones flat, and the rib tubercles with which they articulate have correspondingly rounded or flat facets. Accordingly, when ribs elevate during inspiration, a rotational movement occurs at the upper costotransverse joints and a gliding movement at the lower joints. The primary curvature of the thoracic vertebral column results in the upper thoracic vertebrae leaning forwards, so their transverse processes are tilted up a little. Thus the neck of the first rib slopes backwards and upwards, a feature that enables the side to which it belongs to be determined (see p. 226).

First thoracic vertebra

The body is broad and not heart-shaped. On the body, at its junction with the pedicle, is a large round facet for the single articular surface of the head of the first rib which does not articulate with the body of C7 vertebrae. There is a demifacet for the second rib at the lower border of the body. The pedicle is attached below the upper margin of the body, as in a cervical vertebra, so the body takes part in the formation of the intervertebral foramen above it as well as below it. These are the foramina for the exit of C8 and T1 spinal nerves.

Lower thoracic vertebrae

The tenth, eleventh and twelfth thoracic vertebrae have only single facets on each side of their bodies for articulation with the heads of their same numbered ribs (Fig. 6.93). This facet is at, close to and somewhat below the upper border of the body of the tenth, eleventh and twelfth vertebrae respectively. The last two vertebrae have no costal facets on their small transverse processes. The twelfth vertebra has some lumbar features: the lower articular facet faces laterally and mamillary processes and accessory tubercles are present.

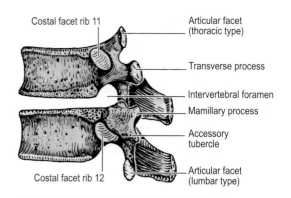

Costal facet rib 11   Articular facet (thoracic type)

Transverse process

Intervertebral foramen
Mamillary process

Accessory tubercle

Costal facet rib 12   Articular facet (lumbar type)

Fig. 6.93   T11 and T12 vertebrae, from the left.

Lumbar vertebrae

The *bodies* of lumbar vertebrae increase in breadth from above down, and this is reflected posteriorly by a progressive widening between the articular processes. Thus in L1 and 2 the four processes as seen from behind make a rectangle set vertically; in L3 they may also make a vertical rectangle, or they may be like those of L4 and make a square; in L5 they make a horizontal rectangle. The body shares with the smaller thoracic vertebrae the characteristics of being concave from above down, of having pedicles attached to its upper half, and of being perforated by a pair of basivertebral veins posteriorly. It differs from the heart-shaped thoracic vertebra in being kidney-shaped, and the posterior surface is flatter, less concave from side to side, so the vertebral canal is somewhat triangular in cross-section (Fig. 6.94).

The *transverse processes* are variable in length, but the fourth is usually the longest (Fig. 6.74). The transverse process of the fifth, however, is quite characteristic. Short, massive, triangular, its base is attached to both the pedicle and the lateral side of the body itself (Fig. 6.95).

The *pedicles* are stout and form the upper and lower margins of the intervertebral foramina. The *laminae* do not show such a downward slope as in the thoracic vertebrae. The quadrangular *spinous process* is roughly horizontal. The upper border is straight but the lower border is concave.

The *articular processes* are characteristic. The upper pair rise up and carry articular facets that face medially (Fig. 6.94). The articular surfaces are concave from front to back. The lower pair of articular processes project down, face laterally and are convex from front to back.

The transverse processes are fused ribs (costal elements). The true transverse element consists of two small elevations with a groove between them occupied by the

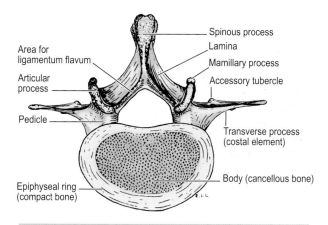

Fig. 6.94   Typical lumbar vertebra, from above.

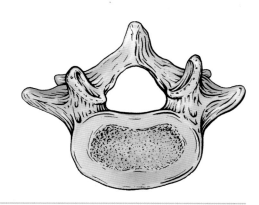

Fig. 6.95   L5 vertebra from above. Compare with Figure 6.94 and note that the transverse process extends well forward on to the side of the body, a feature unique to L5.

medial branch of the posterior ramus of the overlying lumbar nerve (Fig. 6.96). The *mamillary process* is a convexity projecting back from the margin of the superior articular process; the smaller *accessory tubercle* lies below this, at the root of the transverse process (Figs 6.94 and 6.96).

The inferior articular processes of the fifth lumbar vertebra face well forwards, and are received into backward-facing facets on the sacrum, and this locking prevents L5 vertebra from sliding forwards down the slope of S1 vertebra. Furthermore, the adjacent bodies are strongly united by the intervertebral disc. Thus, although the sloping lumbosacral joint carries the whole body weight, it is extremely stable. A strongly contracting erector spinae acts as a supporting strap posteriorly. However, if the neural arch is disrupted between the

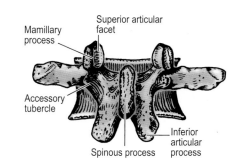

Fig. 6.96   L3 vertebra, from behind.

superior and inferior articular processes, i.e. in the so-called pars interarticularis, the body of L5 tends to slip downwards and forwards (spondylolisthesis).

The fifth lumbar vertebra may be fused on one or both sides to the first sacral vertebra, a condition known as 'sacralization'. More rarely the first sacral vertebra may be partially or completely separate ('lumbarization').

Sacrum

Five progressively smaller sacral vertebrae and their costal elements fuse to make this bone, which is triangular in outline and curved with a concavity towards the pelvis. On its lateral aspect it has an *auricular surface* for articulation with the ilium to make the upper posterior wall of the pelvis. Below the sacroiliac joints the sacrum tapers off down to its apex. The upper surface of the first sacral vertebra forms the base of the sacrum. The body of S1 vertebra is large, and wider transversely; its anterior projecting edge is the *sacral promontory*. Lateral to the body is the wing-like *ala* of the sacrum on each side, consisting of fused costal elements and transverse processes. The ala is crossed anteriorly by the sympathetic trunk, lumbosacral trunk and obturator nerve, in that order from medial to lateral. In the anatomical position the upper surface of the base slopes downwards and forwards at 30° or more. From here the sacrum is directed backwards before curving down over the pelvic cavity.

Pelvic surface

This concave surface is smooth (Fig. 6.97). Across the midline five diminishing bodies are fused, with four ridges persisting to mark the lines of ossification; these transverse lines represent the intervertebral discs. On each side are the four anterior sacral foramina. The rounded bars of bone between adjacent foramina (costal

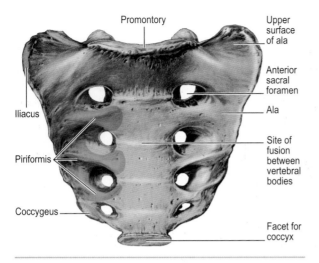

Fig. 6.97   Sacrum: pelvic surface.

elements) represent the heads and necks of ribs. The medial boundaries of the anterior sacral foramina are thus formed by the bodies of the sacral vertebrae, but the other three-quarters of their circumference is costal in origin. The rounded bar of bone above the first sacral foramen continues the arcuate line of the ilium to form the posterior part of the pelvic brim.

The mass of bone lateral to the foramina, the *lateral mass*, is formed by fusion of the costal elements (shafts of ribs) with each other. It is deeply indented by grooves for the anterior rami of the upper four sacral nerves, which pass laterally from the anterior sacral foramina. Piriformis arises from the three ridges (costal elements) that separate the anterior foramina, and from the lateral mass nearby. The sacral anterior primary rami emerging from these foramina lie on piriformis behind its covering fascia (see Fig. 5.56, p. 303). Peritoneum is draped over the front of the upper two bodies and below that level the retroperitoneal rectum lies surrounded by the mesorectum (see p. 302). From the front of the lower sacrum the presacral (rectosacral) fascia passes downwards and forwards to fuse with the mesorectum 3–5 cm above the anorectal junction. Behind this fascia the median sacral artery and vein lie in the midline with some lymph nodes. On each side, the sacral sympathetic trunk lies medial to the sacral foramina, and the lateral sacral vessels lie in front of the piriformis fascia.

Dorsal surface

This convex surface is irregular and rough (Fig. 6.98). In the midline it is closed by fusion of adjacent laminae.

The gap above the first sacral laminae is closed by the ligamenta flava attached to the laminae of L5 vertebra. The *sacral hiatus* below, variable in its extent, indicates failure of fusion of the laminae of S5 and often of S4 vertebrae. This hiatus is closed by fibrous tissue forming the superficial sacrococcygeal ligament. Adjacent spinous processes are fused with each other to produce a midline ridge, the *median sacral crest*, that projects dorsally from the fused laminae. The superior articular process on S1 vertebra carries a backward facing facet for the synovial joint with L5 vertebra. Below this, medial to the posterior foramina is a line of irregular tubercles that represent fusion of adjacent articular processes of the sacral vertebrae. This low ridge forms the *intermediate sacral crest* and it is projected below, alongside the sacral hiatus, to end in the rounded *sacral cornu*. Lateral to the superior articular process is a prominent boss of bone which is the transverse process of S1 vertebra. Below this the transverse processes are fused with each other, making a ridge, the *lateral sacral crest*, lateral to the posterior foramina. It is marked by bosses of bone that represent the tips of the fused transverse processes. The fused costal elements lie lateral to the lateral sacral crest. The gutter between the median and lateral sacral crests is filled by erector spinae, and the posterior layer of the lumbar fascia that covers it is attached to both crests. Between the lateral sacral crest and the auricular surface are deep fossae for the attachment of the posterior sacroiliac ligament.

Sacral canal

This is triangular in cross-section and curves with the sacrum. The sacral canal contains the meninges which extend down to S2 vertebra. From here the filum terminale (pia mater), piercing the dura, runs down to blend with the periosteum on the back of the coccyx. The space around the dura mater and its prolongations is filled with loose fat and the internal vertebral venous plexus. The posterior root ganglia are contained within the sacral canal and the anterior and posterior rami of sacral nerves emerge separately from the anterior and posterior sacral foraminae.

Sex differences are present in the sacrum. The most useful guide is the comparison of the width of the body of S1 vertebra with the width of the lateral mass, or ala. The body is wider than the ala in the male equal to or narrower than the ala in the female (Fig. 6.99). Other differences lie in the curvature of the bone. In the male the anterior surface is gently and uniformly concave; in the female it is flat above and turns forward more prominently below. The auricular surface occupies two and a half vertebrae in the male, but is smaller in the female and may be restricted to two vertebrae.

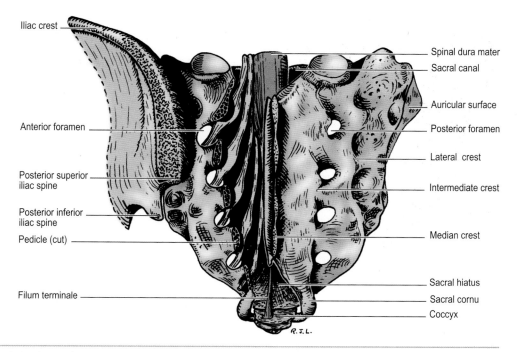

Fig. 6.98   Sacrum from behind. The five pedicles and laminae have been cut through on the left to show the sheaths of dura mater around the nerve roots.

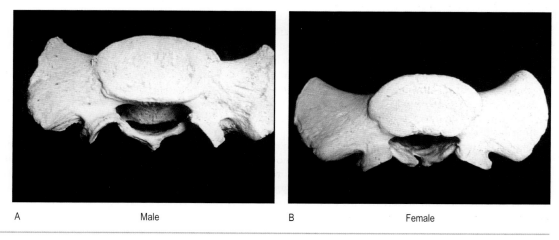

A   Male   B   Female

Fig. 6.99   Male and female sacrum from above. In the male the body of the first sacral vertebra is broad and the alae narrow; in the female the body and the alae broad are of approximately equal width.

Coccyx

This is contracted into four pieces fused together into a small triangular bone joined by its base to the apex of the sacrum at the *sacrococcygeal joint* (see p. 336).

At each side a *lateral sacrococcygeal ligament* joins the transverse process of the first piece of the coccyx to the inferolateral angle of the sacrum and completes the foramen for S5 nerve anteriorly; posteriorly the foramen is closed by the sacral and coccygeal cornua connected by the intercornual ligament. The upper surface of the coccyx is in the pelvic floor, the lower surface is in the buttock, beneath the skin of the natal cleft.

Development of vertebrae

The vertebrae develop from the sclerotome parts of the mesodermal somites (see p. 25). The sclerotomes surround the notochord and neural tube in a sheath of mesoderm. A series of hyaline cartilaginous rings appears in the mesodermal sheath. Each ring is formed by fusion of adjacent halves (caudal and cranial) of the original somites. Thus the vertebrae lie not in segments of the body wall, but in the intersegmental planes.

Each ring ossifies in three centres to form the centrum and the two halves of the neural arch of a vertebra. The centre for the centrum is initially double, but the two areas rapidly fuse; failure of one half results in a hemivertebra; a series of hemivertebrae is one cause of congenital scoliosis (lateral curvature of the spine). By the eighth week of fetal life ossification has commenced in the centrum and the two halves of the neural arch. At birth a vertebra consists of three ossifying parts, centrum and two half arches, united by cartilage. The half arches unite in the first year after birth, first in the lumbar, then thoracic and finally cervical regions. The centra unite with the arches first in the cervical region, about the third year, but in the lumbar region this union is not complete until the sixth year. Failure of fusion of the vertebral arches in the midline results in the condition known as spina bifida. When the overlying skin is intact this is qualified as being occult. A more severe developmental defect results in a cerebrospinal fluid-filled sac (meningocoele) or a sac containing a part of the spinal cord and nerve roots (myelomeningocoele) being exposed on the surface. These defects are more common in the lumbar or lumbosacral region.

The vertical cylindrical surface of the body is covered with compact bone, but the cancellous bone on the flat upper and lower surfaces remains covered with a layer of hyaline cartilage. The epiphyses for the body appear as bony rings, upper and lower, soon after puberty. They are ridged and grooved reciprocally with the margins of the surfaces of the body (Fig. 6.100). Fusion of the epiphyseal ring and body occurs in the early twenties. Soon after puberty secondary centres appear also at the tip of the spinous process (double in the bifid spines of the cervical vertebrae) and at the tips of the transverse processes of all the vertebrae, and in the mamillary processes of T12 and the lumbar vertebrae. These fuse in the early twenties. The costal elements of cervical and lumbar vertebrae do not have a separate bony centre, but ossify by direct extension from the neural arch.

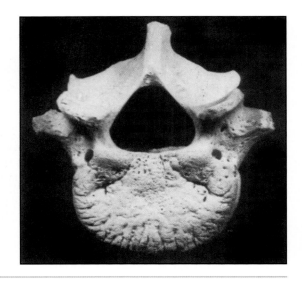

Fig. 6.100   L5 vertebra from above. The neurocentral junction has not yet completely ossified. The radial grooves around the anterolateral convexity of the body indicate that the epiphyseal ring had not united.

An occasional centre in the costal element of C7 or L1 vertebra may lead to the formation of a cervical or lumbar rib. On the other hand the weight-bearing costal elements of the sacrum have primary ossification centres. In general the development of the five segments of the sacrum resembles that of typical vertebrae. After puberty these segments coalesce from below upwards.

The atlas ossifies in the seventh week of fetal life by a centre in each lateral mass. These extend around the posterior arch and unite at the fourth year. In the meantime a centre in the anterior arch has appeared at the first year. Its junction with the bone of the lateral mass cuts across the anterior part of the upper articular surface; these epiphyses fuse at 7 years. This epiphyseal junction may permanently divide the articular surface (as in Fig. 6.89, right side).

Each half of the neural arch of the axis ossifies from a primary centre in the second month; a pair of centres for the centrum, which soon fuse, ossify in the fourth month. The dens is mainly ossified from a pair of centres which appear in the sixth month and join before birth. Thus at birth the axis is in four parts and these fuse with each other in the first few years thereafter; but although the cartilage between the dens and the body ossifies circumferentially, the centre may remain cartilaginous till old age. A secondary centre for the tip of the dens appears at about 6 years and unites with the rest of the dens at about 12 years. As in the case of a typical vertebra, a secondary centre for the lower surface of the body appears at puberty and fuses in the early twenties.

PART TWENTY

Cranial cavity and meninges

The interior of the cranium is lined with dura mater, the surface of the brain is covered with pia mater. Between the two, in contact with the dura mater, lies the arachnoid mater, which is connected to the pia by many fine filamentous processes (hence the name arachnoid: spider-like). These three tissue layers constitute the **meninges**. The cranial meninges are described here; their continuations around the spinal cord as the spinal meninges are considered on page 471.

Pia mater

The pia mater invests the brain and spinal cord as periosteum invests bone. Like periosteum it contains blood vessels, and nowhere does any structure intervene between pia mater and the underlying nervous tissue. It closely invests the surface of the central nervous system to the depths of the deepest fissures and sulci. It is made of thin vascular fibrous tissue and can be stripped away from the brain surface. It is prolonged out over the cranial nerves and spinal nerve roots to fuse with their epineurium, and it is invaginated into the substance of the brain by the entering cerebral arteries. The arteries lie loose in these sheaths of pia, surrounded by a narrow perivascular space containing cerebrospinal fluid.

The region between the pia and the arachnoid is the **subarachnoid space**, filled with cerebrospinal fluid.

Arachnoid mater and subarachnoid space

The **arachnoid mater** consists of an impermeable delicate membrane that everywhere is supported by the inner surface of the inner layer of the dura mater with only a thin film of tissue fluid between them in the **subdural space**. Vessels and nerves pierce the dura and arachnoid mater both at the same place; they cross the subdural space, but do not run along between the two membranes.

In certain areas the arachnoid herniates through little holes in the dura mater into the venous sinuses. Such herniae are the *arachnoid villi*; through their walls the cerebrospinal fluid 'oozes' back into the blood. The arachnoid villi are most numerous in the superior sagittal sinus and its laterally projecting blood lakes. In the child the villi are discrete; as age progresses they become aggregated into visible clumps, the *arachnoid granulations* (*Pacchionian bodies*). These latter leave indentations on the inner table of the cranial vault mainly alongside the superior sagittal sinus, at the site of the blood lakes (see Fig. 7.16, p. 493).

Between the base of the brain and the base of the skull several larger spaces exist as a result of the incongruities in the contours of bone and brain. These spaces form the **subarachnoid cisterns**.

The *cerebellomedullary cistern* (*cisterna magna*) is the largest. It occupies the angle between the undersurface of the cerebellum and the posterior surface of the medulla. Cerebrospinal fluid flows into it from the midline aperture (foramen of Magendie) in the roof of the fourth ventricle (see p. 502). The lateral part of the cistern contains the vertebral artery and its posterior inferior cerebellar branch on each side (see Fig. 7.19, p. 495). The cisterna magna can be tapped in the midline by a needle passed above the posterior arch of the atlas, through the posterior atlanto-occipital membrane and spinal dura.

The *pontine cistern* lies between the clivus (see p. 532) and the front of the pons and medulla. Cerebrospinal fluid flows into it from the lateral apertures (foramina of Luschka) of the fourth ventricle (see p. 502). The cistern contains the basilar artery and its pontine and labyrinthine branches and the fifth to twelfth cranial nerves.

The *interpeduncular cistern* lies between the dorsum sellae of the sphenoid and the cerebral peduncles; it is roofed in by the floor of the third ventricle (mamillary bodies and posterior perforated substance). The floor of the cistern, on the dorsum sellae, is formed by the arachnoid membrane passing across, in contact with the dura mater, between the right and left temporal lobes. The cistern contains the terminal branches of the basilar artery (including the posterior part of the circle of Willis), the stalk of the pituitary gland, and the third and fourth cranial nerves (see Fig. 7.19, p. 495).

The *chiasmatic cistern* lies above the optic chiasma, beneath the rostrum of the corpus callosum (see Fig. 7.3A, p. 476). It contains the anterior communicating artery and the intracranial part of the optic nerves.

Dura mater

The dura mater consists of an outer endosteal layer, and an inner meningeal layer. The two layers are united except where they separate to enclose the venous sinuses of the dura. The *outer layer* is the *periosteum* which invests the surface of any bone, and blood vessels pass through it to supply the bone. Around the margins of every foramen in the skull it lies in continuity with the periosteum on the outer surface of the cranial bones (pericranium). It is not prolonged into the dura mater of the vertebral canal nor is it evaginated by any cranial nerve. The *inner layer* consists of a dense, strong fibrous membrane, which is really the dura mater proper. Over the vault of the skull the fused layers are easily stripped away from the bone as a single sheet, a fact which makes removal of the vault relatively easy. Over the base of the skull the fused layers are so firmly attached that they can only be stripped off with difficulty. Although theoretically structures such as the middle meningeal vessels (see p. 459) lie between the two layers, they appear to be on the outer surface of this single sheet (as when the bone of the skull vault is removed leaving the dura intact), and so are usually described as being extradural. The vessels are thicker than the outer layer and so bulge out to make impressions on the bone with a negligible amount of intervening tissue. Haemorrhage from these vessels is described as extradural (see p. 464).

Folds of the inner layer project into the cranial cavity. One such fold, the tentorium cerebelli, roofs in the posterior cranial fossa; another forms the falx cerebri, lying in the midline between the two cerebral hemispheres. The falx cerebelli and diaphragma sellae are smaller derivatives of the inner dural layer. These fibrous flanges or septa minimize rotary displacement of the brain. Concussion is caused more readily by rotary movement of the brain rather than by mass displacement of the head. At the foramen magnum the inner layer leaves the outer layer and is projected down the vertebral canal as the spinal dura mater (see p. 471). The inner layer is likewise evaginated around the cranial nerves and spinal nerve roots.

The **tentorium cerebelli** is a flange of the inner layer which projects from the margins of the transverse sinuses and the margins of the superior petrosal sinuses (Fig. 6.101). It is attached to the posterior clinoid processes, along the upper borders of the petrous temporal bones and horizontally along the inner surface of each

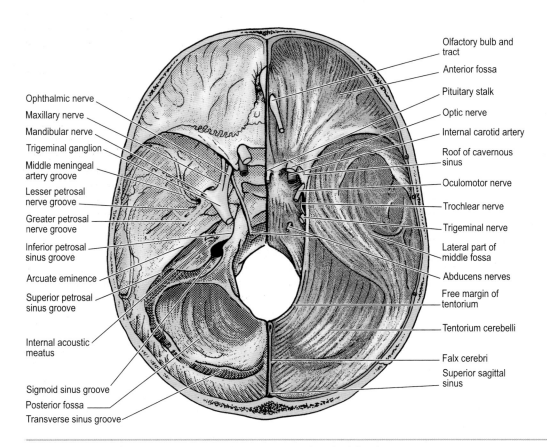

Fig. 6.101   Cranial fossae. The dura mater has been removed on the left side.

side of the skull to the internal occipital protuberance; this is the attached margin of the tentorium. Its upper and lower layers are separated at their bony attachments by the superior petrosal and transverse sinuses, but elsewhere are intimately fused with each other. The free margin of the tentorium is U-shaped and lies at a higher level than the bony attachment. The large central gap is the *tentorial notch* (*incisure*), through which passes the upper part of the brainstem (midbrain). The membrane slopes concavely upwards as it converges from the attached to the free margin, in conformity with the shape of the upper surface of the cerebellum and the undersurface of the posterior part of the cerebral hemisphere. The concave free margin is traceable forwards to the anterior clinoid process on each side. Over the superior petrosal sinus it overlies the attached margin, and from this point forwards to the anterior clinoid process it lies as a ridge of dura mater on the roof of the cavernous sinus. To the medial side of the ridge is the concave triangular roof of the cavernous sinus (see p. 461), which is pierced by the third and fourth nerves.

The midline attachment of the falx suspends the tentorium and the straight sinus lies in the midline at the junction of the two.

The **falx cerebri** is a sickle-shaped flange of the inner layer in the midline between the cerebral hemispheres. Its anterior margin is attached to the crista galli of the ethmoid bone and to the cavity of the foramen caecum (see p. 531), into which it projects like a peg, an enlarged Sharpey's fibre. The posterior margin is attached to the upper surface of the tentorium cerebelli in the midline, from the attached to the free margin of the tentorium; here its layers separate to enclose the straight sinus. Its convex upper border is attached alongside the midline to the whole length of the concave inner surface of the skull, from the foramen caecum to the internal occipital protuberance. Its two layers are separated a short distance above the foramen caecum to accommodate the superior sagittal sinus, which becomes progressively broader from this point to the internal occipital protuberance. The concave lower border of the falx cerebri is free and contains the inferior sagittal sinus within its two layers; this border lies just above the corpus callosum (see Fig. 7.15, p. 492). Between superior and inferior sagittal sinuses the two layers of the falx are firmly united to form a strong inelastic membrane.

The **falx cerebelli** is a low elevation of the inner layer in the midline of the posterior cranial fossa, extending from the internal occipital protuberance along the internal occipital crest to the posterior margin of the foramen magnum. It lodges the small occipital sinus between its layers, and it projects a little into the sulcus between the cerebellar hemispheres.

The **diaphragma sellae** is a horizontal sheet of the inner layer that forms a roof for the pituitary fossa (see p. 465). The dura of the floor of the fossa is prolonged up the sides of the fossa, hitched between the middle and posterior clinoid processes, to form a flange lying between the fossa and the cavernous sinus. From this the dura extends medially to form the diaphragma, which is perforated centrally for the passage of the pituitary stalk, and is continuous laterally with the roof of the cavernous sinus.

Blood supply

The inner layer of the dura mater requires very little blood to nourish it. The outer layer, on the other hand, is richly supplied, with the adjacent bone. In the supratentorial part it is supplied by the middle meningeal artery. The dura is supplied, in the anterior cranial fossa, by meningeal branches of the ophthalmic and anterior and posterior ethmoidal arteries and a branch of the middle meningeal artery, in the middle cranial fossa by the middle and accessory meningeal arteries and by meningeal branches of the internal carotid and ascending pharyngeal arteries and in the posterior cranial fossa by meningeal branches of the vertebral artery (Fig. 6.109). All these meningeal arteries are chiefly distributed to bone.

The **middle meningeal artery**, a branch of the maxillary, arises in the infratemporal fossa and passes upwards between the two roots of the auriculotemporal nerve to enter the foramen spinosum. It thus enters the middle cranial fossa, accompanied by its own plexus of sympathetic nerves. It is accompanied throughout all its ramifications by veins which lie between it and bone. It courses laterally on the floor of the middle cranial fossa and turns upwards and forwards on the greater wing of the sphenoid, where it divides into anterior and posterior branches.

The *frontal (anterior) branch* courses up towards the pterion (see p. 526) and then curves back to ascend towards the vertex, lying over the precentral gyrus. Haemorrhage from the vessel thus causes pressure on the motor area. In the region of the pterion the artery frequently lies in a tunnel in the parietal bone for a centimetre or more.

The *parietal (posterior) branch* courses horizontally backwards, on a groove in the squamous part of the temporal bone, and ramifies over the posterior part of the skull. It lies along the superior temporal gyrus; haemorrhage here may cause contralateral impaired hearing through pressure on the auditory area (see p. 482).

The main purpose of the middle meningeal artery is to supply the bones of the vault of the skull; it does not supply the brain. These bones receive very little blood from the vessels of the scalp; scalping produces no necrosis of the underlying bones. Only where the bones give attachment to muscles (temporal fossa and sub-occipital region) is any substantial supply received from the exterior.

Much of the blood from the marrow is drained by large *diploic veins*, which emerge on the exterior. Other diploic veins drain into the venous sinuses, especially the superior sagittal. The remaining blood drains into the middle meningeal veins.

The **middle meningeal veins** are sinuses in the dura mater and accompany the branches of the artery. They lie between the artery and the bone, grooving the latter. Some converge to two veins which leave the skull through the foramen spinosum and foramen ovale to join the pterygoid plexus. Some join the sphenoparietal and superior sagittal sinus.

The *surface marking* of the middle meningeal artery as it enters the skull lies just above the midpoint of the zygomatic arch. The frontal branch can be *surgically approached* through a burr hole made in the region of the pterion, about 3 cm above the zygomatic arch and 3 cm behind the zygomatic process of the frontal bone; a position that is above the midpoint of the zygomatic arch and behind the palpable frontozygomatic suture. The posterior branch runs backwards parallel with and above the upper border of the zygomatic arch and the supramastoid crest; it is usually exposed vertically above the mastoid process on a level horizontal with the upper margin of the orbit.

Nerve supply

Most of the supratentorial part of the dura mater is supplied from the ophthalmic division of the trigeminal nerve; the tentorial nerves course up and back from the anterior end of the cavernous sinus to supply the falx, the dura of the vault, and the upper surface of the tentorium cerebelli.

The anterior cranial fossa is supplied by the anterior and posterior ethmoidal nerves and receives some twigs from the maxillary nerve. The middle fossa is supplied, in its anterior portion by a branch of the maxillary nerve, and in its posterior part by the meningeal branch of the mandibular nerve (nervus spinosus). The posterior fossa is supplied by meningeal branches of the vagus and hypoglossal nerves; these are C1 and C2 fibres carried by the cranial nerves. They innervate the undersurface of the tentorium cerebelli and the upper part of the bony fossa. The dura around the foramen magnum is supplied directly by the second and third cervical nerves. Clinical experience suggests that this cervical supply extends farther afield than the posterior cranial fossa; cervical spondylosis, for example, may be associated with deep-seated pain in the orbit, presumably referred from spinal nerves.

Venous sinuses of the dura mater

All the venous sinuses, except the inferior sagittal and straight sinuses, lie between the inner and outer layers of the dura. They receive all the blood from the brain, and with the above exceptions they receive blood also from the adjacent bone. Several of them have important communicating branches with veins outside the skull. Like all vascular channels the venous sinuses are lined by endothelium. They do not contain valves.

The **superior sagittal sinus** lies between the two layers of the falx cerebri along the convexity of its attached margin. It commences just above the foramen caecum and grows progressively larger as it passes back to the internal occipital protuberance. It grooves the bones along the midline of the vault of the skull. Three or four lakes of blood project laterally from it, between the inner dura and the endosteum; into these lakes the arachnoid granulations project to return cerebrospinal fluid to the bloodstream (see Fig. 7.16, p. 493).

The superior sinus does not drain the frontal pole of the hemisphere, but receives veins from the upper and posterior parts of both medial and lateral surfaces of both hemispheres. These superior cerebral veins enter the sinus obliquely, against the flow of the bloodstream (see Fig. 7.15, p. 492). The superior sagittal sinus turns at the internal occipital protuberance, generally to the right, and becomes the transverse (lateral) sinus.

The **inferior sagittal sinus** begins some little distance above the crista galli and lies between the folds of the free margin of the falx cerebri. It drains the lower parts of the medial surface of each hemisphere. At the attachment of falx cerebri and tentorium cerebelli it flows into the straight sinus (see Fig. 7.15, p. 492).

The **straight sinus** lies between the folds of the fibrous dura at the junction of falx cerebri and tentorium cerebelli. It commences anteriorly by receiving the inferior sagittal sinus and the great cerebral vein (of Galen) (see p. 493). The straight sinus also receives veins from the adjoining occipital lobes and from the upper surface of the cerebellum. It slopes down steeply and ends at the internal occipital protuberance by turning into the transverse (lateral) sinus, generally the left (see Fig. 7.15, p. 492).

The **transverse sinus** commences at the internal occipital protuberance and runs laterally between the two layers of the attached margin of the tentorium cerebelli (Fig. 6.101). It courses horizontally forwards, grooving the occipital bone and the mastoid angle of the parietal bone. Reaching the junction of petrous and mastoid parts of the temporal bone it curves downwards, deeply grooving the inner surface of the mastoid bone, as the sigmoid sinus. One sinus is larger than the other, namely that which receives the superior sagittal sinus; this is usually the right.

The two transverse sinuses communicate at their commencement at the internal occipital protuberance (*confluence of the sinuses*). Each receives tributaries from the nearby surfaces of cerebral and cerebellar hemispheres and, at its termination at the commencement of the sigmoid sinus, the superior petrosal sinus enters.

The *surface marking* of the transverse sinus is a horizontal line from the external occipital protuberance to the top of the mastoid, that is, at the upper limit of the neck muscles where they join the skull, along the superior nuchal line.

The **sigmoid sinus** commences as the termination of the transverse sinus, deeply grooving the inner surface of the mastoid part of the petrous bone. It curves downwards and then forwards to the posterior margin of the jugular foramen, through which it passes, and expands into the superior jugular bulb, from which emerges the internal jugular vein (see p. 356). The sigmoid sinus is connected with the exterior in its upper part by the mastoid emissary vein which joins the posterior auricular vein, and in its lower part by a vein which passes through the posterior condylar foramen (when present) to join the suboccipital plexus of veins.

As the superior petrosal sinus drains into the termination of the transverse sinus, it could be said that the sigmoid sinus receives the superior petrosal sinus at its upper end and the occipital sinus at its lower end. Cerebellar veins drain to it, and it receives veins also from the mastoid air cells. Thrombophlebitis in these veins may lead to cerebellar abscess from mastoid infection.

The **occipital sinus** runs downwards from the beginning of the transverse sinus to the foramen magnum, skirts the margin of the foramen and drains into the sigmoid sinus. The two sinuses, lying along the attachment of the falx cerebelli, are often fused into a single trunk. Around the margins of the foramen magnum the sinuses communicate with the veins outside the spinal dura (the internal vertebral plexus). The occipital sinus receives tributaries from the cerebellum and medulla and drains the choroid plexus of the fourth ventricle.

The **basilar plexus** consist of a network of veins, lying between the two layers of the dura, on the clivus (see p. 532). They connect the two inferior petrosal sinuses and receive veins from the lower part of the pons and from the front of the medulla. Thrombosis in this plexus is therefore usually fatal.

No veins accompany the vertebral and basilar arteries; the vertebral vein itself commences outside the skull below the occipital bone (see p. 447).

Cavernous sinus

The cavernous sinus lies alongside the body of the sphenoid bone in the middle cranial fossa. Each contains the internal carotid artery (Figs 6.102 and 6.103) and transmits some cranial nerves; each receives blood from three sources (orbit, vault bones, and cerebral hemisphere); each drains by the superior and inferior petrosal sinuses to the sigmoid sinus and internal jugular vein respectively, and each is connected to the pterygoid plexus by emissary veins.

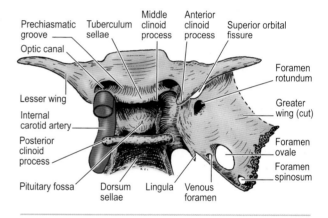

Fig. 6.102 Pituitary fossa, from above.

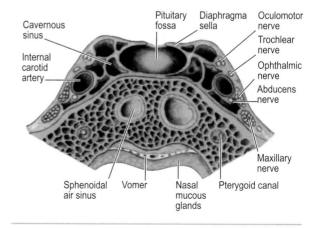

Fig. 6.103 Pituitary fossa and cavernous sinuses in coronal section.

The cavernous sinus lies in a space between the periosteum of the body of the sphenoid (outer layer of the dura mater) and a fold of the inner layer of the dura, which forms the upper part of the medial wall, the roof and the lateral wall of the sinus (Fig. 6.103). Medially the roof is continuous with the diaphragma sellae. At its lower edge the lateral wall is continued laterally as the inner layer of dura across the middle cranial fossa (Fig. 6.101). Anteriorly the roof is attached to the anterior and middle clinoid processes of the sphenoid bone; it is perforated between these processes by the emerging internal carotid artery. Posteriorly the roof has a triangular depression between the attached edge of the tentorium cerebelli (to the posterior clinoid process) and the ridge raised by the free edge of the tentorium, as it extends forwards to the anterior clinoid process. The third and fourth cranial nerves invaginate the roof here (Fig. 6.104), and then run forwards in the lateral wall (i.e. between the dura and the endothelial lining) above the ophthalmic and maxillary branches of the fifth

nerve. Further back the lateral wall is medial to the anterior parts of the trigeminal ganglion and the trigeminal (Meckel's) cave (see p. 467). The rest of the cave and ganglion are posteroinferior to the lateral wall. The floor of the sinus is a narrow strip of periosteum along the base of the greater wing of the sphenoid.

The cavernous sinus extends from the apex of the orbit back to the apex of the petrous temporal bone. Each end is pointed, so that the sinus is spindle-shaped in lateral view. It is about 2 cm long and 1 cm wide. Despite its name, the cavernous sinus is usually a plexus of veins and not a trabeculated venous space, like the corpora cavernosa of the penis.

Medial to the sinus lies the fibrous lateral wall of the pituitary fossa and the body of the sphenoid, with the sphenoid air sinus within it (Fig. 6.103). The air sinus lies towards the front of the pituitary fossa at a lower level; its extent is very variable and tends to increase posteriorly with advancing years. Lateral to the cavernous sinus lies the medial surface of the temporal lobe of

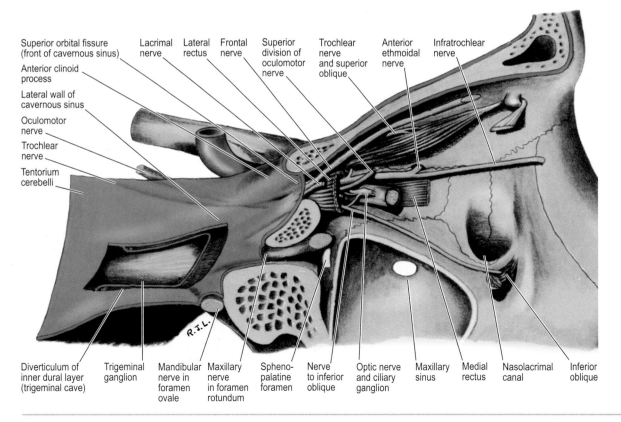

Fig. 6.104   Longitudinal section through the right orbit and middle cranial fossa, viewed from the right (lateral) side.

the hemisphere. Superiorly, the emerging internal carotid artery lies in contact with the forepart of the roof of the sinus as the artery passes backwards a little before turning up towards the anterior perforated substance of the brain (Fig. 6.102). Further back and somewhat above the roof lies the uncus of the temporal lobe.

The *contents* of the cavernous sinus include the structures lying within the cavity (the internal carotid artery and sixth nerve) and those embedded within the lateral wall (the third and fourth nerves and the ophthalmic and maxillary branches of the fifth nerve) (Fig. 6.103).

The **internal carotid artery** curves upwards from the foramen lacerum to enter the posterior part of the sinus and runs forwards within the sinus, deeply grooving the body of the sphenoid and the base of its greater wing. The artery then curves upwards again to pierce the roof of the sinus, medial to the anterior clinoid process, and turns backwards (Figs 6.102 and 6.105). The artery is accompanied by a plexus of postganglionic sympathetic fibres from the superior cervical ganglion.

The **abducens nerve** (see p. 468) enters the back of the cavernous sinus after passing over the apex of the petrous part of the temporal bone. It runs forwards on the inferolateral side of the internal carotid artery (Fig. 6.105). At the anterior end of the sinus it enters the superior orbital fissure (Fig. 6.53).

The **oculomotor nerve** (see p. 467) enters the roof between the free and attached margins of the tentorium cerebelli (Fig. 6.101), and then passes forward in the lateral wall. As it does so it inclines downwards medial to the other nerves, namely, the trochlear nerve and the branches of the ophthalmic nerve (Fig. 6.104), and at the anterior end of the sinus it breaks into its superior and inferior divisions which enter the superior orbital fissure. In its course it picks up sympathetic fibres from the internal carotid plexus; these are for the smooth muscle part of levator palpebrae superioris.

The **trochlear nerve** (see p. 467) enters the roof of the sinus behind the oculomotor nerve, alongside the ridge raised by the free margin of the tentorium, and courses horizontally forwards in the lateral wall of the sinus to enter the superior orbital fissure at a higher level and lateral to the oculomotor nerve.

The **trigeminal ganglion**, in its anterior part, lies forward of Meckel's cave. Its **mandibular division** passes downwards to the foramen ovale and does not come in contact with the lateral wall of the cavernous sinus (Fig. 6.101). The **maxillary division** runs horizontally forwards in the lateral wall and leaves the middle fossa through the foramen rotundum. The **ophthalmic division** runs forwards above the maxillary division and divides into its three branches towards the anterior end of the lateral wall; these enter the orbit through the superior orbital fissure. At the anterior end of the sinus the ophthalmic division gives off its tentorial branches to the dura mater (see p. 460). In its course through the

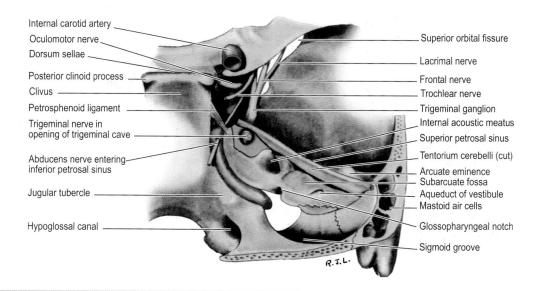

Internal carotid artery
Oculomotor nerve
Dorsum sellae
Posterior clinoid process
Clivus
Petrosphenoid ligament
Trigeminal nerve in opening of trigeminal cave
Abducens nerve entering inferior petrosal sinus
Jugular tubercle
Hypoglossal canal

Superior orbital fissure
Lacrimal nerve
Frontal nerve
Trochlear nerve
Trigeminal ganglion
Internal acoustic meatus
Superior petrosal sinus
Tentorium cerebelli (cut)
Arcuate eminence
Subarcuate fossa
Aqueduct of vestibule
Mastoid air cells
Glossopharyngeal notch
Sigmoid groove

R.J.L.

Fig. 6.105 Part of the posterior and middle cranial fossae seen from behind after sectioning the skull coronally through the mastoid process. All dura mater has been removed except for that over the superior and inferior petrosal sinuses, the dura around the opening of the trigeminal cave and the cut edge of the tentorium cerebelli at its attachment to the petrous temporal bone.

sinus the ophthalmic division picks up sympathetic fibres from the internal carotid plexus; these eventually enter the long ciliary nerves to reach the dilator pupillae muscle.

Veins of the cavernous sinus

Although it is customary to think of venous blood as entering the cavernous sinus at the front and leaving from behind and below, blood can flow in either direction in the sinus, depending on local venous pressures. There are no valves in the cavernous sinus or its connected veins.

The **superior ophthalmic vein** passes back directly into the anterior end of the sinus at the superior orbital fissure. The **inferior ophthalmic vein** drains into both the pterygoid plexus and the cavernous sinus.

The **superficial middle cerebral vein** traverses the subarachnoid space and drains into the sinus by piercing its roof near the emerging carotid artery. Some inferior cerebral veins also drain through the roof of the sinus.

The **sphenoparietal sinus** runs beneath the edge of the lesser wing of the sphenoid, lying between the two layers of the dura mater, and enters the sinus through its roof.

The **superior petrosal sinus** leaves the top of the posterior end and, bridging the groove made by the underlying trigeminal nerve, runs back along the upper border of the petrous bone between the two layers at the attached margin of the tentorium cerebelli (Fig. 6.105). It enters the commencement of the sigmoid sinus, at the termination of the transverse sinus.

The **inferior petrosal sinus** is larger and empties the bulk of the blood from the cavernous sinus. It leaves the posterior end of the sinus beneath the petrosphenoid ligament, a fibrous band stretched between the apex of the petrous part of the temporal bone and the side of the dorsum sellae (Fig. 6.105); it is occasionally partly ossified. The abducens nerve may enter the sinus and pass through it into the cavernous sinus. The inferior petrosal sinus runs down between the two layers of the dura along the suture between the apex of the petrous bone and the side of the clivus (occipital bone), enters the anterior compartment of the jugular foramen medial to the glossopharyngeal nerve, and joins the internal jugular vein as its first (highest) tributary.

The cavernous sinus communicates with the **pterygoid venous plexus** by emissary veins which usually pass through the foramen ovale and the foramen lacerum. When the venous foramen (of Vesalius) is present medial to the foramen ovale (Fig. 6.102), it too transmits a vein.

The cavernous sinuses communicate with each other through the **intercavernous sinuses**, which form a small plexus that lies between the two layers of the dura of the floor of the pituitary fossa. An anterior and a posterior intercavernous sinus lie also in the diaphragma sellae.

The cavernous sinus is in venous connection with the skin of part of the face whence infection may produce thrombosis (see p. 368). By the superficial middle cerebral vein such thrombosis can spread to the cerebral hemisphere. The 'danger area of the face' comprises the upper lip and nose and medial part of the cheek. It lies between the two veins which communicate with the cavernous sinus, namely, the angular vein (via superior ophthalmic vein) and the deep facial vein (via pterygoid plexus and emissary veins). Thrombosis of the cavernous sinus causes ophthalmoplegia from ocular nerve interruption. Spread of thrombosis to the inferior petrosal sinus and medullary veins is usually fatal.

Rupture of the internal carotid artery within the cavernous sinus, following a fracture of the skull base, produces a pulsating exophthalmos (bulging eyeball) from suffusion of the ophthalmic veins with arterial blood.

Extradural, subdural and subarachnoid haemorrhage

Fractures of the side of the skull may rupture the middle meningeal artery (especially its frontal branch) causing **extradural haemorrhage** which leads to the formation of a haematoma between the bone of the skull and the dura. The resultant swelling may cause (apart from the clinical features of raised intracranial pressure, namely headache, drowsiness and a slow pulse) pressure on the cerebral hemisphere in the region of the motor area (see p. 481), giving contralateral hemiparesis (commencing usually in the face and then spreading to the upper limb), and the medial edge of the temporal lobe may be displaced over the free edge of the tentorium, compressing the oculomotor nerve and causing dilatation of the pupil on the injured side.

Subdural haemorrhage may be caused by rupture of a superior cerebral vein as it crosses the subdural space to enter the superior sagittal sinus; the venous blood escapes into the (potential) space between the dura and arachnoid. There may be similar pressure symptoms to those caused by extradural haemorrhage, but because venous rather than arterial blood is involved they are slower to develop and less severe (chronic subdural haematoma). As the haematoma tends to be located near the vertex the contralateral hemiparesis usually commences in the lower limb.

Subarachnoid haemorrhage is usually caused by rupture of arteries that lie within the space, such as aneurysms of the arterial circle at the base of the brain (see p. 490). This causes blood to contaminate the cerebrospinal fluid.

PART TWENTY-ONE

Cranial fossae

Anterior cranial fossa

The anterior cranial fossa is formed by the frontal bone, the cribriform plate of the ethmoid, the lesser wings and anterior part of the body of the sphenoid. The floor of the fossa roofs in the orbits, ethmoidal sinuses and the nose.

The gyri and sulci of the undersurface of the frontal lobes cause grooves and ridges on the orbital parts of the frontal bone. From the nose up to 20 **olfactory nerve** filaments (on each side) perforate the dura and arachnoid mater over the cribriform plate and pass upwards through the subarachnoid space to enter the olfactory bulb, from which the olfactory tract passes back on the inferior surface of the frontal lobe (see Fig. 7.4, p. 477).

The **anterior ethmoidal nerve** and **artery** have a very short course in the fossa. Coming in from the orbit they lie beneath the dura at the edge of the cribriform plate, where they run forwards in a slit and pass down into the nose at the side of the crista galli.

The posterior border of the lesser wing of the sphenoid lies at the boundary between the anterior and middle cranial fossae. The sphenoparietal sinus runs between the two layers of the dura at this edge, which fits into the stem of the lateral cerebral sulcus (see p. 474); a branch of the middle meningeal artery crosses over the sinus to reach the anterior cranial fossa.

Middle cranial fossa

The middle cranial fossa consists of a median part, formed by the sphenoid body, and right and left lateral parts, formed by the cerebral surfaces of the greater wings of the sphenoid and the squamous and petrous parts of the temporal bones. The median part (Fig. 6.102) contains the pituitary gland, optic nerves and chiasma, and the intercavernous sinuses. The right and left lateral parts each contain the cavernous sinus, the third to the sixth cranial nerves and trigeminal ganglion, internal carotid artery, middle and accessory meningeal vessels, and the greater and lesser petrosal nerves. The temporal lobes lie on the right and left lateral parts.

The superior border of the petrous temporal bone lies at the boundary between the middle and posterior cranial fossae; the superior petrosal sinus lies here between the two layers of the dura.

Pituitary gland

The pituitary gland (hypophysis cerebri) lies in its fossa (sella turcica) with the diaphragma sellae above it. Intercavernous sinuses lie in the diaphragma and in the dural floor of the fossa. On each side is a flange of dura mater separating the gland from the upper part of the cavernous sinus. The pia and arachnoid blend with the capsule of the gland. Below the fossa lies the body of the sphenoid bone containing the sphenoidal air sinuses. When small the sinuses lie anteroinferior to the fossa, but when large one or both extend back beneath the fossa.

The *pituitary stalk* slopes downwards and forwards to the perforation in the diaphragma, connecting the posterior part of the gland to the hypothalamus (see p. 489). The upper, or infundibular, part of the stalk is hollowed out (continuous with the third ventricle). The optic chiasma lies above the diaphragma sellae, anterosuperior to the pituitary stalk. A pituitary tumour, rising upwards, presses on the lower anterior part of the chiasma and the medial sides of the optic nerves (so causing hemianopia of the temporal fields; see p. 521).

Structure. The gland is a composite structure consisting essentially of two main parts, the *anterior and posterior lobes*; these terms are not entirely synonymous with the terms adenohypophysis and neurohypophysis, which indicate different developmental origins. The *adenohypophysis*, developed from an ectodermal saccule (Rathke's pouch) of the stomodeum (see p. 26), consists of the pars anterior (distalis), pars tuberalis and the rudimentary pars intermedia. The *neurohypophysis*, developed as a neuroectodermal downgrowth from the floor of the third ventricle, consists of the pars posterior (nervosa), the infundibular stalk and the median eminence (see p. 489). The pars anterior and the pars posterior form the anterior and posterior lobes respectively.

The *pars anterior* accounts for 75% of the whole gland. It is highly vascular, and its cells consist of 50% chromophobes, 35% acidophils and 15% basophils. The acidophils (eosinophils) secrete growth hormone and prolactin, with the basophils producing ACTH, TSH, FSH and LH (adrenocorticotropic, thyroid-stimulating, follicle-stimulating and luteinizing hormones). The pars tuberalis is a small extension of the pars anterior along the pituitary stalk, but its cells are different and their function not known. The pars anterior lies in front of a narrow cleft (the remains of the pharyngeal downgrowth), behind which is the small pars intermedia. It consists of a number of colloid-filled vesicles and secretes MSH (melanocyte-stimulating hormone). Its cells contain endorphins.

The *pars posterior* consists largely of about 100 000 unmyelinated nerve fibres whose cell bodies are in the supraoptic and paraventricular nuclei of the hypothalamus. Neurosecretory material manufactured in the cell bodies (mainly oxytocin from the paraventricular cells and vasopressin—antidiuretic hormone—from the supraoptic cells) migrates at the rate of about 3 mm/day along their axons which run in the pituitary stalk and end in the pars nervosa. Both hormones are combined with a carrier protein, neurophysin. Scattered among the nerve fibres are the rather scanty pituicytes which resemble astrocytes.

Blood supply and the hypophyseal portal system. A single inferior and several superior *hypophyseal arteries* arise from the internal carotid artery. Venous blood enters the adjacent cavernous and intercavernous sinuses. In addition to these vessels there is a *hypothalamo-hypophyseal portal venous system* connecting the hypothalamus and neurohypophysis with the adenohypophysis. These fine vessels form a plexus on the stalk and pars anterior. Into them in the upper part of the stalk are secreted the various hypophysiotropic hormones (hormone-releasing factors) derived from cells of the median eminence and possibly other parts of the hypothalamus. The portal vessels then transport these substances to their target cells which are the chromophils of the anterior lobe. Thus the anterior lobe cells are controlled by hypothalamic messengers delivered to them by a portal venous system. Reverse blood flow in this system and venous drainage from the hypophysis to the hypothalamus has also been suggested. There is no blood–brain barrier (see p. 491) in the posterior pituitary or median eminence.

Surgical approach. The gland can be approached through the anterior cranial fossa by elevating the frontal lobe of the brain, the subfrontal approach, or by the trans-sphenoidal approach, entering the pituitary fossa from below through a sphenoidal air sinus. This is entered either via the ethmoidal air cells after raising the periosteum from the medial wall of the orbit, or by elevating the nasal mucosa from the nasal septum and removing the septum (the nasal cavity itself is not entered).

The **internal carotid artery** emerges from the roof of the cavernous sinus medial to the anterior clinoid process and curves immediately backwards, lying on the roof of the sinus before curving upwards lateral to the optic chiasma. At the anterior perforated substance it divides into its terminal branches (Fig. 6.106). The curve of the internal carotid artery in and above the cavernous sinus as seen in a lateral carotid arteriogram (like a U on its side, opening backwards) is commonly called the *carotid siphon* (Fig. 6.107).

The **ophthalmic artery** branches from the internal carotid immediately above the roof of the cavernous sinus. The internal carotid arteries come from below and laterally, the optic nerves come from above and medially (i.e. from the chiasma), and this is the relationship of nerve and artery in the optic canal.

The **optic nerve** passes forward, down and laterally from the chiasma to the optic canal. Clad only in pia mater, it receives its tube of arachnoid and dura mater at the optic canal. Its intracranial part, in the chiasmatic cistern, is here supplied by branches of the anterior cerebral artery that run down from the chiasma.

Fig. 6.106   Right carotid arteriogram: anteroposterior view.

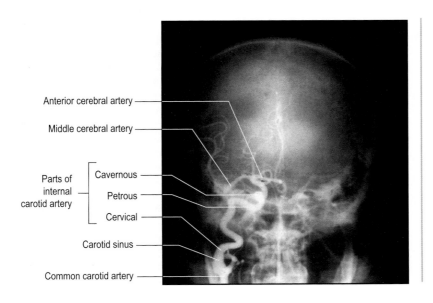

Anterior cerebral artery

Middle cerebral artery

Parts of internal carotid artery — Cavernous

Petrous

Cervical

Carotid sinus

Common carotid artery

Fig. 6.107 Right carotid arteriogram: lateral view.

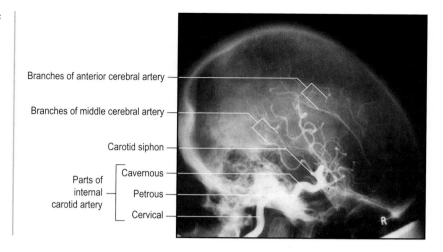

Branches of anterior cerebral artery

Branches of middle cerebral artery

Carotid siphon

Parts of internal carotid artery — Cavernous / Petrous / Cervical

The **oculomotor nerve** leaves the medial side of the crus of the cerebral peduncle (see Fig. 7.18, p. 494). The nerve passes forwards between the posterior cerebral and superior cerebellar arteries (see Fig. 7.19, p. 495), just below the free margin of the tentorium cerebelli, below the posterior communicating artery; aneurysms may damage the nerve here. It crosses the interpeduncular cistern and enters the roof of the cavernous sinus in the middle fossa.

The **trochlear nerve**, after emerging from the dorsal surface of the brainstem below the inferior colliculus (see p. 497), curls around the cerebral peduncle below the posterior cerebral artery and runs forward above the superior cerebellar artery, lateral to the oculomotor nerve in the interpeduncular cistern, just below the free margin of the tentorium cerebelli (i.e. in the posterior fossa). It enters the middle fossa just behind the oculomotor nerve and enters the roof of the cavernous sinus, near where the free and attached margins of the tentorium cerebelli cross each other.

The **abducens nerve** enters the middle cranial fossa by passing over the apex of the petrous temporal and then runs round the lateral side of the ascending part of the internal carotid artery (Fig. 6.105) as it enters the cavernous sinus.

The **posterior communicating artery**, joining the internal carotid and posterior cerebral artery in the circle of Willis, lies in the interpeduncular cistern, above and lateral to the pituitary gland (see Fig. 7.19, p. 495).

Trigeminal ganglion

The trigeminal ganglion lies beneath the dura mater in the floor of the middle cranial fossa alongside the cavernous sinus, and occupies the trigeminal impression, a small fossa on the front of the apex of the petrous temporal bone posterolateral to the foramen lacerum (Figs 6.101 and 8.4, p. 529). The trigeminal nerve leaves the pons in the posterior fossa and runs forwards to cross the upper border of the petrous bone, upon which it leaves a shallow groove some 5 mm wide; it is accompanied by the small motor root, which lies below the sensory root. They pass beneath the superior petrosal sinus at this point (Fig. 6.105). As they do so, with their covering of pia, they evaginate a diverticulum of the inner layer of the dura and the arachnoid, the **trigeminal cave** (of Meckel), which passes forwards with them to lie in the trigeminal impression beneath the dural floor of the middle cranial fossa, the sensory root now enlarged to form the ganglion, with the motor root still below it. The evaginated inner layer of dura and the arachnoid fuse with the pia mater at the middle of the trigeminal ganglion, so the sensory and motor roots of the nerve and the posterior half of the ganglion are bathed in cerebrospinal fluid (Fig. 6.104).

Blood supply. The accessory meningeal artery enters through the foramen ovale and runs up along the mandibular division to reach the ganglion, a similar arrangement to that in the spinal nerves. Small ganglionic branches are also given off by the internal carotid artery in the cavernous sinus.

The *surgical approach* to the sensory root and posterior half of the ganglion, in Meckel's cave, traverses the subarachnoid space. The anterior half of the ganglion and the three divisions of the trigeminal nerve lie in front of Meckel's cave. The upper part of the anterior half of the ganglion, with the ophthalmic and maxillary divisions, lies in the fibrous lateral wall of the cavernous sinus; the lower part of the ganglion and the mandibular division lie in the middle fossa between the otherwise fused two layers of dura mater. An extradural approach is therefore possible across the floor of the middle fossa by stripping the dura from the bone, avoiding entry into the subarachnoid space.

Transient facial palsy sometimes follows the latter approach. The explanation is thought to be that in stripping up the dura from the floor of the middle fossa tension is exerted on the greater petrosal nerve (which lies below the trigeminal ganglion; see below) and therefore on the geniculate ganglion. Subsequent oedema here causes pressure on the motor fibres of the facial nerve with paralysis of the muscles until the oedema subsides and the nerve recovers.

The **mandibular division** of the trigeminal nerve passes laterally to descend through the foramen ovale (Fig. 6.101). It is joined just below the foramen ovale by the small *motor root* to form the (mixed) mandibular nerve, a similar arrangement to that of the spinal nerves in the intervertebral foramina.

The **maxillary nerve** passes forwards within the inner layer of dura to leave the skull through the foramen rotundum (Fig. 6.102). The branches of the **ophthalmic nerve** pass forwards likewise, to leave the skull through the medial end of the superior orbital fissure.

The **greater petrosal nerve** (from the nervus intermedius part of the facial, see p. 518) emerges from its hiatus in the petrous bone (see Fig. 8.4, p. 529) and runs obliquely forwards, between the two layers of the dura mater and beneath the trigeminal ganglion to the foramen lacerum. Here it is joined by the **deep petrosal nerve**, a branch from the carotid plexus of sympathetic nerves. The two join to form the **nerve of the pterygoid canal** (Vidian nerve). This nerve enters the posterior end of the pterygoid canal at the front of the foramen lacerum and runs along the canal to join the pterygopalatine ganglion (see p. 384).

The **lesser petrosal nerve** (from the glossopharyngeal) leaves its hiatus in the petrous bone (see Fig. 8.4, p. 529) and runs forwards between the two layers of the dura mater to emerge through the foramen ovale to join the otic ganglion (see p. 379).

The middle meningeal artery is considered on page 459.

Posterior cranial fossa

The posterior cranial fossa lies behind the clivus (see p. 532) and in front of the squamous part of the occipital bone which extends laterally to where the fossa is bounded anterolaterally by the petrous and mastoid parts of the temporal bone. It lodges the convexities of the cerebellar hemispheres as well as the pons and medulla oblongata. In it the fifth to twelfth cranial nerves inclusive pierce the dura mater (Fig. 6.109).

The **trigeminal nerve** leaves the middle of the anterolateral surface of the pons by two roots, a *large sensory* and a *small motor* (see Fig. 7.18, p. 494). They lie close together. The motor root emerges somewhat above and medial to the sensory root, but spirals to enter the mouth of Meckel's cave below it. The sensory root itself shows a spiral arrangement of its fibres. At the junction with the pons the mandibular fibres lie superior, the ophthalmic inferior with the maxillary fibres between, but in Meckel's cave the mandibular fibres lie most laterally and the ophthalmic fibres most medially.

The **abducens nerve** leaves the brainstem near the ventral midline at the junction of the pons and the pyramid of the medulla (see Fig. 7.18, p. 494) and runs upwards through the pontine cistern. It enters the dura mater of the clivus some distance above its origin from the brainstem, and runs thence upwards between the two layers of the dura, passing over the apex of the petrous bone, to enter the posterior end of the cavernous sinus. The relatively long intracranial course of this delicate nerve renders it particularly vulnerable to increase of intracranial pressure; paralysis of the lateral rectus may be an early sign in such cases.

The **facial** and **vestibulocochlear nerves**, with the intervening **nervus intermedius** part of the facial nerve, leave the lateral end of the junction of pons and medulla (see Fig. 7.6, p. 479) and pass upwards to enter the internal acoustic meatus, accompanied by the labyrinthine artery. This vessel is a branch of the basilar artery, or arises from the anterior inferior cerebellar artery.

The **internal acoustic meatus** is a foramen directed laterally in the posterior surface of the obliquely set petrous bone. Its fundus consists of a plate of bone divided by a horizontal crest into an upper and lower semicircle (Fig. 6.108). The facial nerve and its nervus intermedius part pierce the front of the upper part, the cochlear nerve the front of the lower part (by many branches in spiral arrangement). The vestibular nerve pierces the plate posteriorly, by upper and lower divisions that lie behind the facial nerve foramen (separated by a vertical bar of bone) and the spiral cochlear foramina respectively. Each division of the vestibular nerve is connected to the vestibular ganglion deep in the meatus. Behind the vestibular area is a single foramen (the foramen singulare) for the passage of the branch of the inferior division to the posterior semicircular duct. The labyrinthine artery divides in the meatus and its branches accompany the nerves through the bony plate.

The **subarcuate fossa** lies lateral to the internal acoustic meatus (Fig. 6.105). It is a very shallow fossa against which the flocculus of the cerebellum lies.

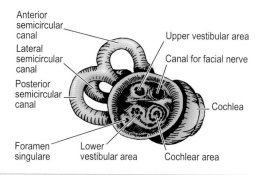

Anterior semicircular canal
Lateral semicircular canal
Posterior semicircular canal
Upper vestibular area
Canal for facial nerve
Cochlea
Foramen singulare
Lower vestibular area
Cochlear area

Fig. 6.108   Left internal acoustic meatus with the osseous labyrinth.

Further laterally on the posterior surface of the petrous bone is the orifice of the **aqueduct of the vestibule**, a narrow slit overhung by a sharp scale of bone (Fig. 6.105). The endolymphatic sac (see p. 437) hangs down from this slit beneath the inner layer of the dura.

The **glossopharyngeal, vagus** and **accessory nerves** arise from the side of the medulla oblongata as a series of rootlets lying vertically between the olive and the inferior cerebellar peduncle (see Fig. 7.6, p. 479). The three nerves run laterally across the occipital bone and pass through the jugular foramen (Fig. 6.109).

The **spinal root of the accessory nerve** enters the posterior fossa through the foramen magnum (Fig. 6.109). It arises by a series of rootlets that emerge from the lateral surface of the upper five or six segments of the cervical cord posterior to the denticulate ligament. These rootlets unite into a single trunk that passes forwards over the top of the ligament and ascends lateral to the vertebral artery to unite with the cranial root medial to the jugular foramen.

The **jugular foramen** is divided by two transverse septa of the inner layer of dura into three compartments. These septa may ossify. The glossopharyngeal nerve and inferior petrosal sinus share the anterior compartment, vagus and accessory nerves lie in the middle compartment, while the large posterior compartment is occupied by the termination of the sigmoid sinus. The inferior border of the petrous bone shows a deep notch immediately below the internal acoustic meatus (Fig. 6.105). This notch is indented by the inferior ganglion of the glossopharyngeal nerve; the aqueduct of the cochlea (see p. 436) opens into the depths of the notch and by this means perilymph drains into the subarachnoid space. The groove made by the inferior petrosal sinus is seen to enter the jugular foramen medial to the notch.

The **hypoglossal nerve** leaves the medulla by a vertical series of rootlets between the pyramid and the olive (see Fig. 7.18, p. 494). The rootlets unite into two roots

Fig. 6.109 Posterior cranial fossa and the vertebral canal opened from behind.

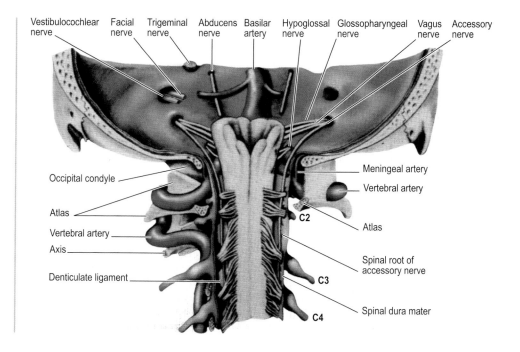

Vestibulocochlear nerve
Facial nerve
Trigeminal nerve
Abducens nerve
Basilar artery
Hypoglossal nerve
Glossopharyngeal nerve
Vagus nerve
Accessory nerve
Occipital condyle
Atlas
Vertebral artery
Axis
Denticulate ligament
Meningeal artery
Vertebral artery
C2
Atlas
Spinal root of accessory nerve
C3
Spinal dura mater
C4

which enter the hypoglossal canal separately, divided from each other by a septum of dura mater which occasionally ossifies.

The **arteries** in the posterior fossa comprise the two vertebral and the basilar arteries with their branches. After piercing the posterior atlanto-occipital membrane the vertebral arteries give off meningeal branches which enter the posterior fossa between the two layers of the dura mater at the foramen magnum (Fig. 6.109).

The **vertebral artery** then pierces the spinal dura mater and arachnoid and gives off the small *posterior spinal artery* (which may arise instead from the posterior inferior cerebellar branch). This fourth part of the vertebral artery runs forward in front of the highest denticulate ligament, in front of or between the rootlets of the hypoglossal nerve. It gives off the *anterior spinal artery* and the *posterior inferior cerebellar artery* and spirals up to meet its opposite fellow at the lower border of the pons to form the *basilar artery*. The posterior and anterior spinal arteries pass downwards through the foramen magnum on the spinal cord (see p. 511). The posterior inferior cerebellar artery is perhaps the most tortuous artery in the body. Its coils insinuate themselves between the rootlets of the hypoglossal, accessory and vagus nerves and the vessel is distributed to the cerebellum and medulla (see pp 500 and 506).

The **basilar artery** runs up in front of the pons. It is not responsible for the ventral median groove in the pons; indeed, the artery is usually curved to one side of the midline (see Fig. 7.19, p. 495). It gives off the *anterior inferior cerebellar artery* and many *pontine branches*. The *labyrinthine artery* arises from the anterior inferior cerebellar or directly from the basilar trunk. The basilar artery ends at the upper border of the pons by dividing into the **posterior cerebral arteries** (see p. 491), immediately after giving off the *superior cerebellar branches*.

PART **TWENTY-TWO**

Vertebral canal

The vertebral canal (spinal canal) is a smooth-walled tubular space formed by the whole series of vertebral foramina lying one above the other (see p. 438). Its anterior boundaries are the bodies of the vertebrae, intervertebral discs and the posterior longitudinal ligament. Posteriorly are the vertebral laminae and ligamenta flava, while at the sides are the pedicles of the vertebrae and the large intervening spaces, the intervertebral foramina. The canal contains the spinal meninges and the spinal

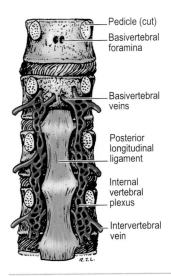

Fig. 6.110 Anterior aspect of vertebral canal exposed by removal of neural arches to show the internal vertebral venous plexus. The posterior longitudinal ligament is usually narrower behind the vertebral bodies than seen here.

cord with its nerve roots. Its lower end becomes continuous with the sacral canal (see p. 454).

The bony walls of the canal are separated from the contained meninges by the **epidural space** (*extradural space*) which contains loose connective tissue, fat and veins. The adipose tissue is mainly in the posterior part of the epidural space and extends laterally into the intervertebral foramina with the nerve roots and their dural sheaths. The veins form the **internal vertebral venous plexus** (Fig. 6.110). The plexus receives its tributaries mostly from the large **basivertebral veins** draining the active red marrow in the bodies of the vertebrae (see p. 445). The plexus lies mainly in the anterior part of the epidural space and comprises a collection of longitudinally aligned veins with numerous transverse connections. The internal vertebral plexus sends its efferent veins (the *intervertebral veins*) through the intervertebral foramina and between adjacent ligamenta flava to drain into the *external vertebral venous plexus* and thence into the segmental veins. The internal vertebral plexus provides a venous bypass of the diaphragm. It functions when the inferior vena cava cannot cope with a sudden flush of blood resulting from a sudden increase of intra-abdominal pressure (e.g. in coughing or abdominal straining). Thus pelvic and abdominal venous blood is momentarily squirted up the plexus above the diaphragm, into posterior intercostal veins, and thereby into the superior vena cava.

Spinal meninges

The **spinal dura mater**, or *theca*, is a prolongation of the inner layer of the dura mater of the posterior cranial fossa. It extends downwards through the foramen magnum to the level of S2 vertebra. It is attached rather firmly to the margin of the foramen magnum, to the tectorial membrane and to the posterior longitudinal ligament on the body of the axis vertebra. Elsewhere it lies free in the spinal canal, apart from five fibrous bands to the posterior longitudinal ligament in places, especially towards the caudal end of the canal. The spinal dura is pierced segmentally by the anterior and posterior roots of the spinal nerves and is prolonged over these roots as sleeve-like projections which enter the intervertebral foramina and fuse with the epineurium of the mixed spinal nerves.

The **spinal arachnoid mater** lines the inner surface of the spinal dura, with only a potential space between these two membranes. Below the level of the spinal cord (i.e. over the cauda equina) the arachnoid is nothing but a delicate membrane that is supported by the dura mater, but over the spinal cord itself the arachnoid sends many delicate processes across the subarachnoid space to the pia mater on the cord, forming a lace-like arrangement.

The **spinal pia mater**, as in the cranium, invests the surface of the central nervous system. It clothes the spinal cord and lines the anterior median sulcus. It is prolonged over the spinal nerve roots until where the dura blends with the epineurium of the mixed spinal nerves. It is projected below the apex of the conus medullaris, whence it extends as the **filum terminale** to perforate the spinal theca at the level of S2 vertebra. It then descends to the back of the coccyx (Fig. 6.98). The filum terminale lies centrally in the cauda equina, but is not part of the cauda which consists of nerve roots only. A lateral projection of pia mater on each side forms the **denticulate ligament**. This flange crosses the subarachnoid space between the anterior and posterior nerve roots and, piercing the arachnoid, connects the side of the spinal cord to the dura mater. It is attached in an unbroken line along the spinal cord from the foramen magnum to the conus medullaris, but its lateral edge has a series of teeth-like projections, which are attached to the dura between successive nerve roots (Fig. 6.111). There are usually 21 such dentate ligaments on each side. The highest is attached to the dura just above the foramen magnum, behind the vertebral artery and in front of the spinal root of the accessory nerve. The lowest dentate ligament lies between the twelfth thoracic and first lumbar nerve roots.

The **spinal subarachnoid space** is relatively large, accommodating about half of the total volume of

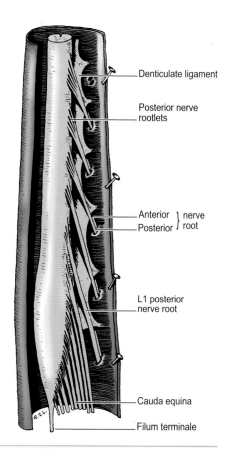

Fig. 6.111 Lower end of the spinal cord exposed by opening the dura and arachnoid mater from behind. On the left the nerve roots and denticulate ligament have been removed. The nerve roots on the right are shown devoid of their pial covering.

cerebrospinal fluid (75 mL out of 150 mL). It communicates through the foramen magnum with the subarachnoid space of the posterior cranial fossa. Some cerebrospinal fluid percolates away along the meningeal sheaths of the spinal nerves.

Below the level of the conus medullaris the space contains only the cauda equina and filum terminale, in addition to cerebrospinal fluid, and it ends at the level of S2 vertebra.

Lumbar puncture and spinal and epidural anaesthesia

In **lumbar puncture** the needle is generally inserted between the spines of L3 and L4 or L4 and L5 vertebrae when the patient's back is flexed, usually when curled up lying on one side. The needle passes through the supraspinous and interspinous ligaments and through or between ligamenta flava before penetrating the dura. Since the spinal cord ends at the level of L1 vertebra, it is in no danger.

In **spinal anaesthesia**, the anaesthetic solution is injected into the subarachnoid space (with the needle in a similar position to that used for lumbar puncture), so mixing with the cerebrospinal fluid surrounding the nerve roots and percolating into them.

In **epidural anaesthesia** the solution is injected at the clinically indicated level into the epidural (extradural) space without penetrating the dura, and the solution infiltrates through the meningeal sheaths containing the nerve roots. The approach is similar to that for lumbar puncture, but in the thoracic region a paramedian route, through the muscles of the back, may have to be used on account of the overlap of long thoracic spinous processes. An alternative less-used approach is through the sacral hiatus into the sacral canal. Through any of these routes a catheter may be inserted for the continuous infusion of an analgesic solution.

Central nervous system 7

General plan

The **central nervous system** consists of the **brain** and **spinal cord** (spinal medulla). The central nervous system is hollow; it develops from a neural tube whose cavity persists. Developmentally the brain consists of the forebrain, midbrain and hindbrain. The *forebrain* is composed of the cerebrum (the two cerebral hemispheres, each with a cavity, the lateral ventricle), and a deeper central portion, the diencephalon, whose main parts are the thalamus and hypothalamus and whose cavity is the third ventricle. The *midbrain* is a small region whose cavity is the aqueduct and which connects the forebrain with the *hindbrain*, consisting of the pons, medulla oblongata and cerebellum and whose cavity is the fourth ventricle. The midbrain, pons and medulla collectively form the brainstem. All parts of the brain are contained within the cranial cavity; the medulla passes through the foramen magnum of the skull and changes its name to spinal cord where the first cervical nerve roots emerge; the spinal cord has a central canal. Cerebrospinal fluid (CSF) is produced by the choroid plexuses within the ventricles, which it fills; it exits through the midline and lateral apertures of the fourth ventricle to cover the surface of the brain and spinal cord.

PART ONE

Forebrain

Cerebral hemispheres

The cerebral hemispheres occupy the greater part of the cranial cavity—above the floors of the anterior and middle cranial fossae, and above the tentorium cerebelli. One hemisphere, usually the left in right-handed people, is slightly larger than the other and constitutes the *dominant hemisphere*. The medial surface of each hemisphere is flat and lies against the falx cerebri; below the falx the two hemispheres are joined by the corpus callosum. The undersurface of the hemisphere is more irregular than the medial surface; the orbital surface of the frontal lobe is slightly concave from the impression of the anterior cranial fossa, the temporal pole is boldly convex in conformity with the middle cranial fossa while the undersurface of the occipital lobe slopes downwards and outwards to conform with the shape of the tentorium. The superolateral surface of the hemispheres is boldly convex in conformity with the shape of the skull.

All surfaces of the cerebral hemisphere are covered with a **cortex** of grey matter (the cells of the cerebral cortex), and internally there are further groups of cells that form such structures as the basal nuclei and thalamus. The cortex is thrown into a complicated series of tortuous folds, the *gyri*; the grooves between them are the *sulci* (Fig. 7.1). All the gyri and sulci are named but only the most important are described here. Although the configurations of no two brains are identical, there is always an underlying similarity and this general pattern is common to all.

Some of the larger sulci are used to divide the surface of the hemisphere into **lobes** which are named according to the cranial bones that lie adjacent when the brain is in situ: frontal, temporal, parietal and occipital lobes. The **frontal lobe** lies in front of the central sulcus and above the lateral sulcus; the **parietal lobe** is behind the central sulcus and above the lateral sulcus; the **temporal lobe** is below the lateral sulcus; and the **occipital lobe** lies below and behind the parieto-occipital sulcus.

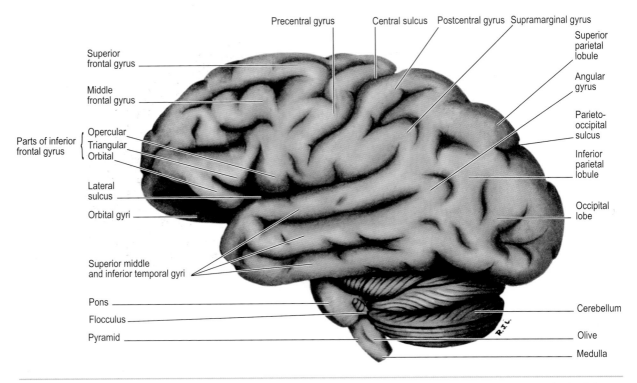

Fig. 7.1   Left side of the brain, with the gyri somewhat simplified. The curved lunate sulcus (unlabelled) is seen in front of the occipital pole.

Superolateral surface

A deep fissure that separates the frontal and temporal lobes on the undersurface of the brain is continued to the superolateral surface and passes backwards, above the temporal lobe. This is the **lateral sulcus** (fissure of Sylvius) (Fig. 7.1), although strictly speaking the part on the lateral surface is the *posterior ramus* of the lateral sulcus, for, at the front end of this part, there are short *anterior* and *ascending rami* that branch off from it to penetrate the inferior frontal gyrus. The areas of cortex bounding the short sulci are the orbital, triangular and opercular parts of the inferior frontal gyrus. The parts of the frontal, parietal and temporal lobes that bound the lateral sulcus form the *opercula*, which overlie a buried part of the cortex, the *insula* (Fig. 7.2), composed of various *long* and *short gyri* almost completely surrounded by the *circular sulcus*.

From just behind the midpoint of the superior border of the hemisphere, an oblique sulcus runs downwards and forwards to end a little above the lateral sulcus; it is the only long sulcus to pass over on to the medial surface of the hemisphere. This is the **central sulcus** (fissure

of Rolando) and it separates frontal and parietal lobes (Fig. 7.1). The **precentral** and **postcentral gyri** lie in front of and behind it; they contain the primary motor and sensory cortical areas.

In front of the precentral gyrus the frontal lobe is divided by two horizontal sulci into three gyri, the superior, middle and inferior *frontal gyri*. A similar arrangement divides the temporal lobe below the lateral sulcus into superior, middle and inferior *temporal gyri*. The parietal lobe is divided by a transverse sulcus into superior and inferior parietal lobules. Into the latter project the lateral sulcus and the superior temporal sulcus; the posterior ends of these sulci are closed by the curved *supramarginal* and *angular gyri* respectively.

An imaginary line divides the occipital lobe from the parietal and temporal lobes. It extends from the small part of the parieto-occipital sulcus visible on this lateral surface, downwards in a 45° slope to the inferior border where there is often a slight *preoccipital notch* (Fig. 7.2) indented in the border by a fold of dura mater over the transverse sinus. A further arbitrary line, carried backwards from the main direction of the lateral sulcus

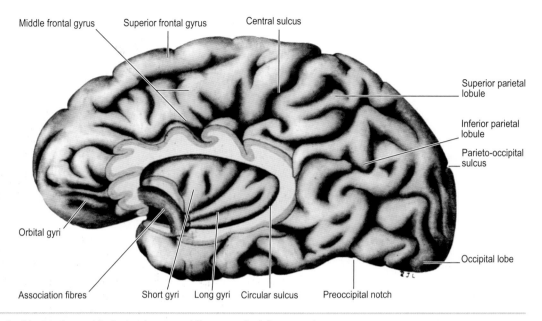

Fig. 7.2 Left cerebral hemisphere with the insula exposed by removal of the opercula.

until it meets the occipital demarcation line, indicates where the parietal and temporal lobes join.

Medial surface

The two medial surfaces are flat and lie close together; they can be inspected only when their midline connections are divided by sagittal section (Fig. 7.3). Such a section severs the corpus callosum and the roof and floor of the third ventricle, as well as the brainstem and cerebellum. The medial surface of the hemisphere above the corpus callosum forms the *cingulate gyrus*, above which is the *cingulate sulcus*. The *medial frontal gyrus* lies above the anterior part of the sulcus and extends to the superior border of the hemisphere where it is continuous with the superior frontal gyrus. Just behind the midpoint of the superior border the central sulcus turns on to the medial surface; it is enclosed in the paracentral lobule.

At the posterior part of the hemisphere, the oblique *parieto-occipital sulcus* separates the parietal from the occipital lobe and extends over the superior border. The medial surface of the occipital lobe is wedge-shaped and is named the *cuneus*. Between the parieto-occipital sulcus and the paracentral lobule is the *precuneus*.

The cuneus is limited inferiorly by the **calcarine sulcus** which runs forward from the occipital pole to the medial surface of the temporal lobe. The visual area of the cortex occupies the lips of the sulcus (see p. 482).

The parieto-occipital sulcus runs into it and the parieto-occipital and calcarine sulci form a pattern like the letter Y on its side; the common stem of the Y is the anterior part of the calcarine sulcus, and the two limbs are the parieto-occipital sulcus and the posterior part of the calcarine sulcus. The *lingual gyrus* lies below the posterior part of the calcarine sulcus and is limited at the border between the medial and inferior surfaces of the occipital lobe by the collateral sulcus.

Inferior surface

This shows the orbital surfaces of the frontal lobes and the sloping inferior surface of the temporo-occipital part of the brain (Fig. 7.4).

The orbital surface of the frontal lobe has the straight *gyrus rectus* along its medial margin. The olfactory bulb and the olfactory tract lie on the olfactory sulcus alongside the gyrus rectus. Lateral to the olfactory bulb and tract this surface is gently concave and is divided into a series of orbital gyri and sulci which leave prominent impressions on the orbital part of the frontal bone.

The temporal pole is boldly convex; the temporal lobe merges posteriorly with the occipital lobe and the continuous surface so formed is oblique in conformity with the slope of the tentorium cerebelli, against which it lies. Hence much of the medial surface of the temporal lobe can be seen from the inferior view. It is characterized

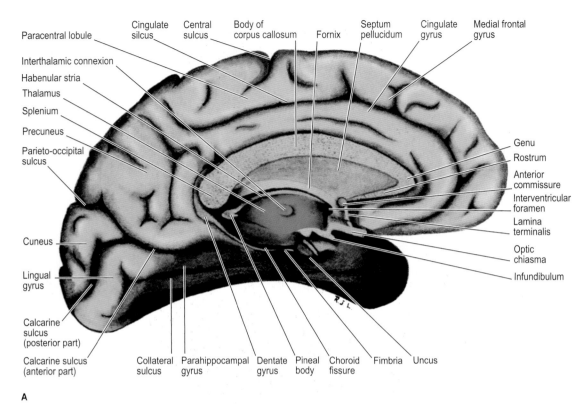

Paracentral lobule

Interthalamic connexion

Habenular stria

Thalamus

Splenium

Precuneus

Parieto-occipital sulcus

Cuneus

Lingual gyrus

Calcarine sulcus (posterior part)

Calcarine sulcus (anterior part)

Cingulate silcus

Central sulcus

Body of corpus callosum

Fornix

Septum pellucidum

Cingulate gyrus

Medial frontal gyrus

Genu

Rostrum

Anterior commissure

Interventricular foramen

Lamina terminalis

Optic chiasma

Infundibulum

Collateral sulcus

Parahippocampal gyrus

Dentate gyrus

Pineal body

Choroid fissure

Fimbria

Uncus

A

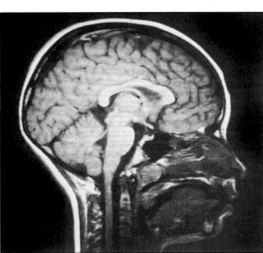

B

Fig. 7.3 Brain and brainstem in sagittal section: **A** the medial surface of the left cerebral hemisphere, with the cerebellum and brainstem removed to expose the choroid fissure and the undersurface of the hemisphere; **B** magnetic resonance image of the head. Compare with **A** and note the corpus callosum, fornix, thalamus and interventricular foramen. The triangular fourth ventricle is seen between the cerebellum and the pons and medulla. The midbrain, with the superior and inferior colliculi on its posterior surface, is also seen.

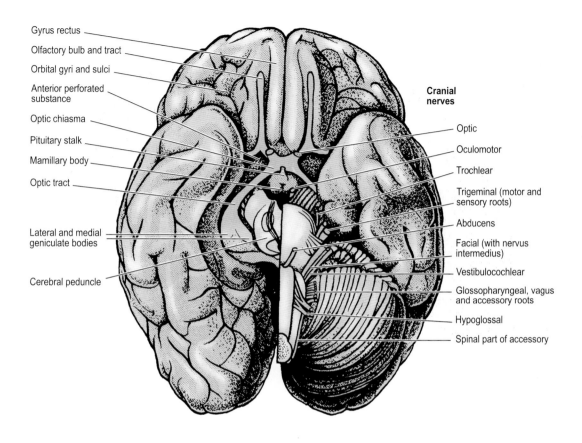

Gyrus rectus
Olfactory bulb and tract
Orbital gyri and sulci
Anterior perforated substance
Optic chiasma
Pituitary stalk
Mamillary body
Optic tract
Lateral and medial geniculate bodies
Cerebral peduncle

Cranial nerves

Optic
Oculomotor
Trochlear
Trigeminal (motor and sensory roots)
Abducens
Facial (with nervus intermedius)
Vestibulocochlear
Glossopharyngeal, vagus and accessory roots
Hypoglossal
Spinal part of accessory

Fig. 7.4 Inferior surface of the brain. All the cranial nerves are intact on the left side. The right half of the brainstem and cerebellum have been removed, together with part of the temporal lobe.

by two long parallel sulci, the *occipitotemporal sulcus* laterally and the *collateral sulcus* medially (Fig. 7.3A). They run anteroposteriorly between the temporal and occipital poles. Medial to the collateral sulcus is the *parahippocampal gyrus*, confined to the temporal lobe and recurved at its anterior end to form the *uncus* (Fig. 7.3A); at the back it may appear to become continuous with the front of the lingual gyrus.

Internal structure

The interior of the forebrain is characterized by the presence within the white matter of large masses of **grey matter** and also by cavities which contain the CSF. The largest such mass of cells is the thalamus; it belongs to the diencephalon and is described on page 489.

Other cell groups lie lateral to the thalamus within the cerebral hemisphere and some of them constitute the **basal nuclei** (also called *basal ganglia*). They are usually classified anatomically as consisting of the caudate nucleus, lentiform nucleus (which has an outer part, the putamen, and an inner part, the globus pallidus), amygdaloid body and claustrum. The caudate nucleus and the lentiform nucleus are separated by the internal capsule (see below). The caudate nucleus and the putamen part of the lentiform nucleus are joined by many inter-connecting fibres, which pass through the anterior part of the internal capsule, giving the area a striated appearance. The caudate nucleus and lentiform nucleus together with the intervening internal capsule are hence referred to as the **corpus striatum.**

The **caudate nucleus** has the shape of a highly curved comma (Figs 7.5 and 7.6) with a head, body and tail. The bulbous *head* tapers back to the *body* which, curving back round the lateral part of the thalamus, bends sharply forwards into the long thin *tail* that joins the

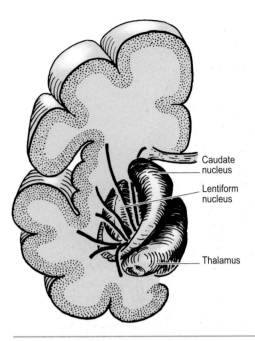

Caudate
nucleus

Lentiform
nucleus

Thalamus

Fig. 7.5 Left thalamus and basal nuclei, viewed from above and behind. The heavy lines indicate the disposition of fibres of the internal capsule and corona radiata.

amygdaloid body. The caudate nucleus is curled snugly round the internal capsule like a hand holding a bunch of flowers. The whole length of its convexity projects into the lateral ventricle.

The **lentiform nucleus** is the shape of a biconvex lens, completely buried in the hemisphere (Figs 7.6 and 7.7). It is oval in outline and has two parts: the large lateral *putamen* and the small medial *globus pallidus* (or pallidum).

The **amygdaloid body** (or amygdala) consists of several groups of neurons and is connected with the tip of the tail of the caudate nucleus in the roof of the inferior horn of the lateral ventricle. The amygdala is functionally part of the limbic system (see p. 484). It has connections with the frontal and temporal lobes, including the olfactory cortex. An efferent bundle of axons, the *stria terminalis*, runs posteriorly following the curvature of the tail of the caudate nucleus, in the roof of the inferior horn and the floor of the body of the lateral ventricle, to the septal area and anterior hypothalamus.

The **claustrum** is a thin lamina, circular in outline and curved into a saucer-shape. It lies lateral to the putamen, and although easy to identify in horizontal or coronal sections (Fig. 7.7) its significance is unknown.

Functionally the basal nuclei exert a supraspinal control over skeletal muscle movements by influencing their rate, range and coordination. The corpus striatum receives fibres mainly from the cerebral cortex, thalamus and substantia nigra. The globus pallidus is the main efferent pathway from the corpus striatum and sends fibres to the thalamus, subthalamic nucleus, substantia nigra and the reticular formation. Different pathways involve different transmitters which include acetylcholine, dopamine, glutamate, serotonin and γ-aminobutyric acid (GABA). The most common disease of the basal nuclei is parkinsonism, characterized by tremor, rigidity and abnormal slowness of movements (bradykinesia); there is a decrease of dopamine in the nigrostriatal pathway.

The **white matter** of the cerebral hemisphere is made up of fibres belonging to three main groups.

Commissural fibres join the cortices of the two hemispheres. Most of them are gathered together in the *corpus callosum*; a few lie in the *anterior and posterior commissures*. They radiate widely and symmetrically through the white matter of the hemispheres.

Association (arcuate) fibres are confined to their own hemisphere, in which they connect different parts of the cortex.

Projection fibres are those which join the grey matter of the hemisphere with subcortical nuclei in the hemispheres and with nuclei in the brainstem and spinal cord. In the base of the hemisphere a major collection of projection fibres lies lateral to the thalamus and the head of the caudate nucleus, forming the internal capsule. The lentiform nucleus lies lateral to the internal capsule. The tail of the caudate nucleus curls around the capsule and runs down to lie lateral to it (Fig. 7.5). From the internal capsule the fibres radiate upwards and outwards in the shape of a curved fan to reach the cortex and similarly pass from the cortex down to the capsule; this fan-shaped arrangement is the *corona radiata*. Fibres of the corpus callosum intersect it.

Internal capsule

The internal capsule consists of afferent fibres passing up to the cortex from cell bodies in the thalamus, and of efferent fibres passing down from cell bodies in the cortex to the cerebral peduncle of the midbrain. It lies within the concavity of the C-shaped caudate nucleus, which separates it from the C-shaped concavity of the lateral ventricle (Figs 7.5 and 7.7).

The internal capsule is seen in a typical horizontal section through the hemisphere (e.g. at a level through the interventricular foramen and the pineal gland) as a band of white matter that is not a straight line but bent into a lateral concavity by the convex medial border

Fig. 7.6 Left basal nuclei and the brainstem from the left. The left half of the cerebellum has been removed by transecting the left cerebellar peduncles.

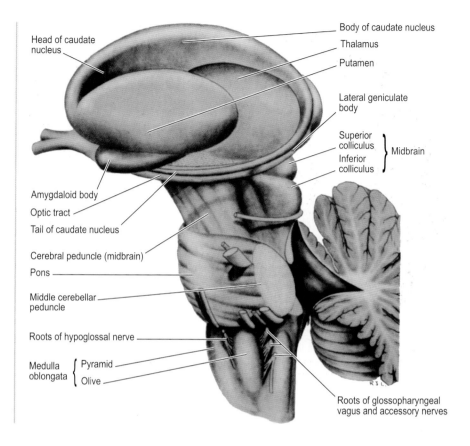

Head of caudate nucleus

Amygdaloid body

Optic tract

Tail of caudate nucleus

Cerebral peduncle (midbrain)

Pons

Middle cerebellar peduncle

Roots of hypoglossal nerve

Medulla oblongata { Pyramid
Olive

Body of caudate nucleus

Thalamus

Putamen

Lateral geniculate body

Superior colliculus } Midbrain
Inferior colliculus

Roots of glossopharyngeal vagus and accessory nerves

of the lentiform nucleus (i.e. by the globus pallidus). The internal capsule is thus described as having an anterior limb, genu and posterior limb, and there are also two other portions posteriorly: the sublentiform and retrolentiform parts.

The **anterior limb** lies between the head of the caudate nucleus medially and the lentiform nucleus laterally. It contains frontopontine fibres from cell bodies in the frontal cortex. They pass down below the thalamus into the cerebral peduncle, where they occupy the medial part of the base of the peduncle. They arborize round the pontine nuclei. The anterior limb also probably contains fibres running from the frontal eye field to the oculomotor nucleus, concerned with the accommodation–convergence reflex (see p. 423).

The **genu** is the region of the bend in the capsule (as seen in horizontal section), at the apex of the globus pallidus. Its principal constituents are the *corticonuclear fibres* which pass from the cerebral cortex to the motor nuclei of cranial nerves in the brainstem (see p. 501).

The **posterior limb** lies between the thalamus medially and the lentiform nucleus laterally. Occupying the

anterior two-thirds of the posterior limb are the *corticospinal fibres*. From cell bodies in the cortex the fibres pass down through this part of the capsule, then through the brainstem to the lower medulla (Fig. 7.8) where most of them decussate to form the lateral corticospinal *tract* and eventually arborize with the anterior horn cells that innervate skeletal muscle. Thus passing through small parts of the internal capsules—genu and anterior two-thirds of the posterior limbs—are the motor fibres that control all the skeletal muscle in the body. The head (corticonuclear) fibres lie most anteriorly and immediately behind them are corticospinal fibres for the arm, hand, trunk, leg and perineum in that order from front to back. (In the cerebral peduncle of the midbrain the head fibres lie medially and the fibres for the perineum laterally, in the same order.) It is in this part of the internal capsule that haemorrhage or thrombosis of a striate artery commonly occurs. The muscles of the opposite side of the body are thus paralysed; they become spastic with increased stretch reflexes, the signs of an upper motor neuron lesion (see p. 511). Fibres from the speech (Broca's) area are interrupted in lesions of the

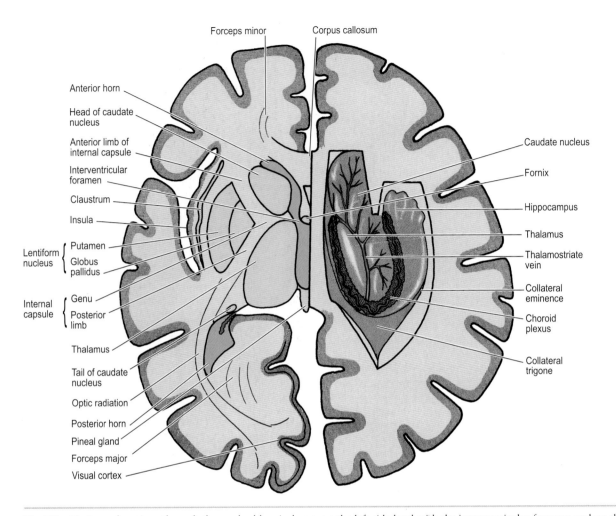

Fig. 7.7 Horizontal sections through the cerebral hemispheres, on the left side level with the interventricular foramen and on the right at a slightly higher level with dissection to open up the lateral ventricle.

left internal capsule; thus loss of speech accompanies hemiplegia of the right side of the body.

Beside and behind the corticospinal fibres in the posterior limb of the capsule there are *thalamocortical fibres* passing from cell bodies in the thalamus to the cerebral cortex. These include sensory fibres mediating impulses derived from the opposite side of the body which run upwards through the corona radiata to the sensory cortex. There are also some frontopontine fibres.

In the **retrolentiform part** of the capsule, at the posterior end of the lentiform nucleus, are parieto-, occipito- and temporopontine (corticopontine) fibres which will occupy the lateral part of the base of the cerebral peduncle. This part of the capsule also contains visual fibres passing from cell bodies in the lateral geniculate body to the visual area of the cortex as the *optic radiation* (Fig. 7.7). A further group of fibres runs from the medial geniculate body below the posterior end of the lentiform nucleus, so forming the **sublentiform part** of the capsule. These are the fibres of the *auditory radiation* which reach the auditory area of the cortex in the superior temporal gyrus (see p. 482).

Corpus callosum

The corpus callosum (Fig. 7.3) consists of a mass of 100 million commissural fibres, each of which extends from cortex to cortex between symmetrical parts of the

Fig. 7.8   Coronal section of the brain and brainstem. The section is not quite vertical but passes downwards and backwards to show the continuity of the corticospinal and corticonuclear fibres which run through the internal capsule to the brainstem.

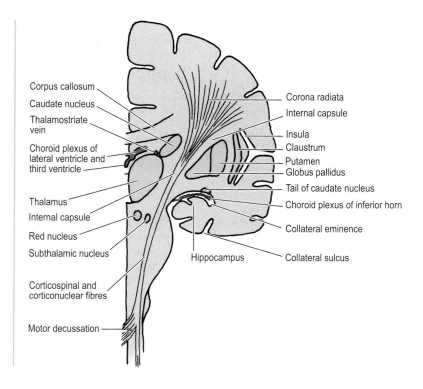

Corpus callosum
Caudate nucleus
Thalamostriate vein
Choroid plexus of lateral ventricle and third ventricle
Thalamus
Internal capsule
Red nucleus
Subthalamic nucleus
Corticospinal and corticonuclear fibres
Motor decussation

Corona radiata
Internal capsule
Insula
Claustrum
Putamen
Globus pallidus
Tail of caudate nucleus
Choroid plexus of inferior horn
Collateral eminence
Hippocampus
Collateral sulcus

two hemispheres. It commences at the anterior commissure, at the upper end of the lamina terminalis of the diencephalon and, traced from here to its termination, it becomes increasingly thicker. It is described as having four parts: the rostrum, genu, body and splenium. From the anterior commissure the mass passes upwards and forwards as the *rostrum*. It now takes a sharp bend backwards as the *genu*. From here it is gently convex upwards (the *body*) and it ends posteriorly as a thick rounded free border, the *splenium*. The corpus callosum can be seen by separating the two hemispheres, and its cut surface is exposed in a midline sagittal section through the brain (Fig. 7.12).

The fibres of the corpus callosum extend to all parts of the cerebral cortex. In a horizontal section the fibres of the genu are seen arching forwards on each side to the frontal cortex; this appearance gives them the name *forceps minor*. Similarly, the fibres of the massive splenium curve backwards symmetrically to the occipital cortex, forming the *forceps major* (Fig. 7.7).

Between forceps minor and forceps major the fibres of the corpus callosum spread out to the cortex on the lateral surface of the hemisphere. They pass over the anterior horn and body of the lateral ventricle, for each of which they form the roof. As they turn down into the

temporal lobe they form the lateral wall of the inferior and posterior horns of the lateral ventricle, where they are known as the *tapetum*.

Cortical areas

Certain areas of the cerebral cortex have long been identified with specific functions. Although these areas are still clinically relevant, modern investigations are modifying traditional concepts as far as the separation of motor and sensory functions is concerned. Many motor fibres, for example, have their origin outside the traditional motor cortex and some arise from what were previously regarded as purely sensory areas. A new terminology has emerged, and it is now customary to refer to a combined '*sensorimotor cortex*', subdividing it into four areas designated by the letters Ms and Sm (the capital M or S indicating whether the association is predominantly with motor or sensory functions). Thus the area MsI (first or primary motosensory area) includes the old 'motor and premotor' regions of the precentral and other gyri of the frontal lobe (corresponding to areas 4 and 6 as described by Brodmann in his now classical study of cortical histology). The area MsII (the supplementary motor area) is on part of the medial surface of the frontal lobe (part of areas 6 and 8). Similarly SmI (first sensorimotor area) includes most of the postcentral gyrus (areas 3, 1 and 2) and its extension on to the medial surface of the parietal lobe, and SmII is the lowest part of the postcentral gyrus (areas 40 and 43). These four main motor and sensory areas have many interconnections, both within their own and with the opposite hemisphere.

The **area MsI** is where movements of the various parts of the body are initiated, and it receives its main inputs from the cerebellum and thalamus. Some of the cortical cells send their axons down as the cortico-nuclear and corticospinal (pyramidal) tracts (see p. 501). **MsII** receives many fibres from thalamic nuclei which in turn have received fibres from the basal nuclei; its role in the control of movements is mainly with the mental processes that precede the effecting of a movement. In the precentral gyrus of MsI the body is represented upside down along this cortex, although the face itself is represented the right way up. The face lies lowest, then the hand (a very large area), then arm, trunk and leg. The leg overlaps the superior border and the foot and perineum extend down on the medial surface of the hemisphere into the paracentral lobule. In MsII the body is represented with the face anterior, the lower limbs posterior and the upper limbs in between.

The **motor (anterior) speech area** (of Broca, areas 44 and 45) is usually situated in the inferior frontal gyrus on the left side (in right-handed and in most left-handed people), below and in front of the face area and centred on the triangular part between the anterior and ascending rami of the lateral fissure. Damage to it produces motor aphasia: difficulty in finding the right words but not paralysis of laryngeal musculature.

The **posterior speech area** (of Wernicke) is in the posterior parts of the superior and middle temporal gyri and extends into the lower part of the parietal lobe. Its integrity is necessary for the understanding of speech.

The **frontal eye field**, involved in voluntary eye movements and the accommodation pathway (see p. 423), is in the centre of the middle frontal gyrus (parts of areas 6, 8 and 9).

The **areas SmI** and **SmII** receive a large thalamic input. SmI is for the appreciation of touch, kinaesthetic and vibration sense, and the parts of the body are represented in roughly the same way as in MsI and MsII. SmII appears to be associated with pain and temperature sensations. Although the conscious appreciation of pain may occur at the thalamic level, the cortex is necessary for its localization.

The **gustatory area** for the conscious appreciation of taste lies in the inferior part of the postcentral gyrus (frontoparietal operculum), near the tongue area of SmI.

The **auditory area** (areas 41 and 42) is mostly in the floor of the lateral sulcus, in the anterior transverse temporal gyrus. It extends into the superior temporal gyrus below the sulcus, and is here surrounded by the auditory association area (area 22). These regions receive fibres from the medial geniculate body via the auditory radiation. The cochleae are bilaterally represented, so a lesion of one cortex does not cause unilateral deafness.

The **olfactory area** is in the uncus at the front of the parahippocampal gyrus (Fig. 7.3A) and adjacent parts of the cortex.

The **visual area** (area 17) is mainly on the medial surface of the occipital lobe on the lips of the posterior part of the calcarine sulcus, and extends for a short distance on to the lateral surface of the occipital lobe as far as the lunate sulcus, a small curved sulcus in front of the occipital pole (Fig. 7.1). The true visual area is characterized by a white line (stria of Gennari) which bisects the grey matter of the cortex; in cortical sections it is easily seen with the naked eye, hence the name 'striate cortex' often given to this area. The cortex adjacent to the striate part on the medial and lateral surfaces of the hemisphere forms the visual association area (areas 18 and 19).

Each visual area receives from its own half of each retina, i.e. it registers the opposite visual field, on account of the curved configuration of the retina and the crossing of the medial fibres of the optic nerve at the optic chiasma. The temporal (lateral) half of the visual field of one eye conveys its impressions to the nasal (medial) half of the retina of that eye; similarly the temporal half of the retina receives its impressions from the nasal half of the visual field. In each cortex the upper half receives from the upper half of each half-retina, the lower half from the lower half of each half-retina; accordingly the representation of the upper and lower halves of the visual fields is reversed on the cortex. The macula registers at the posterior end of the visual area over a disproportionately large area, while more peripheral parts of the retina register progressively more anteriorly.

Cortical structure

The **cerebral cortex** is composed of layers of cells which vary in their characteristics in different regions. In most parts of the cortex six layers of nerve cells can be distinguished, and are conventionally numbered from the surface inwards by Roman numerals. Layer I has an abundance of fibres with relatively few cells, the plexiform layer. Then follow the external granular (II), external pyramidal (III), internal granular (IV), internal pyramidal (ganglionic) (V) and multiform (VI) layers, roughly named from the density and shapes of their cells. In layer IV there are often prominent strands of horizontal fibres, and in the visual cortex they form the stria of Gennari.

Changes in the relative distribution of these layers are most pronounced in the known sensory and motor areas. The postcentral gyrus (touch), the superior temporal gyrus (hearing), and the calcarine sulcus (sight) are covered by cortex in which granular cells predominate, while motor areas typically have larger numbers of pyramidal cells. Among the cells of layer V of the precentral gyrus are the giant pyramidal cells (of Betz), which resemble large anterior horn cells of the spinal cord; they give rise to no more than 2% of corticospinal fibres.

The **white matter** is composed of myelinated nerve fibres bound together by the fibres of the neuroglia. Myelin within the central nervous system is derived from the oligodendrocytes (in contrast to the peripheral nervous system where it comes from Schwann cells).

Visual pathways

The peripheral nerves of ordinary sensation, with their cell bodies in posterior root ganglia, are represented in the visual pathway by the *bipolar cells* of the retina (Fig. 7.9A). These cells receive impulses from the *retinal rods and cones*. The bipolar cells synapse with *ganglion cells* in the inner part of the retina (next to the vitreous body, 1 cell for each cone, 1 cell for 80 rods). These are homologous with the second neuron cell bodies in the central nervous system in the other sensory pathways. Their axons run on the inner surface of the retina and enter the optic disc and so pass to the optic nerve.

The **optic nerve** is not a nerve in the sense of other cranial and spinal nerves; it is an elongated tract of white matter stretched out from the brain and enclosed in the meninges thereof as far forward as its attachment to the sclera. Histologically it is identical with white matter of the central nervous system, and there is no effective regeneration when divided. In the orbit it is surrounded by a tube of dura mater and arachnoid, with CSF in the subarachnoid space. At the optic foramen the dura and arachnoid leave it and the nerve, still sheathed in pia mater, passes up to meet its fellow at the **optic chiasma**, which is attached to the anterior part of the floor of the third ventricle.

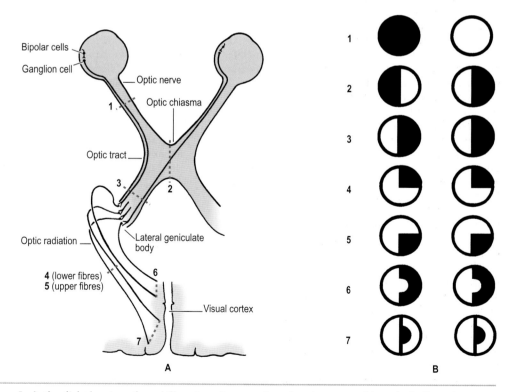

Fig. 7.9 Visual pathways. In **A**, the slight looping of nasal fibres into the contralateral optic nerve and into the ipsilateral optic tract, described on page 484, is not shown. In **B**, the numbers refer to the sites of lesions discussed on page 521.

In the chiasma the nasal fibres of each optic nerve decussate and pass into the optic tract of the opposite side; as they do so, some crossing fibres loop forwards slightly into the contralateral optic nerve before entering the optic tract, while some fibres loop backwards slightly into the ipsilateral optic tract before crossing the midline. The temporal fibres from each retina pass directly to the optic tract of their own side (Fig. 7.9A). Thus the right optic tract contains fibres from the right half of each retina, i.e. it carries impressions from the nasal field of the right eye and the temporal field of the left eye. Likewise, the left optic tract contains fibres which carry impressions from the right half of each visual field.

Cortical pathways for common sensation consist of three neurons. They reach the opposite hemisphere by a complete decussation of the second order neurons. The visual pathway by the half decussation of its second order neurons at the chiasma achieves the same object. One hemisphere registers common sensation from the opposite half of the body and also from the opposite half of the visible environment.

The **optic tract** passes from the chiasma around the cerebral peduncle, high up against the temporal lobe, and, reaching the side of the thalamus, divides into two branches. The larger of these enters the lateral geniculate body, in which the fibres synapse. These are visual fibres. The smaller branch (superior brachium) passes down medially, between the lateral and medial geniculate bodies, and synapses in the superior colliculus and the pretectal nuclei; these are fibres mediating light reflexes (see p. 423).

Blood supply. The optic tract is supplied chiefly by the anterior choroidal and posterior communicating arteries, the chiasma and intracranial part of the optic nerve by the anterior cerebral. In the orbit the nerve is supplied by the ophthalmic artery and, distally, by the central artery on its way to the retina.

The **lateral geniculate body**, which is a part of the thalamus, is a small rounded elevation on the posterior surface of the thalamus (Figs 7.4 and 7.20). It has six layers of neurons numbered 1–6 from the ventral to the dorsal surface. Crossed optic tract fibres end in layers 1, 4 and 6; uncrossed fibres end in layers 2, 3 and 5. The neurons of the geniculate body send their axons through the optic radiation to the occipital cortex (Fig. 7.9). The axons from the lateral part of the geniculate body, carrying impressions from the upper part of the opposite side of the visual fields, fan out laterally and inferiorly around the anterior tip of the inferior horn of the lateral ventricle (Meyer's loop) before swinging posteriorly to reach the inferior lip of the calcarine sulcus; axons from the medial part, carrying impressions from the corresponding inferior part of the visual fields, pass directly backwards to the superior lip of the calcarine sulcus.

The *superior brachium* is the small (medial) branch of the optic tract. It passes down to the tectum of the midbrain, (see p. 494), where its fibres synapse with cells in the superior colliculus. Tectobulbar and tectospinal tracts from the superior colliculus pass to motor nuclei in the brainstem and spinal cord for the mediation of *general light reflexes* (e.g. reflex blinking and jumping or turning away from a flash of bright light). The superior colliculi are united by the posterior commissure and thus general body reflexes to light are usually bilateral. The fibres concerned in the *pupillary light reflex* (see p. 423) do not synapse in the colliculus, but pass bilaterally to each pretectal nucleus. The **pretectal nucleus** is a small group of cells in the tegmentum of the midbrain, just cranial to the superior colliculus. It passes light impulses to each Edinger–Westphal nucleus and so to the sphincter pupillae. A lesion here produces the Argyll Robertson pupil; contraction to light is lost, but the pupil still contracts to accommodation and convergence.

Limbic system and olfactory pathways

Surrounding the corpus callosum and diencephalon are a number of features that have come to be known collectively as the **limbic system**. Because the olfactory tracts and its associated structures were originally included in this descriptive concept, much of its function was thought to be concerned with olfaction. This view is no longer tenable and it is now known to play a role in such abstract functions as emotion, behaviour, mood and memory; thus lesions of one of its major constituents, the hippocampus, result in loss of memory for recent events, although the memory of distant events is retained. However, much remains to be discovered about the form and function of the limbic system.

Limbic system

Apart from the olfactory nerves, bulb and tract, the following are among the major components of the limbic system:

- the hippocampus, fimbria, fornix, dentate gyrus and mammillary body (see below)
- the uncus (see p. 477), and the cingulate and parahippocampal gyri (see pp 475 and 477)
- the amygdaloid body (see p. 478)
- the septal and piriform areas of cerebral cortex, near the lamina terminalis (anterior boundary of the third ventricle; see p. 488), and the anterior thalamic nucleus.

Olfactory pathways

The **olfactory tract**, which is an elongated extension of the white matter of the brain (like the optic nerve), lies in the olfactory sulcus beside the gyrus rectus on the inferior surface of the frontal lobe (Fig. 7.4). Its anterior end is expanded as the **olfactory bulb**. After passing through the cribriform plate of the ethmoid, the olfactory nerve filaments synapse with the cells of the second order neuron in the bulb. The axons of these cells run back in the tract to the *anterior perforated substance*, which lies on the inferior surface of the frontal lobe immediately lateral to the optic chiasma. Here the tract divides into lateral and medial striae. The lateral stria runs along the anterolateral margin of the anterior perforated substance to the region of the uncus, at the front of the parahippocampal gyrus (Fig. 7.3). The medial stria passes in front of the lamina terminalis and makes connections with other parts of the limbic system.

Thus the olfactory pathway reaches the olfactory cortex without relay in the thalamus, unlike other sensory pathways (light, sound, taste, touch). However, the olfactory cortex projects directly and via the thalamus to areas of the orbitofrontal cortex that are involved in olfactory information processing. Furthermore, connections with the hypothalamus and brainstem mediate visceral and somatic effects distinct from conscious perception.

Hippocampus

Just above the anterior part of the parahippocampal gyrus of the temporal lobe lies the hippocampal sulcus, which is projected into the floor of the inferior horn of the lateral ventricle as the **hippocampus**. The transitional zone between the cortex of the parahippocampal gyrus and that of the hippocampus is known as the *subiculum*. Viewed from above the anterior part of the hippocampus (the *pes hippocampi*) has the appearance of the knuckles of a clenched fist (Fig. 7.7). On its ventricular surface is a thin film of white matter, the *alveus*; its cell bodies are in the hippocampus and subiculum. The fibres of the alveus thicken medially to form the *fimbria*. This breaks free from the hippocampus as the *crus (posterior pillar) of the fornix* (Fig. 7.10). The *dentate gyrus* is a small part of the hippocampus which, as seen from the medial side, lies between the fimbria and the parahippocampal gyrus.

Fornix

The fornix is the great efferent pathway from the hippocampus. As a flat band continuous with the *fimbria*, it curves up behind the thalamus to join its fellow in a partial decussation across the midline, the *commissure of the fornix*. It is really a chiasma, and is an association tract as well as a commissure. The conjoined mass of white matter, lying beneath the corpus callosum, is the *body of the fornix*. From it the conjoined *anterior columns* arch down in front of the anterior poles of the thalami and diverge, forming the anterior margins of the interventricular foramina (Fig. 7.12).

The columns of the fornix pass both anterior and posterior to the anterior commissure. The anterior fibres pass mainly to the *septal nuclei* near the lamina terminalis. The posterior fibres pass directly to the thalamus or into the *mamillary body*. From the mamillary body fibres pass in the lateral wall of the third ventricle as the *mamillothalamic tract* to the anterior nucleus of the thalamus. Here they relay and the thalamic neurons send their fibres through the internal capsule to the cingulate gyrus, which has connections with the parahippocampal gyrus and thus to the hippocampus.

Lateral ventricles

Each lateral ventricle is a C-shaped cavity, lined with ependyma, lying within the cerebral hemisphere. It consists of the body of the ventricle and anterior, posterior and inferior horns (Figs 7.7 and 7.11). On its medial side the pia mater and ependyma come into contact with each other. This line of contact is narrow, and curves around the top of the thalamus and the tail of the caudate nucleus, forming a C-shaped slit on the medial surface of the hemisphere, the **choroid fissure** (Fig. 7.3). The choroid fissure should be regarded as the medial wall of the body and inferior horn of the ventricle. A mass of blood capillaries enters through the choroid fissure, invaginating the pia mater and ependyma before it. This combination of capillaries, pia and ependyma constitutes the **choroid plexus**, which secretes *CSF*. The lips of the choroid fissure meet around the invaginated plexus, which thus lies hidden within the body and inferior horn of the ventricle. The choroid plexuses of the lateral ventricles are large and highly vascular; this pair secretes the bulk of the CSF. Each lateral ventricle opens into the third ventricle by the interventricular foramen, and the choroid plexus of the lateral ventricle is continuous through this foramen with the very small amount of plexus in the third ventricle.

In other places the grey matter at the bottom of a sulcus indents the cavity of the lateral ventricle. Such sulci are the parahippocampal, calcarine and collateral, which show as convexities within the cavity of the ventricle. The caudate nucleus and thalamus also project

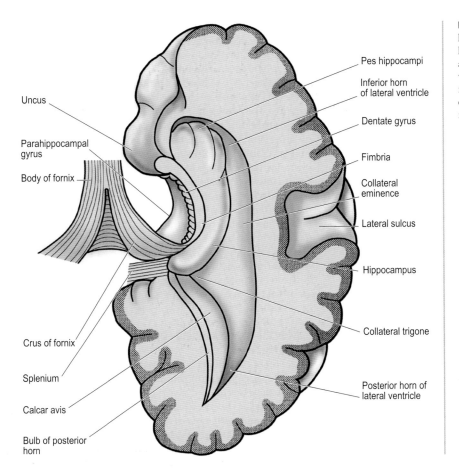

Uncus

Parahippocampal gyrus

Body of fornix

Crus of fornix

Splenium

Calcar avis

Bulb of posterior horn

Pes hippocampi

Inferior horn of lateral ventricle

Dentate gyrus

Fimbria

Collateral eminence

Lateral sulcus

Hippocampus

Collateral trigone

Posterior horn of lateral ventricle

Fig. 7.10 The right cerebral hemisphere has been divided horizontally to expose the inferior and posterior horns of the lateral ventricle. The posterior part of the fornix has been preserved. The ependyma of the ventricle has been removed.

into the cavity. Elsewhere the walls of the cavity are formed by white matter of the cerebral hemisphere.

The **anterior horn** is bounded by the fibres of the corpus callosum that run laterally from the genu (forceps minor). The bulbous head of the caudate nucleus lies in the floor, meeting the roof at an angle on the lateral side (Fig. 7.7), but separated from the roof medially by a thin partition between the fornix and corpus callosum, the *septum pellucidum* (Fig. 7.12). Behind the anterior column of the fornix, between it and the anterior pole of the thalamus, is a small aperture, the **interventricular foramen** (of Monro), which leads from the lateral into the third ventricle. The choroid plexus in the body of the ventricle does not extend into the anterior horn but passes through the interventricular foramen into the third ventricle.

The **body** of the lateral ventricle lies behind the level of the interventricular foramen. Its floor is the thalamus and body of the caudate nucleus, with the thalamostriate

groove between them. The stria terminalis lies in the groove (see p. 478). Also in the groove is the thalamostriate vein (Figs 7.7 and 7.17). The roof of the body is the corpus callosum with, on the medial side, the body and crus of the fornix (Fig. 7.12). Through the medial wall of the body of the ventricle, between roof (fornix) and floor (thalamus) the choroid plexus is invaginated, thrusting pia mater and ependyma before it. This is the upper part of the choroid fissure which is limited anteriorly by the interventricular foramen.

From the body the cavity of the lateral ventricle arches downwards and then forwards into the temporal lobe as the inferior horn, and backwards into the occipital lobe as the posterior horn.

The **posterior horn** is the most variably developed and may even be absent. The floor is a convexity, the *collateral eminence*, produced by the collateral sulcus. The medial wall consists of two slight convexities: the upper is the *bulb of the posterior horn*, formed by fibres

Fig. 7.11 Cast of the cerebral ventricles:
A from the right; **B** from above.

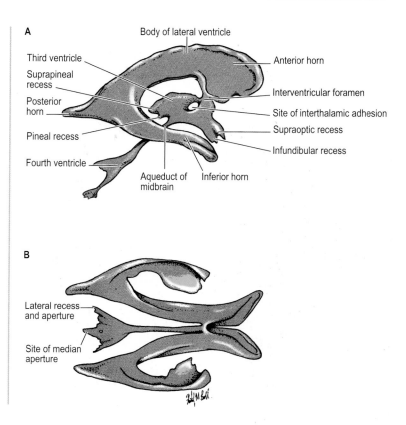

A

Third ventricle

Suprapineal recess

Posterior horn

Pineal recess

Fourth ventricle

Aqueduct of midbrain

Inferior horn

Body of lateral ventricle

Anterior horn

Interventricular foramen

Site of interthalamic adhesion

Supraoptic recess

Infundibular recess

B

Lateral recess and aperture

Site of median aperture

of the forceps major (from the splenium of the corpus callosum), and the lower is the *calcar avis*, formed by the calcarine sulcus. It is the calcar which, if well developed, obliterates the posterior horn. The roof and lateral wall is formed by the tapetum of the corpus callosum, with the optic radiation lying against the tapetum in the lateral wall (Fig. 7.7).

The **inferior horn** is the largest. Its floor consists medially of the hippocampus with, laterally, the collateral eminence, which expands posteriorly into the *collateral trigone* where the posterior and inferior horns diverge (Fig. 7.7). In the roof is the tail of the caudate nucleus. The fimbria forms the lower lip of the choroid fissure in the inferior horn just as its continuation the fornix forms the upper lip of the fissure in the body of the lateral ventricle; they lie in continuity around the convexity of the C. Similarly, within the concavity of the C the caudate nucleus lies in continuity. Its bulbous head in the anterior horn and its thinner body in the floor of the body of the ventricle are continued into the roof of the inferior horn as an ever-diminishing tail of the caudate nucleus. At the extremity of the tail of the caudate nucleus is an expansion of grey matter, the amygdaloid body,

which lies to the lateral side of the anterior perforated substance. It produces a shallow convexity on the roof at the tip of the inferior horn, just above the pes hippocampi. These two projections often lie together, separated only by the choroid plexus. The inferior horn is closed laterally by the white matter of the tapetum.

Diencephalon and third ventricle

That part of the brain cranial to the midbrain is the forebrain. Developed as a single tube (the fore-end of the neural tube) its cranial end is formed by a thin plate of grey matter, the lamina terminalis. Just to the caudal side of this lamina the side walls of the forebrain blow out into two enormous balloons, or vesicles, which become the cerebral hemispheres, already described. The remainder of the forebrain, relatively unexpanded, becomes the **diencephalon**, still closed anteriorly by the lamina terminalis. The cavity within its substance is the third ventricle, into which the lateral ventricles of the cerebral hemispheres open through the interventricular foramina. The diencephalon, enclosing this cavity, has two side walls, a floor and a roof. The floor and roof

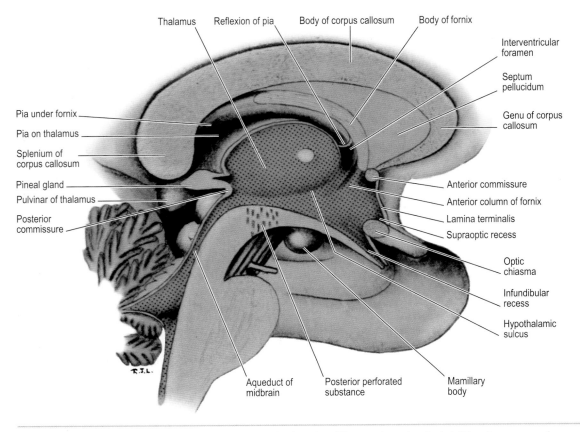

Thalamus   Reflexion of pia   Body of corpus callosum   Body of fornix

Interventricular foramen

Septum pellucidum

Genu of corpus callosum

Pia under fornix

Pia on thalamus

Splenium of corpus callosum

Pineal gland

Pulvinar of thalamus

Posterior commissure

Anterior commissure

Anterior column of fornix

Lamina terminalis

Supraoptic recess

Optic chiasma

Infundibular recess

Hypothalamic sulcus

Aqueduct of midbrain   Posterior perforated substance   Mamillary body

Fig. 7.12   Third ventricle and adjacent structures in sagittal section. The ependyma is stippled. The pia mater on the upper surface of the thalamus is reflected on to the lower surface of the fornix to form the roof of the interventricular foramen.

converge towards each other posteriorly, where they join the midbrain; and the cavity of the third ventricle is continued through the midbrain as the narrow aqueduct.

The anterior wall of the diencephalon is the **lamina terminalis**, a thin sheet which extends between the two hemispheres from the rostrum of the corpus callosum to the top of the optic chiasma (Fig. 7.12). The floor, seen from below as the floor of the third ventricle, extends from the optic chiasma, tuber cinereum and infundibulum, and mamillary bodies to the posterior perforated substance, where the floor joins the tegmentum of the cerebral peduncles (Fig. 7.18).

In a median sagittal section through the third ventricle a thin partition, the **septum pellucidum**, is seen connecting the rostrum, genu and front of the body of the corpus callosum to the anterior column of the fornix (Fig. 7.12). The septum consists of two layers that may be adherent; when they lie apart the closed space between

them is the cavity of the septum pellucidum, which is lined with pia mater and has no connection with the ventricular system.

The **third ventricle** (Fig. 7.12) is a slit-like space, lying in the sagittal plane below the fornix and the corpus callosum. Much of the lateral wall is occupied by the thalamus, a rounded mass of grey matter that bulges convexly into the ventricle. The two thalami often (60% of brains) become gummed together at the *interthalamic adhesion*. It is not a commissure and there is no interchange of fibres between the two sides. The adhesion, when present, gives a fenestrated shadow in images of the third ventricle. The *hypothalamic sulcus* curves down from the interventricular foramen below the thalamus towards the aqueduct of the midbrain.

Below the hypothalamic groove the side wall slopes down to the floor. This region, including the floor, is the **hypothalamus** (Fig. 7.12). The caudal part of this area that merges with the midbrain is the subthalamus, one of whose principal features is the *subthalamic nucleus* which belongs functionally to the basal nuclei.

The hypothalamus contains various cell groups, in particular the *supraoptic* and *paraventricular nuclei* whose axons run in the pituitary stalk into the posterior lobe of the pituitary (see p. 466), and other cells whose processes enter the pituitary stalk to deliver their neurosecretory material to the hypothalamo–hypophyseal portal system of blood vessels for the control of the anterior lobe. Yet other cells have long axons that pass through the brainstem and spinal cord to preganglionic sympathetic cells in the lateral horn of the thoracic and upper lumbar parts, and to preganglionic parasympathetic cells in the lateral horn of the sacral segments, of the spinal cord (see p. 19).

Behind the optic chiasma the (hollow) infundibulum projects downwards to become the (solid) pituitary stalk. Behind the infundibulum the upper surface of the floor slopes smoothly upwards and backwards to the aqueduct, but the external surface is marked by the pair of *mamillary bodies* and behind them by the *posterior perforated substance*. The part of the floor between the optic chiasma and the mamillary bodies is the *tuber cinereum*. The part of the tuber cinereum at the base of the infundibulum is the *median eminence* which is the site of the neurosecretory cells that control the anterior pituitary, and one of the few regions with no blood–brain barrier (see p. 491).

The anterior wall of the third ventricle is the lamina terminalis which extends up from the optic chiasma to the rostrum of the corpus callosum. The tiny angle between the lamina terminalis and the chiasma is the *supraoptic recess*, and the hollow in the infundibulum is the *infundibular recess* (Fig. 7.12). Attached behind the upper end of the lamina terminalis is a rounded cord, the *anterior commissure*, which joins the inferior parts of the temporal lobes. Behind this the conjoined anterior columns of the fornix lie in contact before they diverge to sink down into the lateral wall of the ventricle. Behind each anterior column is an *interventricular foramen*, ependyma-lined and roofed in by bare pia mater sweeping from the under-surface of the body of the fornix to the upper surface of the anterior pole of the thalamus.

The roof of the third ventricle is slack towards its posterior end and bulges back as the *suprapineal recess* (Fig. 7.11). The whole length of the roof is invaginated by the pair of (small) *choroid plexuses of the third ventricle*, which hang down as slender fringes inside the cavity.

The **pineal gland** projects back from the posterior wall of the third ventricle, lying above the superior colliculi of the midbrain, between the posterior parts of the thalami,

just below the splenium (Figs 7.12 and 7.20). It is a soft conical body, less than half a centimetre long, and is one of the few regions with no blood–brain barrier (see p. 491). It contains a number of *corpora arenacea*. These calcify, and to such an extent that after the age of 40 years they may throw a tiny shadow in radiographs of the skull. A displaced calcified pineal indicates a space-occupying lesion above the tentorium. Pineal secretions, including melatonin, have an inhibitory effect on other endocrine organs and gonads. The stalk of the pineal is attached also to the posterior commissure, which connects the two superior colliculi above the entrance to the aqueduct. The pineal stalk is hollowed out as the *pineal recess* (Fig. 7.11).

The **thalamus** is seen in horizontal and coronal sections buried in the cerebral hemisphere (Figs 7.7 and 7.8), and by its connections with the sensory parts of the internal capsule it appears to be part of the hemisphere. Nevertheless, it is part of the wall of the diencephalon.

The mass of grey matter making up the thalamus is roughly wedge-shaped. The medial walls of the two thalami lie parallel, near each other across the third ventricle, where in two-thirds of cases they are joined by the *interthalamic adhesion*. Behind this the medial surface diverges from the midline and expands into a large posterior convexity, the *pulvinar*; the lateral geniculate body (see p. 484) bulges down from its lateral part (Figs 7.4 and 7.20). The *medial geniculate body*, a thalamic nucleus which relays auditory impulses, is separated from the main mass of the thalamus and lies on the midbrain. It receives fibres from the cochlear nerves by way of the nuclei of the nerves and the lateral lemniscus, and relays them through the sublentiform part of the internal capsule to the auditory cortex in the temporal lobe.

The superior surface of the thalamus is convex and triangular in outline, tapering forward from the large pulvinar to the small blunt anterior pole. The superior surface and the posterior surface (pulvinar) of the thalamus are on the external surface of the diencephalon itself. They are covered in pia mater. An oblique strip along the lateral margin of the superior surface lies in the lateral ventricle, covered with ependyma. The body and tail of the caudate nucleus are in contact here with the lateral margin of the thalamus (Fig. 7.6).

The lateral surface of the thalamus is bevelled by the internal capsule (Fig. 7.8), whose descending fibres lie in contact anteriorly. The ascending fibres of the internal capsule arise further back from numerous nuclei in this lateral part.

The inferior surface of the thalamus is narrower than the superior surface. Medially it joins the hypothalamus. Lateral to this, and posterior too, the lemnisci of the tegmentum (see p. 497) enter the thalamus and attach it to the top of the midbrain.

All four surfaces (medial, inferior, lateral and superior) of the thalamus converge to the small blunt anterior pole, which lies at the interventricular foramen, covered in ependyma.

Structurally the thalamus consists of a large number of cell groups, the *thalamic nuclei*, which receive inputs from the medial, spinal and trigeminal lemnisci and the reticular formation and project to sensory areas of the cerebral cortex. Other nuclei receive fibres from the dentate nucleus of the cerebellum and the globus pallidus and project to the motor areas of the cortex, so contributing to motor control. Some nuclei receive fibres from the hypothalamus and corpus striatum and have reciprocal connections with the frontal lobes; they appear to be concerned with emotional responses and memory. Via the mamillothalamic tract the hypothalamus also sends fibres to the anterior pole of the thalamus, which project to the cingulate gyrus and are part of the limbic system. The medial and lateral geniculate bodies are specialized parts of the thalamus concerned with hearing and vision respectively.

Blood supply of the forebrain

The cerebral hemispheres and the walls of the diencephalon are supplied from both the internal carotid and vertebral systems. The arteries are directed in essence to the grey matter, which needs more blood than the white matter. Superficial cortical arteries supply the grey matter on the surface, perforating arteries supply the subcortical nuclei. Both sets of arteries send branches to the adjacent white matter.

An artery that has entered the surface of the brain from either of these sets is always an end artery (i.e. it has no precapillary anastomosis with its fellows), and thus cerebral softening follows its obstruction. Entering arteries invaginate a tubular prolongation of pia mater around them, forming a *perivascular space* that extends to the fine branches of the vessel.

The internal carotid and vertebral systems anastomose with each other around the optic chiasma and infundibulum of the pituitary stalk, forming the **arterial circle** of Willis (the French call it, more accurately, the polygon of Willis). The communicating vessels allow equalization of blood flow between the two sides of the brain, and can allow anastomatic circulation if parts are occluded; however, this is not always effective due to the small size of some vessels. The circle is formed in the following way. The *basilar artery* from the vertebral system divides at the upper border of the pons into right and left *posterior cerebral arteries*. Each posterior cerebral receives

a small *posterior communicating artery* that runs backwards through the interpeduncular cistern from the *internal carotid artery* at the anterior perforated substance on the same side. Each internal carotid artery gives off an *anterior cerebral artery*; the circle of Willis is completed by the *anterior communicating artery*, a small vessel that unites the anterior cerebrals in the chiasmatic cistern, below the rostrum of the corpus callosum. The optic chiasma and the pituitary stalk are encircled by the circle of Willis (Fig. 7.19). Rupture of an aneurysm of the arterial circle accounts for 90% of subarachnoid haemorrhages. Congenital aneurysms are more commonly found on the carotid part of the circle than the basilar part, and are most frequent at sites where vessels branch (e.g. anterior cerebral with anterior communicating, internal carotid with posterior communicating or middle cerebral) because here the tunica media is weakest.

Blood supply of the cerebral hemispheres

The arterial supply of the cerebrum is by the three cerebral arteries, anterior, middle and posterior and there is also a contribution from the anterior choroidal (although, unlike the other three, it does not supply the cerebral cortex). The first two and the last are branches of the internal carotid, the posterior cerebral is the terminal branch of the basilar. The branches of the three cerebral arteries anastomose across the frontiers of their respective territories (Figs 7.13 and 7.14), on the surface of the pia mater, but sparsely and only by arterioles. Their perforating branches are invariably end arteries. The larger surface vessels have a sympathetic innervation, but after becoming intracortical they are not innervated.

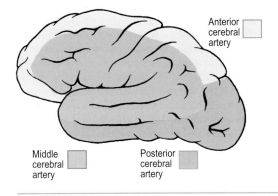

Anterior cerebral artery

Middle cerebral artery

Posterior cerebral artery

Fig. 7.13   Areas of arterial distribution on the lateral surface of the left cerebral hemisphere.

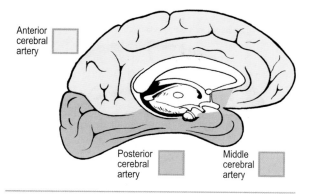

Fig. 7.14   Areas of arterial distribution on the medial surface of the left cerebral hemisphere.

Capillaries in the brain (and spinal cord) are characterized by lack of fenestrations and by abundant tight junctions (zonulae occludentes) between endothelial cells. This is the principal structural reason for the *blood–brain barrier* which operates to protect the internal environment of neural tissue by allowing only selected substances (amino acids, amines and sugars) to be transported across the endothelial cells. This protective mechanism is possibly assisted by a basal lamina that is thicker than usual and by the enveloping foot processes of astrocytes. Among the more important parts of the brain that have no blood–brain barrier are the posterior pituitary, median eminence of the hypothalamus and pineal gland.

The **internal carotid artery** emerges from the roof of the cavernous sinus, gives off the ophthalmic artery, then curls back to lie on the front half of the roof. It then turns vertically upwards to the anterior perforated substance where it divides into middle and anterior cerebral branches for the supply of the cortex (see Figs 6.106 and 6.107, pp 466 and 467). It here gives off also the striate arteries, the anterior choroidal artery, and the posterior communicating artery (Fig. 7.19).

The **middle cerebral artery** is the largest and most direct branch of the internal carotid (Fig. 7.19) and therefore most subject to embolism. It passes deep into the lateral sulcus to supply the cortex of the insula and overlying opercula. It reaches the lateral surface of the hemisphere by continuing in the lateral sulcus, from which its branches emerge and ramify over an area that falls short of the borders of the lateral surface by one gyrus or its equivalent breadth (Fig. 7.13). In its area of cortical distribution lie the motor and sensory areas for the opposite half of the body, excluding leg, foot and perineum (which are in anterior cerebral territory), and the auditory and speech areas.

The **anterior cerebral artery** leaves the internal carotid artery at the anterior perforated substance and passes forwards above the optic nerve (Fig. 7.19). It is connected to its fellow of the opposite side by the *anterior communicating artery*. It is distributed to the orbital surface of the frontal lobe and to the whole of the medial surface of the hemisphere above the corpus callosum as far back as the parieto-occipital sulcus (see Figs 6.106 and 6.107, pp 466 and 467). Its distribution extends over the superior border to meet the area supplied by the middle cerebral artery (Figs 7.13 and 7.14). The motor and sensory areas for the opposite leg, foot and perineum, including the micturition and defecation centres, lie in its territory. Because of the anastomosis via the anterior communicating artery, it is usually possible for one anterior cerebral to be supplied with blood from the contralateral internal carotid. Very occasionally both anterior cerebrals may arise from one carotid by a common stem.

The fact that the internal carotid gives origin to the anterior and middle cerebral arteries (supplying the sensorimotor cortex and internal capsule; see below) and to the ophthalmic artery (supplying the retina, see p. 419) accounts for the characteristic combination of blindness in one eye with contralateral hemiplegia that may follow stenosis or occlusion of the internal carotid artery. However, occlusion may be 'silent' because of collateral circulation through the arterial circle; the effects are very variable, depending on the state and size of the vessels.

The **posterior cerebral artery** curls back around the cerebral peduncle (Fig. 7.19), supplying it and the optic tract, and passes back above the tentorium to supply the inferomedial surface of the temporal and occipital lobes (Figs 7.13 and 7.14). Its territory meets that of the anterior cerebral artery at the parieto-occipital sulcus. Its branches extend around the borders of the brain to supply the inferior temporal gyrus and a corresponding strip of cortex on the lateral surface of the occipital lobe. The visual area for the opposite field of vision lies wholly within its territory, but the middle cerebral branches can sometimes extend sufficiently far back on the occipital lobe to supply the macular part of the visual area (see p. 482). Thus the macular field of vision may be spared when the rest of the visual area is destroyed by a posterior cerebral thrombosis. The posterior cerebral may receive some or all of its blood from the internal carotid and not the basilar; indeed, this is the primitive embryonic condition where the posterior cerebral is a branch of the carotid. The basilar system is a later development which joins the original posterior cerebral, whose proximal end becomes the posterior communicating. The two posterior communicating arteries are often unequal in size.

The arterial supply of the subcortical nuclei is by branches from the three cerebral vessels, and by the anterior choroidal. Branches from the cerebral vessels enter through the perforated substances.

The *anterior perforated substance* (Fig. 7.18) receives numerous small branches mainly from the commencement of the middle cerebral artery. These are the *striate branches* and they supply the *internal capsule*, as well as the thalamus and basal nuclei. Clinicians give them various names such as perforating, lenticulostriate, thalamostriate and thalamolenticular, but anatomically they are divided into medial and lateral groups. One lateral striate branch, usually the largest, is Charcot's 'artery of cerebral haemorrhage' whose rupture or occlusion are the most common causes of a typical 'stroke' with contralateral hemiplegia.

Branches from the posterior cerebral artery enter the *posterior perforated substance* to reach the thalamus and basal ganglia, penetrating the posterior part of the internal capsule on the way.

The **anterior choroidal artery** supplies the choroid plexus, passing below the optic tract to enter the inferior extremity of the choroid fissure at the tip of the inferior horn of the lateral ventricle, just above the uncus. The artery gives branches to the optic tract and radiation and the lateral geniculate body, as well as to the posterior part of the internal capsule, basal nuclei and limbic system. The choroid plexus also receives a few additional twigs from the posterior cerebral artery, which enter the choroid fissure behind the thalamus.

Effects of arterial occlusion. Obviously the effect of occlusion of the cerebral arteries will vary with the degree and site of obstruction, but the main effects of complete occlusion may be summarized as follows.

Anterior cerebral: contralateral weakness and sensory loss (mainly leg, foot and perineum).

Middle cerebral: contralateral hemiplegia and hemianaesthesia (with aphasia if the lesion is left-sided).

Posterior cerebral: contralateral hemianopia and hemianaesthesia.

Anterior choroidal: contralateral hemianopia and hemianaesthesia, with some degree of hemiplegia.

Cerebral veins

The venous return does not follow the arterial pattern. Unlike the cortical arteries, which tend to travel deep in the sulci, the cortical veins tend to travel superficially, adherent to the deep surface of the arachnoid mater that bridges each sulcus. They then usually cross the subdural space to drain into the nearest available venous sinus of the dura mater, generally entering obliquely against the bloodstream.

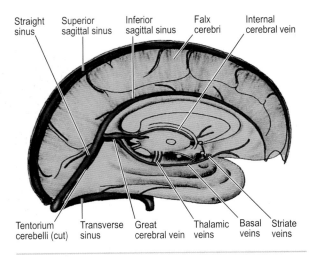

Fig. 7.15 Venous drainage of the cerebral hemisphere, thalamus and basal nuclei, from the medial side. Note that the lower halves of the thalamus and corpus striatum drain via the perforated substances into the basal vein, and their upper halves drain to the internal cerebral vein.

The superolateral and medial surfaces of the hemisphere drain into the superior sagittal sinus (Fig. 7.15) by several **superior cerebral veins**. A few inferior cerebral veins drain into the transverse sinus. In each case the veins mainly enter against the direction of bloodflow. The superior veins, if encountering a blood lake, pass on its cerebral surface beneath the arachnoid (the blood lakes are between the 'two layers' of the dura; Fig. 7.16).

Adherent to the deep surface of the arachnoid mater that bridges the lateral sulcus runs the **superficial middle cerebral vein**, draining the adjacent cortex and emptying into the cavernous sinus. At the posterior end of this vein are *superior and inferior anastomotic veins* which join the superior sagittal and transverse sinuses, respectively. The inferomedial and inferior surfaces of the hemisphere drain by **inferior cerebral veins** into the nearest venous sinus of the dura mater, such as the cavernous, superior petrosal and transverse sinuses.

The depths of the lateral sulcus and the surface of the insula drain into the **deep middle cerebral vein**. The **anterior cerebral vein** returns around the genu of the corpus callosum alongside the anterior cerebral artery; it is the only vein of the brain to have a similar name and course to its companion artery. The anterior cerebral vein drains also the orbital surface of the frontal lobe. At the anterior perforated substance **striate veins** draining the corpus striatum emerge through the perforations. They join the deep middle cerebral vein and the anterior

Fig. 7.16 Superior sagittal sinus, meninges and associated vessels in coronal section of the cranial vault.

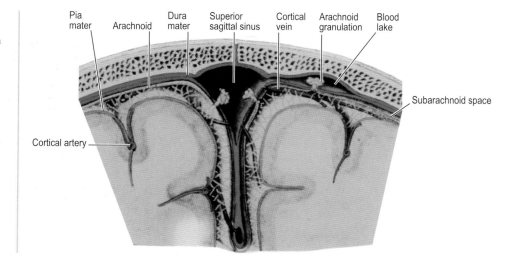

cerebral vein to form the **basal vein** (Figs 7.15 and 7.17). This passes around the cerebral peduncle below the optic tract with the posterior cerebral artery. Just below the splenium the two basal veins join the great cerebral vein (see below). The lower parts of the basal ganglia drain through the perforated substances into the basal vein; their upper parts drain into the internal cerebral vein.

The **internal cerebral vein** (Fig. 7.17) is formed at the interventricular foramen by the *choroidal vein*, draining the choroid plexus of the lateral ventricle, and the *thalamostriate vein*, which lies in the groove between the thalamus and caudate nucleus and receives blood from both. The *veins of the septum pellucidum* which bring blood from the corpus callosum and adjacent cortex and the head of the caudate nucleus usually join the thalamostriate vein.

The internal cerebral vein so formed runs back in the roof of the third ventricle. It receives the veins from the choroid plexus of the third ventricle and then joins its fellow to make the **great cerebral vein** (of Galen) just beneath the splenium. This vein is joined by the two basal veins, and with the inferior sagittal sinus it enters the straight sinus (Fig. 7.15).

PART TWO

Brainstem

The brainstem is the part of the brain connecting the cerebrum and diencephalon with the spinal cord, and consists of the midbrain, pons and medulla oblongata

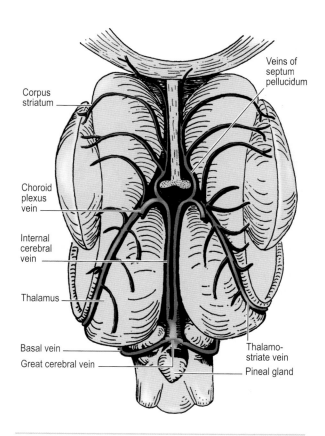

Fig. 7.17 Inferior view of the basal nuclei and thalamus with their draining veins.

(Figs 7.3B, 7.6 and 7.18–7.20). It extends from just above the aperture in the tentorium cerebelli to C1 vertebra below the foramen magnum. The cerebellum projects from its dorsal surface.

The brainstem consists of fibres and cells. Most of the fibres in the brainstem ascend or descend longitudinally, as in the spinal cord, and most of the cells are aggregated into nuclei. These **nuclei** consist of three groups:

- The nuclei of the third to the twelfth cranial nerves.
- Other named nuclei which are demonstrable, such as the colliculi, the red nucleus, the substantia nigra, the pontine nuclei and the olivary nucleus.
- The reticular formation, a diffuse system of cells and fibres which is intermingled with the named nuclei and tracts, continues into the spinal cord, and is described further on page 500. Some of its cells form the so-called 'vital centres'—cardiac, respiratory, vasomotor, etc.—which are not anatomically demonstrable as distinct 'nuclei', but are of great physiological importance.

The levels of the cranial nerve nuclei are as follows.

Those of the third and fourth are in the midbrain.

The motor nucleus of the fifth, and the sixth and seventh, are in the pons. The three sensory nuclei of the fifth are distributed between the midbrain, pons, medulla and upper spinal cord. The salivary (parasympathetic) and sensory (taste) nuclei of the seventh are in the lower pons and upper medulla, respectively.

The eighth nerve nuclei overlap the junction of pons and medulla and lie partly in each.

The nuclei of the ninth to the twelfth are in the medulla (with the eleventh having a spinal part derived from the cervical region of the cord).

Midbrain

The midbrain connects the diencephalon and cerebrum to the pons (Figs 7.3B and 7.18). It is the shortest segment of the brainstem, being not more than 2 cm in length. Most of it lies in the posterior cranial fossa, with its upper part passing through the tentorial notch.

The midbrain consists of right and left halves, each half forming a **cerebral peduncle** made up of a ventral part, the *base* (basis pedunculi) and a dorsal part, the *tegmentum*. Running through the tegmentum is the **aqueduct of the midbrain** (aqueduct of Sylvius), joining the third and fourth ventricles. The part of the tegmentum dorsal to the aqueduct is the *tectum*.

On the ventral surface are seen the bases of the peduncles (often called the crura), which lie in V-shaped manner cranial to the pons, enclosing the posterior

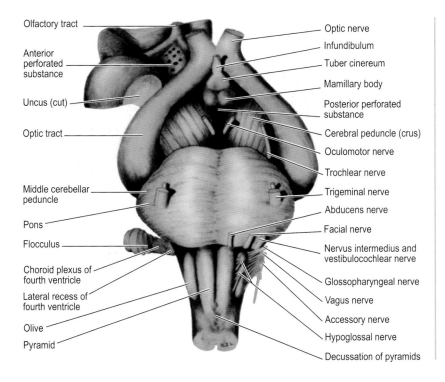

Olfactory tract
Anterior perforated substance
Uncus (cut)
Optic tract
Middle cerebellar peduncle
Pons
Flocculus
Choroid plexus of fourth ventricle
Lateral recess of fourth ventricle
Olive
Pyramid

Optic nerve
Infundibulum
Tuber cinereum
Mamillary body
Posterior perforated substance
Cerebral peduncle (crus)
Oculomotor nerve
Trochlear nerve
Trigeminal nerve
Abducens nerve
Facial nerve
Nervus intermedius and vestibulocochlear nerve
Glossopharyngeal nerve
Vagus nerve
Accessory nerve
Hypoglossal nerve
Decussation of pyramids

Fig. 7.18 Ventral surface of the brainstem, with all vessels removed. On the left side the cranial nerves are intact; on the right all except the oculomotor and trigeminal have been removed.

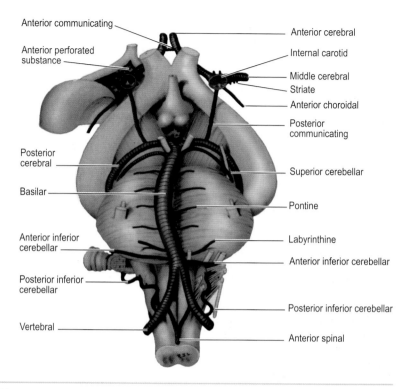

Anterior communicating

Anterior cerebral

Anterior perforated substance

Internal carotid

Middle cerebral

Striate

Anterior choroidal

Posterior communicating

Posterior cerebral

Superior cerebellar

Basilar

Pontine

Anterior inferior cerebellar

Labyrinthine

Anterior inferior cerebellar

Posterior inferior cerebellar

Posterior inferior cerebellar

Vertebral

Anterior spinal

Fig. 7.19 Ventral surface of the brainstem with arteries intact. Although not apparent in a drawing, the arterial circle lies horizontally, at right angles to the basilar artery which is vertical.

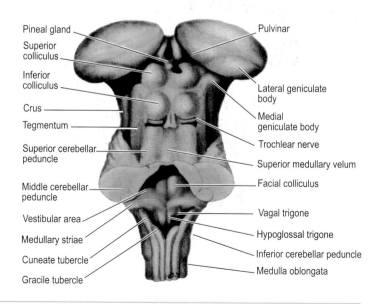

Pineal gland

Pulvinar

Superior colliculus

Inferior colliculus

Lateral geniculate body

Crus

Medial geniculate body

Tegmentum

Trochlear nerve

Superior cerebellar peduncle

Superior medullary velum

Middle cerebellar peduncle

Facial colliculus

Vestibular area

Vagal trigone

Medullary striae

Hypoglossal trigone

Cuneate tubercle

Inferior cerebellar peduncle

Gracile tubercle

Medulla oblongata

Fig. 7.20 Dorsal surface of the brainstem, after removal of the cerebellum and the roof of the fourth ventricle.

perforated substance of the diencephalon between them (Fig. 7.18). They converge down towards the upper border of the pons from their point of emergence below the thalamus.

Dorsally the midbrain shows two pairs of low rounded eminences, the *superior* and *inferior colliculi* (formerly called corpora quadrigemina, Fig. 7.20). The superior colliculi lie below the pineal body and the splenium of the corpus callosum, overlapped by the pulvinar of the thalamus. Lateral to each superior colliculus is the *medial geniculate body* which, although appearing to belong to the brainstem, is part of the thalamus (see p. 489). Below the inferior colliculi the *superior cerebellar peduncles* converge into the dorsal surface of the midbrain from the cerebellum.

The third and fourth cranial nerves leave the brainstem at the midbrain (Figs 7.19, 7.21 and 7.22). The oculomotor nerve leaves through the medial surface of the crus, on the ventral surface of the midbrain, and passes forwards between the posterior cerebral and superior cerebellar arteries in the interpeduncular cistern to reach the roof of the cavernous sinus. The trochlear nerve leaves the dorsal surface of the midbrain just below the inferior colliculus. This nerve is unique in three respects: it is the smallest cranial nerve, the only one to emerge from the dorsal surface of the brainstem, and the only one to decussate within the brainstem. The nerve curls round the lateral side of the peduncle and passes forwards between the same two arteries as the third nerve (posterior cerebral and superior cerebellar) but farther laterally, to reach the roof of the cavernous sinus. The optic tract and the basal vein also curl round the peduncle and the posterior communicating artery lies on the medial surface of the peduncle.

Internal structure

Sections of the midbrain are recognized by the colliculi of the tectum on the dorsal surface, the aqueduct, and the rectangular crura on the ventral surface, delimited by a dark line of pigmented cells, the substantia nigra. Other naked-eye features at superior colliculus level are the red nucleus with fibres of the third nerve sweeping though it, while at inferior colliculus level is the centrally placed decussation of the superior cerebellar peduncles (Figs 7.21 and 7.22).

Each crus contains corticospinal, corticonuclear and corticopontine fibres; the first two occupy the middle two-thirds of the crus. The medial sixth of the crus is occupied by frontopontine fibres and the lateral sixth by temporopontine and other corticopontine fibres (see p. 480).

The **superior colliculus** contains cells involved in *general light reflexes*, while the **inferior colliculus** is concerned with *sound reflexes*. They receive inputs from the retina and cochlea respectively and project to the motor nuclei of cranial and spinal nerves (via tectobulbar and tectospinal tracts) for reflex movements of the eyes, head, body and limbs away from or towards light and sound stimuli. The *pupillary light reflexes* (see p. 423) involve the **pretectal nuclei**, which lie just cranial to the superior colliculi at the junction of the midbrain and diencephalon.

The **oculomotor nucleus** lies close against the midline ventral to the aqueduct at superior colliculus level (Fig. 7.21), in line vertically with the other cranial somatic motor nuclei (fourth, sixth and twelfth). The parasympathetic part (**Edinger–Westphal** or accessory oculomotor nucleus) lies near the midline in the cranial part of the nucleus; its axons run out with the third nerve and relay in the ciliary ganglion, from which postganglionic fibres innervate the sphincter pupillae and ciliary muscles (see p. 423). The third nerve passes ventrally through the red nucleus to emerge from the brainstem on the medial side of the base of the peduncle.

The **trochlear nucleus** lies caudal to the oculomotor nucleus, ventral to the aqueduct at inferior colliculus

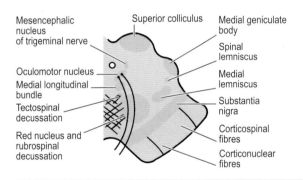

Mesencephalic nucleus of trigeminal nerve

Oculomotor nucleus

Medial longitudinal bundle

Tectospinal decussation

Red nucleus and rubrospinal decussation

Superior colliculus

Medial geniculate body

Spinal lemniscus

Medial lemniscus

Substantia nigra

Corticospinal fibres

Corticonuclear fibres

Fig. 7.21   Cross-section of the midbrain at the level of the superior colliculi.

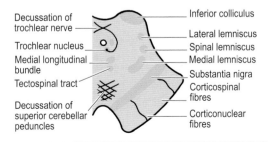

Decussation of trochlear nerve

Trochlear nucleus

Medial longitudinal bundle

Tectospinal tract

Decussation of superior cerebellar peduncles

Inferior colliculus

Lateral lemniscus

Spinal lemniscus

Medial lemniscus

Substantia nigra

Corticospinal fibres

Corticonuclear fibres

Fig. 7.22   Cross-section of the midbrain at the level of the inferior colliculi.

level (Fig. 7.22). The nerve proceeds dorsally and crosses the midline, where it decussates with its fellow dorsal to the aqueduct. It emerges through the superior medullary velum (see p. 502) on the dorsal aspect of the midbrain, below the inferior colliculus (Fig. 7.20).

The **red nucleus** lies in the tegmentum just ventral to the third nerve nucleus (Fig. 7.21). It is slightly larger than a full-sized pea. It receives fibres coming from the dentate nucleus in the opposite cerebellar hemisphere via the superior cerebellar peduncle. Its efferent fibres decussate and descend to motor nuclei of cranial and spinal nerves, as part of the extrapyramidal system (see p. 509).

Although in the midbrain at the junction of the tegmentum and crus, the **substantia nigra** belongs functionally to the basal nuclei (see p. 478). Many of its cells contain melatonin, responsible for its naked-eye dark appearance. Some of its cells give rise to *nigrostriatal fibres* which are dopaminergic and project to the caudate nucleus and putamen. The loss of about 80% of its dopaminergic cells is the fundamental defect in parkinsonism.

The **mesencephalic nucleus** of the trigeminal nerve lies in the central grey matter, lateral to the aqueduct, throughout the whole length of the midbrain. This long slender nucleus receives proprioceptive fibres from the muscles supplied by the mandibular branch of the trigeminal (muscles of mastication) and from the muscles of the orbit and face and, perhaps, the muscles of the tongue (see p. 397). It is unique in being a collection of first neuron cells buried in the central nervous system (see p. 508).

The spinal lemniscus and the medial lemniscus, which are ascending sensory tracts (see p. 502), lie in the lateral part of the tegmentum. Between the medial lemniscus and the central grey matter the tegmentum contains fragments of grey matter broken up by criss-cross bundles of white fibres. The 'network' appearance so produced gives it the name **reticular formation**. It is traceable through the pons (see p. 498) and medulla into the upper spinal cord, and is described further on page 500.

Blood supply

The midbrain is supplied by the *posterior cerebral* and *superior cerebellar arteries* as they curl around the cerebral peduncle. The veins drain for the most part into the basal vein as it passes around the peduncle. From the colliculi some blood enters the great cerebral vein.

Pons

The pons is a broad transverse mass between the midbrain and medulla (Fig. 7.18), curving at the sides into the *middle cerebellar peduncle* (Fig. 7.6). The only cranial nerve to emerge from the pons, the fifth, does so by a large sensory and small motor root. They emerge laterally from the middle of the ventral aspect of the pons, with the motor root slightly cranial and medial to the sensory root. The two nerve roots pass forwards together in the posterior cranial fossa (i.e. below the tentorium) to run over the groove on the apex of the petrous bone into the trigeminal cave in the middle cranial fossa (see Fig. 6.105, p. 463).

The ventral surface of the pons shows a shallow midline groove with a bulge on either side. The bulge is due to the underlying mass of pontine nuclei, intermingled with corticospinal and corticonuclear fibres (see below). This ventral surface lies along the clivus (see p. 532), separated from the bone by the subarachnoid pontine cistern, in which the basilar artery runs upwards. The artery may or may not lie in the midline groove; usually it has a gentle curve to one side. The superior cerebellar artery curls round the upper margin of the pons. The labyrinthine artery passes laterally to reach the internal acoustic meatus. Emerging from the junction of pons and medulla, the sixth nerve runs upwards across the ventral surface to enter the dura on the clivus. The seventh and eighth nerves emerge more laterally at the junction of pons and medulla, in the region often referred to as the cerebellopontine angle; the nervus intermedius part of the seventh nerve lies separately between the main part of the seventh and eighth nerves. Most laterally in this region lies the flocculus of the cerebellum (see p. 505) and the choroid plexus that has emerged from the lateral recess of the fourth ventricle (Fig. 7.18).

The dorsal surface of the pons is concealed by the attached cerebellum. The aqueduct of the midbrain opens out at the upper border of the pons into the cavity of the fourth ventricle, which is mostly pontine but medullary at its lower end (see p. 502). The pontine part of the roof of the ventricle consists only of a thin sheet of white matter, the *superior medullary velum* (Figs 7.20 and 7.29), upon which lies the lingula of the cerebellum. The velum is attached at each side to the superior cerebellar peduncles.

Internal structure

In the ventral part of the pons are the **pontine nuclei**, from which fibres emerge to cross to the opposite side and form the middle cerebellar peduncle. With the various corticopontine fibres that have travelled down in the cerebral peduncles to synapse with the pontine nuclei, they complete an extensive corticopontocerebellar pathway.

In the dorsal part of the pons are the nuclei of the fifth to eighth nerves and the salivary nuclei.

The **motor nucleus of the trigeminal nerve** is in the upper pons below the lateral part of the floor of the fourth ventricle. The fibres pass ventrally and laterally to emerge as already noted as a small *motor root* at the junction of the pons and the middle cerebellar peduncle.

Lateral to the motor nucleus is the **main sensory nucleus of the trigeminal nerve**. It receives those incoming fibres of the *sensory root* subserving touch. Its caudal continuation into the lower pons, medulla and upper cervical spinal cord is the **spinal nucleus**, which receives pain and temperature fibres, while its upward continuation is largely a small bundle of fibres but with some cell bodies, the mesencephalic tract of the trigeminal, leading to the mesencephalic nucleus for proprioception (Figs 7.21 and 7.23).

In the lower part of the pons the **abducens nucleus** lies near the midline just below the floor of the fourth ventricle, but with fibres of the facial nerve overlying it. The abducens nucleus plus the overlying facial nerve fibres form a small swelling, the facial colliculus, in the ventricular floor (Figs 7.20 and 7.24). The **facial nucleus** itself lies deeper and farther from the midline.

A collection of cells alongside the facial nucleus forms the **superior salivary nucleus** (parasympathetic). It provides axons which pass out in the nervus intermedius part of the facial nerve and reach the pterygopalatine and submandibular ganglia. The lower part forms the **inferior salivary nucleus**, just above the pontomedullary junction; its fibres join the glossopharyngeal nerve to reach the otic ganglion.

The **nuclei of the vestibulocochlear nerve** lie beneath the floor of the lateral angle of the fourth ventricle

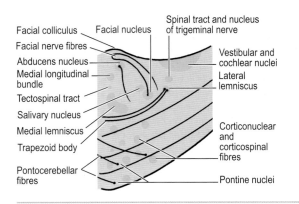

Fig. 7.24   Cross-section of the lower pons.

(the vestibular area, see Fig. 7.20) in both the pons and medulla. The vestibular fibres that emerge from the internal acoustic meatus pass anterior to the inferior cerebellar peduncle of the medulla and synapse in the **vestibular nuclei**, many of whose fibres pass back into that peduncle. Other fibres join the medial longitudinal bundle and connect with extraocular nuclei and cervical anterior horn cells. Some of these connections provide the basis for vestibulo-ocular reflexes.

The spiral ganglia of the cochlea send their axons to **dorsal** and **ventral cochlear nuclei** on the corresponding aspects of the inferior cerebellar peduncle, which are continuous medially with the vestibular area. Axons from these nuclei form the decussating trapezoid body (see p. 502), part of the auditory pathway.

The very uppermost ends of the dorsal nucleus of the vagus and the nucleus of the tractus solitarius also extend into the pons but essentially belong to the medulla, where they are described.

The pontine part of the **reticular formation** (see p. 500) lies dorsal to the pontine nuclei and their intermingled fibres.

Blood supply

The pons is supplied mainly by pontine branches from the *basilar artery*, with contributions from the superior cerebellar and anterior inferior cerebellar vessels. Venous return is into the inferior petrosal sinuses and the basilar plexus.

Medulla oblongata

The medulla oblongata is the part of the brainstem between the pons and spinal cord and it extends through the foramen magnum to the level of the atlas. Above the

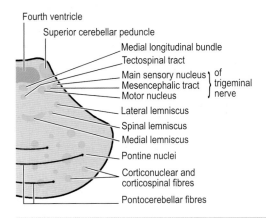

Fig. 7.23   Cross-section of the upper pons.

foramen magnum it is embraced dorsally by the cerebellar hemispheres. The lower end which contains the upward continuation of the central canal of the spinal cord is the 'closed part of the medulla', while the upper end, where the canal comes to the surface as the lower part of the floor of the fourth ventricle, is the 'open part'.

Ventrally (Fig. 7.18) the upper part of the medulla is deeply grooved in the midline, with a bold convexity on either side, the **pyramid**, due to the contained cortico-spinal fibres. Lateral to the pyramid is another convexity, the **olive**, due to the underlying inferior olivary nucleus. Lateral to the olive the lateral surface of the medulla is formed by the *inferior cerebellar peduncle*, which enters the cerebellum medial to and below the middle peduncle.

The sixth, seventh and eighth cranial nerves emerge between the pons and the medulla, the sixth nerve between the pons and the pyramid, the main part of the seventh nerve between the pons and the olive, and the nervus intermedius part of the seventh and the eighth nerve between the pons and the inferior cerebellar peduncle (Fig. 7.15). The rootlets of the ninth, tenth and cranial part of the eleventh nerves emerge lateral to the olive, and those of the twelfth by two small groups of rootlets between the pyramid and the olive (Fig. 7.6).

Dorsally the lower part of the floor of the fourth ventricle forms the upper part of the medulla (Fig. 7.20). Here the roof of the ventricle is ependyma and pia mater. At the lower corner of the diamond-shaped floor the hypoglossal trigone is adjacent to the midline, with the vagal trigone lateral to it. Higher up and at the lateral corners of the diamond is the vestibular area and the medullary striae (see p. 502).

In the lower or closed part of the medulla, the fourth ventricle has become narrowed to the tiny central canal, and the external dorsal surface shows small elevations, the *gracile* and *cuneate tubercles*, the former being medial to the latter.

Internal structure

Decussation of the pyramids characterizes the lowest part of the medulla, and at a slightly higher level is seen the central decussation of the fibres forming the medial lemnisci (Figs 7.25 and 7.26; see also p. 502).

Most of the nuclei of the medulla are below the floor of the fourth ventricle. The hypoglossal nucleus underlies the hypoglossal trigone and the dorsal nucleus of the vagus is under the vagal trigone; more laterally are the nucleus of the tractus solitarius and the spinal nucleus and tract of the trigeminal nerve. At a deeper level is the nucleus ambiguus, with the inferior olivary nucleus ventrally.

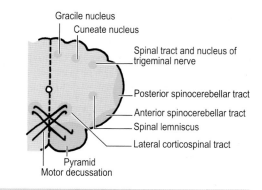

Fig. 7.25   Cross-section of the lower part of the closed medulla.

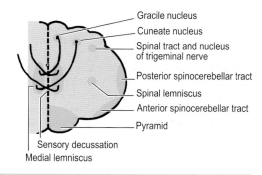

Fig. 7.26   Cross-section of the upper part of the closed medulla.

The **hypoglossal nucleus** adjacent to the midline gives rise to the hypoglossal nerve fibres which pass ventrally to emerge between the pyramid and olive (Fig. 7.27).

Lateral to the hypoglossal nucleus is the **dorsal nucleus of the vagus**, which contains motor cell bodies for cardiac and visceral muscle and the cells of secretomotor fibres for glands. The corresponding afferent cell bodies lie in the **nucleus of the tractus solitarius** lateral to the dorsal nucleus; the afferent fibres form the *tract* which is almost surrounded by cells of the nucleus. The upper part of the nucleus receives taste fibres from the chorda tympani (nervus intermedius part of the facial nerve), glossopharyngeal nerve and internal laryngeal branch of the vagus. The rest of the nucleus receives many afferent fibres of the glossopharyngeal and vagus nerves from thoracic and abdominal viscera, as well as those from the baroreceptors and chemoreceptors of the carotid sinus and carotid body and the aortic arch and aortic bodies (see pp 355 and 198). It has extensive connections

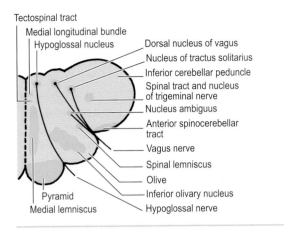

Tectospinal tract
Medial longitudinal bundle
Hypoglossal nucleus
Dorsal nucleus of vagus
Nucleus of tractus solitarius
Inferior cerebellar peduncle
Spinal tract and nucleus of trigeminal nerve
Nucleus ambiguus
Anterior spinocerebellar tract
Vagus nerve
Spinal lemniscus
Olive
Inferior olivary nucleus
Hypoglossal nerve
Pyramid
Medial lemniscus

Fig. 7.27   Cross-section of the open part of the medulla.

with the dorsal nucleus of the vagus and the reticular formation.

The **nucleus ambiguus** contains motor cell bodies for the skeletal muscle of the larynx, soft palate, pharynx and upper oesophagus, all distributed by branches of the vagus except for the supply to stylopharyngeus which is by the glossopharyngeal nerve. The cells of the upper end of the nucleus send their fibres to the glossopharyngeal nerve, while those from the lower part send theirs to the cranial root of the accessory nerve, which joins the vagus below the skull.

The **spinal nucleus** (and tract) **of the trigeminal nerve** continues down into the medulla from the pons (see p. 498) and lies lateral to the nucleus of the tractus solitarius. It receives somatic sensory fibres from the glossopharyngeal and vagus nerves.

The **inferior olivary nucleus** is a crenated C-shaped lamina of grey matter, in section like a wrinkled sac with an open end facing towards the opposite inferior cerebellar peduncle. Its fibres (*olivocerebellar*) decussate across the midline to enter this peduncle (see p. 505).

The cochlear and vestibular nuclei extend into the medullary part of the floor of the fourth ventricle, and have been considered with the pons.

The **gracile** and **cuneate nuclei** underlie the corresponding tubercles of the dorsal surface of the lower medulla. They contain the cell bodies on which the incoming fibres of the gracile and cuneate tracts of the spinal cord terminate, and the nuclei give origin to the medial lemniscus (see p. 502).

The medullary **reticular formation**, continuous upwards with that of the pons and downwards into the spinal cord at the lateral margin of the central grey matter, is the irregular mass of cells and fibres occupying much of the area between the inferior olivary nucleus and the floor of the fourth ventricle, intermingled with other cell groups and tracts. Although they are not anatomically demonstrable as distinct nuclei, pools of neurons of the reticular formation ('centres') are functionally associated with vasoconstrictor, cardioaccelerator, cardiopressor, inspiratory and expiratory effects.

Although anatomically such a diffuse entity, the brainstem reticular formation is responsible for the 'alert' or 'wakeful' component of consciousness. It plays a part in the control of many other functions, including motor activity (as part of the extrapyramidal system, see p. 509), sensory function (by modifying sensory input to the thalamus), autonomic activity (via the medullary centres), circadian rhythms and endocrine secretion (via the hypothalamus). Among its connections are those from the cerebral cortex of the same side via the corpus striatum (see p. 477), from the opposite cerebellar hemisphere via the dentate nucleus (see p. 505), and from the hypothalamus and other components of the limbic system (see p. 484). Some reticular formation cells give origin to the reticulospinal tracts (see p. 511) which are part of the extrapyramidal system, and others receive spinoreticular fibres which are part of the pain pathway from the spinal cord (see p. 510). Other cells provide communications between cranial nerve nuclei, e.g. for eye movements, the corneal reflex, swallowing, etc. However, the conduction paths of the reticular formation are difficult to define, complex, and partly crossed and uncrossed; unilateral stimulation often results in bilateral responses.

Blood supply

The medulla is supplied ventrally by branches of the *vertebral* and *basilar arteries*, and laterally and dorsally by the *posterior inferior cerebellar artery* (Fig. 7.19). The *anterior spinal* branch of the vertebral gives penetrating branches which supply the region next to the midline, i.e. the part containing the pyramid, medial lemniscus and hypoglossal nucleus. Damage to these vessels produces the *medial medullary syndrome*—paralysis of the tongue on the same side and hemiplegia with loss of touch and kinaesthetic sense on the opposite side. Damage to the vessels of the lateral and dorsal part gives rise to the *lateral medullary syndrome* or 'syndrome of the posterior inferior cerebellar artery'. The loss of nucleus ambiguus function paralyses the vocal fold and palatal and pharyngeal muscles on that side, giving dysphonia and dysphagia. Loss of the uncrossed spinal tract of the trigeminal and of the crossed spinal lemniscus results in loss of pain and temperature sensation on the same side of the face and opposite side of the body.

There will also be a Horner's syndrome (see p. 423) on the ipsilateral side due to interruption of descending hypothalamospinal fibres of the sympathetic pathway. Involvement of the vestibular nuclei causes vertigo and nystagmus with nausea and vomiting.

The veins drain dorsally to the occipital sinus and ventrally into the basilar plexus of veins and the inferior petrosal sinus. The medullary veins communicate with the spinal veins.

Brainstem tracts

Some tracts in the brainstem begin from cell groups therein, but most are passing through from the rest of the brain to the spinal cord or vice versa. The most important of the long *descending tracts* are the cortico-nuclear and corticospinal fibres concerned with voluntary movement, supplemented for posture and coordination of movement by reticulospinal and vestibulospinal tracts which begin in the brainstem. The main *ascending tracts* are the medial lemniscus for fine touch and kinaesthetic sensations, beginning in the medulla, and the spinal lemniscus and spinoreticulothalamic fibres for pain, temperature and crude touch, beginning in the cord and brainstem.

Descending tracts

Cells in layer V of the sensorimotor area MsI (see pp 481 and 483) give rise to **corticospinal** (pyramidal) and **corticonuclear fibres**. However, only 40% of such fibres come from this motor area (though they appear to be the ones that matter most); the remainder come from widely scattered areas of the cortex and not just other parts of the frontal lobes. They pass through the corona radiata, and the corticonuclear fibres then run down through the genu of the internal capsule into the brainstem. Some will go straight to the oculomotor and trochlear nuclei, and the others collect in the most medial part of the central two-thirds of the crus of the midbrain. From there they run down to reach the motor nuclei of the rest of the brainstem. Cranial nerve nuclei which send their fibres to skeletal muscle are mostly bilaterally innervated (i.e. from the cortex of both hemispheres, although there are individual variations). The most important exception is the lower part of the facial nucleus, which is only supplied by the opposite cortex.

The corticospinal fibres lie in the anterior two-thirds of the posterior limb of the internal capsule. Continuing down to the brainstem, they occupy the central and lateral parts of the central two-thirds of the crus of the midbrain peduncle, with the 'arm' fibres medial to the 'leg' fibres. In the pons the fibres become broken up into small bundles among the pontine nuclei. Passing on to the medulla the bundles collect into a single large mass forming the bulging pyramid adjacent to the midline. Each pyramid contains about 1 million nerve fibres of which 700 000 are small and myelinated (1–4 µm diameter). In the lowest part of the medulla 75–90% of the fibres cross to the opposite side in the *pyramidal decussation* to form the *lateral corticospinal tract* of the cord (see p. 510). Some of the decussating fibres may be seen on the surface. The few uncrossed fibres continue downwards as the *anterior corticospinal tract*, but they also eventually cross in the spinal cord, where all fibres end in the anterior horn (see p. 511).

After arising from many areas of all four lobes of the cortex, **corticopontine fibres** pass through the internal capsule to the crus of the midbrain peduncle. Fronto-pontine fibres occupy the anterior limb of the capsule and the medial one-sixth of the crus; temporo-, parieto- and occipitopontine fibres occupy the retrolentiform part of the capsule and the lateral one-sixth of the crus. All end by synapsing with cells of the pontine nuclei (see p. 497) whose axons decussate to form the ponto-cerebellar fibres of the middle cerebellar peduncle. This is one of the pathways by which the cerebral cortex communicates with the cerebellar cortex.

The superior cerebellar peduncles (see p. 505) enter the midbrain tegmentum and decussate at the level of the inferior colliculi on their way to the red nuclei (at superior colliculus level), whose efferent fibres form the *rubrospinal tracts* which immediately decussate. Just dorsal to this is the similar decussation of the *tectospinal tracts*.

The **medial longitudinal bundle** lies immediately ventral to the grey matter round the aqueduct, and remains adjacent to the midline at lower levels. It extends from the upper border of the midbrain to the upper cervical part of the spinal cord. It links the vestibular nuclei with the oculomotor, trochlear, abducent, spinal accessory and reticular nuclei, to help coordinate head and eye movements as required for fixation of the gaze and maintaining equilibrium.

The **lateral** and **medial reticulospinal tracts** arise from the medullary and pontine parts of the reticular formation. They are rather ill-defined in the brainstem, and their fibres become largely mixed with corticospinal fibres in the spinal cord. The **lateral** and **medial vestibulospinal tracts** originate from the vestibular nuclei. All these extra-pyramidal tracts end in the anterior horn (see p. 511).

Hypothalamospinal fibres from the hypothalamus run in the region of the spinal lemniscus to sympathetic and parasympathetic neurons in the thoracolumbar and sacral lateral horns (see p. 511).

Ascending tracts

The **medial lemniscus**, the main ascending pathway of the brainstem for touch and its associated sensations (see p. 509), begins in the lower medulla, formed by the axons of the gracile and cuneate nuclei of the opposite side which have crossed (as *internal arcuate fibres*) in the *sensory decussation*. At first the medial lemniscus lies longitudinally adjacent to the midline, but as it passes up through the pons and midbrain it deviates laterally before reaching the thalamus. On its upward path it is joined by the **trigeminal lemniscus**, fibres from the main sensory and spinal nuclei of the trigeminal nerve.

The **spinal lemniscus** is the upward continuation of the lateral spinothalamic (anterolateral) tract of the cord (pain, temperature and crude touch; see p. 509). It lies near the middle of the lateral part of the medulla, and runs up the brainstem at first lateral and then dorsal to the medial lemniscus. It quickly becomes very much smaller, since most of its fibres end in the reticular formation rather than continuing all the way to the thalamus.

The **lateral lemniscus** is formed by the upgoing fibres of the *trapezoid body*, the name given to transversely decussating fibres from the cochlear nuclei at the ponto-medullary junction. Some of the fibres of this lemniscus terminate on cells of the inferior colliculus for auditory reflexes, while the majority relay in the medial geniculate body for passage via the internal capsule to the auditory area of the cerebral cortex. Both the trapezoid body and lateral lemniscus contain cell stations which make connections with the extraocular and spinal accessory nuclei via the medial longitudinal bundle to help coordinate audiovisual reflexes involving the head and neck.

The **anterior** and **posterior spinocerebellar tracts** lie at the lateral margin of the lower medulla. The posterior tract enters the inferior cerebellar peduncle but the anterior tract continues up the lateral part of the brainstem to enter the superior peduncle.

Fourth ventricle

The aqueduct within the midbrain is continuous below with the fourth ventricle, which lies behind the pons and the upper medulla. The dorsal aspects of these parts of the brainstem form the diamond-shaped floor. The roof, or posterior wall, is projected backwards, like that of a tent lying on its side, and is covered by the cerebellum (Fig. 7.6). Hence the cavity of the ventricle is triangular in sagittal section. The caudal part of each lateral boundary is formed by the gracile and cuneate tubercles and the inferior cerebellar peduncle (Fig. 7.20); the cranial part is formed by the superior cerebellar peduncle. A thin sheet of white matter, the *superior medullary vellum*, stretched between the superior cerebellar peduncles, forms the cranial part of the roof. The caudal part of the roof is mostly devoid of neural tissue, and is formed only by ependyma and pia mater. This part of the roof is perforated by a midline slit, the **median aperture** (foramen of Magendie), by which CSF escapes into the cerebellomedullary cistern. The cavity is prolonged laterally as a narrow **lateral recess** behind and around the inferior cerebellar peduncle. The narrow, tubular lateral recess has a patent extremity, the **lateral aperture** (foramen of Luschka), which opens anteriorly, just behind the eighth nerve, into the pontine cistern (Figs 7.11 and 7.18). Through these three apertures (one median and two lateral) the CSF escapes from the ventricular system into the subarachnoid space for absorption by the arachnoid villi. These are the only exits from the system and if blocked, e.g. following meningitis, hydrocephalus results.

The **choroid plexus** of the fourth ventricle is a small T-shaped structure which indents the medullary part of the roof. It receives its blood supply from a branch of the posterior inferior cerebellar artery, which enters through the lateral aperture on each side and passes medially to meet its fellow, and the two turn down towards the median aperture making the vertical part of the T double. The veins from the plexus drain back into the occipital sinus.

The floor of the fourth ventricle is known as the *rhomboid fossa* (Fig. 7.20). The upper boundaries are the superior cerebellar peduncles, the lower are formed by the gracile and cuneate tubercles and their underlying nuclei and, above them, by the inferior cerebellar peduncles. A midline groove, the *median sulcus*, runs from the aperture of the aqueduct of the midbrain above to the commencement of the central canal below. On each side of the groove the floor is symmetrical.

The pontine part of the floor is characterized by an elevation adjacent to the median sulcus, the *facial colliculus*, formed by recurving fibres of the facial nerve over the underlying abducent nucleus. At its widest part, the floor is crossed transversely by glistening white fibres, the *medullary striae*. They are aberrant fibres from pontine nuclei, which emerge from the median sulcus and run transversely into the inferior peduncle. At the lateral angle of the floor, spanning the lower pons and upper medulla, is the *vestibular area*, overlying the vestibular nuclei.

The medullary part of the floor is smaller than the pontine part. On each side, from the inferior angle, a faint groove passes up towards the vestibular area, dividing the floor on each side into two small triangular regions. The medial one, with its apex down, is the *hypoglossal trigone*, overlying the twelfth nerve nucleus; the lateral triangle, apex upwards, is the *vagal trigone*, overlying the dorsal nucleus of the vagus.

Cerebrospinal fluid

Cerebrospinal fluid (CSF) is largely produced by the choroid plexuses of the lateral third and fourth ventricles, but about 30% comes from other brain capillaries and seeps into the system via the extracellular fluid. The total volume of CSF is about 130 mL (at a pressure of approximately 130 mm of water), of which about 30 mL are within the ventricular system and 100 mL in the subarachnoid space (75 mL in the spinal part and 25 mL in the cranial part). The total production is over 500 mL per day, but there is constant circulation and resorption which takes place mainly through the arachnoid granulations (see p. 457). There is also some drainage through the cribriform plate of the ethmoid bone in the anterior cranial fossa (see p. 465) into the tissues of the nose and so into the cervical lymphatics. Changes in arterial pressure have little effect on CSF pressure, but increases in venous pressure, with the accompanying distension of veins and venous sinuses within the skull, are quickly reflected in CSF pressure rises.

The CSF provides a protective buffer for neural tissue and a waterbath in which the brain can float, thus effectively reducing the 1500 g weight of the brain to 50 g. It is also an important pathway for the removal of brain metabolites; there is no 'brain–CSF barrier', but the ependymal cells of the ventricles, which cover the choroid plexuses, have selective transport mechanisms and tight junctions between adjacent cells that provide a 'blood–CSF barrier' (similar to the blood–brain barrier; see p. 491).

Summary of cranial nerve nuclei

Oculomotor nerve nuclei

Two motor.
Somatic efferent: oculomotor nucleus in midbrain level with superior colliculi, for superior, medial and inferior rectus, inferior oblique and levator palpebrae superioris.
General visceral efferent: Edinger–Westphal, or accessory oculomotor nucleus, cranial to somatic part, for sphincter pupillae and ciliary body, via ciliary ganglion.

Trochlear nerve nucleus

Somatic efferent: trochlear nucleus in midbrain level with inferior colliculi, for superior oblique.

Trigeminal nerve nuclei

One motor and three sensory.
Branchial efferent: motor nucleus of trigeminal in upper pons, for mastication muscles, mylohyoid and tensor palati.
Somatic afferent: three sensory nuclei of trigeminal, continuous throughout the brainstem and extending into upper spinal cord. Mesencephalic nucleus in midbrain, for proprioception from muscles of mastication, face, tongue and orbit. Main sensory nucleus in upper pons, lateral to motor nucleus, for touch from trigeminal area. Spinal nucleus in lower pons, medulla and upper cervical spinal cord, for pain and temperature from trigeminal area; also receives afferent fibres from glossopharyngeal and vagus nerves.

Abducens nerve nucleus

Somatic efferent: abducent nucleus in pons deep to facial colliculus in floor of fourth ventricle, for lateral rectus.

Facial nerve nuclei

Two motor and one sensory.
Branchial efferent: facial nerve nucleus in pons. *General visceral efferent*: superior salivary nucleus adjacent to facial nucleus, secretomotor to pterygopalatine and submandibular ganglia, mainly for lacrimal and salivary secretion. *Special visceral afferent*: nucleus of tractus solitarius, lateral to dorsal nucleus of vagus in upper medulla, for taste fibres of chorda tympani from tongue and of greater petrosal nerve from soft palate.

Vestibulocochlear nerve nuclei

Six sensory.
Special somatic afferent: two cochlear nuclei in inferior cerebellar peduncle, for hearing.
Special somatic afferent: four vestibular nuclei in pons and medulla, in lateral angle of floor of fourth ventricle, for equilibrium.

Glossopharyngeal nerve nuclei

Two motor and two sensory.
Branchial efferent: nucleus ambiguus in upper medulla, for stylopharyngeus. *General visceral efferent*: inferior salivary nucleus in lower pons, secretomotor to otic ganglion for parotid secretion.
Special visceral afferent: nucleus of tractus solitarius, lateral to dorsal nucleus of vagus in upper medulla, for taste fibres from posterior third of tongue and for

baroreceptors of carotid sinus and chemoreceptors of carotid body; *somatic afferent*: spinal nucleus of trigeminal nerve for ordinary sensation from mucous membrane of tongue, palate, pharynx and tonsil.

Vagus nerve nuclei

Two motor and two sensory.

Branchial efferent: nucleus ambiguus in upper medulla, for skeletal muscle of pharynx and upper oesophagus, and for cricothyroid. *Special visceral efferent*: dorsal motor nucleus of vagus in upper medulla, for cardiac muscle and visceral muscle of thoracic and abdominal viscera.

Special visceral afferent: nucleus of tractus solitarius, lateral to dorsal nucleus of vagus in upper medulla, for afferent fibres from heart, lungs and abdominal viscera, for baroreceptors of aortic arch and chemoreceptors of aortic bodies, and taste fibres from epiglottis; *somatic afferent*: spinal nucleus of trigeminal nerve, for skin of external acoustic meatus and auricle, and mucous membrane of pharynx and larynx.

Accessory nerve nuclei

Two motor.

Branchial efferent: nucleus ambiguus in upper medulla, for cranial part, fibres joining vagus for skeletal muscle of palate and larynx.

Branchial efferent: anterior horn cells of upper five or six cervical segments of spinal cord, for spinal part, for sternocleidomastoid and trapezius.

Hypoglossal nucleus

Somatic efferent: hypoglossal nucleus in upper medulla, for muscles of tongue.

PART THREE

Cerebellum

The cerebellum accounts for about 10% of the total weight of the brain and occupies the posterior cranial fossa. It consists of two *hemispheres* united in the midline by the *vermis* (Fig. 7.28). Three *peduncles* connect each hemisphere to the three parts of the brainstem (Fig. 7.20). The superior peduncle enters the midbrain, the middle peduncle consists of the transverse fibres of the pons and the inferior peduncle connects with the medulla. The ventral surface of the vermis lies on the superior medullary velum and the roof of the medullary part of the fourth ventricle.

The cerebellum is bounded posteriorly by a convex border that lies below the attached margin of the tentorium cerebelli. From this border the superior surface slopes concavely upwards, in conformity with the shape of the tentorium. The posteroinferior surface is boldly convex below the posterior border and occupies the concavity of the occipital bone.

The surface of the cerebellum is indented by fine slitlike *sulci*, between which lie more or less parallel folds or *folia*. In the main the folia and sulci lie transversely from side to side across the whole extent of the cerebellum.

A well-marked groove, the *horizontal fissure* (of no functional significance), extends around the posterolateral border of each hemisphere and divides the cerebellum into superior and inferior halves. On the superior surface, is a much shallower groove, the *primary fissure*. The hemispheres consist of a small *anterior lobe* on the superior surface in front of the primary fissure and a large *posterior lobe* comprising the rest of the hemisphere behind the primary fissure (Fig. 7.28). The *tonsil*

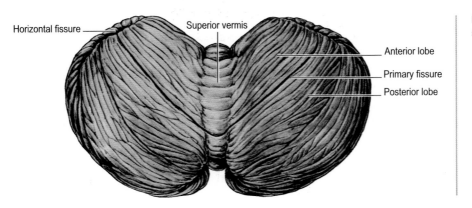

Fig. 7.28 Cerebellum: superior aspect.

Horizontal fissure — Superior vermis — Anterior lobe — Primary fissure — Posterior lobe

is a roughly spherical lobule on the inferior aspect of the posterior lobe. The tonsil may be displaced down through the foramen magnum in conditions of severe raised intracranial pressure or in congenital craniovertebral and hindbrain malformations.

The vermis consists of superior and inferior parts. The superior vermis forms a ridge between the hemispheres (anterior lobe) on the superior surface. Its anterior part, the lingula, lies in contact with the superior medullary velum (Fig. 7.29). On the inferior surface of the posterior lobe there is a deep groove, the vallecula, between the hemispheres. The inferior vermis lies in the groove and consists of the *tuber vermis, pyramid, uvula* and *nodule*. The nodule lies on the roof of the fourth ventricle and projecting laterally from each side of the nodule is a slender band of white matter whose bulbous extremity, capped with grey matter, can be seen from in front, lying in the angle between cerebellum and pons. This is the *flocculus*; the choroid plexus of the fourth ventricle projects just below it (Fig. 7.18). The two flocculi and the nodule form the *flocculonodular lobe*.

In functional terms the cerebellum is divided into a corpus cerebelli (which has afferents from the spinal cord and trigeminal nuclei, and inputs from the pontine nuclei) and a flocculonodular lobe (which, with the lingula, has connections with the vestibular nuclei). Lesions of the latter part lead to disturbances of equilibrium with no alteration of spinal reflexes. The anterior lobe and the pyramid are the main recipients of spinal and trigeminal afferents. Lesions of this part cause disturbances of postural mechanisms with increased muscle reflexes. Cerebropontine connections are relayed by the pontine nuclei via the middle peduncle to the posterior lobe, tuber vermis and uvula. Lesions of these regions result in hypotonia, diminished or pendulum muscle jerks,

intention tremor, clumsy movements and nystagmus (oscillatory movement of the eye).

The essential function of the cerebellum is the co-ordination of movement. Cerebellar lesions do not cause paralysis, but disturbances of movement and balance.

Like the cerebrum, the cerebellum is surfaced with a cortex of grey matter, with the white matter internal. Unlike the cerebral cortex, the cerebellar cortex consists of three layers. Embedded within the white matter are four pairs of nuclei. The most lateral, the *dentate nucleus*, is the largest. It forms a crenated crescent, resembling the inferior olivary nucleus in the medulla, open towards the superior peduncle. Its main connections are cerebro-pontocerebellar, and its efferent fibres leave the hilum and pass to the contralateral red nucleus, thalamus and cerebral cortex.

Cerebellar peduncles and connections

The superior and middle peduncles are simple; the inferior peduncle contains a great mixture of fibres.

The **superior peduncle** contains efferent fibres, passing from the dentate nucleus to the red nucleus, thalamus and cortex of the opposite side. It also contains the afferent anterior spinocerebellar tract, and tectocerebellar fibres from the midbrain.

The **middle peduncle** contains afferent fibres from the pontine nuclei of the opposite side.

The **inferior peduncle** contains the efferent cerebello-vestibular tract and the afferent vestibulocerebellar tract, both connected to the vestibular nuclei of the same side. It also contains the afferent posterior spinocerebellar and cuneocerebellar tracts (the latter consisting of proprioception fibres from the upper limb), and the olivocerebellar tract from the olivary nuclei of the opposite side.

Fig. 7.29 Sagittal section of the cerebellum.

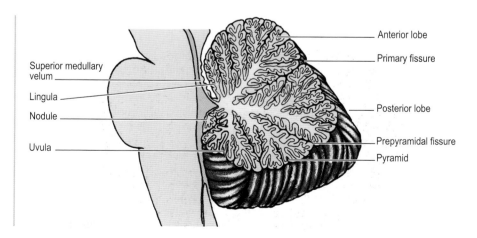

Superior medullary velum

Lingula

Nodule

Uvula

Anterior lobe

Primary fissure

Posterior lobe

Prepyramidal fissure

Pyramid

Blood supply

Two arteries supply the large convex posteroinferior surface and one artery supplies the small upper surface of each cerebellar hemisphere. They anastomose with each other on the cerebellar surface, but their perforating branches into the cerebellum are, as elsewhere in the nervous system, end arteries.

The **posterior inferior cerebellar artery** is one of the most tortuous arteries in the body, and is the largest branch of the vertebral artery. It arises ventrally from the vertebral artery, near the lower end of the olive, and spirals back around the medulla below the hypoglossal rootlets and then between the rootlets of the glosso-pharyngeal and vagus nerves. It supplies the choroid plexus of the fourth ventricle and is distributed to the inferior vermis and the back of the cerebellar hemispheres. It supplies, in passing, the adjacent part of the medulla as described on page 500.

The **anterior inferior cerebellar artery** arises from the basilar artery at the lower part of the pons and passes back on the inferior surface of the cerebellar hemisphere, supplying this surface and the adjacent flocculus. It may give rise to the labyrinthine artery if it has not arisen from the basilar.

The **superior cerebellar artery** arises near the termination of the basilar and passes laterally to wind around the cerebral peduncle below the fourth nerve. It is distributed over the superior surface of the cerebellum.

Venous drainage is from the surface of the cerebellum into the nearest available venous sinus of the dura mater. Thus the superior and posterior surfaces drain into the straight and transverse sinuses, inferior surfaces into the inferior petrosal, sigmoid and occipital sinuses.

PART **FOUR**

Spinal cord

The spinal cord, or spinal medulla, is a cylinder, somewhat flattened from front to back, whose lower end tapers into a cone. Ventrally it possesses a deep midline groove, the *anterior median fissure*, and dorsally it shows a shallow *posterior median sulcus*, from which a *posterior median septum* of neuroglia extends into its substance.

In the fetus the spinal cord extends to the lower limit of the spinal dura mater at the level of S2 vertebra. The spinal dura remains attached at this level throughout life, but the spinal cord becomes relatively shorter, which is to say that the bony spinal column and the dura mater grow more rapidly than the spinal cord. Thus at birth the conus medullaris lies opposite L3 vertebra and does not reach its permanent level opposite L1 or L2 until about the age of 20 years. The spinal nerve roots, especially those of the lumbar and sacral segments, thus come to slope more and more steeply downwards.

The spinal cord possesses two symmetrical enlargements which occupy the segments of the limb plexuses: as the **cervical enlargement** (C5 to T1) for the brachial plexus and the **lumbosacral enlargement** (L2 to S3) for the lumbar and sacral plexuses. Their levels measured by vertebrae are, of course, quite different; the cervical enlargement is approximately opposite vertebrae C3 to T1, but the lumbosacral extends only from T9 to L1. Both enlargements are due to the greatly increased mass of motor cells in the anterior horns of grey matter in these situations.

The spinal meninges have been described on page 471.

Spinal nerve roots

The **anterior** and **posterior roots** of the spinal nerves unite within the intervertebral foramina. Within the subarachnoid space the nerve roots are attached to the spinal cord each by a series of *rootlets*. Each anterior root is formed by three or four rootlets which emerge irregularly along the anterolateral surface of the spinal cord. Each posterior root is formed by several rootlets, attached vertically to the posterolateral surface of the cord. A short distance from the cord the rootlets are combined into a single root (see Fig. 6.111, p. 471). The anterior and posterior roots pass from the cord to their appropriate intervertebral foramina, where each evaginates the dura mater separately before uniting to form the mixed spinal nerve. The **ganglion** on the posterior nerve root lies in the intervertebral foramen, within the tubular evagination of dura and arachnoid immediately proximal to the point of union of anterior and posterior nerve roots. However, the posterior root ganglia of cervical nerves lie partly lateral to the intervertebral foramina, behind and in contact with the vertebral artery (see Fig. 6.109, p. 469). For all levels from C1 to L1 vertebrae the anterior and posterior nerve roots pass in front of and behind the denticulate ligament respectively, and evaginate the dura mater between the denticulations (see Fig. 6.111, p. 471). In conformity with the shortness of the spinal cord, the lower a nerve root the more steeply it slopes down to the intervertebral foramen. The upper cervical roots are horizontal, the upper thoracic roots first slope down to their point of evagination of the meninges only to become kinked upwards at an angle to reach their foramen (Fig. 7.30). Below L1 vertebra the roots pass almost vertically downwards through the subarachnoid space, forming the

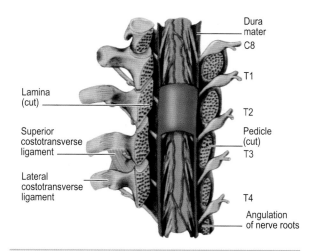

Fig. 7.30   Upper thoracic spinal nerve roots, from behind, showing the upward angulation of the roots as they emerge from the spinal theca.

cauda equina. The *filum terminale* (pia mater, see p. 471) extends down from the tip of the conus medullaris among the nerve roots of the cauda.

The roots of the **spinal part of the accessory nerve** emerge from the lateral surface of the upper five or six segments of the cord, behind the denticulate ligament. They unite into a single trunk which passes upwards through the foramen magnum into the cranium to join the cranial root (see Fig. 6.109, p. 469).

Internal structure

The spinal cord consists of a central mass of **grey matter** (cell bodies), in the form of a vertically grooved column surrounding the central canal, enclosed in a cylindrical mass of **white matter** (fibres) (Fig. 7.31). It is almost divided into two halves by the anterior median fissure and the posterior median septum. The septum extends forwards as far as the *grey commissure* (the central limb of the H in cross-section) which connects the grey matter of the right and left halves of the cord, and contains the *central canal*. This is the tiny downward continuation of the cavity of the fourth ventricle and like it lined by ependyma. It extends into the upper few millimetres of the filum terminale. The anterior fissure does not completely separate the white matter—a narrow *white commissure* lies anterior to the grey. On account of the shape of the grey matter and the attachment of nerve roots, the grey and white matter of the right and left halves is divisible into *anterior*, *lateral* and *posterior* parts, referred to as *horns* for the grey matter and *columns* for the white matter.

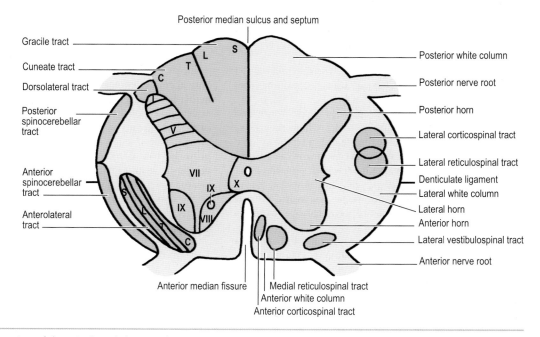

Fig. 7.31   Cross-section of the spinal cord showing the main tracts and laminae of grey matter. The small medial vestibulospinal tract (not shown) lies close to the anterior median fissure.

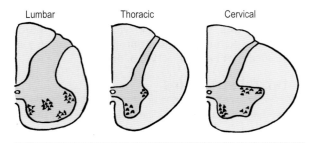

Fig. 7.32 Cross-section of the spinal cord in the lumbar, thoracic and cervical regions.

The shapes of the grey horns and white columns in sections enables the three regions to be distinguished (Fig. 7.32). The anterior grey horns are largest in the cervical and lumbar regions and the posterior white columns largest in the cervical regions.

Grey matter

The **posterior horn** stretches to the surface of the cord, but the **anterior horn** falls short of it. The cervical and lumbosacral enlargements are due to a great increase in the number of anterior horn cells, to provide fibres for the great nerve plexuses. The more *medial* anterior horn cells are concerned with the innervation of *trunk* musculature, with the more *lateral* cells supplying the *limbs*. The more *ventral* cells of the lateral group supply *proximal* limb muscles, and the more *dorsal* cells innervate the more *distal* limb muscles.

Between the limb enlargements, from *segments T1 to L2*, there is a small **lateral horn**, containing preganglionic *sympathetic* cell bodies (see Fig. 1.13C, p. 19). Their axons pass out in the anterior nerve roots and enter the spinal nerves from T1 to L2 which they leave in the white rami communicantes passing to the sympathetic trunk (see p. 21). A similar group of cells forms the small lateral horn in *sacral segments 2–4*; these are preganglionic *parasympathetic* cell bodies whose axons leave in those sacral anterior nerve roots and emerge distally from the sacral nerves as pelvic splanchnic nerves (see p. 292).

The cells of the grey matter in each half of the cord lie in specific functional groups or laminae, designated by the Roman numerals I to X (Fig. 7.31). Among the more important cell groups in the various laminae are those of lamina II which constitute the gelatinous substance; the cells of lamina V are a main source of anterolateral tract (spinothalamic and spinoreticular) fibres; lamina VII contains in its medial part the thoracic nucleus and laterally the thoracolumbar (sympathetic) and sacral

(parasympathetic) lateral horn cells; other cells of lamina VII, together with those of lamina VIII, are interneurons involved in coordinating motor activity and projecting to lamina IX; lamina IX contains the α and γ motor neurons which innervate skeletal muscle.

White matter

In each half of the cord the **posterior white column** lies between the posterior median septum and the posterior grey horn. It is wholly occupied by the ascending fibres of the gracile and cuneate tracts, the pathways for touch and some associated sensations (see below).

The rest of the white matter forms the **lateral** and **anterior white columns**, the emerging anterior nerve roots providing a convenient dividing line between the two. Both these columns contain long ascending and descending tracts. In addition, short intersegmental fibres run up and down adjacent to the central grey matter, forming communications between segments. Except in the posterior columns, there is much intermingling of fibres and there are no sharp boundaries to tracts.

Afferent pathways

There are three possible destinations for all incoming fibres: the cortex of the opposite cerebral hemisphere, via thalamic relay, for conscious sensation; the cerebellum, for muscular coordination; and the brainstem or spinal cord, for reflex actions.

As a guiding principle it is usually stated that afferent impulses are conveyed to the cerebral cortex by three groups of neurons. While this is a convenient concept and accurate enough for the main long-fibre components, it takes no account of the vast numbers of short interneurons in the neuronal pathways. The cell bodies of the first group of neurons (*first neurons* or *first order neurons*) lie outside the central nervous system: in the posterior root ganglia of spinal nerves or the equivalent ganglia of cranial nerves. The cell bodies of the *second neurons* are in the spinal cord or brainstem, and those of the *third neurons* are in the thalamus.

Efferent pathways

For the control of the skeletal muscles supplied by spinal nerves, two main systems of neurons are involved. One can be called the *direct corticospinal pathway*, consisting essentially of two groups of neurons. The cell bodies of the first are in the cerebral cortex, and their fibres extend through the internal capsule and brainstem to the anterior horn cells of the cord; these are the corticospinal fibres. The corresponding corticonuclear fibres go to the motor nuclei of cranial nerves. These fibres (often called *pyramidal*; see p. 501) with their cortical cell bodies are known as the **upper motor neurons**. The second neurons are the anterior horn cells and their axons which end as the motor endplates on skeletal muscle fibres. These neurons (and those of the motor nuclei of cranial nerves) are called the **lower motor neurons**. This sequence does not take account of interneurons that participate in this pathway.

The other system involves a whole series of neurons on the way to anterior horn cells. For example, cortical cells may send their axons to pontine nuclei, from which fibres run to the cerebellum which in turn may project to the red, reticular, vestibular and olivary nuclei, all of which can communicate with the same anterior horn cells as pyramidal fibres. Other cortical fibres run to the basal nuclei (corpus striatum) and thalamus, with projections from them to the red, reticular and subthalamic nuclei and the substantia nigra. These brainstem nuclei can also be activated by reflex sensory pathways (e.g. light and sound). From some of these brainstem groups fibres descend to synapse with the same anterior horn cells that have received corticospinal fibres. None of these fibres has passed through the pyramid of the medulla (hence the name **extrapyramidal**) and because none has passed uninterruptedly from the cortex to anterior horn cells they are also called *indirect corticospinal pathways*.

Ascending tracts

The most important ascending tracts fall into two groups. Those in the lateral and anterior white columns are concerned with pain (nociception) and temperature sensations, crude touch, and the sensations of itch, tickle and sexual orgasm. Here also are tracts to the cerebellum, for muscular coordination.

The posterior white column is wholly occupied by ascending fibres of the **gracile** and **cuneate tracts**. They are concerned with light (discriminative) touch, vibration sense, proprioception (muscle joint or kinaesthetic sense, the conscious appreciation of body position and movement), and the sense of fullness of the bladder and rectum. Their cell bodies lie in the posterior root ganglia of spinal nerves, and the fibres enter the cord from the medial side of the posterior nerve roots. Some branches from the incoming posterior root fibres are short and take part in segmental reflex arcs, but it is the long ascending fibres that form the tracts. The fibres from the lowest parts of the body lie nearest the midline, and incoming fibres are added progressively laterally, i.e. the column is laminated. In this way fibres from the perineum, lower limb and lower trunk form the gracile tract, and those from the upper trunk and upper limb

form the more lateral cuneate tract. The two tracts end in the lower part of the medulla by synapsing with the cells of the gracile and cuneate nuclei respectively. The axons from these (second order) nuclei immediately decussate to form the medial lemniscus which runs through the brainstem to the thalamus. After relay there, the axons of the third group of neurons pass via the internal capsule to area SmI of the cerebral cortex.

Tests for the types of sensation transmitted by the posterior columns include those for light touch, such as gentle stroking of the skin with the fingers or cotton wool. Position sense is tested by the examiner passively moving finger or great toe joints with the patient's eyes closed, to see whether the direction of movement can be appreciated. If upper limb position sense is disturbed the patient cannot hold the outstretched limb and fingers steady with the eyes closed, nor perform the finger-nose test accurately. Similarly, lower limb position sense is tested by standing upright with the feet together and then closing the eyes. Without the visual sense to relate to the environment, there will be loss of balance with the eyes shut (*Romberg's sign*) if there is loss of this posterior column sense. For the same reason there will be difficulty with walking in the dark, or keeping the balance when washing the face with the eyes shut. These are examples of sensory ataxia. (With labyrinthine lesions or cerebellar ataxia there is little difference whether the eyes are open or shut.) Vibration sense, which is also conducted by the posterior columns, is tested by applying a vibrating tuning fork (128 Hz, middle C) to a bony prominence such as the lateral malleolus.

The two-point discrimination test is important because it not only involves the peripheral and central pathways, but the cerebral cortex as well. Two points 3 mm apart are normally distinguishable on the finger pads. Stereognostic sense (ability to appreciate the size and shape of objects in the hand) also requires the intact cortex.

The main ascending tract of the lateral and anterior white columns is the **anterolateral tract**. It is concerned with pain (nociception) and temperature sensations, crude touch, and the sensations of itch, tickle and sexual orgasm. It is a large bundle lying in front of the level of attachment of the denticulate ligament and extending into the anterior white column.

The pain fibres in peripheral nerves are of two kinds: small C fibres, unmyelinated and slow-conducting, for the dull, aching type of pain ('slow pain'), and Aδ fibres, thinly myelinated and fast-conducting, for the sharp, pricking type of pain ('fast pain') and also for temperature conduction (see p. 11). On entering the cord from the posterior nerve roots (cell bodies in the posterior root ganglia), the fibres form the **dorsolateral tract** (of Lissauer), and run up or down at the tip of the posterior horn for one or two segments before synapsing with cells of the **gelatinous substance**.

Through various interneurons in the region of the tip of the posterior horn, the impulses are passed on to the second order neurons whose fibres, mainly from cell bodies in laminae I and V, cross to the opposite side of the cord in front of the central canal and form the anterolateral tract. Although in the lowest part of the cord the fibres from any one segment cross transversely, the crossing takes place more and more obliquely at higher levels so that in the cervical region the decussation may require the height of four or five segments before it is completed. The track is laminated, with fibres subserving impulses from the sacral segments lying most laterally, while those from cervical segments are the most deeply placed (Fig. 7.31). The fibres for crude touch occupy the more medial part of the tract, and have crossed less obliquely than the pain and temperature fibres.

Only about 10% of anterolateral tract fibres pass directly to the thalamus, via the spinal lemniscus of the brainstem (see p. 502). The other 90% of fibres synapse with cells of the brainstem reticular formation, where there may be multiple connections before the onward transmission of impulses to the thalamus; this is the *spinoreticulothalamic pathway*. Third order neurons then pass from the thalamus to the sensory cortex.

The extent to which the anterolateral tract cells are stimulated to pass on impulses from spinal cord to brain is subject to control and modification by both spinal and supraspinal influences. For example, fibres from mechanoreceptors, apart from passing up in the posterior white columns, give branches that synapse with anterolateral tract cells, and their effect is to inhibit transmission from the tract cells ('closing the gate' to nociceptive impulses); hence the effectiveness of rubbing an injured part to reduce the pain. Other inhibitory influences come from supraspinal levels via the reticular formation, so that cerebral and limbic activities such as memory, past experience and emotion can depress or even completely suppress pain, as happens in battle casualties who may feel no pain at the time of severe injury. Certain areas of the nervous system (e.g. the thalamus, limbic system and gelatinous substance) produce their own morphine-like substances (endogenous opioid peptides), such as endorphins and enkephalins, which can inhibit pain by binding to receptors on parts of the pain pathway. Some of these substances may act as modulators of the transmission of pain impulses or may themselves be transmitters. They do not pass the blood–brain barrier and so cannot be given intravenously.

The common tests for pain sensation are by pinprick for superficial pain (spinothalamic) and by pinching or squeezing a fold of skin, muscle or tendon, such as the Achilles tendon, for deep pain (spinoreticulothalamic). Temperature sense can be estimated by touching the skin with a cold metal object and a test-tube of warm water.

In the operation of *anterolateral cordotomy* for the relief of persistent pain, the lateral part of the anterolateral tract is severed to block upward transmission through the tract. The knife is inserted in front of the line of attachment of the denticulate ligament, so avoiding damage to the corticospinal tract which lies behind this. Because of the obliquity of the crossing of fibres, the cut must be made several segments above the desired level of analgesia. Although cordotomy should theoretically result in permanent pain relief, it rarely lasts for more than a few months (2 years at the most), an example of the plasticity of the nervous system and the way new pathways can develop.

The **anterior** and **posterior spinocerebellar tracts** convey unconscious proprioceptive information from cord to cerebellum. Some fibres from posterior root ganglion cells enter the cord through the posterior roots and synapse with the cells of the *thoracic nucleus* (Clarke's column) at the base of the posterior horn in all the thoracic and first two lumbar segments of the cord. The axons of these cells move to the lateral edge of their own side of the cord as the posterior spinocerebellar tract, which runs up into the medulla to reach the cerebellum by the inferior peduncle. Other incoming fibres synapse with other posterior horn cells in lumbar and sacral segments; these give rise to fibres which mostly cross to the opposite side to form the anterior spinocerebellar tract, at the margin of the cord behind the anterior nerve roots. It takes an unexpectedly long route to the cerebellum, running through the brainstem to the midbrain and doubling back into the superior cerebellar peduncle of the opposite side. From cervical nerves, impulses destined for the cerebellum do not travel by these spinocerebellar tracts (since the thoracic nucleus does not extend above T1 level); they reach the *accessory cuneate nucleus* in the medulla by the cuneate tract, and thence by the cuneocerebellar tract enter the inferior peduncle.

A number of ill-defined groups of ascending fibres such as spinoreticular, spino-olivary, spinotectal, spinovestibular and spinospinal provide further connections between the cord and brainstem and between different parts of the cord for reflex activities.

Descending tracts

The **lateral corticospinal tract** is formed from the motor decussation in the lower medulla, and the cortical origin of the fibres has already been described (see p. 501). The tract lies in the lateral white column at a level behind the attachment of the denticulate ligament. Almost all (98%) of the fibres end by synapsing with interneurons which in turn project to the α and γ motor neurons of the anterior horn. (The 2% of fibres that synapse directly with motor neurons are those originating from the giant Betz cells.) About 55% of corticospinal fibres end on cervical and first thoracic anterior horn cells, i.e. more than half of the corticospinal fibres are concerned with the motor supply of the upper limb, leaving 20% for trunk supply and 25% for the lower limb. Because of the medullary decussation, the cerebral cortex of one side controls the muscles of the contralateral side.

The relatively unimportant uncrossed fibres in the medulla continue as the **anterior corticospinal tract**, adjacent to the anterior median fissure, but it goes no lower than the upper thoracic part of the cord. The fibres eventually cross to the opposite anterior horn.

The most important extrapyramidal tracts are the reticulospinal and the vestibulospinal tracts. The **lateral reticulospinal tract** arises from the medullary part of the reticular formation and the fibres run down in the lateral white column, largely intermingled with corticospinal fibres. Its influence on anterior horn cells is facilitatory. The **medial reticulospinal tract** comes from cells in the pontine reticular formation and descends in the anterior white column, to have an inhibitory action on motor neurons. The **lateral vestibulospinal tract** arises from the lateral vestibular nucleus of the medulla and runs down the cord approximately through the anterior nerve root region. The reticulo- and vestibulospinal fibres synapse with interneurons which in turn project to the motor neurons. The vestibulospinal tract primarily affects trunk and limb girdle musculature, and is of great importance for posture and balance.

The **hypothalamospinal tract** provides a link between the hypothalamus and the thoracolumbar (sympathetic) and sacral (parasympathetic) lateral horn cells. The fibres lie adjacent to the lateral horn.

Clinically it is important to distinguish between upper and lower motor neuron lesions. The lower motor neuron lesion produces a flaccid paralysis of muscles with decreased or absent reflexes. Spastic paralysis with increased relexes, clonus and an extensor plantar response (see p. 18) is regarded as evidence of an upper motor neuron lesion. However, it should be noted that a pure pyramidal lesion (rare, but possible from a lesion confined to the pyramid of the medulla) produces a flaccid paralysis. The reason why pyramidal lesions induce spasticity is that there is concomitant involvement of extrapyramidal pathways as well; the responsiveness of the α motor neurons is altered, possibly because they have been released from the inhibition normally exerted by supraspinal levels. Since most of the pyramidal tract is intermingled with extrapyramidal fibres, most pyramidal lesions present as spasticity.

In the brainstem and spinal cord the motor tracts of each side are quite close together so that a single lesion may easily affect both sides, but in the hemispheres the tracts of the two sides are much farther apart and so unlikely to be damaged together. A single lesion that does affect both sides together is a parasagittal meningioma pressing on the leg areas of both hemispheres.

Blood supply

The spinal cord is supplied by the (single) anterior and (right and left) posterior spinal arteries which descend from the level of the foramen magnum and form three longitudinal channels from which branches enter the cord. They are supplemented at variable levels by anastomoses with a variable number of radicular arteries.

The **anterior spinal artery** is a midline vessel that lies on the anterior median fissure (Fig. 7.19). It is formed at the foramen magnum by the union of the two anterior spinal branches, each given off by a vertebral artery above the foramen magnum. Although it is usually larger than the posterior spinal arteries and runs the whole length of the cord, the anterior spinal may become so small in places, especially in the thoracic region, that it may be considered absent. It supplies the whole cord anterior to the posterior grey columns, i.e. the lateral grey and white columns and the anterior grey and white columns of both sides.

The **posterior spinal artery** on each side arises from the posterior inferior cerebellar or vertebral artery above the foramen magnum. It is usually double, forming longitudinal trunks that run through and behind the posterior nerve rootlets for the whole length of the cord. There is some anastomosis between the vessels of the two sides, with rather scanty connections with the anterior spinal artery, except at the lower end of the cord where there are often good anastomoses. The posterior spinal artery supplies the grey and white posterior columns of its own side.

The **radicular arteries** make highly important contributions to reinforce the longitudinal trunks. At one stage during embryonic development every segment of the cord receives a radicular vessel on both sides; they enter through the intervertebral foramina as spinal arteries to penetrate the meninges and run along the nerve roots, and are derived from various parent vessels depending on the level: vertebral, costocervical, posterior intercostals, lumbar, and lateral sacral. As fetal growth proceeds, most of the radicular arteries disappear. Those that remain form anastomoses with the anterior and posterior spinal arteries. Their most characteristic feature is their variability in number and position; blood from them may flow up and/or down the cord. Because of the frequently small size of the longitudinal trunks, considerable lengths of the cord may be largely dependent on the radicular supply. The largest of the feeder vessels, the *arteria radicularis magna* (of Adamkiewicz), usually arises from a lower intercostal or upper lumbar branch of the aorta on the left side. Operations on the vertebral column or adjacent structures (such as aortic aneurysms) that interfere with the parent stem of a major radicular vessel may seriously impair the blood supply to the cord.

The anastomotic connections on the surface of the cord (deep to the pia mater) between the anterior and posterior spinal and radicular vessels provide very small pial arteries that are capable of supplying peripheral areas of the cord. This is important with respect to the lateral corticospinal and anterolateral tracts whose fibres are laminated, with sacral fibres lying nearest to the surface. Interference with the anterior spinal supply may eliminate the function of these tracts, except for the sacral fibres which remain supplied by the pial vessels ('sacral sparing').

The *spinal veins* form loose-knit plexuses in which there are an anterior and a posterior midline longitudinal vein, and on each side a pair of longitudinal veins posterior to the anterior and posterior nerve roots. These veins drain to the internal vertebral venous plexus, and thence via the external vertebral venous plexus to the segmental veins: vertebral in the neck; azygos in the thorax; lumbar in the lumbar region; and lateral sacral in the sacral region. At the foramen magnum they communicate with the veins of the medulla.

Spinal cord injury

In *complete transection* there is loss of movement and all sensation below the level of the injured segment. The paralysis, which is at first flaccid, becomes spastic after a few weeks, and bladder and rectal sphincter control is lost, although reflex emptying will occur provided the sacral part of the cord is intact. In lesions above T10 segment there is no effective cough because of abdominal and lower intercostal paralysis. In suspected transection, examination for sensation in the perianal skin will establish whether or not there is conduction throughout the length of the cord. Perianal pinprick will also establish whether the anal reflex is intact (see p. 18).

In *hemisection* (Brown-Séquard syndrome) there is paralysis and loss of touch and kinaesthetic sense below the level of the lesion on the same side (lateral corticospinal tract and posterior column interruption), and loss of pain and temperature sensation on the opposite side (because of interruption of the crossed anterolateral tract).

In the *central cord syndrome*, commonly due to a crush injury (without transection) following a sudden hyperextension of the cervical spine, there is flaccid (lower motor neuron) paralysis and loss of pain and temperature sensation in the upper limbs (due to anterior horn damage and interruption of the more deeply placed cervical fibres of the anterolateral tracts). The lower limbs may show spasticity if the lumbar fibres of the lateral corticospinal tract are involved (the sacral fibres are more superficial).

In the *anterior spinal artery syndrome*, the posterior white columns (and therefore touch sensation) remain intact, but most of the rest of the cord below the level of the lesion is affected with loss of all motor and sensory functions, except perhaps for the 'sacral sparing' mentioned above.

PART FIVE

Development of the spinal cord and brainstem nuclei

The cranial end of the neural tube (see p. 25) becomes dilated into vesicles and its walls thicken by proliferation of cells; the cerebral hemispheres, brainstem and cerebellum are so developed. More caudally the neural tube enlarges in a simple manner by proliferation of cells, to form the spinal cord. In all regions these proliferating cells arrange themselves regularly in functional groups. Despite the apparent random arrangement of the nuclei in the brainstem, there is a logical pattern to their positions which can be correlated with the rather simpler disposition of cell groups in the spinal cord that results from this development.

Spinal cord

The central canal, relatively very large at first, is not rounded in cross-section, but is projected laterally into a groove on the inner wall of the spinal cord, as the **sulcus limitans** (Fig. 7.33A). The developing nerve cells of the spinal cord form thickenings dorsal and ventral to the sulcus, the alar lamina and basal lamina respectively. The **alar lamina** contains sensory (afferent) cells and the **basal lamina** contains motor (efferent) cells. In each lamina the cells are of two kinds; near the sulcus limitans lie the autonomic (**visceral**) cells, while further away lie the body wall and limb (**somatic**) cells.

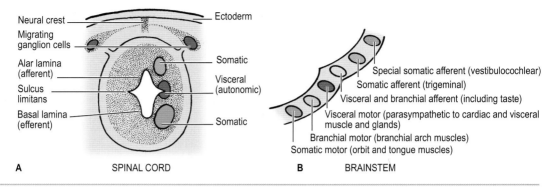

Fig. 7.33 Cell groups of the spinal cord and brainstem: **A** in the developing spinal cord, where motor cells are ventral and sensory cells dorsal with autonomic cells in between; **B** in the brainstem (floor of the fourth ventricle) which resembles an 'opened out' spinal cord, with motor cells now lying medially and sensory cells laterally with autonomic cells in between.

Brainstem

A similar arrangement holds in the brainstem as in the spinal cord. But here a third type of cell appears in each lamina, namely the **branchial** afferent and efferent cells of cranial nerves supplying the derivatives of the branchial arches (see p. 26). These branchial cells theoretically lie between the autonomic and somatic cells of each lamina. They are the central cell stations of the nerves of the pharyngeal arches (trigeminal, facial, glossopharyngeal and vagus). The branchial group or column is also known as the *special visceral* group, and the visceral as the *general visceral* group.

In the **fourth ventricle** the central canal is opened out, and basal and alar laminae lie roughly in the same plane; the dorsal afferent and ventral efferent cells thus become lateral and medial respectively (Fig. 7.33B). The order of the cell groups is similar, but migration of certain cell groups (neurobiotaxis) in the developing brainstem alters, in places, the relatively simple basic arrangement.

Motor nuclei of the brainstem

The motor nuclei are arranged according to the type of muscle they supply (Fig. 7.34). The ordinary skeletal muscle of the head (*somatic* muscle) consists of the muscles of the orbit and the muscles of the tongue. In line with the anterior horn cells of the spinal cord, the brainstem nuclei supplying these muscles (*oculomotor*, *trochlear*, *abducent* and *hypoglossal*) lie near the midline ventral to the 'central canal' (i.e. ventral to the aqueduct or floor of the fourth ventricle as the case may be).

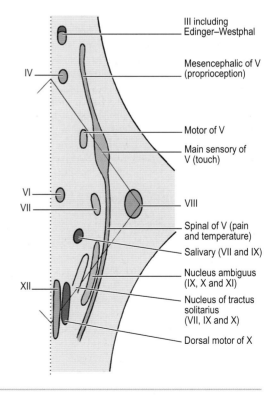

Fig. 7.34 Sites of cranial nerve nuclei in the right half of the brainstem. See text for the correlation between the information in this diagram with that in Figure 7.33B.

Developed from the region of the embryonic pharynx are the striated muscles of mastication, of the face, and of the pharynx and larynx. Their motor nuclei (*branchial*) lie slightly more laterally: the *motor nucleus of the trigeminal nerve*, the *facial nucleus* and the *nucleus ambiguus* (for the glossopharyngeal and vagus nerves and the cranial part of the accessory nerve).

The *general visceral efferent*, parasympathetic motor, nuclei are represented by the *accessory oculomotor* (Edinger–Westphal) *nucleus*, the *salivary nucleus* (whose secretomotor fibres join the nervus intermedius part of the facial nerve and the glossopharyngeal nerve), and the *dorsal motor nucleus of the vagus* (for cardiac muscle and the smooth muscle of the alimentary tract). These nuclei migrate medially.

Afferent nuclei of the brainstem

These follow the general plan outlined above, and from medial to lateral form *visceral*, *branchial* and *somatic* afferent groups (the reverse order of the motor efferent columns). But unlike the motor groups, which consist of interrupted columns forming individual nuclei, each of these afferent 'columns' consists of a single nuclear mass (Fig. 7.34). The *general visceral* and *branchial* (*special visceral*) afferent cell groups merge as the *nucleus of the tractus solitarius*, which receives not only taste fibres from the facial, glossopharyngeal and vagus nerves but also afferents from the heart, lungs and other viscera from the vagus nerve. The *somatic* afferent column is represented by the *sensory nuclei of the trigeminal nerve*, really one elongated nucleus extending throughout the brainstem to the upper spinal cord. The brainstem has a fourth column of sensory nuclei that has no counterpart in the spinal cord; these are the *cochlear* and *vestibular nuclei* of the vestibulocochlear nerve, and they form a *special somatic* afferent group lying farthest laterally.

PART SIX

Summary of cranial nerves

The first two cranial nerves are not really nerves, but rather outdrawn parts of the central nervous system. Only the peripheral bipolar nerve cells correspond with an ordinary nerve.

Olfactory nerve (i)

The first neurons are bipolar cells in the neuroepithelium in the upper part of the nose. Their central processes gather themselves into about 20 olfactory nerve filaments (for each olfactory nerve) that pass through foramina in the cribriform plate of the ethmoid bone, piercing the dura and arachnoid mater of the anterior cranial fossa. They enter the olfactory bulb from where the central processes of the second neuron pass in the olfactory tract to the region of the anterior perforated substance, from where they proceed laterally to the uncus and medially to parts of the limbic system. The arrangement is unique and 'primitive': the second order neuron directly activates the conscious cortex, bypassing the thalamus. Other olfactory pathways, by polysynaptic junctions, activate hypothalamic and brainstem nuclei (as is the case with all sensory pathways) for visceral and somatic effects, distinct from conscious appreciation.

Optic nerve (ii)

The rods and cones, near the choroidal surface of the retina, activate the **bipolar cells** of the retina; these are the first sensory neurons. Their central processes synapse on the large **ganglion cells** that lie on the vitreous surface of the retina. The central processes of these second neurons emerge from the back of the eyeball as the optic nerve surrounded by CSF and the meninges. The optic nerve enters the middle cranial fossa through the optic canal and passes to the chiasma, where the nasal fibres from each retina decussate, above the pituitary gland. From the chiasma the optic tract passes around the midbrain (cerebral peduncle) to three destinations: (1) the lateral geniculate body (thalamus) for relay to the visual cortex; (2) the pretectal nuclei for pupil constriction to light; and (3) the superior colliculus for body reflexes to light.

From the lateral geniculate body fibres of the third neurons of the visual pathway pass through the retrolentiform part of the internal capsule and backwards by the optic radiation to the visual (striate) cortex on the medial surface of the occipital lobe.

Oculomotor nerve (iii)

The nerve emerges from the midbrain on the medial surface of the base of the cerebral peduncle above the pons. It passes forwards and laterally between the posterior cerebral and superior cerebellar branches of the basilar artery, then below and lateral to the posterior communicating artery and just below the free margin of the tentorium cerebelli. It enters the roof of the cavernous sinus and continues forward in the lateral wall of the sinus. It slants down medial to the trochlear nerve and the ophthalmic branch of the trigeminal (see Fig. 6.104, p. 462). At the anterior pole of the cavernous sinus it splits into a superior and an inferior division which enter the tendinous ring at the medial end of the superior orbital fissure.

The **superior division** supplies superior rectus and levator palpebrae superioris. While in the lateral wall of the cavernous sinus, the oculomotor nerve picks up sympathetic fibres from the internal carotid plexus; they supply the smooth muscle part of levator (their loss accounts for the partial ptosis characteristic of Horner's syndrome; see p. 423).

The **inferior division** supplies medial rectus, inferior rectus and inferior oblique. The parasympathetic fibres in the oculomotor nerve pass from the branch to the inferior oblique to the ciliary ganglion, where they relay. Postganglionic fibres then run in the short ciliary nerves to supply the sphincter pupillae (for pupil constriction) and the ciliary muscle (for accommodation).

Trochlear nerve (iv)

The nerve crosses the midline within the midbrain and emerges from its dorsal aspect below the inferior colliculus. It then passes around the cerebral peduncle between the posterior cerebral and superior cerebellar arteries. Clinging to the undersurface of the free edge of the tentorium cerebelli it is directed thereby to the roof of the cavernous sinus, which it enters and then runs forwards in the lateral wall, first below the third nerve, and then above it at the anterior end of the sinus. It enters the superior orbital fissure lateral to the tendinous ring and passes medially over levator palpebrae superioris to supply superior oblique.

Trigeminal nerve (v)

The fibres of the trigeminal nerve that reach the main sensory and spinal nuclei come from cell bodies in the **trigeminal ganglion**. Together with the direct fibres that reach the mesencephalic nucleus they form a single, large, sensory root attached to the ventral aspect of the pons, well lateral and just above centre. The motor root emerges separately, slightly cranial and medial to its companion. Together they pass, below the tentorium cerebelli, to the mouth of the trigeminal cave (see Fig. 6.105, p. 463). This is a tubular prolongation of arachnoid-lined fibrous dura mater around the sensory and motor roots, and it crosses the upper border of the petrous bone near its apex, i.e. it passes from the posterior into the middle cranial fossa. The dural sheath containing the two nerve roots passes forwards, peeling apart the two layers of dura that floor the middle cranial fossa, just lateral to where the same two layers peel apart to enclose the cavernous sinus. The sensory root then expands into the large, flat, crescentic trigeminal ganglion;

the motor root remains separate below the ganglion. The dural sheath obliterates the subarachnoid space by fusing with the pia mater halfway along the ganglion. The posterior half of the ganglion and both roots are thus bathed in CSF. The anterior half of the ganglion, beyond the subarachnoid space, gives off its three sensory divisions, ophthalmic, maxillary and mandibular. The first two pass forwards in the lateral wall of the cavernous sinus; they are wholly sensory. The mandibular division, likewise sensory, passes straight down from the lower part of the ganglion to the foramen ovale. The motor root also passes through the foramen ovale and joins the mandibular division just outside the skull to form the (mixed) mandibular nerve.

Ophthalmic nerve

As the ophthalmic division runs forward in the lateral wall of the cavernous sinus below the trochlear nerve it picks up sympathetic fibres from the cavernous plexus; these are for the dilator pupillae muscle. At the anterior end of the sinus it gives off a *meningeal branch* and divides into three branches that pass through the superior orbital fissure: the lacrimal; frontal; and nasociliary nerves.

The **lacrimal nerve**, passing lateral to the tendinous ring, proceeds along the upper part of the lateral wall of the orbit, there picking up a secretomotor branch from the zygomatic nerve which it gives to the lacrimal gland. It is sensory to a small area of skin at the lateral end of the upper eyelid and to both palpebral and ocular surfaces of the corresponding conjunctiva.

The **frontal nerve** traverses the superior orbital fissure just lateral to the tendinous ring. A large nerve, it runs forward above levator palpebrae superioris, and behind the superior orbital margin it divides into a large supra-orbital and a small supratrochlear branch. The *supra-orbital nerve* supplies the frontal sinus, notches or perforates the orbital margin, supplies the upper eyelid (skin and both surfaces of conjunctiva), all the forehead except a central strip, and the frontal scalp up to the vertex. The *supratrochlear nerve* supplies the upper lid and conjunctiva and a narrow strip of forehead skin alongside the midline.

The **nasociliary nerve** is sensory to the whole eyeball, to the paranasal sinuses along the medial wall of the orbit, to some mucous membrane of the nasal cavity and to the skin of the external nose. It carries hitch-hiking sympathetic fibres for the dilator pupillae muscle.

The nerve runs through the tendinous ring between the two divisions of the oculomotor nerve. It passes forwards and medially above the optic nerve, below superior rectus and superior oblique. At the medial wall of the orbit it passes into the anterior ethmoidal foramen, between the orbital plate of the ethmoid bone and the frontal bone, as the *anterior ethmoidal nerve*. Running in the roof of the middle and anterior ethmoidal air cells, it reaches the lateral edge of the cribriform plate, beneath the dura of the anterior cranial fossa. It then runs forwards and descends through a slit alongside the crista galli into the nose, where it grooves the internal surface of the nasal bone. It supplies the mucous membrane of the anterosuperior part of the lateral wall and septum of the nose, and emerges at the lower margin of the nasal bone as the external nasal nerve, to supply the skin of the ala, tip and vestibule of the nose.

The *infratrochlear nerve* branches off the nasociliary before it the enters the anterior ethmoidal foramen, and continues forward below the trochlea of the superior oblique tendon to supply skin and conjunctiva of the medial end of the upper eyelid and skin over the bridge of the nose.

The *posterior ethmoidal nerve* branches off the nasociliary proximal to the infratrochlear nerve, enters the posterior ethmoidal foramen and supplies the posterior ethmoidal air cells and the adjacent sphenoidal sinus.

In the orbit the nasociliary nerve gives off a communicating branch to the ciliary ganglion and the long ciliary nerves. The *communicating branch* is the sensory root of the ganglion; its fibres pass through the ganglion and via the short ciliary nerves to provide sensory fibres to the eye including the cornea (but not the conjunctiva). The *long ciliary nerves*, usually two, run forward to enter the sclera independently. They carry sympathetic fibres to the dilator pupillae muscle and (like the short ciliary nerves) are also sensory to the eye, including the cornea (but not the conjunctiva).

Maxillary nerve

This nerve runs forward in the lateral wall of the cavernous sinus, below the ophthalmic nerve, gives off a *meningeal branch* and passes through the foramen rotundum into the upper part of the pterygopalatine fossa. It has a short course in the fossa, and turns laterally as it passes through the inferior orbital fissure to enter the orbit as the infraorbital nerve.

Two *ganglionic branches* connect the maxillary nerve and the pterygopalatine ganglion. Most of the fibres of the trunk pass through the ganglion into its branches, where they mingle with the postganglionic fibres of the greater petrosal and deep petrosal nerves (i.e. fibres of the nerve of the pterygoid canal; see p. 384). The branches of the ganglion are nasal (nasopalatine and posterior superior nasal), palatine (greater and lesser), pharyngeal and orbital. Postganglionic parasympathetic fibres

destined for the lacrimal gland pass into the maxillary nerve and enter its zygomatic branch.

The **nasopalatine nerve** (long sphenopalatine) enters the sphenopalatine foramen, crosses the roof of the nose and slopes down along the nasal septum, supplying its posteroinferior part. It goes through the incisive canal and fossa into the hard palate and supplies the gum behind the two incisor teeth.

The **posterior superior nasal nerves** (lateral and medial) enter the sphenopalatine foramen and supply the posterosuperior part of the lateral wall of the nose and nasal septum respectively.

The **greater palatine nerve** runs down in the greater palatine canal, between the perpendicular plate of the palatine bone and the body of the maxilla. Multiple branches supply the posteroinferior part of the lateral wall of the nose and the adjacent floor of the nose. The nerve emerges from the greater palatine foramen and supplies all the hard palate except the incisor gum.

The **lesser palatine nerves** also descend through the greater palatine canal but emerge from the lesser palatine foramina in the palatine bone and pass back to supply the mucous membrane on both surfaces of the soft palate and on the tonsil.

The **pharyngeal nerve** passes back through the palato-vaginal canal to supply the mucous membrane of the nasopharynx.

The **zygomatic nerve** arises from the maxillary in the pterygopalatine fossa and passes through the inferior orbital fissure into the orbit, where it divides into two branches. The *zygomaticofacial nerve* perforates the facial surface of the zygomatic bone and supplies the skin over the bone. The *zygomaticotemporal nerve* perforates the temporal surface of the zygomatic bone, pierces the temporalis fascia, and supplies skin above the zygomatic arch. Through a connection between this nerve and the lacrimal nerve in the orbit secretomotor fibres are transmitted to the lacrimal gland.

The **posterior superior alveolar nerve** (posterior superior dental) arises from the maxillary in the pterygopalatine fossa and divides into two or three nerves which emerge through the pterygomaxillary fissure. They run in or on the posterior wall of the maxilla to supply the maxillary sinus, upper molar teeth and the adjacent gum of the vestibule.

The **infraorbital nerve** passes forward along the floor of the orbit, sinks into a groove, then enters a canal and emerges on the face through the infraorbital foramen. It supplies the maxillary sinus directly and via the *middle superior alveolar* and *anterior superior alveolar nerves*. The former nerve supplies the premolar teeth and the latter nerve supplies the canine and the two incisors, and reaches the anterior inferior part of the lateral wall and the adjacent floor of the nose. It ends on the nasal septum. All the alveolar nerves link up to form a dental plexus; the middle nerve may be absent.

Emerging on the face the infraorbital nerve lies between levator labii superioris and levator anguli oris. It has many communications with branches of the facial nerve. It supplies both surfaces of the lower lid conjunctiva, as well as the skin of the lower lid, mid-face, nose and the skin and mucous membrane of the whole upper lip and adjacent gum.

Mandibular nerve

The mandibular division passes down through the foramen ovale, accompanied by the small motor root of the trigeminal nerve. Just below the foramen they join to form the mixed nerve in the infratemporal fossa, between the upper head of the lateral pterygoid and tensor palati, where the otic ganglion lies on the medial aspect of the nerve. The nerve soon divides into a small anterior and a large posterior branch.

There are two branches from the short trunk before it divides. A *meningeal branch* (nervus spinosus) passes up through the foramen ovale or through the foramen spinosum.

The **nerve to the medial pterygoid** sinks into the deep surface of the muscle. It has a branch that passes through the otic ganglion and supplies the two tensor muscles, tensor palati and tensor tympani.

Anterior division. The branches are all motor except one. They are as follows.

The **nerve to the lateral pterygoid**; this may be double, one to each head.

Two **deep temporal nerves** pass above the upper head of the lateral pterygoid and sink into the deep surface of temporalis.

The **nerve to masseter** passes above the upper head of the lateral pterygoid and proceeds laterally through the mandibular notch to sink into masseter. It gives a branch to the mandibular joint.

The **buccal nerve** is the only sensory branch of the anterior division. It emerges between the two heads of the lateral pterygoid and passes down on the lower head to reach the buccinator. It supplies a small area of cheek skin and pierces the buccinator to supply the mucous membrane adherent to the deep surface of the muscle and the vestibular gum of the three mandibular molar teeth. The buccal nerve carries secretomotor fibres from the otic ganglion for mucous glands in the mouth.

Posterior division. The three branches are all sensory except for motor fibres in the inferior alveolar nerve, which pass to its mylohyoid branch.

The **auriculotemporal nerve** has two roots that pass back around the middle meningeal artery. The nerve picks up postganglionic secretomotor fibres from the otic ganglion for the parotid gland. It passes back deep to the neck of the mandible, and gives the major sensory supply to the mandibular joint. It then ascends behind the joint and the superficial temporal vessels, in front of the ear and in contact with the parotid gland to which it gives the secretomotor fibres. The nerve supplies the external acoustic meatus, the external surface of the auricle above this and the skin of the temporal region.

The **inferior alveolar nerve** (inferior dental) passes down deep to the lower head of the lateral pterygoid, on the lateral surface of the medial pterygoid. Lying between the mandible and the sphenomandibular ligament, it enters the mandibular foramen in front of the inferior alveolar artery and vein, after giving off the *nerve to mylohyoid*. This pierces the sphenomandibular ligament and lies on the mylohyoid groove with its accompanying small vessels. The mylohyoid nerve passes forwards below the mylohyoid muscle accompanied by the submental branches of the facial artery and vein. It supplies mylohyoid and the anterior belly of the digastric, and frequently a small area of submental skin.

The inferior alveolar nerve runs forwards in the mandibular canal and supplies the three molars and two premolars. Then it divides into its two terminal branches. The *incisive branch* goes on to supply the canine and both incisors, and overlaps to the opposite central incisor. The *mental nerve* passes from the mental foramen to supply the lower lip (both surfaces) and the adjacent gum. It carries a few fibres from the otic ganglion to the labial glands of the lower lip.

The **lingual nerve** is joined by the chorda tympani (carrying nervus intermedius fibres) about 2 cm below the base of the skull, deep to the lower border of the lateral pterygoid muscle. It curves down on the medial pterygoid in front of the inferior alveolar nerve. It then passes under the free lower border of the superior constrictor and goes forward above the mylohyoid muscle (i.e. in the mouth). It grooves the thin lingual plate of the mandible just below the last molar tooth, and here the nerve is characteristically flat. Dipping down lateral to the submandibular duct, the nerve turns medially below the duct and ascends on hyoglossus to the anterior two-thirds of the tongue, which it supplies with common sensation and taste, the latter mediated by the chorda tympani fibres. The secretomotor fibres of the chorda tympani are given off to the submandibular ganglion, which is suspended from the lingual nerve; they relay in the ganglion for the submandibular gland, and some postganglionic fibres rejoin the lingual nerve for transport to the salivary glands in the floor of the mouth. The lingual nerve supplies all the mucous membrane of the floor of the mouth and the lingual gum.

Abducens nerve (vi)

The nerve emerges at the lower border of the pons, above the pyramid of the medulla. It enters the pontine cistern and turns upwards, between the anterior inferior cerebellar artery and the pons, to pierce the arachnoid and dura mater on the clivus. Running up now between the two layers of the dura on its own, or within the inferior petrosal sinus, it passes over the apex of the petrous temporal bone to enter the cavernous sinus. It passes forwards in the sinus, inferolateral to the internal carotid artery, and reaches the medial end of the superior orbital fissure. It enters the orbit through the tendinous ring to supply lateral rectus.

Facial nerve (vii)

The main facial nerve emerges at the lower border of the pons above the olive.

The nervus intermedius emerges between the pons and the inferior cerebellar peduncle, near the vestibulocochlear nerve. With the main part of the facial nerve it passes laterally in the cerebellopontine angle through the pontine cistern and, with the eighth nerve, they enter the internal acoustic meatus. In the meatus the main part of the facial nerve lies on the upper surface of the eighth nerve, with the nervus intermedius in between. The whole facial nerve passes into the anterosuperior quadrant of the meatus. Running laterally in the petrous bone, above the vestibule of the internal ear, the two parts of the nerve share a common tube of arachnoid and dura mater. The meninges then fuse with the nerves as they merge into a single trunk. Near the middle ear the nerve makes a sharp posterior bend, the geniculum, which is enlarged by the cell bodies of the afferent (taste) fibres to form the **geniculate ganglion**. From here the nerve runs back in the medial wall of the middle ear, above the promontory and just below the bulge of the lateral semicircular canal. It now curves downwards behind the middle ear, deep to the aditus to the antrum, and passes vertically down the facial canal. After shedding all the nervus intermedius fibres, the nerve emerges from the stylomastoid foramen as a purely motor nerve and passes through the parotid gland. The face muscles supplied by the facial nerve receive their proprioceptive supply from the cutaneous nerves of the overlying skin (trigeminal nerve branches).

The *intracranial branches* of the facial nerve that arise within the petrous bone include the greater petrosal nerve, the nerve to stapedius and the chorda tympani.

The **greater petrosal nerve**, consisting of nervus intermedius fibres, leaves the ganglion and travels forwards and medially at a 45° slant through the petrous bone. It emerges from the anterosuperior surface of the petrous bone and runs forwards in a groove on the bone, between the two layers of the dura mater. Here in the middle cranial fossa it may be pulled on in extradural operations and so cause small haemorrhage or oedema at the geniculate ganglion with consequent pressure on the facial nerve and a temporary facial paresis. The nerve passes beneath the trigeminal ganglion and reaches the foramen lacerum, where it is joined by the deep petrosal nerve from the sympathetic plexus on the internal carotid artery. The two unite and pass forwards through the pterygoid canal. This **nerve of the pterygoid canal** emerges into the pterygopalatine fossa and enters the pterygopalatine ganglion. Here the secretomotor fibres relay. Taste fibres from the soft palate and sympathetic fibres pass straight through the ganglion. Postganglionic secretomotor fibres are distributed with the branches of the ganglion to the nose, paranasal sinuses, hard and soft palates, and nasopharynx. Lacrimatory postganglionic fibres join the maxillary nerve and enter the orbit in its zygomatic branch.

The **nerve to stapedius** is given off in the facial canal and reaches the muscle by a minute canaliculus.

The **chorda tympani**, consisting of nervus intermedius fibres, leaves the facial nerve in the facial canal 6 mm above the stylomastoid foramen and passes through the posterior wall of the middle ear. It runs forward between the mucous membrane and the tympanic membrane, crossing the neck of the malleus. It leaves through the anterior wall of the middle ear and emerges at the medial end of the petrotympanic fissure. It then grooves the medial side of the spine of the sphenoid and slopes downwards and forwards to join the lingual nerve in the infratemporal fossa. By the lingual nerve its taste fibres are taken to the anterior part of the tongue. Its secretomotor fibres relay in the submandibular ganglion for the submandibular gland and glands in the floor of the mouth cavity.

The *extracranial branches* include the posterior auricular nerve (for the occipital belly of occipitofrontalis), the nerves to the posterior belly of digastric and stylohyoid, and the five groups of branches given off within the parotid gland for the facial muscles and platysma.

Vestibulocochlear nerve (viii)

Cochlear nerve

The receptors for hearing are the hair cells of the spiral organ in the internal ear. The cell bodies of the first neurons are in the **spiral ganglion**, in the base of the bony spiral lamina. Their central processes run along the modiolus of the cochlea and join into many small nerves that pierce dura and arachnoid mater at the base of the modiolus in a spiral pattern, at the anteroinferior quadrant of the internal acoustic meatus. They join together in the subarachnoid space and enter the pontine cistern combined with the vestibular part. Together with the nervus intermedius and the main facial nerve, the vestibulocochlear nerve passes through the cerebello-pontine angle in front of the flocculus of the cerebellum and the lateral aperture of the fourth ventricle. The eighth nerve enters the inferior cerebellar peduncle at the lower border of the pons.

Vestibular nerve

The receptors consist of the hair cells in the maculae of utricle and saccule (for static balance) and the ampullae of the semicircular ducts (for kinetic balance). From the posterosuperior quadrant of the fundus of the internal acoustic meatus emerges the superior division of the vestibular nerve from anterior and lateral semicircular ducts and the utricle. Through the posteroinferior quadrant comes the inferior division of the vestibular nerve from the saccule. Alongside it, through the foramen singulare, its branch emerges from the posterior semicircular duct. Having pierced the fibrous dura and arachnoid mater the upper and lower divisions lie in the internal acoustic meatus and are here together distended into the **vestibular ganglion** by the cell bodies of these first order neurons. From the ganglion the vestibular nerve joins the cochlear nerve and passes through the pontine cistern.

Glossopharyngeal nerve (ix)

The nerve emerges from the surface of the medulla between olive and inferior cerebellar peduncle in a series of rootlets which join to make a single nerve that runs laterally in the pontine cistern and enters the anterior compartment of the jugular foramen. Here it lies lateral to the inferior petrosal sinus, and together they are separated from the vagus and accessory nerves by a septum of fibrous dura mater. The glossopharyngeal nerve has a small *superior ganglion* and a large *inferior ganglion* which deeply notches the inferior border of the petrous bone, just below the internal acoustic meatus. The cell bodies of the nerve's afferent fibres are in these ganglia.

The **tympanic branch** passes into the middle ear through the tympanic canaliculus, between the jugular fossa and the carotid canal, to form the tympanic plexus, from which emerges the lesser petrosal nerve, in the middle cranial fossa. This runs through the foramen ovale to join the otic ganglion for the supply of the parotid gland.

The glossopharyngeal nerve passes laterally between the internal jugular vein and internal carotid artery and then passes forwards between the latter and the external carotid artery. The **nerve to stylopharyngeus**, given off as the nerve winds round the muscle, is the only muscular branch.

The **carotid branch** runs down to innervate the carotid sinus and body.

Pharyngeal branches take part (with the vagus) in forming the pharyngeal plexus; the fibres are afferent.

The glossopharyngeal nerve enters the pharynx between the superior and middle constrictors. The **tonsillar branch** provides afferent fibres for the tonsillar mucosa, and the **lingual branch** conveys common sensation and taste from the posterior part of the tongue, as well as secretomotor fibres for lingual glands.

Vagus nerve (x)

Vagal nerve fibres leave the surface of the medulla in a series of rootlets below those of the glossopharyngeal nerve in the sulcus between olive and inferior cerebellar peduncle. These unite into a single nerve that enters the middle compartment of the jugular foramen, with the accessory nerve, sharing an arachnoid and dural sheath. The vagus has a small **superior ganglion** just above the long **inferior ganglion**, which lies in the jugular fossa below the skull base. The superior ganglion has cell bodies for the auricular branch. The inferior ganglion lodges the cell bodies of all the other sensory fibres in the vagus nerve. The cranial root of the accessory nerve is attached to the vagus just above the inferior ganglion and the accessory nerve gives its nucleus ambiguus fibres to the vagus.

In the neck the vagus lies vertical, like a plumb line, in the carotid sheath, deep in the gutter between the internal/common carotid artery and the internal jugular vein.

The small *meningeal, auricular* and *carotid body branches* are all afferent. The meningeal branch carries C1 and C2 fibres which join the vagus at its exit from the skull.

The **pharyngeal branch** passes between the internal and external carotid arteries and provides both motor and sensory fibres for the pharyngeal plexus. The **superior laryngeal branch** runs deep to the carotids and divides into the *internal laryngeal nerve*, which pierces the thyrohyoid membrane to supply mucosa in the pharynx and larynx, and the *external laryngeal nerve* which runs to cricothyroid. **Cervical cardiac branches**, upper and lower on the right and upper on the left, join the deep part of the cardiac plexus; the lower one on the left joins the superficial part of the plexus.

The **right recurrent laryngeal nerve** hooks under the subclavian artery at the root of the neck and runs up near the tracheo-oesophageal border to pass under the inferior constrictor of the pharynx just behind the cricothyroid joint, to supply muscles of the larynx and laryngeal mucosa of the vocal folds and below; it also supplies cricopharyngeus. The **left recurrent laryngeal nerve** hooks round the ligamentum arteriosum, below the aortic arch and ascends in a groove between the trachea and oesophagus to a corresponding destination. Both recurrent laryngeal nerves give *cardiac branches*.

In the superior mediastinum, the left vagus lies between the left common carotid and subclavian arteries, and not in contact with the trachea; it then crosses the left side of the aortic arch. The right vagus comes into contact with the trachea, posterior to the superior vena cava. Both vagi pass behind the lung roots, contributing branches to the *anterior* and *posterior pulmonary plexuses*. Both vagi then break up into branches that form the **oesophageal plexus**.

From the oesophageal plexus the **anterior** and **posterior vagal trunks** emerge, to enter the abdomen through the oesophageal opening in the diaphragm, and supply the stomach. The anterior vagus gives *hepatic branches* and the posterior vagus *coeliac branches*. Through these branches the vagi supply the foregut and midgut as well as their derivatives, the biliary tract and pancreas.

Accessory nerve (xi)

The **spinal root** of the accessory nerve is formed by fibres from cell bodies (the 'spinal accessory nucleus') in the anterior horn of the upper five or six segments of the cervical cord (mainly 2, 3 and 4). Unlike other anterior horn cell axons, they do not leave the cord via the anterior nerve roots, but emerge as a series of rootlets from the lateral surface of the cord behind the denticulate ligament. Joining together, they form a single nerve that ascends behind the uppermost tooth of the denticulate ligaments to join the **cranial root**. The latter emerges from the medulla as a series of rootlets below those of the vagus between the olive and inferior cerebellar peduncle. The spinal and cranial roots unite and the accessory nerve passes through the middle compartment of the jugular foramen, sharing the same arachnoid and dural sheath as the vagus. Outside the skull the accessory gives all its cranial root fibres to the vagus, and these are distributed by vagal branches to the striated muscle of the soft palate and larynx. The nerve then runs backwards and downwards across the internal jugular vein, as it lies in front of the transverse process of the atlas. The accessory nerve supplies sternocleidomastoid, and passes through its substance to reach the posterior triangle, which it crosses to supply trapezius.

Hypoglossal nerve (xii)

Hypoglossal nerve fibres emerge from the surface of the medulla as a vertical line of rootlets between pyramid and olive. These join into two roots that enter the hypoglossal (anterior condylar) canal in the occipital bone, where they are separated by a flange of fibrous dura mater that sometimes ossifies. They join in the canal and emerge as a single nerve.

The hypoglossal nerve passes downwards between the internal jugular vein and the internal carotid artery, until it is crossed laterally by the occipital artery and its lower sternocleidomastoid branch, as they pass backwards. The nerve then swings forwards crossing (laterally) both carotid arteries and the loop at the commencement of the lingual artery. The nerve and the lingual artery part company as they pass superficial and deep, respectively, to hyoglossus, on their way forwards to the tongue, where the nerve supplies all the muscles of the tongue except palatoglossus.

The branches of the hypoglossal nerve before it reaches the tongue are all derived from C1 nerve fibres that join the hypoglossal at its exit from the skull. A very small *meningeal branch* supplies dura mater in the posterior cranial fossa.

The *superior root of the ansa cervicalis* (formerly descendens hypoglossi) branches off as the hypoglossal nerve curves forwards from between the internal carotid artery and the internal jugular vein. It is joined by the lower root of the ansa cervicalis (formerly the descendens cervicalis) derived from C2 and C3 nerves of the cervical plexus. Together these nerves make the ansa cervicalis. The ansa usually lies on the internal jugular vein under cover of sternocleidomastoid embedded in the anterior wall of the carotid sheath. Its branches supply omohyoid, sternohyoid and sternothyroid.

The *nerve to thyrohyoid* comes off the hypoglossal nerve as it lies on the lingual artery, and the *nerve to geniohyoid* is given off in the mouth, above mylohyoid; this contains the last of the C1 fibres that travel along the hypoglossal nerve.

PART SEVEN

Summary of cranial nerve lesions

Having relatively short courses, the peripheral parts of cranial nerves are not subject to the kind of injuries that commonly afflict peripheral nerves in the limbs. Those most commonly affected by trauma are the first, second, third, sixth and seventh, but tumours, ischaemia of nerve trunks and aneurysms of adjacent vessels are among the more usual afflictions of these and other cranial nerves.

Olfactory nerve

Head injury may tear olfactory nerve filaments passing through the cribriform plate of the ethmoid, especially if a fracture involves this part of the anterior cranial fossa. Such a fracture usually causes leakage of CSF through the nose (CSF rhinorrhoea), from tearing of the meningeal sleeves that ensheathe the olfactory nerve bundles. If all filaments on one side are torn there will be complete anosmia on that side. Test by closing one nostril (with finger pressure) and sniffing familiar substances like coffee or oranges. Most deficiencies of smell are due to affections of nasal mucosa rather than neurological disease. Smell is an essential component of taste, and complaints about lack of taste may be due to loss of smell. Olfactory hallucinations, which are usually unpleasant, arise from the uncus of the temporal lobe (the cortical centre for smell).

Optic nerve

Assessment of the visual fields tests the integrity of the visual pathways from retina to cortex, and lesions at different points along the path give rise to characteristic defects, as illustrated in Figure 7.9. The defects are conventionally described with reference to the visual fields and not to the retina. The numbers below correspond to the sites of the lesions in Figure 7.9A; clinically the most common lesions are at the chiasma (2) and in the optic radiation (4). The visual field defects are indicated in Figure 7.9B.

1. A complete lesion of the left optic nerve gives rise to complete blindness in the left eye.
2. Compression of the optic chiasma, as by a pituitary tumour, causes bitemporal hemianopia (blindness in the temporal half of both visual fields) because the nasal fibres from both retinas are interrupted. This effectively narrows the outer part of each visual field, so that the patient complains of bumping into the sides of a doorway or into people on each side.
3. A lesion of the left optic tract gives a right homonymous hemianopia, due to interruption of fibres from the same (left) sides of both retinas (hence homonymous, meaning same-sided). The field defects are therefore right-sided.
4. A lesion of the lower fibres in the left optic radiation (as from an abscess in the temporal lobe spreading

upwards from the middle ear) causes a right upper quadrantic homonymous hemianopia, because the lower fibres in the optic radiation are from the lower part of the retina.
5. Similar to (4), a lesion of the upper fibres in the left optic radiation (as from a parietal lobe lesion, and in practice very rare) gives a right lower quadrantic homonymous hemianopia.
6. A lesion of the anterior part of the left visual cortex (as from occlusion of the posterior cerebral artery) gives a right homonymous hemianopia similar to the optic tract lesion in (3), but there may be sparing of the macular (central) vision when the most posterior part of the visual cortex at the very tip of the occipital lobe, where macular vision is represented, is (sometimes) supplied by the middle cerebral artery.
7. Traumatic damage to the tip of the left occipital lobe, i.e. to the macular area, gives a right homonymous macular defect.

Oculomotor, trochlear and abducens nerves

Ocular nerve palsies are described on page 419. The major signs are as follows.

Oculomotor nerve: ptosis. When the lid is lifted up, the eye is looking down and out. The diplopia disappears on looking outwards. The pupil is dilated and does not react to light or on accommodation; ptosis with a large pupil thus suggests an oculomotor nerve lesion (but with a small pupil suggests Horner's syndrome; see p. 423).

Trochlear nerve: the eye cannot look down as far as it should when turned in. The head is tilted towards the opposite shoulder to compensate for extorsion.

Abducens nerve: the eye cannot look outwards.

Trigeminal nerve

Affections of the motor part of the fifth nerve, whose fibres run in the mandibular branch, are very unusual. Test for contraction of masseter.

The most common condition affecting the sensory part of the nerve is trigeminal neuralgia (tic doloureux), characterized by pain in the distribution of the maxillary and/or mandibular branches. The ophthalmic branch is rarely involved. With the maxillary nerve affected the pain is usually felt deeply in the face and nose between the mouth and orbit, and with the mandibular nerve from the mouth up to the ear and the temporal region. Compression of the trigeminal nerve adjacent to the pons by contact with a vessel (usually a branch of the basilar artery, such as the superior cerebellar or anterior inferior cerebellar artery) is considered to be a cause of trigeminal neuralgia, and patients resistant to medical therapy have been relieved of their pain surgically by the placement of a pad between the vessel and the nerve. Injection or electrocoagulation of the trigeminal ganglion have also been utilized to abolish the pain.

The afferent side of the corneal reflex (see p. 422) depends on the ciliary branches of the nasociliary part of the ophthalmic nerve. Disappearance of the reflex is often the first sign of a lesion of the ophthalmic nerve; test by gently touching the cornea (not the conjunctiva) with cotton wool.

Facial nerve

Facial nerve paralysis is the most common of all cranial nerve lesions, and the most frequent type is Bell's palsy, a sudden onset of facial paralysis of uncertain aetiology. Paralysis of facial muscles causes asymmetry of the corner of the mouth, flattening of skin folds and inability to close the eye or wrinkle the forehead on the affected side. Test by asking the patient to show the teeth forcibly, screw up the eyes and wrinkle the forehead.

A lesion higher in the facial canal, above the origin of the chorda tympani, will add to the facial paralysis a loss of taste in the anterior part of the tongue. Test by holding the tongue out and applying sweet, sour and salt substances on cotton wool to the sides of the dorsum, asking the patient to point to the appropriate flavour written on a card. The accompanying interference with secretion from the submandibular and sublingual glands is very difficult to detect or test. A lesion higher still, above the origin of the nerve to stapedius, will give hyperacusis.

The above are all lesions of the lower motor neuron (infranuclear). A typical upper motor neuron lesion (supranuclear) paralyses the lower part of the face but not the upper (forehead and orbicularis oculi) because the upper part of the facial nerve nucleus which innervates the upper musculature is supplied by the cerebral cortex of both sides, whereas the lower part innervating the lower face only receives contralateral cortical fibres. However, emotional (as opposed to voluntary) movements of the lower facial muscles, as in smiling and laughing, are still possible with supranuclear lesions (so presumably there must be alternative pathways through the cerebrum).

Vestibulocochlear nerve

Acoustic neuromas on the extracerebral part of the eighth nerve are among the most common intracranial tumours, but other lesions of this nerve are rare. In any loss of hearing, it must be determined whether it is *conduction deafness* from lesions of the external or middle ear, or *nerve deafness* from a cochlear lesion.

The simple tests for hearing involve asking the patient to listen to whispering, the ticking of a watch, and the rubbing together of a thumb and forefinger (with the opposite ear closed by finger pressure on the tragus, and after examining the external acoustic meatus and tympanic membrane with an auroscope). Both ears are similarly tested. The basis of the two common tuning fork tests is that air conduction, which involves the amplifying effect of the ossicles across the middle ear cavity, is better than solid bone conduction. In Weber's test a vibrating tuning fork is placed on the midline of the forehead; in conduction deafness the sound is heard better in the deaf ear, and in nerve deafness it is better in the good ear. In Rinne's test the vibrating fork is held on the mastoid process until the sound is no longer heard and then quickly transferred to the external acoustic meatus; in a normal ear or with nerve deafness the sound will be heard again, but in conduction deafness further sound will not be heard. For more precise information audiometric tests are necessary.

Diseases of the internal ear or its central connections (as in Ménière's disease where there are degenerative changes in the utricle and saccule) form one group of causes of muscular incoordination or ataxia (labyrinthine ataxia; the other varieties of ataxia are cerebellar and sensory; see p. 509). The semicircular ducts of the vestibular apparatus can be tested with the head in different positions by irrigating the external acoustic meatus alternately with warm (44°C; 110°F) and cool (30°C; 86°F) water (caloric tests); this stimulates convection currents in the endolymph causing vertigo (giddiness) and nystagmus (an involuntary oscillatory movement of the eyes, which may be horizontal, vertical or rotatory). Internal ear disease gives an exaggerated response with the head in a particular position, whereas vestibular nerve damage gives an exaggerated response in any head position.

Glossopharyngeal nerve

Isolated glossopharyngeal nerve lesions are extremely rare, as the last four cranial nerves are not often damaged and even if they are, they are commonly affected together (e.g. by a posterior cranial fossa tumour). Since the motor part of the glossopharyngeal nerve supplies only one small muscle, stylopharyngeus, it is impossible to test. If necessary, taste sensation on the posterior part of the tongue can be tested, with difficulty. The gag reflex (palatal elevation and pharyngeal contraction on tactile stimulation of the posterior tongue or oropharynx) tests both glossopharyngeal (afferent arc) and vagal (efferent arc) function.

Vagus nerve

Through its pharyngeal and laryngeal branches the motor component of the vagus nerve (nucleus ambiguus) supplies the pharynx, palate and larynx. Recurrent laryngeal nerve palsies are most commonly due to malignant disease (25%) and surgical damage (20%) during operations on the thyroid gland, neck, oesophagus, heart and lung. Because of its longer and partly intrathoracic course, lesions of the left nerve are more frequent than those of the right. Test the motor innervation of the vocal cords by listening to the patient's speech and cough and by inspecting the cords through a laryngoscope.

High lesions of the vagus nerve which affect the pharyngeal and superior laryngeal as well as the recurrent laryngeal branches cause difficulty in swallowing as well as vocal cord defects. The motor innervation of the soft palate can be tested by asking the patient to say a prolonged 'Ah' and observing the upward palatal movement; if paralysed on one side the unaffected side will rise further and pull the uvula towards the normal side.

Accessory nerve

The spinal part of the accessory nerve may be damaged in the posterior triangle, paralysing the trapezius. Test by asking the patient to shrug the shoulder; the paralysis may not be complete on account of some motor innervation occasionally reaching the muscle through cervical nerves. A lesion higher up before the nerve enters sternocleidomastoid will paralyse that muscle also; test whether the patient can turn the face to the opposite side against resistance.

Hypoglossal nerve

Paralysis of this nerve makes its own half of the tongue immobile and if of long standing the tongue will be wasted on that side. Test by asking the patient to put out the tongue; it will deviate towards the affected side due to the unopposed action of the normal half.

Osteology of the skull and hyoid bone

8

PART ONE

Skull

The term *skull* includes the mandible, and the *cranium* is the skull without the mandible. The cranial cavity has a roof or *cranial vault*, and a floor which is the *base of the skull*. The *facial skeleton* is the front part of the skull and includes the mandible (Figs 8.1 and 8.2).

External features

Superior view

Anteriorly the frontal bone articulates with the pair of parietal bones at the **coronal suture**, which runs transversely. The original two halves of the frontal bone occasionally fail to fuse, leaving a midline *metopic suture*. The midline meeting place of the frontal and parietal bones is the *bregma*, the site of the anterior fontanelle

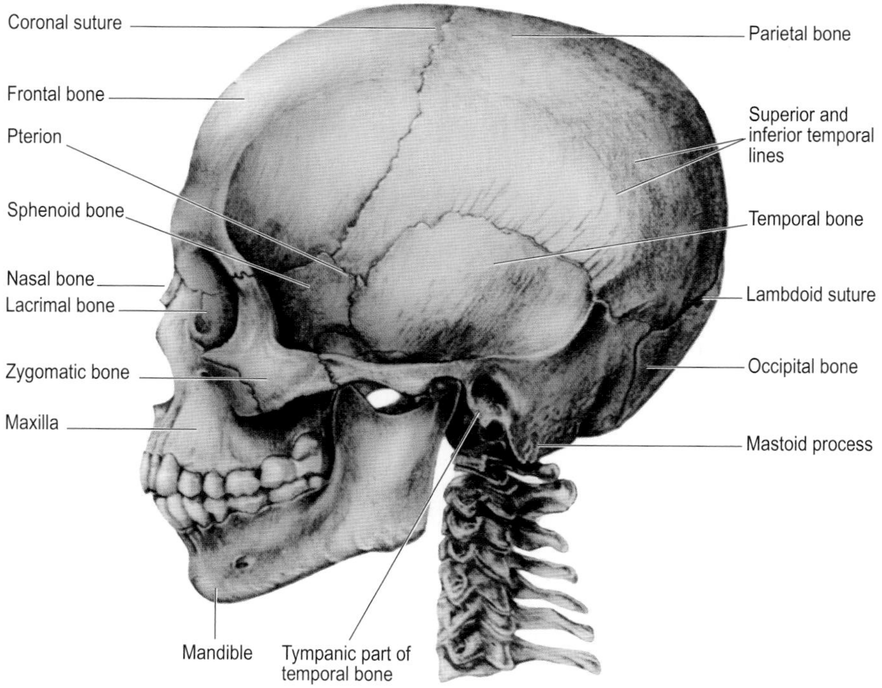

Fig. 8.1 Left side of the skull.

- Coronal suture
- Frontal bone
- Pterion
- Sphenoid bone
- Nasal bone
- Lacrimal bone
- Zygomatic bone
- Maxilla
- Parietal bone
- Superior and inferior temporal lines
- Temporal bone
- Lambdoid suture
- Occipital bone
- Mastoid process
- Mandible
- Tympanic part of temporal bone

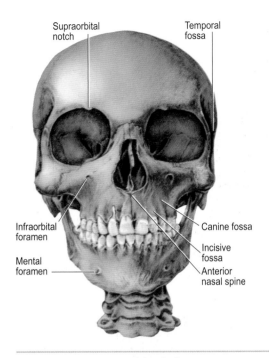

Supraorbital
notch

Temporal
fossa

Infraorbital
foramen

Mental
foramen

Canine fossa

Incisive
fossa

Anterior
nasal spine

Fig. 8.2 Anterior view of the skull.

(see Fig. 1.28, p. 34). Behind the bregma the parietal bones articulate in the midline **sagittal suture**. On either side of the posterior part of this suture a foramen often perforates each parietal bone, through which an emissary vein connects the superior sagittal sinus with scalp veins. The sagittal suture curves down to the *lambda*, at the apex of the occipital bone.

Posterior view

The lambda is the midline point where the sagittal suture meets the tortuous *lambdoid suture* between the squamous part of the occipital and the parietal bones (see Fig. 6.84, p. 448). Along these sutures small sutural (Wormian) bones are commonly found.

Some 6 cm below the lambda the occipital bone is projected into the **external occipital protuberance**, from which a ridge curves, convex upwards, towards the base of the mastoid process. This is the superior nuchal line (Fig. 8.3); gently convex upwards it lies at the junction of neck and scalp. It is the surface marking of the attachment of the tentorium cerebelli and the transverse sinus. Trapezius (medial third) and sternocleidomastoid (lateral half) are attached along the superior nuchal line. Splenius capitis is inserted into the lateral third of

the line deep to sternocleidomastoid. Above this a faint, often imperceptible, highest nuchal line gives origin to occipitalis and the galea aponeurotica. Below the superior nuchal line the bone that covers the cerebellar hemispheres gives attachment to muscles at the back of the neck (see p. 447).

The mastoid region of the temporal bone articulates with the parietal and occipital bones, and the mastoid process projects down at the side. The suture between the mastoid and occipital bones is commonly perforated by a mastoid emissary foramen, for a vein which connects the sigmoid sinus with the posterior auricular vein.

Lateral view

To the lateral surface of the mastoid process is attached the sternocleidomastoid, with splenius and longissimus capitis lying deep to it. In front of this is the external acoustic meatus. Above the meatus is a horizontal ridge, the *supramastoid crest.*

Above the crest the squamous part of the temporal bone extends up to articulate with the parietal bone. The curved anterior border of the squamous part continues to articulate with the parietal bone by its upper part while the lower part articulates with the greater wing of the sphenoid bone. The coronal suture comes down along the side of the skull to reach the curved upper border of the greater wing of the sphenoid, which thus articulates posteriorly with the parietal bone and anteriorly with the frontal bone. The resulting H-shaped pattern of sutures in this region between frontal, parietal, temporal and sphenoid bones is termed the **pterion** (Fig. 8.1).

The supramastoid crest is projected forwards as the upper border of the zygomatic process of the temporal bone. The zygomatic arch is continued by the zygomatic bone. The frontal process of the zygomatic bone reaches up to meet the frontal bone at the *frontozygomatic suture* which is palpable in the living. The zygomatic bone has a sharp posterior border which continues up across the suture as a ridge on the frontal bone (Fig. 8.1). This ridge arches up and back and diverges into the superior and inferior *temporal lines*. The superior line fades posteriorly; the temporalis fascia is attached to it. The inferior temporal line curves down across the squamous temporal bone and turns forwards to join the supramastoid crest.

The **temporal fossa** is the area bounded by the superior temporal line, zygomatic arch and the frontal process of the zygomatic bone. The temporal fascia is attached above to the superior temporal line and below to the zygomatic arch. Temporalis arises from the inferior temporal line and the whole surface of the temporal fossa

Fig 8.3   External surface of the base of the skull, with survey landmarks.

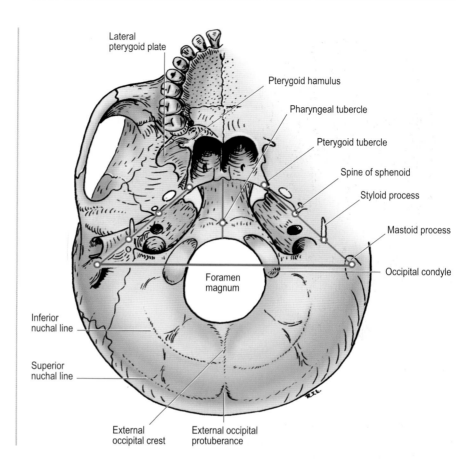

Lateral pterygoid plate

Pterygoid hamulus

Pharyngeal tubercle

Pterygoid tubercle

Spine of sphenoid

Styloid process

Mastoid process

Occipital condyle

Foramen magnum

Inferior nuchal line

Superior nuchal line

External occipital crest

External occipital protuberance

below it. The fossa is walled off anteriorly by the concave surface of the zygomatic bone which is here perforated by the zygomaticotemporal nerve.

The **zygomatic arch** is formed by the zygomatic process of the temporal bone and the temporal process of the zygomatic bone, which meet at an oblique suture near the front end of the arch. (The term 'zygoma' is best avoided; it means the arch, though it is often incorrectly used as a name for the zygomatic bone.) The masseter arises mainly from the lower border of the arch, while its posterior deep fibres arise from the medial surface of the arch. The parotidomasseteric fascia is also attached to the lower border of the arch. The arch is crossed in front of the external acoustic meatus by the auriculo-temporal nerve and the superficial temporal vessels. Further forward the arch is crossed by the temporal and zygomatic branches of the facial nerve.

The posterior part of the zygomatic process of the temporal bone is described as having anterior and poste-rior roots. The latter is the backward extension of the arch above the external auditory meatus, its upper border

continuing into the supramastoid crest. The anterior root runs medially across the front of the mandibular fossa forming the *articular eminence*, which is part of the superior articular surface of the temporomandibular joint. Where the anterior root joins the zygomatic arch, the latter has a triangular projection pointing down-wards. This is the *articular tubercle* to which the lateral ligament of the joint is attached.

The zygomatic bone forms the bony prominence of the cheek; it is perforated by the zygomaticofacial foramen for the zygomaticofacial nerve. Zygomaticus major arises from the surface of the zygomatic bone, and zygomaticus minor from the zygomaticomaxillary suture.

The posterior convexity of the maxilla curves back-wards towards the lateral pterygoid plate, from which it is separated by the *pterygomaxillary fissure*. This is closed inferiorly by the *pyramidal process* (tubercle) of the palatine bone which is wedged between them (see Fig. 6.13, p. 365). The *pterygopalatine fossa* lies deep to the fissure.

The *tuberosity of the maxilla* is a bony prominence above the posterior surface of the last molar tooth. The buccinator arises from a linear strip on the maxilla, running forwards from here above the molar teeth. From the tuberosity a fibrous band, the pterygomaxillary ligament (see Fig. 6.13, p. 365), continues the origin of the buccinator to the tip of the hamulus. Deep to the buccinator is the vestibule of the mouth; superficial to it are the soft tissues of the face. From the tuberosity of the maxilla and the pyramidal process of the palatine bone the small superficial head of the medial pterygoid arises, overlapping the inferior head of the lateral pterygoid, which arises from the whole surface of the lateral pterygoid plate. The posterior convexity of the maxilla above the tuberosity shows two or more foramina for the posterior superior alveolar nerves and vessels.

The zygomatic process of the maxilla articulates with the zygomatic bone and with it forms an anterior pillar for the zygomatic arch. It is palpable through the cheek or the vestibule.

Anterior view

The frontal bone curves down to make the upper margins of the orbits (Fig. 8.2). Medially it goes down to meet the frontal process of each maxilla, between which it articulates with the nasal bones. Laterally it projects down as a zygomatic process to make the frontozygomatic suture with the zygomatic bone at the lateral margin of the orbit. The frontal bone occupies the upper third of the anterior view of the skull, the maxillae and mandible making the other two-thirds.

The nasal bones curve downwards and forwards from their articulation with the frontal bone. Each articulates with the frontal process of the maxilla, and they arch forward to meet in a midline suture. The lower border of each is notched by the external nasal nerve (which also grooves the posterior surface of the nasal bone). These free borders make with the two maxillae a pear-shaped piriform (anterior nasal) aperture (Fig. 8.2). In the nasal cavity the bony septum and the conchae of the lateral wall are visible. The two maxillae meet in a midline intermaxillary suture, and are projected forward as the *anterior nasal spine* at the lower margin of the nasal aperture. The canine root makes a ridge on the anterior surface of the maxilla, on either side of which are slight depressions, the medial one being the incisive fossa and the lateral the canine fossa, from which levator anguli oris arises and above which the anterior surface of the maxilla is perforated by the infraorbital foramen. Levator labii superioris arises from the lower margin of the orbit above the foramen, from which the infraorbital nerve emerges between these muscles. The line of

attachment of buccinator and that of levator anguli oris on the body of the maxilla mark the middle of the maxillary sinus, which lies with its lower half deep to the vestibule and its upper half deep to the soft tissues of the face. The supraorbital notch, infraorbital foramen and mental foramen lie all three in a vertical line, which passes between the two lower premolar teeth. The osteology of the orbital walls and margin is described on page 412.

Inferior view

The area behind the foramen magnum consists of the squamous part of the occipital bone. The **superior nuchal line** lies in a curve concentric with the foramen magnum. Halfway between them the **inferior nuchal line** is concentric with both. The **external occipital crest**, in the midline between the external occipital protuberance and the foramen magnum, bisects this area and gives attachment to the ligamentum nuchae. A rather vague line, radiating back and outwards from the foramen magnum, further bisects each half (Fig. 8.3). Thus four areas are demarcated in each half (Fig. 8.3). There are two alongside the foramen magnum and they receive rectus capitis posterior minor medially, and rectus capitis posterior major laterally (see Fig. 6.84, p. 448). Between superior and inferior nuchal lines semispinalis capitis is attached medially and superior oblique laterally.

One-third of the **foramen magnum** lies in front and two-thirds behind a line joining the tips of the mastoid processes. The occipital condyles have the reverse proportions; two-thirds of the condyle lies in front of the line.

The foramen magnum is in the basilar part of the occipital bone (basiocciput). The fibrous dura mater is attached to the margins of the foramen as it sweeps down from the posterior cranial fossa. Within the tube of dura mater, the lower medulla with the vertebral and spinal arteries and the spinal roots of the accessory nerves traverse the foramen in the subarachnoid space (see Fig. 6.109, p. 469). Anteriorly the margin of the foramen gives attachment to the ligaments sweeping up from the axis. Adherent to dura mater is the tectorial membrane and in front of this is the vertical limb of the cruciform ligament (see Fig. 6.79, p. 444); in front again are the apical and the pair of alar ligaments of the dens of the axis. Most anteriorly is the attachment of the anterior atlanto-occipital membrane. The posterior atlanto-occipital membrane is attached to the posterior margin of the foramen magnum.

The **occipital condyles** are convex kidney-shaped surfaces, covered with hyaline cartilage, beside the front half of the foramen magnum. The two convexities make a ball-and-socket joint with the atlas. But the antero-posterior curve is more pronounced than the combined side to side curvature; so the ball is oval-shaped, like an egg lying on its side, and thus permits nodding and some abduction but no rotation. Behind the condyle is the shallow condylar fossa floored by thin bone, commonly perforated by the *condylar canal*, carrying an emissary vein from the sigmoid sinus to the suboccipital venous plexus. Above the occipital condyle is the *hypoglossal canal* for the hypoglossal nerve, which emerges medial to the jugular foramen.

The basiocciput extends forward from the foramen magnum and fuses with the basisphenoid. The pharyngeal tubercle is a slight bony prominence in front of the foramen magnum, marking the midline attachment of the pharyngobasilar fascia (see Fig. 6.35, p. 398) and the highest fibres of the superior constrictor. The attachment of the fascia extends on either side of the pharyngeal tubercle along a faint ridge, convex forwards. Behind this is the attachment of the prevertebral fascia, longus capitis and rectus capitis anterior in that order from before backwards immediately in front of the occipital condyle (see Fig. 6.8, p. 358).

The mastoid process is grooved on the deep aspect of its base by the digastric notch for the origin of the posterior belly of the digastric (see Fig. 6.35, p. 398). Medial to this notch a groove for the occipital artery indents the bone along the temporo-occipital suture. The length of the styloid process is very variable. The stylo-pharyngeus arises high up medially, the stylohyoid high up posteriorly, and the styloglossus low down in front. The stylohyoid ligament passes on from its tip. Between the bases of the styloid and mastoid processes is the stylomastoid foramen, transmitting the facial nerve and the stylomastoid branch of the posterior auricular artery with its accompanying vein. Medial to the styloid process the petrous bone is deeply hollowed out to form the jugular fossa, which with the shallower jugular notch in the occipital bone forms the **jugular foramen**, and lodges the jugular bulb at the beginning of the internal jugular vein. The inferior petrosal sinus, the glossopharyngeal, vagus and accessory nerves emerge through the foramen anteromedial to the vein.

Anterior to the jugular fossa the petrous part of the temporal bone is perforated by the **carotid canal**. The internal carotid artery enters here and turns forward into the bone. On the ridge of bone between the jugular fossa and the carotid canal is the canaliculus for the tympanic branch of the glossopharyngeal nerve. Antero-lateral to the carotid canal, at the margin of the petrous bone, is the opening of the bony part of the auditory tube. Levator palati arises from the rectangular area at the apex of the petrous within the attachment of the

pharyngobasilar fascia. The tip of the petrous bone forms the posterior boundary of the *foramen lacerum* between the basiocciput and the body and greater wing of the sphenoid. The foramen lacerum is closed here in life by dense fibrous tissue that extends across from the periosteum of the adjacent bones, and is pierced only by a small emissary vein and a meningeal branch of the ascending pharyngeal artery.

Lateral to the jugular fossa, the tympanic part of the temporal bone forms the bony part of the external acoustic meatus. The tympanic part is C-shaped, open above, and the squamous part of the temporal bone completes the bony ring of the external acoustic meatus. The posterosuperior margin of the meatus has a small prominence, the suprameatal spine, and forms one boundary of the (MacEwen's) *suprameatal triangle*; the other boundaries are the supramastoid crest and a vertical line drawn upwards from the posterior margin of the meatus. The tympanic antrum lies 15 mm deep to the surface of the triangle.

Anterior to the tympanic plate, the squamous part of the temporal bone is hollowed into the mandibular fossa which, with the articular eminence in front, forms the upper articular surface of the temporomandibular joint (Fig. 6.19, p. 375). The *squamotympanic fissure* lies between the two parts, but medially they are separated by a thin flange of bone. This is the projecting margin of the *tegmen tympani*, part of the petrous bone that has turned down from the roof of the middle ear (Fig. 8.4). It divides the medial part of the squamotympanic fissure into the *petrosquamous fissure* in front, for the capsule of the jaw joint, and the *petrotympanic fissure* behind

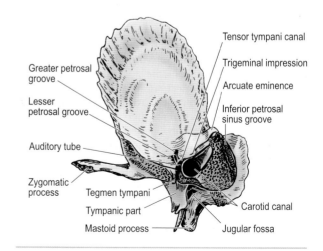

Fig. 8.4 Right temporal bone, looking directly at the apex from the medial aspect.

(see Fig. 6.35, p. 398), through the medial end of which emerges the chorda tympani. The nerve runs down in a groove on the medial surface of the spine of the sphenoid.

A small triangular area of squamous bone in front of the articular eminence and the inferior aspect of the greater wing of the sphenoid form the roof of the infratemporal fossa. The upper head of lateral pterygoid arises from here. Anteriorly the inferior orbital fissure lies between the greater wing and the maxilla. The roof of the infratemporal fossa is pierced medially by the *foramen ovale* through which pass the mandibular nerve, its motor root and meningeal branch, the lesser petrosal nerve, the accessory meningeal artery and an emissary vein that connects the pterygoid plexus with the cavernous sinus. This vein may instead pass through a small venous foramen (of Vesalius) medial to the foramen ovale. The base of the spine of the sphenoid is perforated by the *foramen spinosum* for the middle meningeal vessels. The medial and lateral pterygoid plates project down from a common pterygoid process of the sphenoid at the base of the skull. The pterygoid tubercle projects back towards the foramen lacerum from the attachment of the medial pterygoid plate to the base of the skull. A line joining the tip of the mastoid process, styloid process, spine of the sphenoid and pterygoid tubercle lies at 45° to the sagittal plane (Fig. 8.3). The stylomastoid foramen lies behind the base of the styloid process, and the foramen spinosum perforates the base of the spine of the sphenoid. The spine of the sphenoid overlies the opening in the petrous bone of the bony part of the auditory tube. The cartilaginous part of the tube lies along the above line, below the slit between the greater wing of the sphenoid and the apex of the petrous bone (see Fig. 6.35, p. 398). The foramen ovale perforates the greater wing of the sphenoid just lateral to the line, and the inferior opening of the carotid canal in the petrous temporal bone lies just medial to the line.

The **medial pterygoid plate** forms the most posterior part of the lateral wall of the nose. Its lower end has a small hook-like projection, the *pterygoid hamulus* (Fig. 8.3), around which the tendon of tensor palati turns. To its tip is attached the pterygomandibular raphe where the fibres of buccinator and superior constrictor interdigitate (see Fig. 6.13, p. 365). The expanded medial end of the cartilaginous auditory tube grooves the upper part of the posterior border of the medial pterygoid plate; below this the pharyngobasilar fascia and the superior pharyngeal constrictor are attached down to the hamulus. At its upper end, the posterior border splits into two edges which pass backwards and laterally enclosing the *scaphoid fossa*, that gives attachment to the tensor palati. The small pterygoid tubercle projects backwards medial to the scaphoid fossa, obscuring the

posterior opening of the *pterygoid canal* that lies above it at the anterior end of the foramen lacerum. In the roof of the nose, the medial pterygoid plate has a small medial extension, the vaginal process (see Fig. 6.26, p. 383), which articulates above with the ala of the vomer and below with the sphenoidal process of the palatine bone. A small palatovaginal canal between these processes transmits the pharyngeal branches of the maxillary nerve and artery.

The **lateral pterygoid plate** extends back and laterally into the space of the infratemporal fossa. It gives attachment to the lower head of lateral pterygoid from its lateral surface, and to the deep head of medial pterygoid from its medial surface.

At the lateral and anterior margins of the hard palate the alveolar processes of the maxillae project downwards. Behind this projection in the anterior midline is the *incisive fossa* leading up into bilateral incisive foramina that open into the nasal cavity, and through which pass the greater palatine artery from below and the nasopalatine nerve from above. Medial to the third molar tooth on either side is the *greater palatine foramen*, between the horizontal plate of the palatine bone and the palatine process of the maxilla. Further back are small multiple *lesser palatine foramina* in the pyramidal process of the palatine bone. Through the corresponding palatine foramina pass the greater and lesser palatine nerves and vessels. Medial to the greater palatine foramen is a low transverse crest. The palatine aponeurosis is attached to the smooth part of the palatine bone behind the crest.

Internal features

The inner surface of the cranial vault shows a midline groove, widening as it is traced back, for the superior sagittal sinus. Pits in and lateral to the groove are the indentations of arachnoid granulations, those outside the sinus being in the lateral blood lakes. The grooves for the anterior and posterior branches of the middle meningeal vessels extend on to the side of the skull.

The internal surface of the base of the skull is in three levels, like the steps of a staircase: the anterior, middle and posterior *cranial fossae*. The anterior fossa lodges the frontal lobe and its floor is level with the upper margin of the orbit. The middle fossa lodges the temporal lobe and its floor is level with the upper border of the zygomatic arch. The posterior fossa lodges the brainstem and cerebellum and the attachment of its roof (the tentorium) lies at the upper limit of the neck muscles, attached to the outer aspect of the occipital bone.

The **anterior cranial fossa** extends as far back as the sharp posterior edge of the lesser wing of the sphenoid (see Fig. 6.101, p. 458). The orbital part of the frontal bone is the largest contributor to the anterior fossa. The frontal sinus invades a variable area at the anteromedial part of the roof of the orbit. Medially the frontal bone roofs in the ethmoidal sinuses and articulates with the *cribriform plate*. Anteriorly, a midline crest for the falx cerebri runs backwards from the front wall to a small pit, the foramen caecum, which is plugged by the fibrous tissue of the falx; in only 1% of subjects does a vein pass through the foramen, connecting nasal veins with the superior sagittal sinus. Just behind the foramen, the midline of the cribriform plate is projected up as a sharp triangle of bone, the *crista galli*, also for attachment of the falx. Alongside the anterior end of the crista galli is a slit through which the anterior ethmoidal nerve and vessels pass into the nasal cavity. The perforations in the cribriform plate are for the olfactory nerves. Behind the cribriform plate is the jugam (part of the body) of the sphenoid, which joins the two lesser wings and roofs the sphenoidal sinus.

The **middle cranial fossa** is butterfly-shaped. The small 'body' of the butterfly is the body of the sphenoid between the clinoid processes, while the 'wings' of the butterfly expand hugely into a concavity that extends out to the lateral wall of the skull and back to the upper border of the petrous bone. The body of the sphenoid is centrally hollowed out into the *pituitary fossa*, or sella turcica ('Turkish saddle'), with a hump in front, the *tuberculum sellae*, which has a small elevation, the *middle clinoid process*, at each side (see Fig. 6.102, p. 461). Lateral to this a larger *anterior clinoid process* projects backwards from the medial ends of the lesser wings. At the back is a transverse ledge, the *dorsum sellae* ('back of the saddle'); its upper border ends at each side as the *posterior clinoid process*.

A sheet of fibrous dura mater, the *diaphragma sellae*, sweeps across from the tuberculum sellae to the dorsum sellae, roofing the pituitary fossa. It is continuous laterally with the roof of the cavernous sinus, which lies on each side of the sphenoid body (see Fig. 6.103, p. 461). The diaphragma sellae is perforated centrally for the pituitary stalk, and the roof of each cavernous sinus is pierced anteriorly by the internal carotid artery, between the middle and anterior clinoid processes. A flange of dura mater, attached above to the medial and posterior clinoid processes, descends vertically between the cavernous sinus and the pituitary fossa, and sweeps medially to floor the fossa. The anterior and posterior clinoid processes give attachment to the free and attached margins, respectively, of the tentorium cerebelli (see Fig. 6.101, p. 458).

In front of the tuberculum sellae is the chiasmatic sulcus, a groove on the upper surface of the sphenoid body. Despite the name of the groove, the optic chiasma lies at a higher level well behind it. The optic canals lie at the lateral ends of the groove, bounded by the two roots of the lesser wing and the body of the sphenoid. Each canal transmits an optic nerve, an ophthalmic artery and their meningeal sleeve.

The side of the body of the sphenoid is grooved by the internal carotid artery as it runs in the cavernous sinus from the foramen lacerum to the anterior clinoid process (see Fig. 6.102, p. 461). Lateral to this the floor of the middle fossa is made by the greater wing of the sphenoid and the petrous part of the temporal bone. Between the greater wing, the apex of the petrous bone and the side of the body of the sphenoid bone is the irregular *foramen lacerum*. The internal carotid artery emerges from the apex of the petrous bone to occupy the upper part of the foramen lacerum and then grooves the sphenoid. The posterior end of the lateral ridge of the groove in the sphenoid is often prominent as the *lingula*. Beneath the lingula is the posterior opening of the *pterygoid canal*, which is not visible from the middle cranial fossa. Lateral to the foramen lacerum the anterior surface of the apex of the petrous bone has a fossa, the *trigeminal impression*, occupied by the trigeminal ganglion (Fig. 8.4).

The upper margin of the apex of the petrous bone has a shallow groove made by the sensory root of the trigeminal nerve, with the small motor root below it. Lateral to this the upper border is grooved by the superior petrosal sinus, and to the lips of this narrow groove the tentorium cerebelli is attached, straddling the sinus.

The lateral part of the posterior wall of the middle fossa has a prominence, the *arcuate eminence*, which is made by the underlying anterior semicircular canal (see Fig. 6.105, p. 463). Medial and anterior to the arcuate eminence is the groove for the greater petrosal nerve, which passes obliquely into the foramen lacerum; as it does so, the nerve lies beneath the trigeminal ganglion (see Fig. 6.101, p. 458). Parallel and anterolateral to this is a small groove made by the lesser petrosal nerve; this groove is directed towards the foramen ovale.

Just in front of the petrous part of the temporal bone, the greater wing of the sphenoid is perforated by the small *foramen spinosum* and, anteromedial to this, by the much larger *foramen ovale*. The structures that pass through the foramen ovale have been described on page 530. From the foramen spinosum a groove for the middle meningeal vessels runs anterolaterally and splits into anterior and posterior branches. The anterior groove frequently enters a bony canal in the region of the pterion.

In front of the foramen ovale is the *foramen rotundum*, which opens forwards into the pterygopalatine fossa. It transmits the maxillary nerve.

Anteriorly the greater wing of the sphenoid fails to meet the lesser wing; the slit between them is the *superior orbital fissure.* Lateral to the line of the foramen rotundum this is closed by fibrous dura mater. Medial to the line of the foramen rotundum the medial end of the superior orbital fissure is open for the receipt of venous drainage from the orbit into the cavernous sinus and for the passage of nerves that run along the sinus into the orbit. The sphenoparietal sinus runs medially just below the margin of the lesser wing to enter the roof of the cavernous sinus.

The **posterior cranial fossa**, deeply concave, lies above the foramen magnum. Anteriorly, its upper limit is the upper border of the petrous temporal bone. Posteriorly, at the same horizontal level is a wide groove on the inner surface of the skull, which extends to the midline and is made by the transverse sinus. The two grooves meet at the *internal occipital protuberance*, which lies opposite the external occipital protuberance. Above the internal occipital protuberance (i.e. above the posterior fossa) is the groove made by the superior sagittal sinus. At the internal occipital protuberance the sagittal groove turns to one side (usually the right) into the *transverse groove*. The other transverse groove (usually the left) is narrower; it begins at the internal occipital protuberance by the inflow of the straight sinus. The tentorium cerebelli is attached to the margins of the transverse groove. Anteriorly, the transverse sinus is continuous with the *sigmoid groove*, which indents the cranial surface of the mastoid parts of the temporal bone (see Fig. 6.101, p. 458). Lower down, the sigmoid groove indents the occipital bone, which forms the inferior margin of the *jugular foramen*. The superior margin of the foramen is formed by the sharp inferior edge of the petrous part of the temporal bone, which is notched here by the inferior ganglion of the glossopharyngeal nerve (see Fig. 6.105, p. 463).

Anterior to the foramen magnum, the basiocciput, the posterior part of the sphenoid body and the dorsum sellae form a transversely concave sloping surface, the *clivus*. On each side the clivus is separated from the petrous temporal bone by a fissure in which the inferior petrosal sinus runs down to the jugular foramen. The basilar plexus of veins is lodged in the dura on the clivus and receives blood from the overlying pons and medulla. The plexus drains into the inferior petrosal sinuses.

Medial to the inferior margin of the jugular foramen is a rounded prominence, the *jugular tubercle* (see Fig. 6.105, p. 463). It lies above the occipital condyle, and between them the bone is perforated obliquely by the *hypoglossal canal*. The hypoglossal nerve enters here as two roots (see Fig. 6.109, p. 469). They are separated by a flange of dura mater that often ossifies. The glossopharyngeal, vagus and accessory nerves lie on the surface of the jugular tubercle on their way to the jugular fora-

men. Above the jugular foramen is the *internal acoustic meatus*, through which pass the facial and vestibulo-cochlear nerves, nervus intermedius and labyrinthine vessels.

The *internal occipital crest* runs down in the midline from the internal occipital protuberance; to it is attached the falx cerebelli over the occipital sinus.

Mandible

The mandible (Fig. 8.5) consists of a horizontal U-shaped body, which is continuous at its posterior ends with a pair of vertical rami.

The **body** of the mandible is projected up around the teeth as alveolar bone which forms the walls of the tooth sockets. The alveolar bone is covered by mucoperiosteum to form the inner and outer gums (gingivae). The cavity of the tooth socket gives attachment to the periodontal ligament; loss of this fibrous tissue in the dried skeleton commonly allows the teeth to rattle in the bone. Healthy teeth will not fall out of the dried mandible, for the alveolar bone is constricted somewhat about their necks. After the loss of a tooth, living alveolar bone atrophies and the bottom of the socket fills up with new bone; thus a glance at a gap will tell whether the tooth was lost before or after death.

On the outer surface of the body the sharp anterior border of the ramus extends forward as the *external oblique line*, to which the buccinator is attached opposite the molar teeth (Fig. 8.5A). The *mental foramen* lies halfway between the upper and lower borders of the body, in line with the interval between the two premolars. Its position varies with age (see p. 35). It faces backwards and slightly upwards in the adult, but directly laterally in early childhood; this influences the direction in which a needle is advanced for a mental nerve block. Depressor anguli oris is attached below the mental foramen and depressor labii inferioris anterior to the foramen, deep to the former muscle. Mentalis is attached near the midline. The lower border of the mandible gives attachment to the investing layer of deep cervical fascia, and to the platysma before some of its fibres pass on to the face. The lower border is crossed by the facial vessels and sometimes by the marginal mandibular branch of the facial nerve just in front of the masseter (see Fig. 6.11, p. 363).

The whole of the lateral surface of the **ramus** gives insertion to masseter. The posterior border of the ramus is projected up as the neck, which expands into the head (condyle) of the bone. The sharp anterior border continues up into the pointed *coronoid process*. The medial surface of the coronoid process, adjacent to its margins, is bevelled for the attachment of temporalis (Fig. 8.5B).

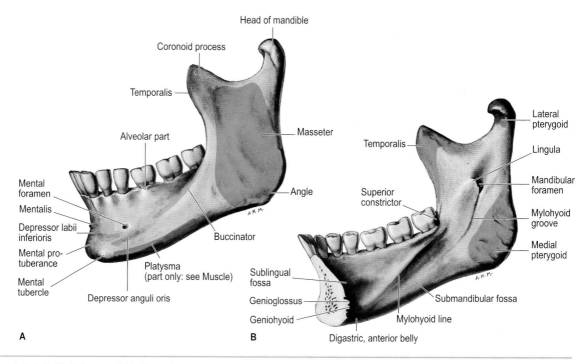

Fig. 8.5 **A** Left half of the mandible: lateral aspect. **B** Right half of the mandible: medial aspect.

The posterior border of this bevelled area is marked by a slight crest which runs downwards and forwards to the medial margin of the socket for the third molar tooth. The anteroinferior part of the temporalis tendon divides into two bands and the deep band is attached to this crest, which accordingly is referred to as the temporal crest. Between the lowest part of this crest and the posterior part of the oblique line is the small triangular retromolar fossa behind the last molar tooth.

The inner surface of the body is characterized by the *mylohyoid line* which forms a ridge that runs downwards and forwards from just below the posterior border of the third molar tooth (Fig. 8.5B). This fades anteriorly although the mylohyoid muscle attachment continues to the midline between the lower mental spine and the digastric fossa. The *mental spines* (previously called genial tubercles) are four small projections low down in the midline; genioglossus arises from the upper pair and geniohyoid from the lower pair of spines. The *digastric fossae* are two oval depressions on either side of the midline, on the inner aspect of the lower border of the mandible, for the attachment of the anterior bellies of the digastric muscles. Above the anterior part of the mylohyoid line is a smooth concavity, the *sublingual fossa*, which lodges the sublingual gland, and below the

line the smooth *submandibular fossa* lodges the superficial part of the submandibular gland. Above the mylohyoid ridge the medial surface of the mandible is grooved below the last molar tooth; the lingual nerve lies here below the attachment of the pterygomandibular raphe, just behind the last molar tooth (see Fig. 6.22A, p. 379).

The medial surface of the ramus is characterized by the *lingula*, a small tongue of bone at the anterior margin of the *mandibular foramen*, which lies halfway between the anterior and posterior borders of the ramus, level with the occlusal surfaces of the teeth (Fig. 8.5B). The inferior alveolar nerve and vessels pass through the foramen. The sphenomandibular ligament is attached to the lingula. The ligament is pierced by the mylohyoid vessels and nerve and these lie in the *mylohyoid groove*, a narrow sulcus that runs forwards from the mandibular foramen below the mylohyoid line. Between the mylohyoid groove and the angle of the mandible the medial pterygoid muscle is inserted, and irregular bony ridges lie in this area for attachment of the fibrous septa that characterize the muscle.

The **neck** of the mandible is hollowed anteriorly by the *pterygoid fovea* for the insertion of the lateral pterygoid muscle. Posteriorly the upper part of the neck is triangular and smooth. This area lies above the attachment of the temporomandibular joint capsule and is lined by synovial membrane. The lateral temporomandibular ligament is attached below this and to the lateral surface of the neck. The auriculotemporal nerve and the maxillary artery and vein cross the medial aspect of the neck, lying between it and the sphenomandibular ligament, together with parotid gland tissue.

The **head** of the mandible is markedly convex from front to back and slightly convex from side to side. The mediolateral axis is longer than the anteroposterior, and projects beyond the neck as medial and lateral poles, the former being more prominent. This axis is directed medially and slightly backwards. The head is bent slightly anteriorly on the neck, such that the articular surface faces upwards and forwards.

Ossification of the skull

Ossification of the skull occurs in both membrane and cartilage. The cranial vault develops in membrane, the skull base mainly in cartilage and the facial bones in membrane. Accordingly, the frontal and parietal bones develop in membrane. At birth the frontal bone is in two parts separated by the metopic suture. Fusion of this suture starts in the second year and is complete by 7 years. But the suture may persist in a small proportion of persons, in whom it must not be mistaken for a fracture line.

The squamous part of the occipital bone above the superior nuchal line ossifies intramembranously and the rest of the bone endochondrally. The skull base component of the occipital bone develops from the sclerotomes of the four occipital somites (see p. 25), and a pair of parachordal cartilages on either side of the cranial end of the notochord. At birth the bone is in four parts: the squamous part, the median basiocciput and a pair of (lateral) exoccipital parts. The squamous and exoccipital parts fuse by the third year and by the sixth year the whole bone is one entity.

The body of the sphenoid bone develops from presphenoidal and postsphenoidal cartilages, the latter forming the sella turcica and dorsum sellae. Endochondral ossification in the adjacent ala orbitalis and ala temporalis give rise to the lesser wing and a part of the greater wing. The rest of the greater wing and the medial and lateral pterygoid plates ossify in membrane. At birth the sphenoid is in three parts: the greater wing being separate from a central part comprising the body and lesser wings. The three parts unite during the first year. At birth the body of the sphenoid is separated from the basiocciput by cartilage. This spheno-occipital synchondrosis (primary cartilaginous joint) begins to fuse between 12 and 14 years of age but ossification is not

complete until 20 to 25 years of age, allowing for backward extension of the hard palate as more teeth erupt and providing space for the growing nasopharynx. Premature fusion between the sphenoid and occipital bones results in a depressed nasal bridge and a flat face.

The squamous and tympanic parts of the temporal bone ossify in membrane, while the petrous and styloid elements ossify in cartilage. The petrous part develops by ossification of the otic capsule that houses the vestibulocochlear apparatus. At birth the temporal bone is in three parts: the squamous and tympanic components have united but are separate from the petrous part and styloid process. All parts unite during the first year. A secondary ossification centre for the styloid fuses with the rest of the process after puberty (see p. 35).

The mandible, maxilla, vomer, inferior concha and the zygomatic, nasal, lacrimal and palatine bones ossify in membrane. The mandible is the second bone (after the clavicle) to start ossifying in the fetus; it does so in the sixth week by an ossification centre situated lateral to Meckel's cartilage (see p. 27). As intramembranous bone formation continues, this first branchial arch cartilage becomes incorporated in the developing mandible. Only the lingula and some occasional ossicles in the chin region of the mandible develop from Meckel's cartilage. A cone-shaped secondary condylar cartilage appears in the tenth week and, although it is largely replaced by bone before birth, growth continues here until 20 to 25 years of age.

PART TWO

Hyoid bone

The hyoid bone lies free, suspended by muscle, and so is very mobile. The floor of the mouth and the tongue are attached to it above, and the larynx below, while behind are attached the epiglottis and the pharynx (see Fig. 6.37, p. 399).

The hyoid bone (Fig. 8.6) has a **body**, which is a curved sheet of bone convex forward and concave behind. On each side a **greater horn** projects back as a long slender process. At the junction of body and greater horn is the **lesser horn**, projecting up as a spike of bone.

At rest the body lies just below the mandible at the level of C3 vertebra. This is the level of the lateral glossoepiglottic folds within the pharynx and marks the junction of oropharynx and laryngopharynx.

The thyrohyoid membrane is attached to the back of the upper border of the body and to the greater horns. Behind the concave posterior surface of the body is a bursa between bone and membrane, and here the

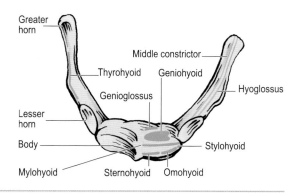

Fig. 8.6 Hyoid bone from above, with muscle attachments on the left side.

thyroglossal duct made an upward detour behind the bone (see Fig. 1.23, p. 28) on its course down the neck. From the rounded upper border of the body a hyoepiglottic ligament passes back to the front of the epiglottis and raises the oral mucous membrane to form the median glossoepiglottic fold. A similar flange of fibrous tissue passes from the greater horn to the side of the epiglottis and raises the lateral glossoepiglottic fold. Attached to the lower border of the body is the upper attachment of the pretracheal fascia. In front of this sternohyoid and omohyoid are attached. Thyrohyoid is attached to the lower border of the greater horn. In front of these muscles the investing layer of deep cervical fascia has a linear attachment to the bone, which is thus subcutaneous and palpable. Just above this line is the linear attachment of mylohyoid to the body of the bone, and above this is the insertion of geniohyoid. A few fibres of genioglossus are attached to the upper border of the body.

The lesser horn gives attachment to the stylohyoid ligament, and the middle constrictor arises from it and from the whole length of the greater horn, thus anchoring the pharynx to the hyoid. Lateral to the constrictor hyoglossus arises from the whole length of the greater horn and the lateral part of the body, thus anchoring the tongue to the hyoid. The fibrous sling, through which the intermediate tendon of digastric glides freely, and the split tendon of stylohyoid are attached to the junction of the greater horn and body.

Biographical notes

ADAMKIEWICZ Albert (1850–1921) Professor of Pathology in the University of Krakow and later, physician in Vienna.

Arterial supply of the spinal cord (see p. 512).

ALCOCK Benjamin (1801–?) Appointed Professor of Anatomy in Queen's College, Cork, in 1849 but was called upon to resign in 1853 in consequence of disputes about the working of the Anatomy Acts. Went to the USA in 1855 and was never heard of again.

Canal for the internal pudendal vessels in the ischioanal fossa (see p. 327).

ARGYLL ROBERTSON (Douglas Moray Cooper Lamb) (1837–1909) Scottish ophthalmologist.

Loss of pupil contraction to light (see p. 484).

ARNOLD Julius (1835–1915) Professor of Pathology in Heidelberg.

Auricular branch of vagus (see p. 381).

AUERBACH Leopold (1828–1897) Professor of Neuropathology in Breslau.

Myenteric nerve plexus of the gut (see p. 256).

BABINSKI Joseph François Felix (1857–1932) Physician in Paris.

Extensor plantar response (see p. 18).

BARRETT Norman Rupert (1903–1979) An Australian from Adelaide, he was educated at Eton and the University of Cambridge in England. He became a surgeon to St Thomas' and the Brompton Hospitals, London.

Extensive columnar epithelial lining of lower oesophagus (see p. 216).

BARTHOLIN Caspar (Secundus) (1655–1738) Succeeded his father, Thomas Bartholin, as Professor of Medicine, Anatomy and Physics at Copenhagen.

Greater vestibular glands of the female perineum (see p. 317).

BEEVOR Charles Edward (1854–1968) London neurologist.

Sign of upward displacement of the umbilicus in lower abdominal paralysis (see p. 18).

BELL Sir Charles (1774–1842) Surgeon, anatomist and artist who taught in Edinburgh and London. Founded the Middlesex Hospital Medical School. Returned to Edinburgh to be Professor of Surgery.

Palsy of the facial nerve (see p. 522).

BERRY Sir James (1860–1946) A Canadian from Kingston, Ontario, he became a surgeon at the Royal Free Hospital, London.

Suspensory ligament of the thyroid gland (see p. 351).

BETZ Vladimir Aleksandrovich (1834–1894) Professor of Anatomy in Kiev from 1868 to 1889.

Giant pyramidal cells of the motor cortex (see p. 483).

BIGELOW Henry Jacob (1818–1890) Professor of Surgery at Harvard University from 1849 to 1882.

Iliofemoral ligament of the hip joint (see p. 132).

BOCHDALEK Victor Alexander (1801–1883) Professor of Anatomy in Prague.

Foramen in the diaphragm—site of congenital diaphragmatic hernia (see p. 194).

BOWMAN Sir William Paget (1816–1892) Professor of Anatomy and Physiology at King's College, London, from 1848 to 1856. Leading ophthalmic surgeon in England.

Capsule surrounding the glomerulus in the kidney (see p. 295), and anterior limiting membrane of the cornea (see p. 422).

BROCA Pierre Paul (1824–1880) Professor of Clinical Surgery and Director of the Anthropological Laboratories in Paris.

Speech area of the cerebral cortex (see p. 479).

BRODMANN Korbinian (1868–1918) German psychiatrist who became Professor of Anatomy at Tübingen.

Areas of the cerebral cortex (see p. 482).

BROWN-SÉQUARD Charles Édouard (1818–1894) Born in Mauritius, he became Professor of Medicine at Harvard University and, later, in Paris.

Syndrome of hemisection of the spinal cord (see p. 512).

BRUNNER Johann Konrad (1653–1727) Professor of Anatomy at Heidelberg and later, at Strasburg.

Submucosal glands of the duodenum (see p. 257).

BUCK Gordon (1807–1877) New York surgeon.

Fascia of the penis (see p. 330).

CALOT Jean-François (1861–1944) French surgeon.

Triangle bounded by the common hepatic and cystic ducts and the liver (see p. 274).

CAMPER Petrus (1722–1789) Professor of Medicine, Anatomy, Surgery and Botany in Gröningen from 1763 to 1773.

Fatty layer of the superficial fascia of the abdomen (see p. 185).

CHARCOT Jean Martin (1825–1893) French neurologist at La Salpêtrière, Paris. He became Professor of Pathology in 1872 and the first Professor of Diseases of the Nervous System in 1882.

Artery of cerebral haemorrhage (see p. 492).

CHASSAIGNAC Charles Marie Édouard (1805–1879) Surgeon in Paris.

Carotid tubercle on the sixth cervical vertebra (see p. 450).

CLARKE Jacob Augustus Lockhart (1817–1880) Physician to the Hospital for Epilepsy and Paralysis, London. FRS 1854.

Dorsal nucleus of the spinal cord (see p. 510).

CLOQUET Jules Germain (1790–1883) Professor of Anatomy and Surgery in Paris.

Lymph node in the femoral canal (see p. 122).

COLLES Abraham (1773–1843) Professor of Anatomy and Surgery in Dublin from 1804 to 1836. FRS 1802.

Fracture of the lower end of the radius (see p. 110), and superficial perineal fascia (see p. 328).

COOPER Sir Astley Paston (1768–1841) Surgeon to St Thomas' and Guy's Hospitals, London. President of the Royal College of Surgeons of England.

Ligaments of the breast attached to the skin (see p. 59), and the pectineal ligament (see p. 231).

CORTI Alfonso (Marquis) (1822–1888) Italian anatomist and eminent histologist.

Organ of hearing (see p. 437).

COWPER William (1666–1709) London surgeon. FRS 1698.

Bulbourethral glands (see p. 328).

DENONVILLIERS Charles Pierre (1808–1872) Professor of Anatomy and Surgery in Paris.

Rectovesical fascia (see p. 303).

DESCEMET Jean (1732–1810) Professor of Anatomy and Surgery in Paris.

Posterior limiting membrane of the cornea (see p. 422).

DOUGLAS James (1675–1742) Anatomist and 'man-midwife' of London. Physician to Queen Caroline, wife of George II. FRS 1706.

Rectouterine peritoneal pouch (see p. 303); semicircular line of the rectus sheath (see p. 232).

DRUMMOND Hamilton (1882–1925) Surgeon in Newcastle upon Tyne.

Marginal artery of anastomoses between the ileocolic, right colic, middle colic, left colic and sigmoid arteries (see p. 267).

DUCHENNE Guillaume Benjamin Amand (1806–1875) An early specialist in neurology, he practised in Paris but held no hospital or university appointments.

Erb–Duchenne birth palsy of the upper brachial plexus (described by Erb) (see p. 100).

DUPUYTREN Guillaume (Baron) (1777–1835) Professor of Surgery in Paris.

Contracture of the palmar aponeurosis (see p. 83).

EDINGER Ludwig (1855–1918) Anatomist and neurologist at Frankfurt am Main. **WESTPHAL Karl Friedrich Otto** (1833–1890) Professor of Psychiatry in Berlin.

Accessory nucleus of the oculomotor nerve (see p. 496).

ERB Wilhelm (1840–1921) Professor of Medicine and eminent neurologist at Leipzig and later, at Heidelberg.

Erb's palsy due to traction injury of the upper brachial plexus (see p. 100).

EUSTACHIO (EUSTACHI; EUSTACHIUS) Bartolomeo (1513–1574) Professor of Anatomy in Rome and physician to the Pope.

Auditory tube (see p. 434).

FABRICIUS Hieronymus (Girolamo Fabrizi of Aquapendente) (1533–1619) Professor of Surgery and Anatomy in Padua.

Bursa in chickens, giving the name to B lymphocytes (see p. 9).

FALLOT Étienne-Louis Arthur (1850–1911) French physician. Professor of Hygiene and Legal Medicine in Marseilles.

Tetralogy of congenital heart defects (see p. 214).

FOERSTER Otfried (1873–1941) Neurologist at the Psychiatric Clinic in Breslau.

Dermatomes (see p. 15).

GALEN Claudius (Clarissimus) (AD 130–200) Physician in Rome. Surgeon to the gladiators in Pergamum. Later was for two years physician to the Emperor Marcus Aurelius in Venice.

Great cerebral vein (see p. 493).

GARTNER Hermann Treschow (1785–1827) Surgeon in the Norwegian and later, Danish armies.

Mesonephric duct remnant (see p. 316).

GENNARI Francesco (1750–1790) Physician and anatomist of Parma.

Stria of the visual area of the cerebral cortex (see p. 482).

GEROTA Dumitru (1867–1930) Professor of Surgery, Bucharest. He studied lymphatic injection techniques in Berlin.

Renal fascia (see p. 294).

GIMBERNAT Manuel Louise Antonio don (1734–1816) Professor of Anatomy in Barcelona from 1762 to 1774. Surgeon to King Charles III of Spain.

Lacunar ligament (see p. 231).

GIRALDÉS Joachim Albin Cardozo Cazado (1808–1875) Surgeon to the Hospital Beaujou in Paris and then Professor of Surgery. Died of a wound sustained while performing a postmortem.

Paradidymis (see p. 240)

GRAAF Regnier de (1641–1673) Anatomist and physician at Delft.

Maturing ovarian follicle (see p. 316).

GUYON Félix Jean Casimir (1831–1920) Genitourinary surgeon and Professor of Surgical Pathology in Paris.

Canal for the ulnar nerve beside the pisiform bone (see p. 85).

HARRIS Henry Albert (1886–1968) Professor of Anatomy in Khartoum and then at the University of Cambridge.

Mnemonic for facts about the spleen (see p. 280).

HARTMANN Henry Albert Charles Antoine (1860–1952) Professor of Surgery in Paris.

Pouch in the neck of the gallbladder (see p. 273).

HASSALL Arthur Hill (1817–1894) Physician and botanist. Practised in London and later, on the Isle of Wight.

Thymic corpuscles (see p. 10).

HAVERS Clopton (1657–1702) London physician. FRS 1685.

Canals in bone (see p. 5); fat pads of joints (see p. 8).

HEAD Henry (1861–1940) Neurologist. Physician to the London Hospital. FRS 1899.

Dermatomes (see p. 15).

HEISTER Lorenz (1683–1758) Professor of Anatomy and Botany in Altdorf and later, Professor of Surgery and Botany in Helmstadt.

Spiral mucosal fold in the cystic duct (see p. 275).

HENLE Friedrich Gustav Jakob (1809–1885) Professor of Anatomy in Göttingen from 1852 to 1885.

Tubules of the kidney (see p. 295).

HESSELBACH Franz Kaspar (1759–1816) Surgeon and anatomist, Professor of Surgery at Würzburg.

Inguinal triangle (see p. 236).

HIGHMORE Nathaniel (1613–1685) Physician of Sherborne, Dorset.

Maxillary sinus (see p. 390).

HIS Wilhelm (1863–1934) Professor of Anatomy successively at Leipzig, Basle, Göttingen and Berlin.

Atrioventricular bundle (see p. 210).

HORNER Johann Friedrich (1831–1916) Professor of Ophthalmology in Zurich.

Syndrome due to damage to the cervical sympathetic nerve fibres (see p. 423).

HOUSTON John (1802–1845) Lecturer in Surgery in Dublin and physician to the City Hospital.

Internal rectal folds (see p. 302).

HUMPHRY Sir George Murray (1820–1896) Professor of Anatomy at the University of Cambridge until 1883 when he became the first Professor of Surgery there. First President of the Anatomical Society of Great Britain and Ireland.

Anterior meniscofemoral ligament of the knee joint (see p. 143).

HUNTER John (1728–1793) London surgeon and anatomist. Founder of the Hunterian Museum (now in the custody of the Royal College of Surgeons of England).

Adductor canal (see p. 125).

JACOBSON Ludwig Levin (1783–1843) Anatomist and Physician in Copenhagen.

Tympanic branch of the glossopharyngeal nerve (see p. 380).

KIESSELBACH Wilhelm (1839–1902) Professor of Otology at Erlangen.

Arterial anastomosis on the nasal septum (see p. 389).

KILLIAN Gustav (1860–1921) Director of the Rhinolaryngological Clinic in Freiburg and later, Berlin.

Dehiscence between the thyropharyngeus and cricopharyngeus parts of the inferior constrictor (see p. 400).

KLUMPKE Augusta (Madame Dejerine-Klumpke) (1859–1927) An American from San Francisco, she studied in Lausanne and Paris and was one of the first women doctors. Described the birth paralysis while still a student with Joseph Jules Dejerine (later Professor of Neurology), whom she married.

Paralysis due to birth injury of the lower brachial plexus (see p. 100).

KOCHER Emil Theodor (1841–1917) Professor of Clinical Surgery at Berne and winner of the Nobel Prize for Medicine in 1909 for work on the thyroid gland.

Subcostal abdominal incision (see p. 241); mobilization of the duodenum (see p. 279).

KUPFFER Karl Wilhelm von (1829–1902) Professor of Anatomy in Kiel (1867), Königsberg (1875) and Munich (1880).

Phagocytic cells of liver sinusoids (see p. 272).

LANGER Karl (1819–1887) Professor of Anatomy in Vienna.

Cleavage lines of the skin (see p. 2).

LANGERHANS Paul (1847–1888) Professor of Pathological Anatomy in Freiburg.

Endocrine islets of the pancreas (see p. 279).

LATARGET André (1876–1947) Professor of Anatomy at Lyons from 1925.

Branches of the vagal nerve trunks along the lesser curvature of the stomach (see p. 259).

LEYDIG Franz von (1821–1908) Professor of Histology in Würzburg, Tübingen and Bonn.

Interstitial cells of the testis (see p. 238).

LIEBERKÜHN Johann Nathanael (1711–1756) Physician and anatomist of Berlin, noted for his technique of injecting.

Intestinal crypts or glands (see p. 257).

LISSAUER Heinrich (1861–1891) Neurologist in Breslau.

Dorsolateral tract of the spinal cord (see p. 509).

LISTER Joseph (Lord) (1827–1912) Professor of Surgery in Glasgow (1860), Edinburgh (1869) and King's College, London (1877). Pioneer of antiseptic surgery.

Dorsal tubercle of the radius (see p. 109).

LITTLE James Laurence (1836–1885) Professor of Surgery in Vermont.

Site of arterial anastomosis on the nasal septum (see p. 389).

LITTRE Alexis (1658–1726) Surgeon and anatomist of Paris.

Glands of the penile urethra (see p. 331).

LOCKWOOD Charles Barrett (1856–1914) Surgeon to St Bartholomew's Hospital, London. Founder of the *Journal of Anatomy and Physiology*.

Suspensory ligament of the eye (see p. 417).

LOUIS Pierre Charles Alexandre (1787–1872) Physician of Paris.

Angle between manubrium and body of the sternum; named after, not by, him (see p. 196).

LUDWIG Wilhelm Friedrich (1790–1865) Professor of Surgery and Midwifery in Tübingen. Court physician.

Submandibular cellulitis (see p. 343).

LUSCHKA Hubert (1820–1875) Professor of Anatomy in Tübingen from 1849 to 1875.

Aperture in the lateral recess of the fourth ventricle (see p. 502).

McBURNEY Charles (1845–1913) Professor of Surgery at the College of Physicians and Surgeons, New York.

Point indicating the position of the base of the appendix (see p. 265) and abdominal incision (see p. 241).

MACEWEN Sir William (1848–1924) Surgeon at the Royal Infirmary, Glasgow. He trained under Lister.

Suprameatal triangle, surface marking of mastoid antrum (see p. 529).

MACKENRODT Alwin (1859–1925) Professor of Gynaecology in Berlin. Also known as a pathologist.

Transverse cervical ligament of the uterus (see p. 315).

MAGENDIE François (1783–1855) Professor of Pathology and Physiology in Paris and physician to the Hôtel-Dieu.

Median aperture of the fourth ventricle (see p. 502).

MARSHALL John (1818–1891) Fullerian Professor of Physiology at the Royal Institute; Professor of Anatomy at the Royal Academy; Professor of Surgery at University College London.

Oblique vein of the left atrium (see p. 214).

MAYO Charles Horace (1865–1939) With his father and brother, founded a small hospital, which developed into the Mayo Clinic, the world's largest private hospital.

Prepyloric vein (see p. 258).

MECKEL Johann Friedrich (1724–1774) Professor of Anatomy, Botany and Gynaecology in Berlin.

Dural space for the trigeminal ganglion (see p. 468).

MECKEL Johann Friedrich (1781–1833) Professor of Anatomy and Surgery in Halle. Grandson of the preceding.

Cartilage of the first branchial arch (see p. 27), and ileal diverticulum (see p. 263).

MEIBOM Heinrich (1638–1700) Professor of Medicine, History and Poetry in Helmstadt.

Sebaceous glands of the eyelids (see p. 413).

MEISSNER Georg (1829–1905) Professor of Anatomy and Physiology in Basle and later, Professor of Physiology in Göttingen.

Submucosal nerve plexus of the gut (see p. 256).

MÉNIÈRE Prosper (1799–1862) Physician in Paris.

Disease of the inner ear with deafness, tinnitus and vomiting (see p. 522).

MEYER Adolf (1866–1950) Neurologist in the USA.

Loop of optic radiation fibres (see p. 484).

MONRO Alexander (Secundus) (1733–1817) Succeeded his father Alexander Monro (Primus) as Professor of Anatomy in Edinburgh.

Interventricular foramen (see p. 486).

MONTGOMERY William Fetherstone (1797–1859) Professor of Midwifery in Dublin.

Tubercles of the areola of the breast (previously described by and called tubercles of Morgagni) (see p. 59).

MORGAGNI Giovanni Battista (1682–1771) Professor of Anatomy in Padua for 59 years, and considered to be the father of morbid anatomy.

Foramen between sternal and costal parts of diaphragm—site of congenital hernia (see p. 194).

MORISON James Rutherford (1853–1939) Surgeon to the Royal Infirmary, Newcastle upon Tyne. Emeritus Professor of Surgery at the University of Durham.

541

Hepatorenal pouch of peritoneum (see p. 245), and abdominal incision (see p. 241).

MÜLLER Johannes Peter (1801–1858) Professor of Anatomy and Physiology in Berlin.

Paramesonephric duct (see p. 315).

ODDI Ruggero (1845–1906) Physiologist in Perugia.

Sphincter of the hepatopancreatic ampulla (see p. 275).

ONUFROWICZ B (*circa* 1880) Medical Practitioner in Zurich. Later became Lecturer on Nervous and Mental Diseases at the New York Polytechnic and Associate in Pathology at the Pathological Institute of the New York State Hospitals. Abridged his name to Onuf.

Nucleus in sacral segments of the spinal cord (see p. 308).

PACCHIONI Antoine (1665–1726) Professor of Anatomy in Rome and later, Tivoli.

Arachnoid granulations (see p. 457).

PACINI Filippo (1812–1883) Professor of Anatomy and Physiology in Pisa and Professor of Histology in Florence.

Sensory end organs (see p. 457).

PANETH Joseph (1857–1890) Professor of Physiology in the Universities of Breslau and Vienna.

Cells at the base of intestinal crypts (see p. 257).

PARKINSON James (1755–1824) Inherited his father's practice in the East End of London, and was a well-known palaeontologist.

Disease of basal nuclei (see p. 478).

PARKS Sir Alan Guyatt (1921–1982) Surgeon to St Mark's Hospital and the London Hospital, and President of the Royal College of Surgeons of England from 1980 to 1982.

Mucosal suspensory ligament of the anal canal (see p. 325).

PARONA Francesco (1861–1910) Chief Surgeon to the Novara Hospital, Italy.

Deep intermuscular space of the forearm (see p. 72).

PASSAVANT Philipp Gustav (1815–1893) Surgeon in Frankfurt.

Ridge on the posterior pharyngeal wall during swallowing (see p. 404).

PETIT Jean Louis (1664–1750) Began to learn anatomy at the age of 7 and when he was 12 was demonstrator of anatomy for Littre. When he was 16 he was appointed Surgeon to La Charité Hospital in Paris and finally became Director of the Academy of Surgery. FRS 1729.

Lumbar muscular triangle (see p. 231).

PEYER Johann Conrad (1653–1712) Professor of Logic, Rhetoric and Medicine in Schaffhausen, Switzerland.

Aggregated lymphoid follicles in the lower ileum (see p. 263).

PFANNENSTIEL Hermann Johannes (1862–1909) Gynaecologist in Breslau.

Transverse lower abdominal incision (see p. 241).

POUPART François (1661–1709) Surgeon to the Hôtel-Dieu, Paris.

Inguinal ligament (see p. 231).

PURKINJE Jan Evangelista (1787–1869) Czech physiologist.

Subendocardial fibres (see p. 210).

RANVIER Louis Antoine (1835–1922) Physician and histologist in Paris.

Nodes of myelinated nerves (see p. 11).

RATHKE Martin Heinrich (1793–1860) Professor of Zoology and Anatomy in Königsberg.

Ectodermal pharyngeal pouch forming the adenohypophysis (see p. 465).

RAYNAUD Maurice (1834–1881) French physician.

Raynaud's syndrome (see p. 219)

REISSNER Ernst (1824–1878) Professor of Anatomy in Dorpat and, later, Breslau.

Vestibular membrane of the cochlea (see p. 437).

RETZIUS Andreas Adolf (1796–1860) Professor of Anatomy and Physiology in the Carolinska Institute, Stockholm, from 1840 to 1860.

Retropubic space (see p. 306).

RINNE Friedrich Heinrich Adolf (1819–1868) Otologist in Göttingen.

Tuning-fork hearing test (see p. 522).

RIOLAN Jean (1577–1657) Professor of Anatomy and Botany in Paris.

Arc of anastomosis between the middle colic and the ascending branch of the left colic arteries (see p. 267).

ROLANDO Luigi (1773–1831) First Professor of Practical Medicine at Sassari, Sardinia, and later, Professor of Anatomy at Turin.

Central sulcus of the cerebral hemisphere (see p. 474).

ROMBERG Moritz Heinrich von (1795–1873) Professor of Medicine in Berlin and a famous neurologist.

Sign recognizing loss of posterior column sensibility (see p. 509).

ROSENMÜLLER Johann Christian (1771–1820) Professor of Anatomy and Surgery in Leipzig from 1802 to 1820.

Pharyngeal recess (see p. 401).

SANTORINI Giovanni Domenico (1681–1737) Professor of Anatomy and Medicine in Venice. Published a textbook of anatomy.

Accessory pancreatic duct (see p. 278).

SCARPA Antonio (1747–1832) Professor of Anatomy in Pavia. FRS 1791.

Fibrous layer of the superficial fascia of the abdomen (see p. 185).

SCHLEMM Friedrich (1795–1858) Professor of Anatomy in Berlin from 1833 to 1858.

Canal at the junction of the cornea and the sclera (see p. 421).

SCHWANN Theodor (1810–1882) Professor of Comparative Anatomy and Physiology in Liège.

Neurilemmal cells of peripheral nerves (see p. 11).

SERTOLI Enrico (1842–1910) Professor of Experimental Physiology in Milan.

Sustentacular cells of the testis (see p. 238).

SHARPEY William (1802–1880) Professor of Anatomy in Edinburgh and, later, at University College London, from 1836 to 1874.

Connective tissue fibres between periosteum and bone (see p. 6).

SHERRINGTON Sir Charles Scott (1857–1952) Professor of Physiology at the University of Liverpool from 1895 to 1913 and at the University of Oxford from 1913 to 1936. FRS 1893.

Dermatomes (see p. 15).

SHRAPNELL Henry Jones (1761–1834) Surgeon to the South Gloucestershire Regiment; married Edward Jenner's ward and became a surgeon and anatomist in London.

Pars flaccida of the tympanic membrane (see p. 431).

SIBSON Francis (1814–1876) Professor of Medicine at St Mary's Hospital, London.

Fascia—suprapleural membrane—attached to the first rib (see p. 190).

SKENE Alexander John Chalmers (1838–1900) Born in Aberdeen, he studied in the USA and became Professor of Gynaecology in the Long Island College Hospital, Brooklyn, and, later, at the New York Postgraduate Medical School.

Paraurethral glands of the female (see p. 318).

STENSEN Niels (Nicolaus Steno) (1638–1686) Professor of Anatomy in Copenhagen. A pioneer in geology and crystallography, he gave up science to become a priest.

Parotid duct (see p. 372).

STURGE William Allen (1850–1919) and **WEBER Frederick Parkes** (1863–1962) London physicians.

Syndrome including port wine naevus in the trigeminal area (see p. 366).

SYLVIUS François de la Böe (1614–1672) Professor of Practical Medicine in Leiden.

Lateral sulcus of the cerebral hemisphere (see p. 474), and the aqueduct of the midbrain (see p. 494).

TENON Jacques René (1724–1816) Professor of Pathology in the Academy of Sciences, Paris, and Chief Surgeon at La Salpêtrière.

Fascial sheath of the eyeball (see p. 417).

TOLDT Karl (1840–1920) Professor of Anatomy in Prague and later, Vienna.

White line of peritoneal fusion alongside descending colon (see p. 250).

TREITZ Wenzel (1819–1872) Professor of Pathological Anatomy in Krakow and later, Professor of Pathology in Prague.

Suspensory muscle of the duodenum (see p. 262).

TRENDELENBURG Friedrich (1844–1924) Professor of Surgery in Rostock, Bonn and Leipzig.

Test for adductors of the hip (see p. 130).

TREVES Sir Frederick (1853–1923) Surgeon to the London Hospital. With Lord Lister, operated on King Edward VII for appendicitis.

Ileocaecal fold of peritoneum (see p. 266).

TROISIER Charles Émile (1844–1919) Professor of Pathology in Paris.

Sign of enlarged supraclavicular lymph nodes in gastric carcinoma (see p. 259).

VALSALVA Antonio Maria (1666–1723) Professor of Anatomy at Bologna. He studied under Malpighi. Morgagni was his pupil.

Aortic sinuses (see p. 210).

VATER Abraham (1684–1751) Professor of Anatomy, Botany, Pathology and Therapeutics in Wittenberg.

Hepatopancreatic ampulla in the duodenal wall (see p. 275).

VESALIUS Andreas (1514–1564) Professor of Anatomy at Padua and later, Bologna and Pisa. Physician to Charles V and Philip II of Spain. His anatomical atlas *De humani corporis fabrica* (Basle, 1543) is one of the world's greatest books.

Venous foramen medial to the foramen ovale (see p. 464).

VIDUS VIDIUS (Guido Guidi) (1500–1569) Physician to Francis I of France and, from 1548, Professor of Medicine at the University of Pisa.

Nerve of the pterygoid canal (see p. 384).

VOLKMANN Alfred Wilhelm (1800–1877) Professor of Physiology and Anatomy in Dorpat and later, Halle.

Vascular canals in bone (see p. 5).

WALDEYER Heinrich Wilhelm Gottfried (1836–1921) Professor of Pathological Anatomy in Breslau and later, Berlin.

Ring of lymphoid tissue in the mouth and pharynx (see p. 402).

WEBER Ernst Heinrich (1795–1878) Professor of Anatomy and Physiology in Leipzig.

Tuning-fork hearing test (also attributed to Friedrich Eugen Weber, 1832–1891, German otologist) (see p. 522).

WERNICKE Karl (1848–1904) Professor of Neurology and Psychiatry in Breslau and later, in Halle.

Posterior speech area of the cerebral cortex (see p. 482).

WHARTON Thomas (1616–1673) Physician to St Thomas' Hospital, London.

Submandibular duct (see p. 349).

WHITNALL Samuel Ernest (1876–1950) Professor of Anatomy at McGill University, Montreal (1919–1934), and at the University of Bristol (1935–1941).

Marginal tubercle on the zygomatic bone (see p. 413).

WILLIS Thomas (1621–1675) Professor of Natural Philosophy at the University of Oxford and subsequently physician to James II. One of the founders of the Royal Society.

Arterial circle at the base of the brain (see p. 490).

WINSLOW Jacob Benignus (1669–1760) At the age of 74 was appointed Professor of Anatomy, Physic and Surgery in Paris and was considered one of the best anatomical teachers in Europe.

Epiploic foramen (see p. 245).

WIRSUNG Johann Georg (1600–1643) Professor of Anatomy in Padua, where he was assassinated.

Pancreactic duct (see p. 278).

WOLFF Kaspar Friedrich (1733–1794) Professor of Anatomy and Physiology at St Petersburg. One of the founders of modern embryology.

Mesonephric duct (see p. 240).

WORM Ole (1588–1654) Danish theologian and anatomist. Professor of Greek and Philosophy, and later became Professor of Anatomy in Copenhagen.

Sutural bones of the skull (see p. 526).

WRISBERG Heinrich August (1739–1808) Anatomist and gynaecologist. Professor of Anatomy in Göttingen.

Posterior meniscofemoral ligament (see p. 143).

Index

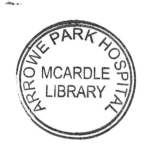